Multiple Sclerosis: An Evidence-Based Approach

Multiple Sclerosis: An Evidence-Based Approach

Edited by Steven Pitts

AMERICAN
MEDICAL PUBLISHERS
www.americanmedicalpublishers.com

American Medical Publishers,
41 Flatbush Avenue,
1st Floor, New York,
NY 11217, USA

Visit us on the World Wide Web at:
www.americanmedicalpublishers.com

ISBN: 978-1-63927-305-8

Cataloging-in-Publication Data

Multiple sclerosis : an evidence-based approach / edited by Steven Pitts.
p. cm.
Includes bibliographical references and index.
ISBN 978-1-63927-305-8
1. Multiple sclerosis. 2. Demyelination. 3. Myelin sheath--Diseases.
4. Nervous system--Diseases. I. Pitts, Steven.
RC377 .M85 2022
616.834--dc23

Table of Contents

Preface

This book has been an outcome of determined endeavour from a group of educationists in the field. The primary objective was to involve a broad spectrum of professionals from diverse cultural background involved in the field for developing new researches. The book not only targets students but also scholars pursuing higher research for further enhancement of the theoretical and practical applications of the subject.

Multiple sclerosis (MS) is a neurological disorder caused by the damage to the insulating covers of nerve cells in the brain and spinal cord. It is a common immune-mediated disorder which directly affects the central nervous system. It results in the disruption of the ability of certain parts of the nervous system to transmit signals, resulting in physical and mental problems. Some of the symptoms of MS are double vision, blindness in one eye, muscle weakness, trouble with sensation and coordination, etc. Multiple sclerosis can be diagnosed depending on the signs and symptoms along with neuroimaging, magnetic resonance imaging, etc. Intravenous as well as oral corticosteroids are used for its management. This book covers in detail some existent theories and innovative concepts revolving around multiple sclerosis. It presents researches and studies performed by experts across the globe. This book will serve as a valuable source of reference for graduate and postgraduate students.

It was an honour to edit such a profound book and also a challenging task to compile and examine all the relevant data for accuracy and originality. I wish to acknowledge the efforts of the contributors for submitting such brilliant and diverse chapters in the field and for endlessly working for the completion of the book. Last, but not the least; I thank my family for being a constant source of support in all my research endeavours.

Editor

1

BAFF Index and CXCL13 levels in the cerebrospinal fluid associate respectively with intrathecal IgG synthesis and cortical atrophy in multiple sclerosis at clinical onset

M. Puthenparampil[1*], L. Federle[1], S. Miante[1], A. Zito[1], E. Toffanin[2], S. Ruggero[2], M. Ermani[2], S. Pravato[2], D. Poggiali[1], P. Perini[1], F. Rinaldi[1] and P. Gallo[1]

Abstract

Background: B lymphocytes are thought to play a relevant role in multiple sclerosis (MS) pathology. The in vivo analysis of intrathecally produced B cell-related cytokines may help to clarify the mechanisms of B cell recruitment and immunoglobulin production within the central nervous system (CNS) in MS.

Methods: Paired cerebrospinal fluid (CSF) and serum specimens from 40 clinically isolated syndrome suggestive of MS or early-onset relapsing-remitting MS patients (CIS/eRRMS) and 17 healthy controls (HC) were analyzed for the intrathecal synthesis of IgG (quantitative formulae and IgG oligoclonal bands, IgGOB), CXCL13, BAFF, and IL-21. 3D-FLAIR, 3D-DIR, and 3D-T1 MRI sequences were applied to evaluate white matter (WM) and gray matter (GM) lesions and global cortical thickness (gCTh).

Results: Compared to HC, CIS/eRRMS having IgGOB (IgGOB+, 26 patients) had higher intrathecal IgG indexes ($p < 0.01$), lower values of BAFF Index (11.9 ± 6.1 vs 17.5 ± 5.2, $p < 0.01$), and higher CSF CXCL13 levels (27.7 ± 33.5 vs 0.9 ± 1.5, $p < 0.005$). In these patients, BAFF Index but not CSF CXCL13 levels inversely correlated with the intrathecal IgG synthesis ($r > 0.5$ and $p < 0.05$ for all correlations). CSF leukocyte counts were significantly higher in IgGOB+ compared to IgGOB– ($p < 0.05$) and HC ($p < 0.01$), and correlated to CSF CXCL13 concentrations (r 0.77, $p < 0.001$).
The gCTh was significantly lower in patients with higher CSF CXCL13 levels (2.41 ± 0.1 vs 2.49 ± 0.1 mm, $p < 0.05$), while no difference in MRI parameters of WM and GM pathology was observed between IgGOB+ and IgGOB–.

Conclusions: The intrathecal IgG synthesis inversely correlated with BAFF Index and showed no correlation with CSF CXCL13. These findings seem to indicate that intrathecally synthesized IgG are produced by long-term PCs that have entered the CNS from the peripheral blood, rather than produced by PCs developed in the meningeal follicle-like structures (FLS). In this study, CXCL13 identifies a subgroup of MS patients characterized by higher leukocyte counts in the CSF and early evidence of cortical thinning, further suggesting a role for this chemokine as a possible marker of disease severity.

Keywords: Multiple sclerosis, BAFF, CXCL13, IL21, Cerebrospinal fluid, IgGOB, FLS, Intrathecal IgG synthesis

* Correspondence: marco.puthenparampil@studenti.unipd.it
[1]Multiple Sclerosis Centre, Department of Neurosciences DNS, University Hospital–Medical School, via Giustiniani 5, 3518 Padova, Italy

Background

Several lines of evidence suggest that B cells play a central role in the pathogenesis and/or the clinical evolution of multiple sclerosis (MS). First, it is well known that the great majority of MS patients have quantitative (increased indexes) and/or qualitative (presence of IgG oligoclonal bands, IgGOB) immunoglobulin changes in the cerebrospinal fluid (CSF), indicating an intrathecal Ig production [1, 2]. Second, histological studies have disclosed the presence of complement deposition and plasma cells (PCs) in white matter (WM) lesions [3]. Third, B cell follicle-like structures (FLS) are observed in the meninges of patients with progressive MS [4] and correlate with the degree of meningeal inflammation and cortical demyelination, and with a higher rate of disability progression [5]. Finally, the treatment of MS patients with anti-CD20 monoclonal antibodies determines a significant reduction in the number of both active brain lesions and in clinical relapses [6–9].

The role of B cells in MS pathology may be multifaceted [7]. Beside autoantibody production [10, 11], B cells may present central nervous system (CNS) antigens with co-stimulatory signals leading to activation and proliferation of effector T cells, may produce pro-inflammatory cytokines (e.g. IL-6, IL-12, and TNF), or may regulate the immune response by providing IL-10, a cytokine that suppresses the T cell functions either directly or indirectly [12] (i.e., differentiation of T regulatory cells and the suppression of dendritic cell function [7, 10–12]).

The presence of meningeal follicle-like structures (FLS) has stimulated the hypothesis of a "germinal center reaction" within the CNS of MS. Briefly, naïve B cells recruited in the CNS (throughout CXCL13 signal) may locally meet and present CNS antigens to T helper lymphocytes. Both B and T cells actively collaborate (respectively as centroblast and follicular T helper, that produce IL-21, the "signature" of an ongoing follicular reaction) to establish a germinal center reaction that leads B cell maturation to IgG-secreting PCs. PCs will survive within the CNS thanks to intrathecally produced B cell survival factors, such as B cell-activating factor (BAFF), as suggested by a recent observation [13]. On the other hand, we cannot exclude that FLS formation may be a mere epiphenomenon of MS, expression of a chronic meningeal inflammation, not directly involved in intrathecal Ig synthesis.

We studied serum and CSF levels of soluble factors involved in naïve B cell recruitment (CXCL13), in follicular reaction (IL-21) and intrathecal B cell survival (BAFF) in MS patients at clinical onset and correlated their intrathecal synthesis with local Ig production and with magnetic resonance imaging (MRI) parameters of white and gray matter damage. The aim of the study was to explore whether, at clinical onset, B cell-related cytokines could serve as immunological markers of MS severity/prognosis.

Methods

Patients

Forty consecutive patients with a diagnosis of clinically isolated syndrome suggestive of MS (CIS) or early-onset relapsing-remitting MS (eRRMS), whose diagnosis was achieved in agreement with the most recent diagnostic criteria [14], were enrolled in the study. Inclusion criteria were as follows: (i) age between 18 and 50 years, (ii) no medical history of steroid therapy in the previous 30 days, (iii) no medical history of immunomodulating or immunosuppressive therapy, and (iv) no gadolinium-enhancing lesion at the MRI performed at the study entry.

Seventeen healthy controls (HC) were also enrolled in the study. These subjects complained tension headache, subjective transient sensory symptoms, psychosomatic disorders, etc. that underwent lumbar puncture for diagnostic purposes having unexpected, subtle, but unspecific white matter lesions at MRI. Immunological and coagulation screenings, microbiological and standard CSF analysis were normal; also upper aortic artery and Transcranic ultrasound EcoColorDoppler and visual evoked potentials were normal.

No differences for age and gender were observed between eRRMS and HC (Table 1). The study was

Table 1 Standard serum and CSF parameters in HC and CIS/eRRMS

	HC	CIS/eRRMS
Gender (F/M)	13/4	26/14
Age at LP (years)	43.2 ± 9.2	37.8 ± 10.0
Disease duration (years)	n.a.	0.5 ± 0.9
CSF [Alb] (mg/dL)	17.0 ± 5.1	22.5 ± 9.8
Serum [Alb] (mg/dL)	4370.6 ± 379.0	4260.0 ± 333.6
Q_{Alb} (10^{-3})	3.9 ± 1.2	5.3 ± 2.3*
CSF [IgG] (mg/dL)	2.2 ± 0.9	3.7 ± 1.8***
Serum [IgG] (mg/dL)	1141.2 ± 215.2	1042.0 ± 197.7
Q_{IgG} (10^{-3})	1.9 ± 0.6	3.6 ± 1.7****
IgG Index	0.5 ± 0.1	0.7 ± 0.3***
IgG Loc (mg/dL)	0.1 ± 0.3	5.9 ± 10.2*
IgIF (%)	0 ± 0	11 ± 17*
IgGOB (%)	0%	65%****
Leukocyte counts (/μL)	2.1 ± 1.1	6.9 ± 7.7*

Disease duration was defined as the time between clinical disease onset and lumbar puncture. For gander, IgIF% and IgGOB chi-square test was applied. For all the other variables, a *t* test was performed

HC healthy controls, *CIS/eRRMS* CIS suggestive of MS or early RRMS, *LP* lumbar puncture, *n.a.* not applicable, *Csf* cerebrospinal fluid, *S* serum, *IgGOB* IgG oligoclonal bands

*$p < 0.05$; **$p < 0.01$; ***$p < 0.005$; ****$p < 0.001$

approved by the local ethics committee and a written informed consent was obtained by all the participants.

CSF and serum routine analysis

CSF was collected by non-traumatic lumbar puncture between 8:00 and 9:00 am. Routine examination on paired CSF and serum specimens included cell count and differentiation, CSF/serum IgG ratio (Q_{IgG}), CSF/serum albumin ratio (Q_{Alb}) to estimate the integrity of the blood-brain barrier (BBB), calculation of intrathecal IgG synthesis by means of quantitative formulae (IgG Index) [2] IgG Reiber's Hyperbolic Function for IgG intrathecal synthesis fraction (IgGIF) [1] and Local Production (IgGLoc) [1], and demonstration of IgGOB by isoelectric-focusing and specific IgG immunofixation. BBB damage was considered when Q_{Alb} was higher than the normal value for patient's age (i.e., age/15 + 4). After cell centrifugation, both CSF and serum were stored at −80 °C until cytokine analysis.

Cytokine determination

CSF and serum levels of BAFF (R&D System, Cat. Numb. DBLYS0B), IL-21 (Bender MedSystems Cat. Numb. BMS2043TEN), and CXCL13 (R&D System, Cat. Numb. DCX130) were measured by a highly sensitive immune-enzymatic assay ELISA according to the manufacturer's instruction. BAFF concentrations (pg/mL) were measured on 1:2 diluted sera and on native CSF. IL-21 and CXCL13 concentrations (pg/mL) were measured on native sera and CSF. Cytokine ratio (CSF/serum cytokine: Q_{BAFF}, Q_{CXCL13}, and Q_{IL-21}) and Index (CSF/serum cytokine/CSF/serum albumin: BAFF Index, CXCL13 Index, IL21 Index) were calculated.

MRI protocol

Images were acquired using a 3T scanner (Ingenia, Philips Medical Systems, Best, The Netherlands) with 33 mT/m power gradient and a 32-channel head coil. No major hardware upgrades occurred during the study, and bimonthly quality-assurance sessions assured measurement stability. The following images were acquired for each subject: (a) three-dimensional (3D) turbo field echo (TFE, 3D-T1): repetition time (RT) 7.8 ms; echo time (ET) 3.6 ms; 180 contiguous axial slices with the off-center positioned on zero with thickness of 1.0 mm; flip angle = 8°; matrix size = 220 × 220; FOV = 220 × 220 × 180 mm^3. This sequence was acquired before and after gadolinium administration. (b) 3D-fluid attenuated inversion recovery (FLAIR): RT 4800 ms; ET 310 ms; inversion time (IT) 1650 ms; 365 contiguous axial slices with thickness of 1.0 mm; matrix size 256 × 256; and FOV = 256 × 256 × 182 mm3; (c) 3D-double inversion recovery (DIR): RT 13,000 ms, ET 10 ms, IT 3400/325 ms; 40 contiguous axial slices, resolution 1 × 1 × 3 mm, FOV 230 × 200 mm, time 3.5 min. Two experienced observers, blinded to the patient's identity, assessed all images. The global cortical thickness (gCTh) was analyzed by means of Freesurfer on 3D-T1 sequences. WM lesions were identified on FLAIR sequences, while cortical lesions (CL) were identified on DIR scans by two blinded evaluators (PD, PS) using published consensus recommendations.

Statistical analysis

For normally distributed variables, the *T* test (when two groups were compared) or the ANOVA (for more than two group comparisons) were performed applying the Bonferroni correction. For ordinal categorical variables, the Mann-Whitney *U* test was performed, while for no ordinal variables, Pearson's chi-square test was used. Linear correlation between variables was tested using Pearson's single or multiple linear model when all variables were normally distributed. The significance level was set at $p < 0.05$.

Results

Intrathecal IgG synthesis in HC and CIS/eRRMS

Table 1 summarizes routine serum and CSF findings in HC and CIS/eRRMS. As expected, all the indexes of intrathecal IgG synthesis (IgG CSF, Q_{IgG}, IgG Index, IgGLoc, and IgGIF) were significantly higher in CIS/eRRMS compared to HC. Higher Q_{Alb} values were observed in CIS/eRRMS ($5.3 \pm 2.3 \times 10^{-3}$) than in HC ($3.9 \pm 1.2 \times 10^{-3}$, $p < 0.05$), but only six CIS/eRRMS patients (15 vs 0% in HC, $p = 0.2$) had BBB damage.

Intrathecal cytokine synthesis in HC and CIS/eRRMS

CXCL13

In HC, CXCL13 was found in all sera and, at very low levels (0.9 ± 1.5 pg/mL), in 8/17 (47%) CSF. In these subjects, no correlation was observed between Q_{CXCL13} and Q_{Alb} (*r* 0.2, $p = 0.4$), even when only CXCL13-positive CSF were included in the analysis (*r* 0.7, $p = 0.1$). Since these data indicated that CXCL13 was intrathecally produced, rather than derived from passive filtration from blood, only the CSF concentrations of this cytokine were considered in further analyses. CXCL13 was detected more frequently (75%, $p < 0.05$) and at higher concentration (19.7 ± 29.3 pg/mL, $p < 0.05$) in the CSF of CIS/eRRMS than HC.

IL-21

In HC, IL-21 was detectable in all CSF (28.1 ± 29.1 pg/mL) but only in one serum, thus suggesting that CSF IL-21 was intrathecally produced. No difference in CSF IL-21 levels was observed between HC (28.1 ± 29.1 pg/mL) and CIS/eRRMS (20.7 ± 22.8 pg/mL, $p = 0.3$).

BAFF

BAFF was detected in all the sera and CSF of HC and CIS/eRRMS. In HC Q_{BAFF} mildly correlated to Q_{Alb} (r 0.4), indicating that CSF BAFF may result from both choroid plexus filtration and active production within the CNS. The BAFF Index was lower in CIS/eRRMS (12.4 ± 5.5 pg/mL) than in HC (17.5 ± 5.2 pg/mL, $p < 0.005$).

IgGOB-based stratification of CIS/eRRMS

Based on the presence of IgGOB in the CSF, CIS/eRRMS patients were divided in IgGOB positive (IgGOB+, 26 patients) and in IgGOB negative (IgGOB–, 14 patients) (Table 2). The analysis based on this stratification disclosed that all the differences previously found between HC and CIS/eRRMS were confirmed for IgGOB+ patients, but not for IgGOB– patients (Fig. 1a). Furthermore, serum IgG concentrations in IgGOB– were lower than in HC ($p < 0.01$) and IgGOB+ ($p < 0.05$).

CSF CXCL13 concentrations were higher in IgGOB+ compared to both IgGOB– ($p < 0.05$) and HC ($p < 0.005$) (Fig. 1b). A higher number of IgGOB+ patients had detectable CXCL13 in the CSF (77%) compared to IgGOB– (50%), but the difference was not significant ($p = 0.2$).

Table 2 Serum and CSF parameters in HC, IgGOB–, and IgGOB + patients

	HC	IgGOB–	IgGOB+
Gender (F/M)	13/4	9/5	17/9
Age at LP (years)	43.2 ± 9.2	37.2 ± 10.7	38.2 ± 9.7
Disease duration (years)	n.a.	0.3 ± 0.6	0.6 ± 1.1
Csf-[Alb] (mg/dL)	17.0 ± 5.1	21.2 ± 8.7	23.1 ± 10.4
S-[Alb] (mg/dL)	4370.6 ± 379.0	4225.0 ± 297.7	4278.8 ± 355.6
Q_{Alb} (10^{-3})	3.9 ± 1.2	5.0 ± 2.0	5.4 ± 2.4*
Csf-[IgG] (mg/dL)	2.2 ± 0.9	2.4 ± 0.8	4.5 ± 1.8**** °°°°
S-[IgG] (mg/dL)	1141.2 ± 215.2	944.6 ± 124.2**	1094.3 ± 211.6°
Q_{IgG} (10^{-3})	1.9 ± 0.6	2.6 ± 1.0	4.2 ± 1.8**** °°
IgG Index	0.5 ± 0.1	0.5 ± 0.1	0.8 ± 0.3**** °°°
IgG Loc (mg/dL)	0.1 ± 0.3	0.2 ± 0.6	9.0 ± 11.5** °
IgIF (%)	0 ± 0	1.1 ± 2.7	16.4 ± 18.5*** °°
Leukocyte counts (/μL)	2.1 ± 1.1	2.9 ± 2.4	9.0 ± 8.6*** °
Csf -[BAFF] (pg/mL)	67.3 ± 21.6	69.9 ± 27.3	50.7 ± 20.5* °
BAFF Index	17.5 ± 5.2	13.2 ± 5.1	11.9 ± 6.1**
Csf-[CXCL13] (pg/mL)	0.9 ± 1.5	5.0 ± 8.2	27.7 ± 33.5*** °
Csf-[IL21] (pg/mL)	28.1 ± 29.1	21.6 ± 25.3	20.2 ± 21.9

IgGOB+ patients differed from both BOIgG– and HC for intrathecal IgG synthesis parameters, CSF CXCL13 concentrations, and BAFF Index values. For gender, IgIF%, and IgGOB, chi square test was applied. For all the other variables, a t test was performed. Abbreviations as in Table 1
P values compared to HC: *$p < 0.5$; **$p < 0.01$; ***$p < 0.005$; ****$p < 0.001$;
p values compared to IgGOB–: °$p < 0.5$; °°$p < 0.01$; °°°$p < 0.005$; °°°°$p < 0.001$

No difference in CSF IL-21 levels was observed between HC, IgGOB–, and IgGOB+ (Fig. 1c).

As expected on the base of previous results, CSF BAFF levels and Index were significantly lower in IgGOB+ (50.7 ± 20.5 pg/ml, $p < 0.05$, and 11.9 ± 6.1, both $p < 0.005$, respectively) but not in IgGOB– (69.9 ± 27.3 pg/ml and 13.2 ± 5.1, respectively, $p = 0.8$ and $p = 0.1$) compared to HC (Fig. 1d).

Correlation analysis

For the correlation analysis, only quantitative continuous variables, namely IgG Index, IgGLoc, and IgGIF, were included as dependent variables. Table 3 shows the correlation between the parameters of intrathecal IgG synthesis and BAFF Index or CSF CXCL13 concentrations in IgGOB+. CSF CXCL13 concentrations correlated with all the parameters of intrathecal IgG synthesis (Fig. 2a–c), while BAFF Index mildly correlated only with IgGLoc values (Fig. 3a–c). In order to avoid the influence of null values on the direct correlation and considering that IgGOB+ presented null values for CSF CXCL13, we focused on patients with quantitatively increased intrathecal IgG synthesis. In 15 IgGOB+ patients having IgG Index, IgGLoc, and IgGIF values above the normal range of reference, only BAFF Index correlated to all these parameters (Fig. 3a'–c'), while CXCL13 concentrations correlated only with IgGLoc (Fig. 2a').

Finally, BAFF Index did not correlate to CSF CXCL13 concentrations in HC (r –0.36, $p = 0.2$), MS patients (r –0.29, $p = 0.1$), IgGOB– (r –0.05, $p = 0.9$), and IgGOB+ (r –0.31, $p = 0.1$).

CSF leukocyte counts in CIS/eRRMS and in IgGOB+ and IgGOB–

CSF leukocyte number was significantly higher in CIS/eRRMS (6.9 ± 7.7/μL) compared to HC (2.1 ± 1.1 μL, $p < 0.05$). CSF CXCL13 concentrations, but not BAFF Index, significantly correlated to leukocyte counts (r 0.77, $p < 0.001$, Table 4).

BOIgG+ had higher CSF leukocyte number (9.0 ± 8.6/μL) than IgGOB– (2.9 ± 2.4/μL, $p < 0.05$) and HC ($p < 0.01$). In IgGOB+, CSF CXCL13 concentrations, but not BAFF Index values, significantly correlated to leukocyte number (r 0.77, $p < 0.001$, Table 4), while no correlation between leukocyte number and all the other CSF parameters was observed in BOIgG–.

MRI parameters in CIS/eRRMS

No difference in gCTh was observed between HC and CIS/eRRMS. However, a higher variability in gCTh was found in CIS/eRRMS (range 2.25–2.67 mm) compared to HC (2.34–2.58 mm). In order to find associations

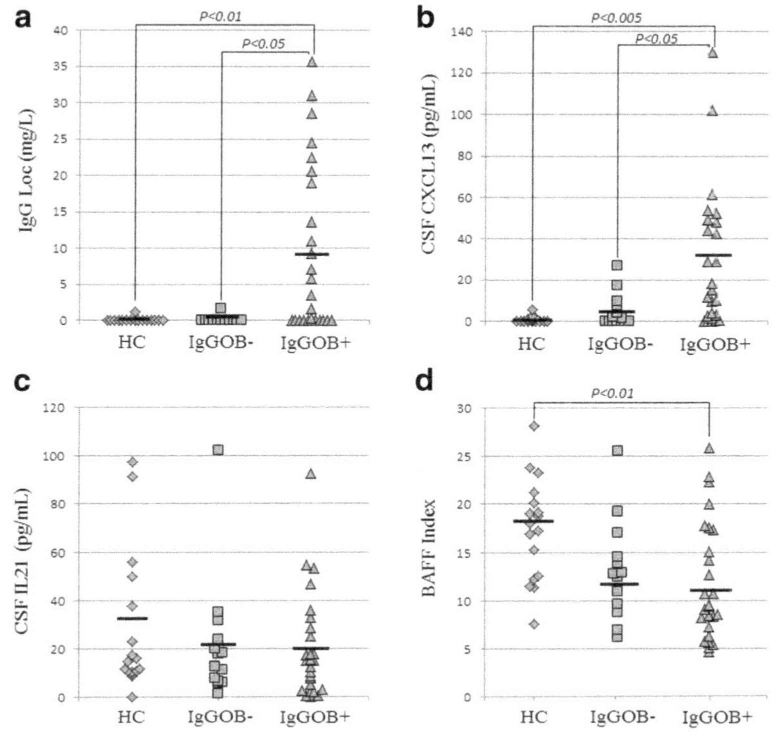

Fig. 1 IgG and cytokine concentrations in the CSF. IgG Loc expressed in mg/dL (**a**), CSF CXCL13 and IL-21 concentrations (pg/mL; **b**, **c**), and BAFF Index values (**d**) in HC and CIS/eRRMS with (IgGOB+) or without (IgGOB−) intrathecal synthesis of IgG oligoclonal bands. IgGOB+ patients had increased CXCL13, normal IL-21, and decreased BAFF Index compared to HC and IgGOB− patients. Only significant comparison is indicated. *Abbreviations: HC* healthy controls, *CIS/eRRMS* CIS suggestive of MS or early RRMS, *LP* lumbar puncture, *n.a.* not applicable, *CSF* cerebrospinal fluid, *S* serum. *IgGOB+*: patients with IgG oligoclonal bands in the CSF; *IgGOB−*: patients without IgG oligoclonal bands in the CSF

between CSF (IgGOB detection, BAFF Index, CSF CXCL13, IgG Index, IgGLoc, IgG IF) and MRI parameters, we performed a subgroup analysis.

On the base CXCL13 concentrations in the CSF of HC, we found a cutoff value of 6.8 pg/mL ($\mu + 4\delta$) that allowed the identification of two groups of CIS/eRRMS patients having CSF CXCL13 values below (CXCL13−, 20 patients) or above (CXCL13+, 20 patients) this limit. All HC had CXCL13 values below this limit.

Table 3 Correlation between intrathecal IgG synthesis parameters and BAFF Index or CXCL13

(A) All patients	BAFF Index	
IgG Loc (mg/dL)	−0.41*	0.59***
IgIF (%)	−0.36	0.45*
IgG Index	−0.38	0.48*
(B) Only IS+	BAFF Index	LCS-CXCL13
IgG Loc (mg/dL)	−0.56*	0.57*
IgIF (%)	−0.52*	0.35
IgG Index	−0.64*	0.43

The correlation was calculating on overall population of BOIgG+ patients (A) or including only patients with quantitatively increased intrathecal IgG synthesis (IS+, B). *R* values derived from Pearson's single linear model are represented. Other abbreviations as in Table 2

*$p < 0.5$; **$p < 0.01$; ***$p < 0.005$

BAFF Index was not applicable in this analysis, since its range did not differ between the two groups and therefore a cut-off value was meaningless.

In as much as the three quantitative indexes of intrathecal IgG synthesis gave highly concordant values, only IgG Loc was considered for further analysis (values ≤0.0 = IgGLoc−; values >0.0 = IgGLoc+).

Interestingly, no difference in any MRI parameter was observed between IgGOB+ and IgGOB− or between IgGLoc− and IgGLoc+. CXCL13+ patients had a significant thinning of gCTh (2.42 ± 0.09 mm) compared to CXCL13− (2.48 ± 0.10 mm, $p < 0.05$; Fig. 4). The results did not change when a different cut-off value ($\mu + 3\delta$, i.e., 5.2 pg/mL) was applied.

No association was found between any CSF parameters and WM or GM lesion number and volume.

Discussion

Intrathecally produced IgGOB can be demonstrated in the great majority of MS patients at clinical onset, persist in the CSF throughout the patient's life, and constitute the major evidence of B lymphocytes and PC involvement in MS

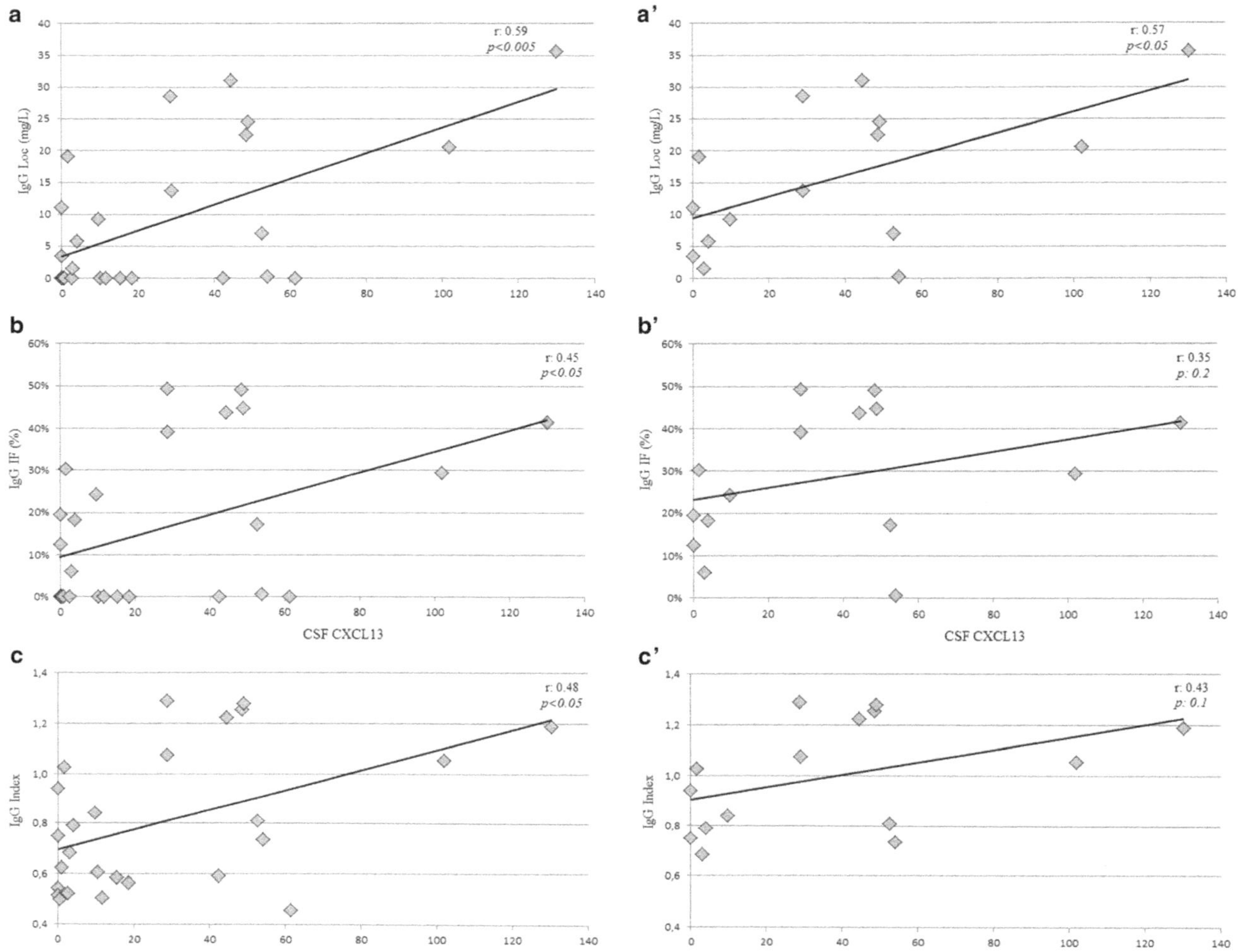

Fig. 2 Correlations between CSF CXCL13 and intrathecal IgG synthesis. A mild correlation was observed between CSFCXCL13 and intrathecal IgG synthesis when all the patients were included in the analysis (**a–c**). When the null values for intrathecal IgG synthesis were excluded, the correlation was weak (**a'**) or lost (**b'**, **c'**)

pathology [3]. The origin of long-term secreting PCs, likely the source of intrathecally synthesized IgG, has not been established yet. Moreover, the progressive colonization of MS meninges by FLS suggests that local B cell maturation to PCs may support the intrathecal synthesis of IgM and IgG [5]. However, since FLS accumulation seems to parallel disease progression (i.e., they were demonstrated in high percentage in progressive MS cases, rarely in RRMS and not at clinical onset), we would expect to observe qualitative modifications of the IgGOB patterns over the course of the disease. On the contrary, longitudinal studies demonstrated that IgGOB are almost qualitatively stable [15–19].

B cells have several other functions than producing antibodies [12]. They may act as efficient antigen-presenting or cytokine-secreting cells, thus enhancing T cell response. Therefore, the pathogenic role of B cells in the FLS may be multifaceted. FLS have been observed in association with cortical inflammation, gray matter demyelination, and various degrees of microglia activation [4]. Moreover, meningeal and cortical inflammation were found to correlate with some clinical parameters, such as median age at disease onset, time to disease progression, time to wheelchair dependence, and age at death [4]. Thus, the analysis of intrathecally synthesized B cell-related cytokines/chemokines may give the opportunity to define the timing of B cell recruitment and FLS formation in the CNS and to explore the role of FLS in the pathogenesis and clinical progression of MS.

In a previous study [13], we observed that BAFF Index correlated to quantitative parameters of intrathecal IgG synthesis in MS at clinical onset and suggested a BAFF-dependent PCs survival within the CNS. In this study, we analyzed the intrathecal production of cytokines involved in B cell recruitment and follicular maturation in order to explore the origin of intracerebral PCs.

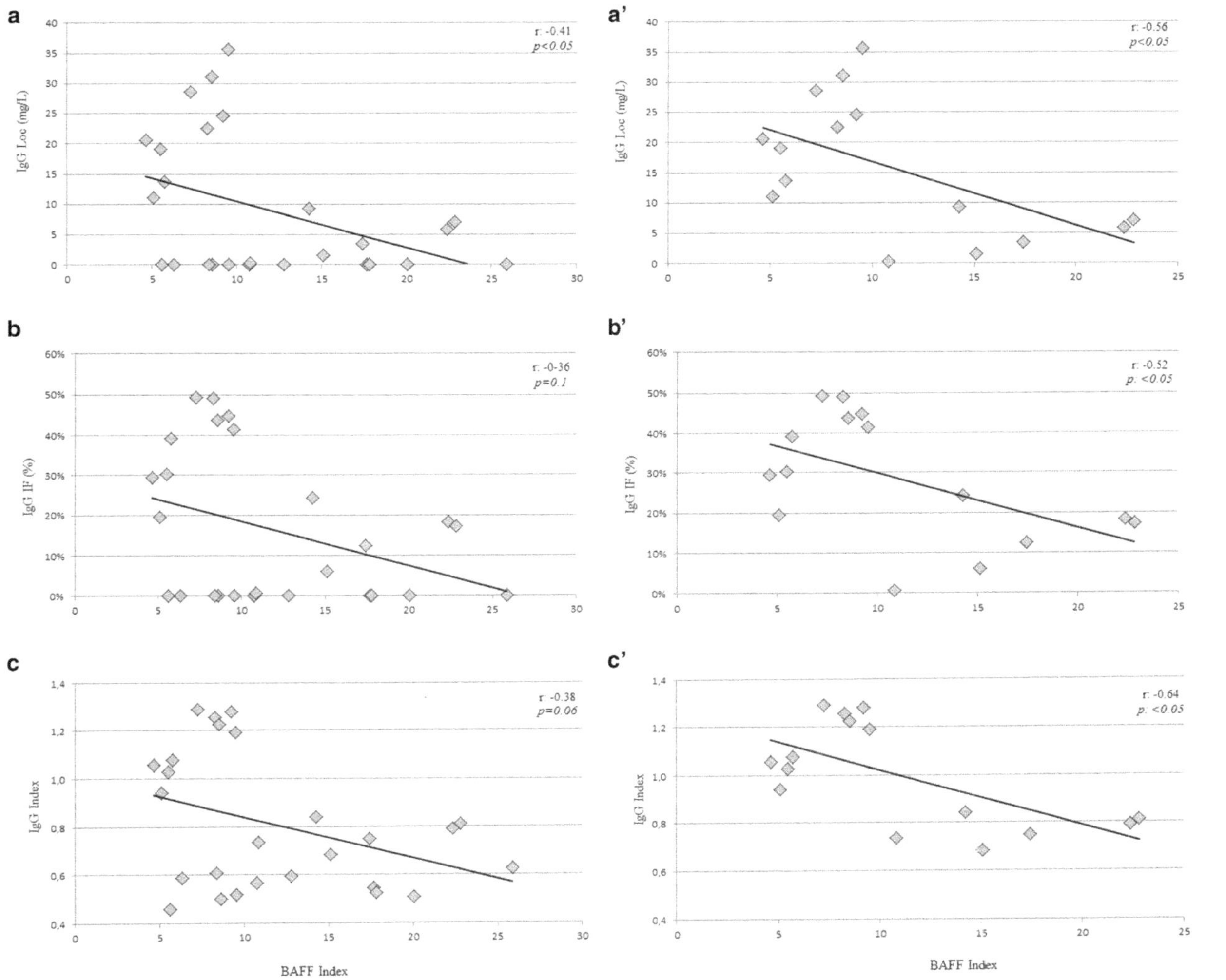

Fig. 3 Correlations between BAFF Index and intrathecal IgG synthesis. A mild correlation between BAFF Index and intrathecal IgG synthesis was observed when all the patients were considered (**a**–**c**). The correlation was strong when the null values of intrathecal IgG synthesis were excluded (**a'**–**c'**)

Table 4 Leukocyte counts in CIS/eRRMS correlates to CSF-CXCL13

	r	r^2	*p* value
CIS/eRRMS			
CSF-[CXCL13] (pg/mL)	0.79	63.2%	<0.001
BAFF Index	−0.21	4.4%	0.2
IgGOB+			
CSF-[CXCL13] (pg/mL)	0.77	59.3%	<0.001
BAFF Index	−0.22	4.7%	0.3
IgGOB−			
Csf-[CXCL13] (pg/mL)	0.34	11.6%	0.3
BAFF Index	0.22	4.8%	0.5

Subgroup analysis revealed that this correlation was confirmed only in IgGOB+ patients. Abbreviations as in Table 2. *R* values derived from Pearson's single linear model are represented

CXCL13, a chemokine that is not physiologically produced within the CNS, was increased in the CSF of CIS/eRRMS, especially in IgGOB+ patients. This finding suggests that CXCL13, produced by activated microgial cells, becomes detectable since the early disease phases, and is responsible for the recruitment of naïve B cells within the CNS. On the other hand, BAFF, constitutively produced in the CNS by astrocytes, is absorbed by local antibody-producing PCs, thus explaining the decreased levels of this cytokine in early MS stages. The previously described increased BAFF levels in the CSF of progressive MS [20] might found an explanation in the more diffuse astroglial proliferation and in the decreased burden of inflammation that characterize the more advanced phase of MS. However, since CSF CXCL13 was detected, although rarely, in patients with no evidence of intrathecal IgG synthesis, is not associated with

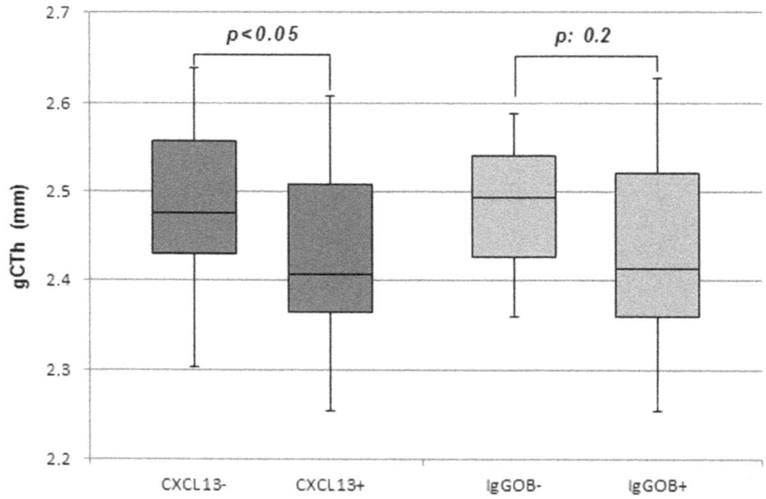

Fig. 4 Global cortical thickness is reduced in patients with higher CSF CXCL13. MS patients with higher CSF CXCL13 (CXCL13+) concentrations presented a significant cortical thinning compared to patients with lower values (CXCL13−)

BAFF Index and correlates only mildly with IgGLoc, we may argue that the majority of naïve B cells recruited in the CNS do not undergo the process of maturation to PCs. Taken all together, these findings do not speak in favor of a germinal center reaction within FLS, at least in early MS phases, and are in line with the qualitative stability of IgGOB patterns during the course of MS.

An interesting finding of our study was the association of CSF CXCL13, but not BAFF Index, with cortical thinning since early MS phases. This observation seems to link a soluble factor that plays a pivotal role in the B cell recruitment in the CNS, to a MRI parameter of neurodegeneration (gray matter atrophy), that is correlated to disability progression in MS.

Our findings are in line with the previous reports on the association of CXCL13 to leukocyte CSF counts [20], higher risk of relapse, and CIS conversion to MS [21], as well as with higher disease activity in the WM [22, 23], further suggesting a possible role of CXCL13 as a soluble marker of disease activity or severity in MS.

Other cytokines were found to increase in MS CSF [24]. Among these, the macrophage/microglia-derived interleukin-1 beta (IL-1β) was also found to correlate with cortical thinning [25]. The finding that both IL-1β and CXCL13 can be found in the CSF of very early MS and both factors associate with cortical thinning further suggests a pivotal role of microglia in MS pathology. Indeed, in vitro, CXCL13 is produced by monocytes, and at much higher levels by macrophages, and CXCL13 mRNA and protein expression is induced by TNFα and IL-1β [26]. All these data suggest that activated and proliferating microglia cells (a characteristic histological feature of cortical pathology) produce large amounts cytokines, such as IL-1β and CXCL13, that attract and maintain T and B cells in the inflamed meninges and in the cortex of MS.

Conclusions

Our findings indicate that intrathecally synthesized IgG are produced by PCs that enter the CNS from the peripheral blood at a given time and are locally retained as long-term PCs. A role for FLS as source of intrathecal IgG in early disease phases is not supported by our observations on CXCL13.

In our study, CXCL13 identifies a subgroup of MS patients characterized by the early evidence of cortical thinning, further suggesting a role for this chemokine as marker of disease severity.

Abbreviations

BAFF: B cell-activating factor; BBB: Blood brain barrier; CIS: Clinical isolated syndrome; CL: Cortical lesions; CNS: Central nervous system; CSF: Cerebrospinal fluid; DIR: Double inversion recovery; eRRMS: Early-onset relapsing-remitting multiple sclerosis; FLAIR: Fluid attenuated inversion recovery; HC: Healthy control; IgGIF: IgG intrathecal fraction; IgGLoc: IgG locally produced; IgGOB: IgG oligoclonal bands; MS: Multiple sclerosis; PCs: Plasma cells; Q_{Alb}: CSF/serum albumin; Q_{BAFF}: CSF/serum BAFF; Q_{CXCL13}: CSF/serum CXCL13; Q_{IgG}: CSF/serum IgG ratio; $Q_{IL\text{-}21}$: CSF/serum IL-21; WM: White matter

Acknowledgements

The authors would like to thank the patients and staff at the Multiple Sclerosis Centre of Padua, especially the nurses Elena Bortolami, Irene Boscariol, and Elisa Quaggia.

Funding

This research was supported by the grants from the Italian Minister of Public Health, Project GR-2010-2313255.

Authors' contributions

PM, FL, and SM contributed to the concept and design of the study and performed clinical data acquisition, analysis, and interpretation and they performed a critical revision of the manuscript for important intellectual content. AZ and ME performed the data analysis and interpretation and they performed a critical revision of the manuscript for important intellectual content. ET and SR performed the CSF and serum analysis and they performed a critical revision of the manuscript for important intellectual content. SP and DP performed the acquisition, analysis, and interpretation of MRI data. RF, PP, and GP contributed to the concept of the study and performed a critical revision of the manuscript for important intellectual content. All authors read and approved the final manuscript.

Competing interests

Puthenparampil Marco received a travel grant from Novartis, Genzyme, Biogen Idec, Teva and Sanofi Aventis; he has been a consultant for Genzyme. Federle Lisa has received funding for travel from Novartis, Merck Serono, Biogen Idec, Sanofi-Aventis, Bayer Schering Pharma, Almirall, Genzyme, Teva and honoraria from MerkSerono, Teva and Almirall. Miante Silvia received a travel grant form Biogen Idec, Novartis, Sanofi Aventis and Teva. Zito Antonio, Toffanin Elisabetta, Ruggiero Susanna, Mario Ermani, and Stefano Pravato have nothing to disclose. Davide Poggiali received a travel grant from Biogen Idec, Novartis, Sanofi Aventis and Teva. Perini Paola has received funding for travel and speaker honoraria from Merck Serono, Biogen Idec, Sanofi-Aventis, and Bayer Schering Pharma and has been a consultant for Merck Serono, Biogen Idec and Teva; Midena Edoardo has nothing to disclose Rinaldi Francesca serves as an advisory board member of Biogen-Idec and has received funding for travel and speaker honoraria from Merck Serono, Biogen Idec, Sanofi-Aventis, Teva and Bayer Schering Pharma. Gallo Paolo has been a consultant for Bayer Schering, Biogen Idec, Genzyme, Merck Serono and Novartis, has received funding for travel and speaker honoraria from Merck-Serono, Biogen Idec, Sanofi-Aventis, Novartis Pharma and Bayer-Schering Pharma, Teva, has received research support from Bayer, Biogen Idec/Elan, MerkSerono, Genzyme and Teva, and has received research grant from the University of Padova, Veneto Region of Italy, the Italian Association for Multiple Sclerosis, the Italian Ministry of Public Health.

Consent for publication

Not applicable.

Author details

[1]Multiple Sclerosis Centre, Department of Neurosciences DNS, University Hospital–Medical School, via Giustiniani 5, 3518 Padova, Italy. [2]Department of Neurosciences DNS, University Hospital–Medical School, via Giustiniani 5, 3518 Padova, Italy.

References

1. Reiber H, Peter JB. Cerebrospinal fluid analysis: disease-related data patterns and evaluation programs. J Neurol Sci. 2001;184:101–22.
2. Link H, Tibbling G. Principles of albumin and IgG analyses in neurological disorders. III. Evaluation of IgG synthesis within the central nervous system in multiple sclerosis. Scand J Clin Lab Invest. 1977;37:397–401.
3. Lucchinetti C, Bruck W, Parisi J, Scheithauer B, Rodriguez M, Lassmann H. Heterogeneity of multiple sclerosis lesions: implications for the pathogenesis of demyelination. Ann Neurol. 2000;47:707–17.
4. Howell OW, Reeves CA, Nicholas R, Carassiti D, Radotra B, Gentleman SM, et al. Meningeal inflammation is widespread and linked to cortical pathology in multiple sclerosis. Brain. 2011;134:2755–71.
5. Magliozzi R, Howell O, Vora A, Serafini B, Nicholas R, Puopolo M, et al. Meningeal B-cell follicles in secondary progressive multiple sclerosis associate with early onset of disease and severe cortical pathology. Brain. 2007;130:1089–104.
6. Hauser SL, Waubant E, Arnold DL, Vollmer T, Antel J, Fox RJ, et al. B-cell depletion with rituximab in relapsing-remitting multiple sclerosis. N Engl J Med. 2008;358:676–88.
7. Krumbholz M, Derfuss T, Hohlfeld R, Meinl E. B cells and antibodies in multiple sclerosis pathogenesis and therapy. Nat Rev Neurol. 2012;8:613–23.
8. He D, Guo R, Zhang F, Zhang C, Dong S, et al. Rituximab for relapsing-remitting multiple sclerosis. Cochrane Database Syst. Rev. 2013.
9. Hauser SL, Comi GC, Hartung HP, Selmaj K, Traboulsee A, Bar-Or A, et al. Oral Presentation n. 190: efficacy and safety of ocrelizumab in relapsing multiple sclerosis—results of the interferon-beta-1a-controlled, double-blind, phase III OPERA I and II studies. Mult Scler J. 2015;21:21.
10. Owens GP, Bennett JL, Lassmann H, O'Connor KC, Ritchie AM, Shearer A, et al. Antibodies produced by clonally expanded plasma cells in multiple sclerosis cerebrospinal fluid. Ann Neurol. 2009;65:639–49.
11. Obermeier B, Lovato L, Mentele R, Brück W, Forne I, Imhof A, et al. Related B cell clones that populate the CSF and CNS of patients with multiple sclerosis produce CSF immunoglobulin. J Neuroimmunol. 2011.
12. Thaunat O, Morelon E, Defrance T. Am"B"valent: anti-CD20 antibodies unravel the dual role of B cells in immunopathogenesis. Blood. 2010;116:515–21.
13. Puthenparampil M, Miante S, Federle L, Zanetta C, Toffanin E, Ruggero S, et al. BAFF is decreased in the cerebrospinal fluid of multiple sclerosis at clinical onset. J Neuroimmunol. 2016;297:63–7.
14. Filippi M, Rocca MA, Ciccarelli O, De Stefano N, Evangelou N, Kappos L, et al. MRI criteria for the diagnosis of multiple sclerosis: MAGNIMS consensus guidelines. Lancet Neurol. 2016;15:292–303.
15. Petzold A, Abraira V, Alvarez-Cermeño JC, Arroyo R, Cámara C, Casanova B, et al. Intrathecal oligoclonal IgG synthesis in multiple sclerosis. J Neuroimmunol. 2013;262:1–10.
16. Link H, Huang Y-M. Oligoclonal bands in multiple sclerosis cerebrospinal fluid: an update on methodology and clinical usefulness. J Neuroimmunol. 2006;180:17–28.
17. Correale J, de los Milagros Bassani Molinas M. Oligoclonal bands and antibody responses in multiple sclerosis. J Neurol. 2002;249:375–89.
18. Confavreux C, Chapuis-Cellier C, Arnaud P, Robert O, Aimard G, Devic M. Oligoclonal "fingerprint" of CSF IgG in multiple sclerosis patients is not modified following intrathecal administration of natural beta-interferon. J Neurol Neurosurg Psychiatry. 1986;49:1308–12.
19. Yu X, Burgoon M, Green M, Barmina O, Dennison K, Pointon T, et al. Intrathecally synthesized IgG in multiple sclerosis cerebrospinal fluid recognizes identical epitopes over time. J Neuroimmunol. 2011;240-241:129–36.
20. Ragheb S, Li Y, Simon K, VanHaerents S, Galimberti D, De Riz M, et al. Multiple sclerosis: BAFF and CXCL13 in cerebrospinal fluid. Mult Scler. 2011;17:819–29.
21. Brettschneider J, Czerwoniak A, Senel M, Fang L, Kassubek J, Pinkhardt E, et al. The chemokine CXCL13 is a prognostic marker in clinically isolated syndrome (CIS). PLoS One. 2010;5:e11986.
22. Sellebjerg F, Bornsen L, Khademi M, Krakauer M, Olsson T, Frederiksen JL, et al. Increased cerebrospinal fluid concentrations of the chemokine CXCL13 in active MS. Neurology. 2009;73:2003–10.
23. Khademi M, Kockum I, Andersson ML, Iacobaeus E, Brundin L, Sellebjerg F, et al. Cerebrospinal fluid CXCL13 in multiple sclerosis: a suggestive prognostic marker for the disease course. Mult Scler. 2011;17:335–43.
24. Kothur K, Wienholt L, Brilot F, Dale RC. CSF cytokines/chemokines as biomarkers in neuroinflammatory CNS disorders: a systematic review. Cytokine. 2016;77:227–37.
25. Seppi D, Puthenparampil M, Federle L, Ruggero S, Toffanin E, Rinaldi F, et al. Cerebrospinal fluid IL-1β correlates with cortical pathology load in multiple sclerosis at clinical onset. J Neuroimmunol. 2014;270:56–60.
26. Krumbholz M, Theil D, Cepok S, Hemmer B, Kivisäkk P, Ransohoff RM, et al. Chemokines in multiple sclerosis: CXCL12 and CXCL13 up-regulation is differentially linked to CNS immune cell recruitment. Brain. 2006;129:200–11.

2

Neurofilament levels, disease activity and brain volume during follow-up in multiple sclerosis

Irene Håkansson[1*], Anders Tisell[2,3], Petra Cassel[4], Kaj Blennow[5,6], Henrik Zetterberg[5,6,7,8], Peter Lundberg[2,3,9], Charlotte Dahle[1,4], Magnus Vrethem[1] and Jan Ernerudh[4]

Abstract

Background: There is a need for clinically useful biomarkers of disease activity in clinically isolated syndrome (CIS) and relapsing remitting MS (RRMS). The aim of this study was to assess the correlation between neurofilament light chain (NFL) in cerebrospinal fluid (CSF) and serum and the relationship between NFL and other biomarkers, subsequent disease activity, and brain volume loss in CIS and RRMS.

Methods: A panel of neurodegenerative and neuroinflammatory markers were analyzed in repeated CSF samples from 41 patients with CIS or RRMS in a prospective longitudinal cohort study and from 22 healthy controls. NFL in serum was analyzed using a single-molecule array (Simoa) method. "No evidence of disease activity-3" (NEDA-3) status and brain volume (brain parenchymal fraction calculated using SyMRI®) were recorded during 4 years of follow-up.

Results: NFL levels in CSF and serum correlated significantly (all samples, $n = 63$, r 0.74, $p < 0.001$), but CSF-NFL showed an overall stronger association profile with NEDA-3 status, new T2 lesions, and brain volume loss. CSF-NFL was associated with both new T2 lesions and brain volume loss during follow-up, whereas CSF-CHI3L1 was associated mainly with brain volume loss and CXCL1, CXCL10, CXCL13, CCL22, and MMP-9 were associated mainly with new T2 lesions.

Conclusions: Serum and CSF levels of NFL correlate, but CSF-NFL predicts and reflects disease activity better than S-NFL. CSF-NFL levels are associated with both new T2 lesions and brain volume loss. Our findings further add to the accumulating evidence that CSF-NFL is a clinically useful biomarker in CIS and RRMS and should be considered in the expanding NEDA concept. CSF-CXCL10 and CSF-CSF-CHI3L1 are potential markers of disease activity and brain volume loss, respectively.

Keywords: Multiple sclerosis, Clinically isolated syndrome, Disease activity, Neurofilament light chain, CHI3L1, CXCL10, Brain volume

Background

Multiple sclerosis (MS) is a chronic disease characterized by inflammation and degeneration of the central nervous system (CNS). Relapses, new T2 lesions, and disability progression are conventional signs of disease activity in MS. To aid personalized treatment, prognostic biomarkers and biomarkers of disease activity are needed. Assessing brain volume loss and biomarkers in cerebrospinal fluid (CSF) or serum (S) could potentially give a more comprehensive evaluation of disease activity [1–4].

Brain atrophy is present early in the disease course [5, 6] and associated with disability progression [7]. Using SyMRI® to determine brain volume as brain parenchymal fraction (BPF) has been reported as a valid and reproducible method with a clinically acceptable scan time and post-processing time [8]. Neurofilament light chain (NFL) in CSF correlates with long-term prognosis in MS [9], is a risk factor for conversion from clinically isolated syndrome (CIS) to relapsing remitting

* Correspondence: irene.hakansson@regionostergotland.se
[1]Department of Neurology and Department of Clinical and Experimental Medicine, Linköping University, Linköping, Sweden

multiple sclerosis (RRMS) [10], and decreases on treatment with fingolimod and natalizumab [11, 12]. We recently reported that CSF-NFL at baseline predicted disease activity during 2 years of follow-up in patients with CIS and RRMS [13]. S-NFL, determined with sensitive single-molecule array (Simoa) technology [14], has been reported to be highly correlated to CSF levels in RRMS [15].

This study aimed to assess the correlation between S-NFL and CSF-NFL, to evaluate NFL levels in relation to other biomarkers and disease activity parameters and to identify parameters associated with number of new T2 lesions and brain volume loss during 4 years of follow-up in a longitudinal cohort of patients with newly diagnosed CIS and RRMS.

Methods

Patients and controls

Forty-one patients with CIS or RRMS were consecutively enrolled in a prospective longitudinal cohort study of CIS and newly diagnosed MS at the Department of Neurology, University Hospital of Linköping, Sweden. All patients fulfilled the revised McDonald criteria from 2010 [16] for CIS or MS. Patients underwent clinical neurological examination including expanded disability status scale (EDSS), blood and CSF sampling as well as MRI at baseline, and at 1, 2, and 4 years of follow-up. Patients received immunomodulatory treatment according to Swedish clinical practice during the study period, from 2009 to 2016. Patient characteristics are presented in Tables 1 and 2. For blood and CSF parameters, 22 age- and sex-matched healthy controls (HC) were recruited from healthy blood donors. Healthy controls were free from past and current neurological and autoimmune disease, and their clinical neurological examinations were normal as were routine findings in CSF (Table 1). No medication, except oral contraceptives, was allowed in healthy controls. The patients and controls were included in a previous study reporting biomarkers in relation to 2 years of follow-up, while in the present study, we report data from 4 years of follow-up and also include BPF and serum NFL.

Disease activity assessment

All clinical assessments regarding relapses and EDSS were performed by the same neurologist (IH), and all MRI examinations were thoroughly reviewed by the same neuroradiologist. Patients that showed no relapses, no brain MRI activity (no new or enlarging T2 lesions or Gadolinium-enhancing lesions), and no sustained disability worsening (EDSS progression) during follow-up were classified as showing "no evidence of disease activity"-3 (NEDA-3) ($n = 20$ at 1 year, $n = 12$ at 2 years, and $n = 7$ at 4 years), while patients with relapses, brain MRI activity, or sustained disability worsening were classified as showing evidence of disease activity (EDA-3) ($n = 21$ at 1 year, $n = 27$ at 2 years, and $n = 32$ at 4 years). All 41 patients were evaluated at 1 year and 39 patients were

Table 1 Patient and healthy control characteristics at baseline

Clinical and laboratory data	Patients $n = 41$	Healthy controls $n = 22$	p value
Women/men (% women)	32/9 (78%)	17/5 (77%)	0.9
Age[a] (years)	31 (24–36)	32 (26–41)	0.3
Diagnosis (CIS/RRMS)	19/22	N/A	
Relapse within last 2 months (yes/no)	23/18	N/A	
Mean disease duration[b] (months)	11.8	N/A	
Median disease duration[b] (months)	3.5	N/A	
Disease duration[b] (number of subjects)		N/A	
0–1 months	*10*		
1.25–2 months	*7*		
2.25–3 months	*3*		
3.25–6 months	*6*		
6.5–12 months	*7*		
13–24 months	*3*		
25–36 months	*2*		
37–48 months	*1*		
49–120 months	*2*		
Median EDSS	2.0	N/A	
EDSS (number of subjects)			
0	*6*	*22*	
1.0	*12*		
1.5	*2*		
2.0	*12*		
2.5	*3*		
3.0	*1*		
3.5	*2*		
4.0	*2*		
4.5	*1*		
CSF mononuclear cell count[a]	4.6×10^6/L (1.8–9.2)	2.1×10^6/L (0.9–2.7)	0.001
Albumin ratio[a]	4.8 (3.4–6.0)	4.7 (3.6–5.3)	0.5
IgG index[a]	0.7 (0.5–1.1)	0.5 (0.5–0.5)	< 0.001
IgG synthesis index[a]	1.3 (1.0–2.1)	0.9 (0.9–1.0)	< 0.001
Oligoclonal CSF IgG bands (pos/neg)	33/8	0/22	< 0.001

p values from chi-square test for sex distribution and oligoclonal bands and from Mann-Whitney U test for age and CSF data
N/A not applicable, *DMT* disease-modifying treatment
[a]Median and within brackets interquartile range
[b]Disease duration refers to time from first symptom suggestive of demyelinating disease

Table 2 Patient diagnoses, relapse status, and treatment status over time

Clinical and laboratory data	Baseline	1 year	2 years	4 years
Number of subjects	41	41	40	39
Diagnosis (CIS/RRMS)	19/22	12/29	9/31	7/32
Relapse within last 2 months (yes/no)	23/18	4/37	2/38	2/37
Treatment (number of subjects)				
No DMT	41	17	18	18
Interferon-β 1b	0	18	12	5
Interferon-β 1a	0	1	1	1
Dimetylfumarate	0	0	0	2
Fingolimod	0	1	2	3
Natalizumab	0	4	7	10

evaluated at 2 and 4 years of follow-up. At 2 years, one pregnant patient did not undergo MRI and one patient had left the study. At 4 years, one additional patient had left the study, while the previously pregnant patient completed 4-year follow-up.

Cerebrospinal fluid and serum analyses

All CSF sampling was carried out by the same neurologist (IH), and CSF was always collected 8–12 a.m. Serum samples were collected directly after CSF collection. One aliquot of the CSF sample was used for cell counting, CSF/serum albumin ratio, IgG index, IgG synthesis index, and isoelectric focusing, all according to clinical routines performed at the Department of Clinical Chemistry, Linköping University Hospital. Within 1 hour, the remaining CSF was centrifuged (300×*g* for 10 min.) and the supernatant was aliquoted and immediately frozen and stored at – 70 °C.

CSF samples were analyzed for chemokine concentrations with a multiplex bead assay (Milliplex® MAP kits, EMD Millipore Corporation, St. Charles, MO, USA) according to the manufacturer's instructions, except that an additional lower standard point was added to the standard curve. The measurements were performed using Luminex®200™ (Invitrogen, Merelbeke, Belgium). For data acquisition, the software program xPONENT 3.1™ (Luminex Corporation, Austin, TX, USA) was used, and for data analysis, MasterPlex® Reader Fit was used. The detection limits were 16 pg/mL for CXCL1, CXCL10, and CCL22; 3.2 pg/mL for CXCL8; and 3.9 pg/mL for CXCL13. Values below the detection limit were assigned half the value of the detection limit.

CSF NFL concentration was measured using the NF-light assay according to instructions from the manufacturer (UmanDiagnostics, Umeå, Sweden). CSF NFH concentration was measured using the Phosphorylated NEFH (Human) ELISA Kit according to instructions from the manufacturer (Abnova, Taipei City, Taiwan). CSF MMP-9 concentration was measured using the Human MMP-9 Base Kit according to instructions from the manufacturer (Meso Scale Discovery, Rockville, MD). CSF GFAP concentration was measured using an in-house ELISA as previously described [17]. CSF CHI3L1 and OPN concentrations were measured using commercially available ELISAs (R&D Systems, Inc. Minneapolis, MN). The lower limits of quantification for the NFH and MMP-9 assays were 31.2 and 122 pg/mL, respectively. For the other analytes, all samples had concentrations within the quantifiable range of the assay. All measurements were performed in one round of experiments using one batch of reagents by board-certified laboratory technicians who were blinded to clinical information. Intra-assay coefficients of variation were below 15%.

S-NFL concentration was measured using the NF-Light kit from UmanDiagnostics (UmanDiagnostics, Umeå, Sweden), transferred onto the Simoa platform using a homebrew kit (Quanterix Corp, Boston, MA, USA), as previously described in detail [18]. The lower limit of quantification (LLoQ), determined by the blank mean signal + 10 SD, was 1.95 pg/mL. Levels in all samples were well above LLoQ. The analyses were performed by board-certified laboratory technicians using one batch of reagents with intra- and inter-assay coefficients of variation below 10 and 15%, respectively.

Magnetic resonance imaging and post processing

All subjects were examined on a 1.5-T Philips Achieve MRI scanner (Philips Healthcare, Best, The Netherlands) using an eight-channel phased array head coil. Quantitative MRI images were acquired using QMAP sequence [19]. BPF was calculated using SyMRI® version 8.0 (SyntheticMR, Linköping, Sweden).

Statistical analyses

Statistical analyses were performed using SPSS for Windows, version 23. Analyzing data sets with non-Gaussian distribution, the Mann-Whitney *U* test was used to compare two groups and non-parametric bivariate correlation analysis (Spearman) was used for correlation analyses. The relationship between NFL in CSF and serum was examined using bivariate linear regression and Spearman correlation analysis, as well as Pearson correlation analysis when sample size was > 50. Friedman's test with Dunn correction for multiple comparisons was used to compare repeated measurements of immunological markers in patients over time. Repeated measures ANOVA with Bonferroni correction for multiple comparisons was used to compare repeated BPF measurements in patients over time. Multiple linear regression analysis was used to evaluate brain volume loss over time and number of new T2 lesions over time. Logistic regression was used when investigating NFL and other markers in relation to NEDA. Receiver operating characteristic (ROC) curves were derived from logistic regression to investigate the discriminatory power of NFL and other markers between patients with and without disease activity during follow-up. Because of multiple testing, a stringent p value of ≤ 0.01 was considered to be significant in Mann-Whitney U tests, t tests, repeated measures ANOVA, and linear regression analyses. In Spearman correlation analyses, a very stringent significance level of Spearman's rho ≥ 0.5 and $p \leq 0.01$ was used, which entailed a maximum type II error of 0.21 when $n = 41$ and 0.27 when $n = 37$. For comparisons within the CIS group, where patient numbers were small and comparisons few, a p value of ≤ 0.05 was considered significant in Mann-Whitney U tests. Area under curve (AUC) values were compared using the DeLong method, in MEDCALC®, with the significance level set at 0.05. All p values were based on two-tailed statistical tests.

Results

S-NFL and CSF-NFL correlate, and both are elevated in patients at baseline

S-NFL and CSF-NFL correlated in HC ($n = 22$, Spearman's rho 0.59, $p = 0.004$), in patients at baseline ($n = 41$, Spearman's rho 0.63, $p < 0.001$), in samples from patients at baseline and HC combined ($n = 63$, Spearman's rho 0.65, $p < 0.001$, and Pearson's r 0.74 ($p < 0.001$). R^2 from bivariate linear regression with S-NFL as dependent variable and CSF-NFL as independent variable ($n = 63$) was 0.54, $p < 0.001$, equation $y = 0.007x + 10.1$. A correlation plot is presented in Fig. 1.

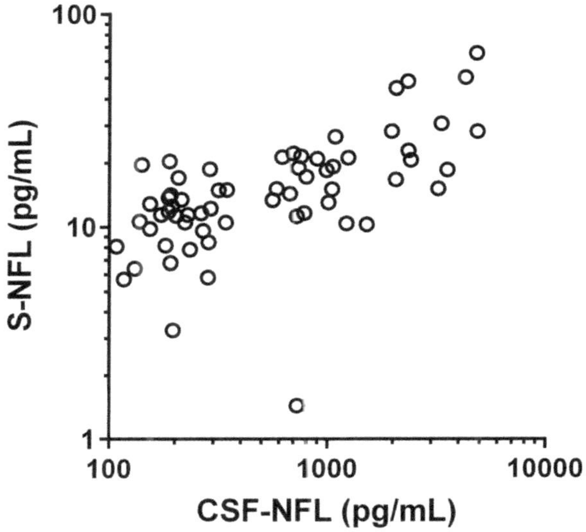

Fig. 1 Correlation between S-NFL and CSF-NFL. Correlation between S-NFL and CSF-NFL, all samples from patients and healthy controls ($n = 63$). Logarithmic scales are used on graph axes for improved visibility (increased separation of data points), whereas statistical analyses were performed on non-transformed linear data. Spearman's rho 0.65 ($p < 0.001$) and Pearson's r 0.74 ($p < 0.001$)

To compare NFL levels in health and disease, patients at baseline (all untreated) were compared with healthy controls. Both S-NFL and CSF-NFL were significantly higher in patients than in controls, see Fig. 2.

In patients, neither CSF nor serum NFL could be explained by age (R^2 0.01, $p = 0.5$ for CSF-NFL and R^2 0.003, $p = 0.7$ for S-NFL in simple linear regression). In healthy controls, on the other hand, age was a significant factor in relation to both CSF-NFL and S-NFL levels (R^2 0.73, $p < 0.001$ for CSF-NFL and R^2 0.30, $p = 0.008$ for S-NFL in simple linear regression). S-NFL levels, just like recently reported for CSF-NFL levels [13] in this cohort, did not differ between CIS patients and RRMS patients ($p = 0.9$ for S-NFL and $p = 0.4$ for CSF-NFL) or between patients with and without a relapse starting within 2 months prior to sample collection at baseline ($p = 0.7$ for S-NFL and $p = 0.1$ for CSF-NFL). However, when including not only baseline samples but also follow-up samples, thereby increasing total n from 41 to 161, RRMS patients had higher CSF-NFL ($p = 0.01$), but not S-NFL ($p = 0.6$), than CIS patients, and NFL levels were higher in relapse patients than in non-relapse patients ($p = 0.004$ for S-NFL and $p \leq 0.001$ for CSF-NFL).

Neuroinflammatory and neurodegenerative markers at baseline and over time

CSF and serum was collected at baseline and after 1, 2, and 4 years. The complete descriptive data are presented in an additional table (see Additional file 1: Table S1) for neuroinflammatory and neurodegenerative markers (NFL, neurofilament heavy chain (NFH), glial fibrillary acidic protein (GFAP), chitinase 3 like 1 (CHI3L1), matrix metalloproteinase 9 (MMP-9), osteopontin (OPN), CXCL1, CXCL8, CXCL10, CXCL13, and CCL22). Data on levels in healthy controls and in patients at baseline have been reported previously [13].

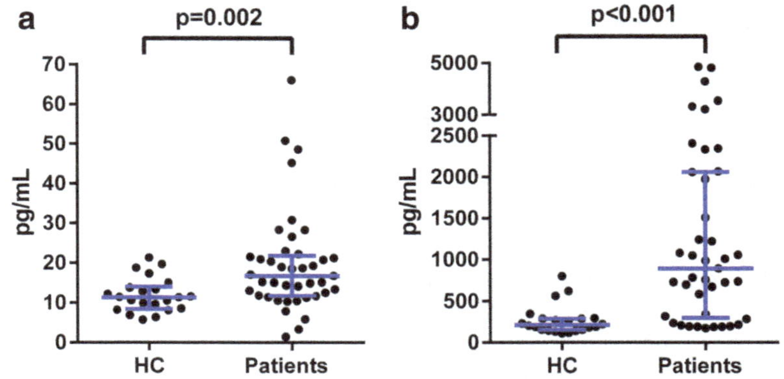

Fig. 2 NFL in serum (**a**) and CSF (**b**) in healthy controls and patients at baseline. Lines show median and interquartile range. For S-NFL, patient group ($n = 41$) median was 17 pg/mL (interquartile range 12–22 pg/mL) and healthy control (HC) ($n = 22$) group median was 11 pg/mL (interquartile range 8–14 pg/mL). For CSF-NFL, patient group median was 895 pg/mL (interquartile range 300–2060 pg/mL) and HC group median was 212 pg/mL (interquartile range 151–289 pg/mL). *P*- values from Mann-Whitney *U* test

NFL levels at baseline, in particular in CSF, predict NEDA-3 status during follow-up

Area under curve (AUC) for baseline levels of NFL in relation to disease activity during 1, 2, and 4 years of follow-up were 0.75, 0.65, and 0.69 for S-NFL, and 0.81, 0.85, and 0.73 for CSF-NFL; ROC curves are presented in Fig. 3. The AUC value was significantly higher at 2 years for CSF-NFL than S-NFL ($p = 0.05$), but did not differ significantly at 1 and 4 years ($p > 0.05$). With a cutoff value of ≥ 450 ng/L for baseline CSF-NFL, the sensitivity of identifying patients with disease activity was 95% at 1 year, 93% at 2 years, and 81% at 4 years, with specificity 50, 67, and 57%, respectively. With a cutoff value of 14.2 ng/L for baseline S-NFL, sensitivity of identifying patients with disease activity was 76% at 1 year, 74% at 2 years, and 72% at 4 years, with specificity 50, 50, and 57%, respectively. Thus, low levels of CSF-NFL entail a high probability of NEDA during follow-up.

Chemokines at baseline predict NEDA-3 status during follow-up

For prediction of NEDA-3/EDA-3 during 1 and 2 years of follow-up, baseline CXCL10 and baseline CSF-NFL had the highest ROC-based AUCs (0.81–0.85) and for prediction of NEDA-3/EDA-3 during 4 years of follow-up, baseline MMP-9, CXCL10, CCL22, and CXCL13 had the highest AUCs (0.80–0.83), see Additional file 2: Table S2 for predictive values (AUCs) of the whole panel of markers. There were no statistically significant differences between AUCs ≥ 0.80 (all $p \geq 0.05$). CXCL10 was the only marker with all three (1, 2, and 4 years) AUCs above 0.8.

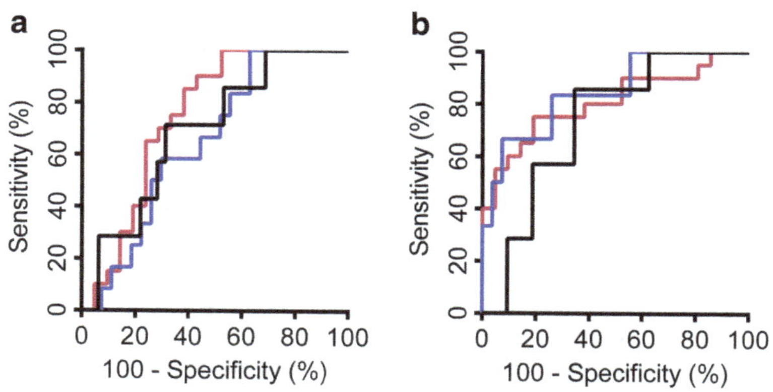

Fig. 3 S-NFL and CSF-NFL and separation of patients with and without disease activity during follow-up. Receiver operating characteristics (ROC) curves for baseline **a** S-NFL and **b** CSF-NFL and separation of patients with and without disease activity during follow-up after 1 (purple), 2 (blue), and 4 (black) years. Disease activity was defined as relapses, brain MRI activity (new or enlarging T2 lesions or Gd-enhancing lesions), or disability worsening. With a cutoff level of 450 ng/L for baseline CSF-NFL, sensitivity for identifying disease activity was 95% at 1 year, 93% at 2 years, and 81% at 4 years, with specificity 50, 67, and 57%, respectively. With a cutoff level of 14.2 ng/L for baseline S-NFL, sensitivity for identifying disease activity was 76% at 1 year, 74% at 2 years, and 72% at 4 years, with specificity 50, 50, and 57%, respectively

NFL levels during follow-up are associated with NEDA-3 status during follow-up

When evaluating associations with disease activity, both in the cross-sectional and the longitudinal perspective, AUCs from follow-up levels as well as mean levels of follow-up levels were assessed, in addition to AUCs from baseline levels (table presented in Additional file 2: Table S2). The marker with the highest AUC for NEDA-3/EDA-3 during 1 year of follow-up was CSF-NFL at 1 year (AUC 0.89), and for 2 years, it was mean CSF-NFL during 2 years of follow-up (AUC 0.88). Regarding NEDA-3/EDA-3 during 4 years of follow-up, the highest NFL AUC (mean CSF-NFL during 4 years of follow-up, AUC 0.76) was surpassed by others in absolute numbers (see Additional file 2: Table S2), although not significantly different ($p \geq 0.05$). These data show that NFL levels in CSF during follow-up, especially mean levels, are highly associated with ongoing disease activity expressed as NEDA-3/EDA-3.

Brain parenchymal fraction decreases over time and is associated with increased disease activity in the early phase

One patient was excluded at all four time points due to very low BPF associated with congenital hydrocephalus. Three patients were excluded due to missing data. BPF data from the 37 patients that completed all four BPF measurements are presented in Fig. 4. BPF mean ± SD was 91.8 ± 2.9 at baseline, 91.3 ± 2.8 at 1 year follow-up, 90.8 ± 3.0 at 2 years follow-up, and 90.5 ± 3.2 at 4 years follow-up. In repeated measures ANOVA with Bonferroni correction for multiple comparisons, BPF at 1, 2, and 4 years of follow-up were significantly lower than at baseline ($p < 0.005$, $p < 0.001$, and $p < 0.001$) and BPF at 2 and 4 years were significantly lower than at 1 year ($p < 0.001$ and 0.004). However, BPF at 4 years was not lower than at 2 years ($p = 0.9$). Time from baseline MRI to follow-up MRI (mean ± SD) was 12 ± 1 months, 24 ± 1 months, and 44 ± 5 months for 1-, 2-, and 4-year follow-up, respectively.

Mean BPF decrease was 0.49/year from baseline to 1 year, 0.50/year from baseline to 2 years, and 0.36/year from baseline to 4 years. Mean BPF decrease from baseline to 4-year follow-up was significantly higher in patients with EDA-3 than in patients with NEDA-3 during 1 year (− 1.6 vs − 0.7, $p = 0.001$), but not two (− 1.4 vs − 0.7, $p = 0.02$) and four (− 1.3 vs − 0.6, $p = 0.06$) years of follow-up.

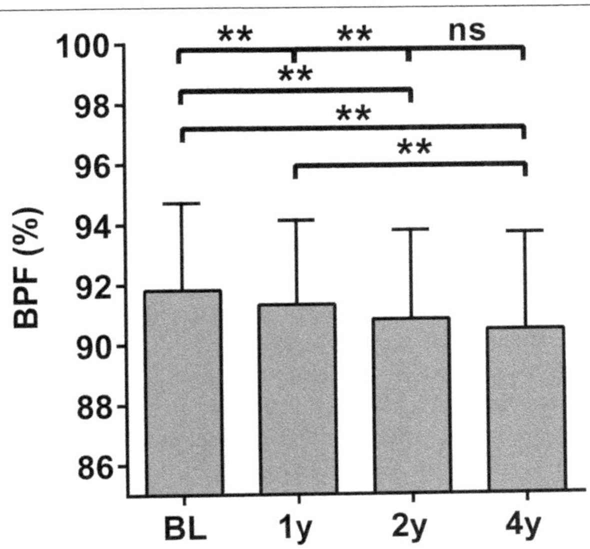

Fig. 4 Brain parenchymal fraction in patients at baseline and during follow-up. Brain parenchymal fraction (BPF) in patients at baseline (BL) and at 1 year (1y), 2 years (2y), and 4 years (4y) of follow-up. $^{**}p \leq 0.01$ in repeated measures ANOVA with Bonferroni correction for multiple comparisons. ns: not significant

Neurofilament levels correlate with both new T2 lesions and BPF decrease, while chemokines correlate with new T2 lesions and CHI3L1 correlates with BPF decrease

Correlations between the panel of biomarkers (listed in Additional file 1: Table S1) and baseline BPF, BPF decrease over time, baseline number of T2 lesions in brain MRI, and number of new T2 lesions over time were examined in 37 patients with complete data sets of BPF and the other parameters. Table 3 shows a map of the significant correlations. Of note, neurofilament levels correlated with both number of new T2 lesions and BPF decrease during follow-up, whereas inflammatory chemokines correlated only with new T2 lesions and CHI3L1 levels correlated only with BPF decrease.

Linear regression modeling indicates CHI3L1 as the strongest predictor of BPF decrease

To identify the most important parameters for prediction (using baseline parameters only) of, and for association (follow-up data included as well) with, BPF decrease and new T2 lesions, linear regression modeling of BPF decrease and new T2 lesions during 4 years of follow-up was performed. Details about these procedures are given in Supplemental data. For prediction of BPF decrease, baseline CHI3L1 was the single parameter that performed best (R^2 0.26, $p = 0.001$) and a peak adjusted R^2 of 0.41 ($p = 0.001$) was noted for a model including age, CSF-mononuclear cells, NFH, MMP-9, CHI3L1, and T2 lesions at baseline. As for association with BPF decrease, adjusted R^2 peaked with a model including baseline T2 lesions, baseline OPN, and 1-year CHI3L1 (adjusted R^2 0.30, $p = 0.002$), and the single parameter that performed best was 1-year CHI3L1 (R^2 0.29, $p =$ 0.001). For prediction of new T2 lesions, no model reached the significance level $p \leq 0.01$, whereas for

Table 3 Correlations between neuroinflammatory and neurodegenerative markers, baseline number of T2 lesions, number of new T2 lesions, and BPF change during follow-up

	T2, BL	New T2, 1 year	New T2, 2 years	New T2, 4 years	BPF change, 4 years
S-NFL, BL	0.33	0.55*	0.43	0.44	− 0.24
S-NFL, 1y	0.45	0.43	0.33	0.34	− 0.56*
S-NFL, 2y mean	0.45	0.52*	0.37	0.37	− 0.37
S-NFL, 4y mean	0.41	0.43	0.32	0.35	−0.42
CSF-NFL, BL	0.29	0.60*	0.64*	0.51*	− 0.20
CSF-NFL, 1y	0.59*	0.59*	0.58*	0.50*	− 0.54*
CSF-NFL, 2y mean	0.43	0.62*	0.65	0.54	−0.33
CSF-NFL, 4y mean	0.41	0.55*	0.60*	0.53*	− 0.35
MMP-9, BL	0.46	0.53*	0.47	0.42	− 0.16
MMP-9, mean	0.38	0.51*	0.51*	0.46	−0.26
CHI3L1, BL	0.49	0.42	0.36	0.26	−0.55*
CHI3L1, 1y	0.45	0.35	0.30	0.30	− 0.60*
CHI3L1, 2y	0.31	0.13	0.11	0.13	− 0.50*
CHI3L1, mean	0.42	0.30	0.24	0.20	− 0.54*
OPN, BL	0.51*	0.34	0.21	0.23	− 0.52*
CXCL1, BL	0.51*	0.56*	0.42	0.23	− 0.34
CXCL10, BL	0.50*	0.58*	0.48	0.41	− 0.26
CXCL10, mean	0.47	0.51*	0.42	0.34	− 0.37
CXCL13, BL	0.37	0.51*	0.52*	0.46	− 0.26
CXCL13, mean	0.40	0.49	0.52*	0.45	− 0.33
CCL22, mean	0.29	0.49	0.57*	0.54*	− 0.31
T2, BL	1.00	0.48	0.39	0.27	− 0.56*
New T2, 1y	0.48	1.00	0.86*	0.66*	− 0.44
New T2, 2y	0.39	0.86*	1.00	0.83*	− 0.47
New T2, 4y	0.27	0.66*	0.83*	1.00	− 0.36
BPF decrease, 4y	− 0.56*	− 0.44	− 0.47	− 0.36	1.00

Magnitude of correlation coefficients (Spearman's rho) from bivariate non-parametric correlation analyses (Spearman) are shown
2y mean refers to the mean of levels at baseline, 1-year, and 2-year follow-up
4y mean refers to the mean of levels at baseline, 1-year, 2-year, and 4-year follow-up
T2, BL: number of T2 lesions in baseline brain MRI
New T2, 1y, 2y and 4y: number of new T2 lesions in brain MRI during 1, 2, and 4 years of follow-up, respectively, compared to baseline MRI
BPF change, 4y: brain parenchymal fraction decrease during 4 years of follow-up
S serum, *CSF* cerebrospinal fluid, *BL* baseline
*Spearman's rho ≥ 0.50 and $p \leq 0.001$

association with new T2 lesions, adjusted R^2 peaked with a model including mean CCL22, 1-year CSF-NFL, and baseline CXCL13 (adjusted R^2 0.40, $p < 0.001$), and the single parameter that performed best was 1-year CSF-NFL (R^2 0.32, $p < 0.001$). Details of linear regression statistics are given in Additional file 3.

CIS converters

Within the CIS group at baseline ($n = 19$), CXCL10, NFL, and MMP-9 in CSF were significantly higher ($p \leq 0.05$ in Mann-Whitney *U* tests) in patients that converted to RRMS during 4 years of follow-up ($n = 12$) than in non-converters ($n = 7$), whereas S-NFL ($p = 0.10$) and the other markers ($p = 0.07$–0.90) did not differ. For the 12 CIS patients that converted to RRMS during the study, multiple regression modeling of time to conversion resulted in a highly significant model (adjusted R^2 0.81, $p = 0.006$) when including baseline CSF levels of CXCL1, CXCL10, CXCL13, and NFL, and number of T2 lesions at baseline).

Discussion

In the present study, we report a correlation between NFL levels in CSF and serum (Pearson's r 0.74) that is in line with what has been reported by others [15, 20]. Although baseline S-NFL was correlated with subsequent disease activity, CSF NFL seems to reflect disease activity better since baseline CSF-NFL predicted NEDA-3 during 2 years of follow-up significantly better than S-NFL, and moreover, CSF-NFL levels showed an overall stronger correlation profile than serum levels with regard to number of new T2 lesions. Our findings confirm CSF-NFL as a prognostic biomarker for conversion from CIS to MS [13, 21], association with disease activity [9, 13], and change in brain volume [22]. The fact that all these findings were significant in our moderately sized cohort, and the finding that CSF-NFL performed well compared with other markers and showed associations with both disease activity and brain volume loss, render further support for CSF-NFL as a clinically useful biomarker in MS.

Interestingly, 1-year CSF-NFL levels correlated significantly with both new T2 lesions and BPF decrease during 4 years of follow-up. For other markers, they were either associated with BPF decrease (CHI3L1 and OPN) or with new T2 lesions (CXCL1, CXCL10, CXCL13, CCL22, and MMP-9). In linear regression modeling of new T2 lesions, the combination of 1-year CSF-NFL, CCL22 (mean level) and CXCL13 (baseline level) performed better than 1-year CSF-NFL alone, suggesting an added value of combining several markers, which was recently shown for chemokines and OPN [23]. Of note, chemokines, in contrast to most cytokines, are present at measurable levels in CSF. We here showed that CXCL10 was able to predict disease activity at all follow-up time points (NEDA-3 status at 1, 2, and 4 years) and that CXCL10 was also higher in CIS-converters than in non-converters, findings that suggest CXCL10 as a biomarker in CIS and RRMS. This has been indicated in other studies as well [24, 25]. As for brain volume loss, CHI3L1 had the highest predictive value, and further studies may confirm its clinical role.

Expanding NEDA-3 to NEDA-4 and NEDA-5 by including brain volume loss and biomarkers could improve assessment of disease activity in MS. Number of T2 lesions and T2 lesion volume in conventional MRI correlate poorly to clinical disease manifestations and disease progression in MS [26], although lesion volume has been reported to predict long-term disability [27]. Measuring brain volume loss as BPF decrease is non-invasive and logistically easy, only marginally extending time in the MRI-scanner. However, the use of BPF measurements and other brain volume quantification methods are hampered by technical limitations, physiological variation, and difficulties in identifying optimal cutoff levels for annual brain volume loss [3, 28]. It has been argued that although suitable for cohort studies, BPF measurements do not seem adequate for assessing changes in individual patients over months or a few years [28]. CSF-NFL, on the other hand, is a biomarker that provides clinically useful information and therefore emerges as a strong candidate for inclusion in the NEDA concept, although cutoff levels need to be settled. As for the more feasible S-NFL, a reasonable correlation with CSF-NFL and an ability to reflect disease activity in MS [15, 29, 30] was here confirmed, reiterating the suggestion of S-NFL as a promising biomarker. Indeed, recently published data from a large MS cohort show that higher S-NFL is clearly associated with worse clinical (EDSS progression) as well as MRI (T2 lesions and atrophy) outcome [31]. CSF-NFL was however not reported, and in our cohort, S-NFL did not perform as well as in that study [31]. It could be that smaller sample size affected our results, but still we noted that CSF-NFL yielded strong results in our single-center cohort. The exciting development of reliable high sensitivity assays has enabled detection of brain-derived markers in serum and plasma, but still these levels constitute a proxy for the levels in CSF. As long as there is no absolute correlation between CSF- and S-NFL, it seems clear that CSF levels should better reflect CNS pathology than blood, as supported by the stronger associations that we see between CSF-NFL and NEDA-3 as well as T2 lesions and brain volume, compared with S-NFL. Also, some markers of inflammation, such as the chemokines CXCL10 and CXCL13, have been reported to be elevated and to correlate with disease activity when measured in the CSF, but not in plasma [13, 32, 33]. Since CSF analysis is recommended in the diagnostic process [34], it is uncontroversial and appropriate to include NFL and other biomarkers in CSF at this stage. Also in monitoring of disease activity and treatment effects, the best possible medical information would be obtained by CSF analyses, which in the future also may include tools to personalized treatment [23, 35]. On the other hand, aspects like patient discomfort and various practical issues limit the use of CSF biomarkers, whereas blood samples can usually be easily obtained. We believe that both CSF- and S-NFL should be part of the initial diagnostic work-up for all patients and that follow-up CSF analyses should be considered when as complete as possible information is required to make a clinical decision. For many patients follow-up CSF analyses may not be motivated, whereas S-NFL could be liberally considered as an addition to NEDA-3 evaluation. As for the other neuroinflammatory and neurodegenerative markers in our panel, we have previously reported that chemokine levels in plasma did not differ significantly between patients and healthy controls [13]. There have been reports by others that e.g. CHI3L1 in serum may be a useful biomarker [36, 37], but so far, S-NFL shows most promise [31].

Limitations of this study include the cohort size, varying treatment and lack of MRI data from healthy controls. Varying treatment regimens in the cohort could lower the prognostic value of baseline biomarker levels. However, despite the fact that some patients received disease modifying drugs during follow-up, baseline levels of some proteins clearly showed prognostic value. We also focused on NEDA status, new T2 lesions, and BPF decrease in relation to follow-up levels and mean levels of NFL, etc., thereby exploring association over time instead of prediction. When examining, for example, the association between mean level of NFL during follow-up and NEDA-3 status during follow-up, the impact of treatment is negligible or small unless treatment affect NFL and NEDA-3 status very unevenly. Study strengths are the control group, consisting of sex- and age-matched healthy individuals, that the patient group consisted of well-characterized CIS and MS patients examined and thoroughly followed up prospectively by the same neurologist in a standardized way and that all patients were untreated at baseline. Also, a broad panel of potential biomarkers was included. The present study provides 4-year follow-up data on CSF-NFL in a patient cohort that we have previously presented 2-year follow-up data from, and in addition, we report S-NFL data as well as brain volume analyses for the entire study period (4 years). Taken together, this is the first study that reports longitudinal data on these markers, including NFL levels in CSF and serum, in relation to both NEDA-3 and brain volume loss in a clinical setting study.

Conclusions

We show that although serum and CSF levels of NFL correlate significantly, CSF-NFL predicts and reflects disease activity better than S-NFL during follow-up in our cohort of patients with CIS and RRMS. CSF-NFL is associated with both new T2 lesions and brain volume loss during follow-up. Our findings further add to the accumulating evidence that CSF-NFL is a useful biomarker in CIS and RRMS and should be considered in the expanding NEDA concept. Our findings also support S-NFL as a potential biomarker in CIS and RRMS. Other biomarkers that need further attention include CXCL10 and CHI3L1 for prediction of NEDA-3 and brain volume loss, respectively.

Abbreviations

AUC: Area under curve; BPF: Brain parenchymal fraction; CHI3L1: Chitinase 3 like 1; CIS: Clinically isolated syndrome; CNS: Central nervous system; CSF: Cerebrospinal fluid; EDA: Evidence of disease activity; EDSS: Expanded disability status scale; GFAP: Glial fibrillary acidic protein; HC: Healthy controls; MMP-9: Matrix metalloproteinase 9; MS: Multiple sclerosis; NEDA: No evidence of disease activity; NFH: Neurofilament heavy chain; NFL: Neurofilament light chain; OPN: Osteopontin; ROC: Receiver operating characteristic; RRMS: Relapsing remitting multiple sclerosis; S: Serum

Acknowledgements

We thank Patrik Fägerstam at the Department of Radiology, Linköping University Hospital, for systematically reviewing MRI scans and detailed MRI reports. We also thank the staff at the Department of Neurology and the Center for Medical Image science and Visualization (CMIV), Linköping University Hospital, for their help in collecting samples and carrying out MRI scans.

Funding

The study was supported by grants from the Swedish Research Council (K2013-61X-22310-01-4) and from Linköping University and the University Hospital of Linköping, Sweden. The study was also supported by an unrestricted grant from Novartis. KB is supported by the Torsten Söderberg Foundation and the Royal Academy of Sciences, Sweden. HZ is a Wallenberg Academy Fellow.

Authors' contributions

IH contributed to the study design, acquisition of data, statistical analysis and interpretation of data, drafting of manuscript, critical revision, and final approval of the manuscript. AT and PC contributed to the study design, acquisition of data, critical revision, and final approval of the manuscript. KB and HZ contributed to the acquisition of data (laboratory analyses), critical revision, and final approval of the manuscript. PL, CD, and MV contributed to the study design, critical revision, and final approval of the manuscript. JE contributed to the study design, interpretation of data, critical revision, and final approval of the manuscript.

Consent for publication

Not applicable

Competing interests

KB has served as a consultant or at advisory boards for IBL International, Roche Diagnostics, Eli Lilly, Fujirebio Europe, and Novartis. Dr. Blennow is a co-founder of Brain Biomarker Solutions in Gothenburg AB, a GU Venture-based platform company at the University of Gothenburg. HZ has served at advisory boards of Eli Lilly and Roche Diagnostics and has received travel support from Teva. Dr. Zetterberg is a co-founder of Brain Biomarker Solutions in Gothenburg AB, a GU Venture-based platform company at the University of Gothenburg. CD has received honoraria for lectures from Biogen, Teva, Genzyme, and Novartis and for advisory boards from Roche, Novartis, and Biogen. MV has received unrestricted research grants from Biogen and Novartis, honoraria for lectures from Biogen and Genzyme and for advisory boards from Roche and Novartis. The other authors declare that they have no competing interests.

Author details

[1]Department of Neurology and Department of Clinical and Experimental Medicine, Linköping University, Linköping, Sweden. [2]Radiation Physics, Department of Medical and Health Sciences, Linköping University, Linköping, Sweden. [3]Center for Medical Image Science and Visualization (CMIV), Linköping University, Linköping, Sweden. [4]Department of Clinical Immunology and Transfusion Medicine and Department of Clinical and Experimental Medicine, Linköping University, Linköping, Sweden. [5]Inst. of Neuroscience and Physiology, Department of Psychiatry and Neurochemistry, The Sahlgrenska Academy at the University of Gothenburg, Gothenburg, Sweden. [6]Clinical Neurochemistry Laboratory, Sahlgrenska University Hospital, Mölndal, Sweden. [7]Department of Molecular Neuroscience, UCL Institute of Neurology, Queen Square, London, UK. [8]UK Dementia Research Institute at UCL, London, UK. [9]Radiology, Department of Medical and Health Sciences, Linköping University, Linköping, Sweden.

References

1. Giovannoni G, Turner B, Gnanapavan S, Offiah C, Schmierer K, Marta M. Is it time to target no evident disease activity (NEDA) in multiple sclerosis? Mult Scler Relat Disord. 2015;4:329–33.

2. Kappos L, De Stefano N, Freedman MS, Cree BA, Radue EW, Sprenger T, Sormani MP, Smith T, Haring DA, Piani Meier D, Tomic D. Inclusion of brain volume loss in a revised measure of 'no evidence of disease activity' (NEDA-4) in relapsing-remitting multiple sclerosis. Mult Scler. 2016;22:1297–305.
3. Sastre-Garriga J, Pareto D, Rovira A. Brain atrophy in multiple sclerosis: Clinical Relevance and Technical Aspects. *Neuroimaging Clin N Am.* 2017;27:289–300.
4. Bodini B, Calabresi PA. From neurofilament research to multiple sclerosis clinical practice: where do we stand? Neurology. 2017;88:816–7.
5. Bermel RA, Bakshi R. The measurement and clinical relevance of brain atrophy in multiple sclerosis. Lancet Neurol. 2006;5:158–70.
6. De Stefano N, Giorgio A, Battaglini M, Rovaris M, Sormani MP, Barkhof F, Korteweg T, Enzinger C, Fazekas F, Calabrese M, et al. Assessing brain atrophy rates in a large population of untreated multiple sclerosis subtypes. Neurology. 2010;74:1868–76.
7. Zivadinov R, Uher T, Hagemeier J, Vaneckova M, Ramasamy DP, Tyblova M, Bergsland N, Seidl Z, Dwyer MG, Krasensky J, et al. A serial 10-year follow-up study of brain atrophy and disability progression in RRMS patients. Mult Scler. 2016;22:1709–18.
8. Vagberg M, Lindqvist T, Ambarki K, Warntjes JB, Sundstrom P, Birgander R, Svenningsson A. Automated determination of brain parenchymal fraction in multiple sclerosis. AJNR Am J Neuroradiol. 2012;
9. Salzer J, Svenningsson A, Sundstrom P. Neurofilament light as a prognostic marker in multiple sclerosis. Mult Scler. 2010;16:287–92.
10. Arrambide G, Espejo C, Eixarch H, Villar LM, Alvarez-Cermeno JC, Picon C, Kuhle J, Disanto G, Kappos L, Sastre-Garriga J, et al. Neurofilament light chain level is a weak risk factor for the development of MS. Neurology. 2016;87:1076–84.
11. Kuhle J, Disanto G, Lorscheider J, Stites T, Chen Y, Dahlke F, Francis G, Shrinivasan A, Radue EW, Giovannoni G, Kappos L. Fingolimod and CSF neurofilament light chain levels in relapsing-remitting multiple sclerosis. Neurology. 2015;84:1639–43.
12. Gunnarsson M, Malmestrom C, Axelsson M, Sundstrom P, Dahle C, Vrethem M, Olsson T, Piehl F, Norgren N, Rosengren L, et al. Axonal damage in relapsing multiple sclerosis is markedly reduced by natalizumab. Ann Neurol. 2011;69:83–9.
13. Hakansson I, Tisell A, Cassel P, Blennow K, Zetterberg H, Lundberg P, Dahle C, Vrethem M, Ernerudh J. Neurofilament light chain in cerebrospinal fluid and prediction of disease activity in clinically isolated syndrome and relapsing-remitting multiple sclerosis. Eur J Neurol. 2017;24:703–12.
14. Kuhle J, Barro C, Andreasson U, Derfuss T, Lindberg R, Sandelius A, Liman V, Norgren N, Blennow K, Zetterberg H. Comparison of three analytical platforms for quantification of the neurofilament light chain in blood samples: ELISA, electrochemiluminescence immunoassay and Simoa. Clin Chem Lab Med. 2016;
15. Kuhle J, Barro C, Disanto G, Mathias A, Soneson C, Bonnier G, Yaldizli O, Regeniter A, Derfuss T, Canales M, et al. Serum neurofilament light chain in early relapsing remitting MS is increased and correlates with CSF levels and with MRI measures of disease severity. Mult Scler. 2016;
16. Polman CH, Reingold SC, Banwell B, Clanet M, Cohen JA, Filippi M, Fujihara K, Havrdova E, Hutchinson M, Kappos L, et al. Diagnostic criteria for multiple sclerosis: 2010 revisions to the McDonald criteria. Ann Neurol. 2011;69:292–302.
17. Rosengren LE, Wikkelso C, Hagberg L. A sensitive ELISA for glial fibrillary acidic protein: application in CSF of adults. J Neurosci Methods. 1994;51:197–204.
18. Rohrer JD, Woollacott IO, Dick KM, Brotherhood E, Gordon E, Fellows A, Toombs J, Druyeh R, Cardoso MJ, Ourselin S, et al. Serum neurofilament light chain protein is a measure of disease intensity in frontotemporal dementia. Neurology. 2016;87:1329–36.
19. Warntjes JB, Leinhard OD, West J, Lundberg P. Rapid magnetic resonance quantification on the brain: optimization for clinical usage. Magn Reson Med. 2008;60:320–9.
20. Novakova L, Zetterberg H, Sundstrom P, Axelsson M, Khademi M, Gunnarsson M, Malmestrom C, Svenningsson A, Olsson T, Piehl F, et al. Monitoring disease activity in multiple sclerosis using serum neurofilament light protein. Neurology. 2017;
21. Martinez MA, Olsson B, Bau L, Matas E, Cobo Calvo A, Andreasson U, Blennow K, Romero-Pinel L, Martinez-Yelamos S, Zetterberg H. Glial and neuronal markers in cerebrospinal fluid predict progression in multiple sclerosis. Mult Scler. 2015;21:550–61.
22. Mellergard J, Tisell A, Blystad I, Gronqvist A, Blennow K, Olsson B, Dahle C, Vrethem M, Lundberg P, Ernerudh J. Cerebrospinal fluid levels of neurofilament and tau correlate with brain atrophy in natalizumab-treated multiple sclerosis. Eur J Neurol. 2016;
23. Hellberg S, Eklund D, Gawel DR, Kopsen M, Zhang H, Nestor CE, Kockum I, Olsson T, Skogh T, Kastbom A, et al. Dynamic response genes in CD4+ T cells reveal a network of interactive proteins that classifies disease activity in multiple sclerosis. Cell Rep. 2016;16:2928–39.
24. Moreira MA, Souza AL, Lana-Peixoto MA, Teixeira MM, Teixeira AL. Chemokines in the cerebrospinal fluid of patients with active and stable relapsing-remitting multiple sclerosis. Braz J Med Biol Res. 2006;39:441–5.
25. Mahad DJ, Howell SJ, Woodroofe MN. Expression of chemokines in the CSF and correlation with clinical disease activity in patients with multiple sclerosis. J Neurol Neurosurg Psychiatry. 2002;72:498–502.
26. Hartel M, Kluczewska E, Pierzchala K, Adamczyk-Sowa M, Karpe J. What you cannot get from routine MRI of MS patient and why—the growing need for atrophy assessment and seeing beyond the plaque. Neurol Neurochir Pol. 2016;50:123–30.
27. Popescu V, Agosta F, Hulst HE, Sluimer IC, Knol DL, Sormani MP, Enzinger C, Ropele S, Alonso J, Sastre-Garriga J, et al. Brain atrophy and lesion load predict long term disability in multiple sclerosis. J Neurol Neurosurg Psychiatry. 2013;84:1082–91.
28. Rocca MA, Battaglini M, Benedict RH, De Stefano N, Geurts JJ, Henry RG, Horsfield MA, Jenkinson M, Pagani E, Filippi M. Brain MRI atrophy quantification in MS: from methods to clinical application. Neurology. 2017;88:403–13.
29. Varhaug KN, Barro C, Bjornevik K, Myhr KM, Torkildsen O, Wergeland S, Bindoff LA, Kuhle J, Vedeler C. Neurofilament light chain predicts disease activity in relapsing-remitting MS. Neurol Neuroimmunol Neuroinflamm. 2018;5:e422.
30. Disanto G, Barro C, Benkert P, Naegelin Y, Schadelin S, Giardiello A, Zecca C, Blennow K, Zetterberg H, Leppert D, et al. Serum neurofilament light: a biomarker of neuronal damage in multiple sclerosis. Ann Neurol. 2017;81:857–70.
31. Barro C, Benkert P, Disanto G, Tsagkas C, Amann M, Naegelin Y, Leppert D, Gobbi C, Granziera C, Yaldizli O, et al. Serum neurofilament as a predictor of disease worsening and brain and spinal cord atrophy in multiple sclerosis. Brain. 2018;
32. Iwanowski P, Losy J, Kramer L, Wojcicka M, Kaufman E. CXCL10 and CXCL13 chemokines in patients with relapsing remitting and primary progressive multiple sclerosis. J Neurol Sci. 2017;380:22–6.
33. Sellebjerg F, Bornsen L, Khademi M, Krakauer M, Olsson T, Frederiksen JL, Sorensen PS. Increased cerebrospinal fluid concentrations of the chemokine CXCL13 in active MS. Neurology. 2009;73:2003–10.
34. Thompson AJ, Banwell BL, Barkhof F, Carroll WM, Coetzee T, Comi G, Correale J, Fazekas F, Filippi M, Freedman MS, et al. Diagnosis of multiple sclerosis: 2017 revisions of the McDonald criteria. Lancet Neurol. 2018;17:162–73.
35. Paul A, Comabella M, Gandhi R. Biomarkers in multiple sclerosis. Cold Spring Harb Perspect Med. 2018;
36. Hinsinger G, Galeotti N, Nabholz N, Urbach S, Rigau V, Demattei C, Lehmann S, Camu W, Labauge P, Castelnovo G, et al. Chitinase 3-like proteins as diagnostic and prognostic biomarkers of multiple sclerosis. Mult Scler. 2015;21:1251–61.
37. Thouvenot E. Multiple sclerosis biomarkers: helping the diagnosis? Rev Neurol (Paris). 2018;174:364–71.

3

Identification of the flotillin-1/2 heterocomplex as a target of autoantibodies in *bona fide* multiple sclerosis

S. Hahn[1†], G. Trendelenburg[2†], M. Scharf[1], Y. Denno[1], S. Brakopp[1], B. Teegen[1,3], C. Probst[1], K. P. Wandinger[4], M. Buttmann[5,6], A. Haarmann[5], F. Szabados[7], M. vom Dahl[8], T. Kümpfel[9], P. Eichhorn[10], H. Gold[11], F. Paul[12,13], S. Jarius[14], N. Melzer[15], W. Stöcker[1,3] and L. Komorowski[1*]

Abstract

Background: Autoantibodies, in particular those against aquaporin-4 and myelin-oligodendrocyte glycoprotein (MOG), aid as biomarkers in the differential diagnosis of demyelination. Here, we report on discovery of autoantibodies against flotillin in patients with multiple sclerosis (MS).

Methods: The target antigen was identified by histo-immunoprecipitation using the patients' sera and cryosections of rat or pig cerebellum combined with mass spectrometrical analysis. Correct identification was ascertained by indirect immunofluorescence and neutralization tests using the target antigens recombinantly expressed in HEK293 cells.

Results: Serum and CSF of the index patient produced a fine-granular IgG indirect immunofluorescence staining of the hippocampal and cerebellar molecular layers. Flotillin-1 and flotillin-2 were identified as target autoantigens. They also reacted with recombinant human flotillin-1/2 co-expressed in HEK293 cells, but not with the individual flotillins in fixed- and live-cell assays. Moreover, neutralization using flotillin-1/2, but not the single flotillins, abolished the tissue reactivity of patient serum. Screening of 521 patients, for whom anti-aquaporin-4 testing was requested and negative, revealed 8 additional patients with anti-flotillin-1/2 autoantibodies. All eight were negative for anti-MOG. Six patients *ex post* fulfilled the revised McDonald criteria for MS. Vice versa, screening of 538 MS sera revealed anti-flotillin-1/2 autoantibodies in eight patients. The autoantibodies were not found in a cohort of 67 patients with other neural autoantibody-associated syndromes and in 444 healthy blood donors.

Conclusions: Autoantibodies against the flotillin-1/2 heterocomplex, a peripheral membrane protein that is involved in axon outgrowth and regeneration of the optic nerve, are present in 1–2% of patients with *bona fide* MS.

Keywords: Autoantibodies, Flotillin, Reggie, Histo-immunoprecipitation, Multiple sclerosis, Optic neuritis

Background

Several immune-mediated inflammatory central nervous system (CNS) disorders are characterized by the presence of autoantibodies against components of neural tissues [1]. Moreover, a significant number of autoantibodies with pathogenic potential, e.g., directed against aquaporin-4, have been described [2–7]. Autoantibodies against aquaporin-4 (AQP4) cause inflammation in the CNS and can be regarded as pathognomonic for neuromyelitis optica spectrum disorder (NMOSD) [2, 8–10]. Lead symptoms are uni- or bilateral optic neuritis (ON) together with longitudinal extensive transverse myelitis [11]. ON and transverse myelitis are also frequent initial symptoms in multiple sclerosis (MS). Most MS patients develop ON at least once during the disease course [12], and conversely, both children and adults with ON have an elevated risk of developing MS [13, 14]. Generally,

* Correspondence: l.komorowski@euroimmun.de
†Equal contributors
[1]Institute of Experimental Immunology, Euroimmun AG, Seekamp 31, 23560 Lübeck, Germany

neuroimaging and laboratory testing help to diagnose and differentiate MS, NMOSD, and other forms of central demyelination [10]. However, intrathecal immunoglobulin synthesis and oligoclonal bands in the CSF, frequently detected in patients with MS, are not disease-specific. Searching for anti-AQP4 has therefore become an important step in the diagnostic work-up of patients under suspicion of having a central demyelinating disease. Broad screening for multiple autoantibodies is justified at this stage because they can be linked to phenotypically diffuse neurological syndromes, especially in early disease stages. Conclusively, *ex ante* unexpected findings are frequent in the serological laboratory.

Here, we report on autoantibodies against the flotillin-1/2 complex detected in patients referred for anti-AQP4 testing, most of whom turned out to suffer from *bona fide* multiple sclerosis presenting with ON. Flotillin-1 and flotillin-2 (reggie-2 and reggie-1) are homologous scaffolding proteins of lipid raft microdomains with a molecular mass of 47 kDa [15, 16]. They are highly conserved and ubiquitously expressed [17]. Membrane association of flotillins depends amongst other factors on palmitoylation at Cys34 of flotillin-1 [18, 19] and Cys4, Cys19, and Cys20 of flotillin-2 [20, 21]. The flotillin proteins form hetero-oligomeric complexes and were originally named reggies due to their upregulation in regenerating axons of goldfish retinal ganglion cells after lesion of the optic nerve [22]. Furthermore, they play an important role in cell proliferation, tumor progression, neurodegenerative diseases, and signaling in T cells. Flotillin microdomains form flotillin cap at one pole of T cells regulating recruitment of signaling molecules to the cap which is important for T cell activation [15].

Methods

Patients were analyzed as part of their diagnostic work-up based on the suspicion of a neuroinflammatory disease by a broad screening for autoantibodies. Serum and CSF samples were initially investigated on the assumption of an autoimmune disorder of the CNS in the accredited Clinical Immunological Laboratory in Lübeck by indirect immunofluorescence assay (IFA) using a combination of brain tissue cryosections and HEK293 cells expressing established neural autoantigens between May 2012 and September 2015.

The six patients revealed in the initial screening were diagnosed and treated at the Departments of Neurology of the contributing Medical Centers and Hospitals. All patients were referred for serology as part of their diagnostic work-up based on the clinical differential diagnosis between MS and NMOSD mostly due to clinical presentation with prominent ON by a broad screening for autoantibodies. The index patient (P1) gave written informed consent for using her serum and CSF samples for autoantigen identification. All six patients for whom detailed data are reported consented to the serological analysis of their samples and the subsequent evaluation of their medical records.

Control collectives included 538 serum samples from random patients with pre-diagnosed MS, 444 healthy blood donors, and 67 patients with defined autoantibody-associated neurological syndromes (5x anti-NMDAR, 5x anti-Hu, 2x anti-Hu/anti-Ri, 3x anti-Yo, 2x anti-Yo/anti-Ri, 3x anti-Ri, 38x anti-AQP4, 5x anti-LGI1, 4x anti-CASPR2).

Reagents were obtained from Euroimmun (Lübeck, Germany) or Merck (Darmstadt, Germany) or Sigma-Aldrich (Heidelberg, Germany) if not specified otherwise.

Histo-immunoprecipitation and identification of the antigen

The cerebellum from rat or pig was dissected and shock-frozen in −160 °C isopentane. The tissue was then cryosected (4 μm) with a SM2000R microtome (Leica Microsystems, Nussloch, Germany), placed on glass slides, dried, and stored at −196 °C. For histo-immunoprecipitation (HIP), the slides were incubated with the patient's serum (diluted 1:100) at 4 °C for 3 h followed by three washing steps with PBS, 0.2% (*w*/*v*) Tween-20 (IFA buffer). The tissue was then extracted with solubilization buffer (100 mmol/l tris-HCl pH 7.4, 150 mmol/l sodium chloride, 2.5 mmol/l EDTA, 0.5% (*w*/*v*) deoxycholate, 1% (*w*/*v*) Triton X-100 containing protease inhibitors) at 4 °C for 1 h. The resulting suspension was homogenized and centrifuged at 16,000×*g* at 4 °C for 15 min. Immunocomplexes were precipitated from the clear supernatant with Protein G Dynabeads (ThermoFisher Scientific, Dreieich, Germany) at 4 °C overnight, washed three times with solubilization buffer, and eluted with NuPAGE LDS Sample Buffer (Thermo Fisher Scientific, Dreieich, Germany) at 70 °C for 10 min. The eluates were analyzed by SDS-PAGE and mass spectrometry or Western blot.

Indirect immunofluorescence assay

Slides with biochip mosaic including brain tissue cryosections (rat hippocampus and rat, pig, and primate cerebellum) and HEK293 cells expressing wild-type and mutated flotillin-1 and flotillin-2 as well as 30 recombinant brain antigens were used for IFA. Each mosaic was incubated with 30 μl of sample diluted in PBS, 0.2% Tween-20 (IFA buffer) at room temperature for 30 min; flushed with IFA buffer; and immersed in IFA buffer for 5 min. Subsequently, polyclonal goat anti-human pan-IgG (Euroimmun, Lübeck, Germany) or monoclonal murine anti-human IgG1, IgG2, IgG3, or IgG4 (Sigma-Aldrich, Heidelberg, Germany), each labeled with fluorescein isothiocyanate (FITC) or Alexa

Fluor 488, were incubated at room temperature for 30 min. The slides were then washed again; embedded in PBS-buffered, DABCO-containing glycerol (approximately 10 µl per mosaic); and examined by two independent observers using an EUROStar microscope (Euroimmun, Lübeck, Germany) and a laser scanning microscope (LSM700, Zeiss, Jena, Germany). Positive and negative controls were included. Samples were categorized based on tissue patterns and fluorescence intensity of transfected cells in direct comparison with non-transfected cells and control samples. Endpoint titers refer to the highest dilution showing visible fluorescence. Live-cell IFA with primary hippocampal neurons or transfected HEK293 cells was conducted as described by Dalmau et al. [3].

Polyclonal rabbit antibodies against flotillin-1 and flotillin-2 (both Sigma-Aldrich, Heidelberg, Germany; dilution 1:250), respectively, were used in some experiments in the first step followed by incubation with anti-rabbit IgG-Cy3 (Jackson Research, Suffolk, UK). Cell nuclei were visualized by DNA staining with TO-PRO-3 iodide (ThermoFisher Scientific, Dreieich, Germany; dilution 1:2000). Recombinant antigens were mixed with diluted serum sample 1 h at room temperature prior to IFA as described in Stöcker et al. for neutralization experiments [23].

See Additional file 1 for further details.

Results

Characterization of the patient's autoantibodies

The IFA analysis of the index patient's (P1) serum and CSF revealed a fine-granular IgG staining of the molecular layer on the rat hippocampus as well as on the rat and primate cerebella (Fig. 1, Additional file 1: Figure e-5). The hippocampal inner molecular layer showed a more intense staining than the outer molecular layer. Serum and CSF titers were 1:320 and 1:32, respectively, and the antibodies were of subclass IgG1, exclusively (see details in Table 1, Additional file 1: Figure e-5). Further monospecific analyses revealed no specific reactivity applying 30 different neural autoantigens recombinantly expressed in HEK293 cells: Hu, Yo, Ri, CV2, SOX1, PNMA1, PNMA2, ITPR1, Homer 3, CARP VIII, ARHGAP26, ZIC4, DNER/Tr, GAD65, GAD67, amphiphysin, recoverin, GABA B receptor, glycine receptor, DPPX, glutamate receptors (types NMDA, AMPA, mGluR1, mGluR5), LGI1, CASPR2, AQP4 (M1 and M23), MOG, and ATP1A3.

Identification of flotillin as the target autoantigen

Immunocomplexes precipitated with the patient's serum from the rat cerebellum contained proteins of approximately 50 kDa, as detected by SDS-PAGE, which were absent in equally prepared controls (Fig. 2A). Using MALDI-TOF, the 50-kDa proteins were identified as flotillin-1 and flotillin-2 from *Rattus norvegicus* (UNIPROT acc. # Q9Z1E1, Q9Z2S9) and *Sus scrofa* (#Q767L6, I3LFS8), respectively.

Western blot analysis of the immunoprecipitates exhibited a strong reaction at 50 kDa applying polyclonal rabbit anti-flotillin-1 and anti-flotillin-2 antibodies, respectively (Fig. 2A and Additional file 1: Figure e-1A). When used in IFA, the anti-flotillin-1 and anti-flotillin-2 antibodies produced fluorescence patterns on rat hippocampus as well as on rat and primate cerebella comparable to those generated by the patient samples (Fig. 2B and Additional file 1: Figure e-1B).

As a proof of correct antigen identification, the patient's samples were then tested by IFA using recombinant HEK293 cells which expressed either flotillin-1, flotillin-2, or both proteins (Fig. 3A). Serum (Additional file 1: Figure e-3) and CSF (Additional file 1: Figure e-5) reacted with the cells co-expressing flotillin-1 and flotillin-2 after acetone fixation and in live-cell IFA (Additional file 1: Figure e-4) but not with those expressing individual flotillin-1 or flotillin-2. Endpoint titers were higher with the recombinant substrates than titers determined on tissue. Mock transfection did not result in any antibody binding.

The congruence of the autoantibody target and flotillin-1/2 was further demonstrated by the proof of a dose-dependent neutralization of antibody binding to brain tissue: An incubation of the patient's samples with HEK293 lysate containing co-expressed flotillin-1 and flotillin-2 abolished the positive IFT reaction which did not happen if separately expressed flotillin-1 or flotillin-2 or lysates from mock-transfected HEK293 were added to the patient's samples (Fig. 3B).

Surface localization of autoantibody-binding recombinant flotillin-1/2

To study the membrane association of flotillins, acylation-deficient mutants were expressed in HEK293 cells. For this purpose, Cys5 and Cys17 of flotillin-1 and Cys4, Cys19, and Cys20 of flotillin-2 were replaced by serine [A: flotillin-1 wild-type + flotillin-2 wild-type; B: flotillin-1 wild-type + flotillin-2 (C4S, C19S, C20S); C: flotillin-1 (C5S, C17S) + flotillin-2 wild-type; D: flotillin-1 (C5S, C17S) + flotillin-2 (C4S, C19S, C20S)] (Additional file 1: Figure e-2). Using non-permeabilized HEK293 cells in a live cell-based assay, the patient serum and the antibodies against flotillin-1 and flotillin-2 only displayed reactions with the wild-type flotillin-1/2. Co-expression of acylation-deficient flotillin-1 (C5S, C17S) and flotillin-2 (C4S, C19S, C20S) impaired antibody binding to the flotillins and abolished the reactivity of patient serum and polyclonal antibodies, indicating that flotillins are not trafficked to the cellular surface without the attachment of fatty acids (Additional file 1: Figure e-4).

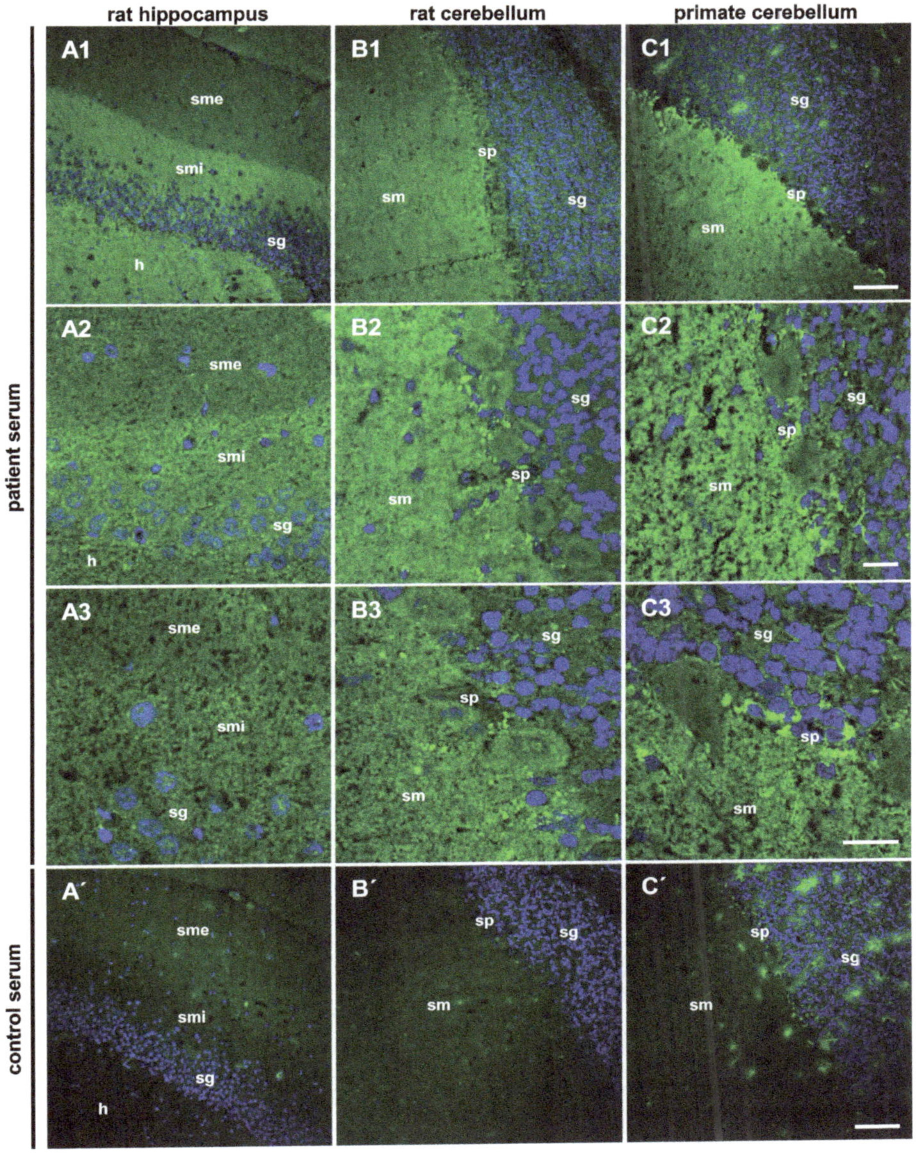

Fig. 1 Immunofluorescence staining of central nervous tissues. Cryosections of rat hippocampus (**A**) and cerebellum (**B**) as well as primate cerebellum (**C**) were incubated with patient serum (**A**–**C**) or with control serum (*A′*–*C′*) (*A*–*C1*, *A′*–*C′* 1:100, *A*–*C2*, *C3* 1:50) in the first step and with Alexa Fluor 488-labeled goat anti-human IgG in the second step (*green*). Nuclei were counterstained by incubation with TO-PRO-3 iodide (*blue*). A fine-granular staining of the stratum moleculare (*sm*) was obtained. On the hippocampus, the sm internum was stained more intensely than the sm externum. *Scale bar.* 100 μm (*A*–*C1*, *A′*–*C′*), 20 μm (*A*–*C2*, *C3*). *h* hilus, *sm* stratum moleculare, *smi* stratum moleculare internum, *sme* stratum moleculare externum, *sg* stratum granulosum, *sp* stratum purkinjense

Estimation of anti-flotillin-1/2 autoantibody prevalence

Anti-flotillin-1/2 status was determined in 521 samples referred for anti-AQP4 testing due to suspected autoimmune inflammatory CNS disorder (1) which had been found to be anti-AQP4-negative; (2) for which a general broad neural autoantibody screening, including the aforementioned parameters, had been conducted in the Clinical Immunological Laboratory, Lübeck (Germany); and (3) for which a neural tissue-reactive IgG autoantibody without known antigen specificity had been reported. Serum anti-flotillin-1/2 was detected in nine patients with titers of up to 1:10,000. For five of these patients, medical records were available (P2–P6 in Table 1). Patients P2, P3, and P5 also showed anti-flotillin-1/2 in CSF (titers 1:3.2, 1:100, and 1:1000). For P4 and P6, CSF was not available. Additional follow-up sera of the patients were analyzed when available and showed that the anti-flotillin-1/2 titers of P1, P2, and P4 were unaltered over a period of 18, 24, and 72 months, respectively, despite initiation of disease-modifying treatment

Table 1 Summary of the clinical and paraclinical features of six patients with anti-flotillin-1/2

	Patient 1 (P1)	Patient 2 (P2)	Patient 3 (P3)	Patient 4 (P4)	Patient 5 (P5)	Patient 6 (P6)
Age (years) at diagnostic testing, gender	34, female	35, female	54, male	40, female	46, female	54, female
Disease duration at time of serum sampling (years)	0	3	0	18	0	8
Diagnosis	RRMS	RRMS	RRMS	RRMS	RRMS	RRMS
ON	Unilateral	No	Unilateral	Bilateral	P100 difference in the VEP	Unilateral
Imaging	Several brain lesions, no spinal lesion	Contrast-enhancing spinal lesion, no brain lesion	One spinal lesion and further brain lesions	Multiple white matter lesions including the temporal lobe, cerebellum, and spinal cord	Several subcortical T2 lesions, one DWI-positive ponto-medullar lesion, and 3 further spinal lesions	Contrast-enhancing lesions at atlanto-occipital level
McDonald's criteria fulfilled	DIS, DIT, positive CSF	Relapses, positive CSF	Relapses, DIS, DIT, positive CSF	Relapses, DIS, DIT, positive CSF	DIS, DIT, positive CSF	Relapses, DIS, positive CSF
Expanded Disability Status Scale	2.0	2.0	2.0	3.5	2.0	2.0
Serum titer (tissue pattern on cerebellum/anti-flotillin-1/2)	1:320/1:3200	1:100/1:1000	1:100/1:1000	1:1000/1:10,000	1:1000/1:10,000	1:100/1:1000
OCB in CSF only	Yes	Yes	Yes	Yes	Yes	Yes
White cell count in CSF (cells/μl)	9	5	7	n.a.	6	2
CSF titer (tissue pattern on cerebellum/anti-flotillin-1/2)	1:32/1:100	Neg./1:3.2	1:10/1:100	n.a.	1:100/1:1000	n.a.
Intrathecal anti-flotillin-1/2 synthesis	Yes	No	Yes	n.a.[b]	Yes	n.a.[b]

Flot-1/2 HEK293-flotillin-1/2, *RRMS* relapsing-remitting multiple sclerosis, *n.a.* not available, *DIS* dissemination over space, *DIS* dissemination over time

[b]CSF not available for anti-flotillin-1/2 testing

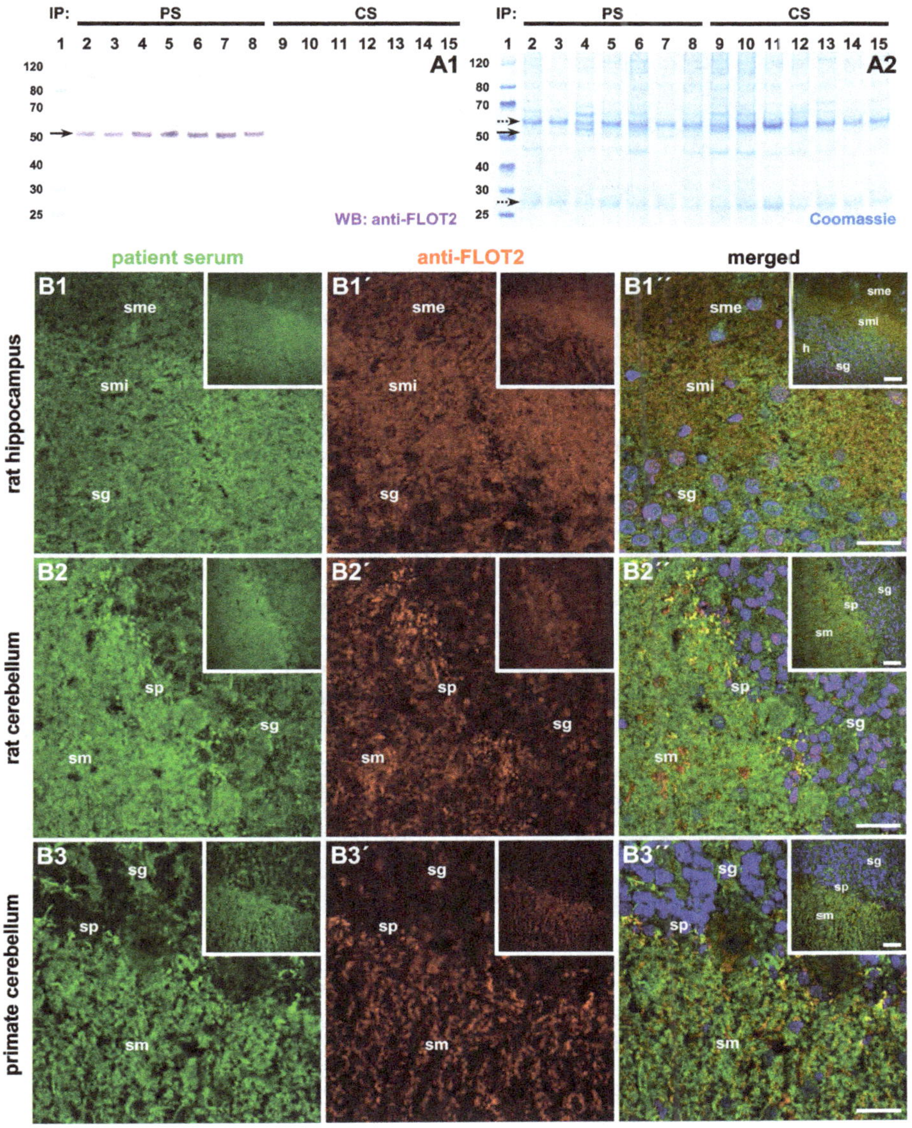

Fig. 2 Histo-immunoprecipitation and antigen identification. Cryosections of rat or pig cerebellum were incubated with the serum (1:100), washed in PBS, and solubilized using detergents. The solution was incubated with protein-G-coated magnetic beads. The immunocomplexes were eluted by SDS and subjected to SDS-PAGE analysis and Western blot. **A** Western blot after incubation with anti-flotillin-2 (*A1*) and enzymatic visualization of antibody binding. Staining of SDS polyacrylamide gel with colloidal Coomassie (*A2*). Lane 1: molecular mass (kDa) marker; lanes 2–8: histo-immunoprecipitates of patient sera from rat cerebellum; lanes 9–15: histo-immunoprecipitates of control samples. The *arrow* indicates the position of the immunoprecipitated antigen 50 kDa while *dotted arrows* indicate the position of IgG heavy and light chain at 52 and 27 kDa, respectively. *PS* patient sample, *CS* control sample. **B** Immunofluorescence staining of rat hippocampus (*B1*) and cerebellum (*B2*) and primate cerebellum (*B3*) tissue sections with patient serum (*green, 1–3*) and anti-flotillin-2 antibody (*red, 1′–3′*). The merged images show localization of the reactivity in the same region including the more intense staining of the sm internum on the hippocampus (*1″–3″*). *Scale bar.* 50 µm (large images), 100 µm (inserts). *PS* patient serum, *CS* control serum, *h* hilus, *sg* stratum granulosum, *sm* stratum moleculare, *smi* stratum moleculare internum, *sme* stratum moleculare externum, *sp* stratum purkinjense

for MS (interferon-β or natalizumab). The serum of P5 showed a reduction from 1:1000 to 1:320 7 weeks after plasma exchange, to which the patient had responded well clinically.

Screening of 538 serum samples from pre-diagnosed MS patients revealed anti-flotillin-1/2 autoantibodies in eight further patients (Additional file 1: Table e-2). All eight patient samples did not contain antibodies against AQP4 and MOG; however, screening of the remaining 530 samples uncovered 3 anti-AQP4- and 10 anti-MOG-positive sera in patients diagnosed with MS. Sera from 67 patients with various neural autoantibodies,

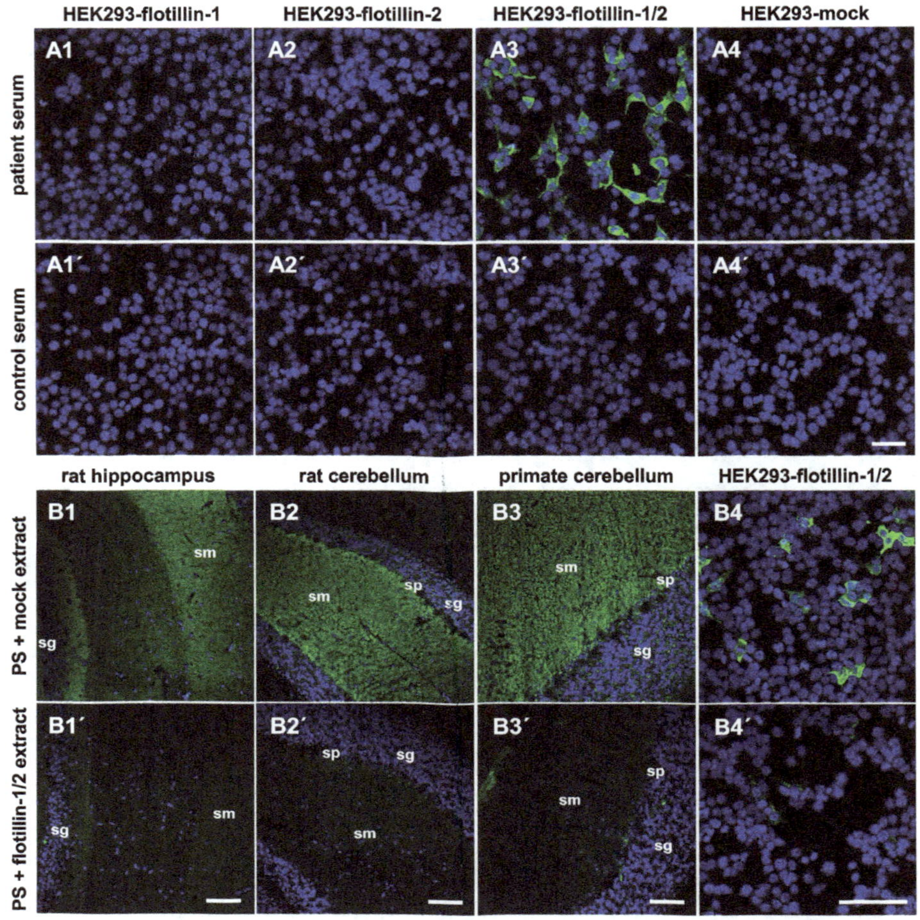

Fig. 3 Immunofluorescence staining of recombinant flotillin and the neutralization of antibody reaction on tissue. **A** Immunofluorescence analysis of transfected HEK293 cells. Acetone-fixed recombinant HEK293 cells expressing flotillin-1 (*1*), flotillin-2 (*2*), flotillin-1 and flotillin-2 (*3*) or a mock-transfected control (*4*) were incubated with patient serum (*1–4*) or with control serum (*1′–4′*) (both 1:100). Cell nuclei were counterstained with TO-PRO-3 iodide (*blue*). Only HEK293-flotillin-1/2 cells reacted with the samples (*green*). *Scale bar*: 50 μm. **B** Neutralization of immunofluorescence reaction on neuronal tissues. Serum was pre-incubated with extracts of HEK293 cells transfected with empty control vector (*1–4*) or with the plasmid harboring flotillin-1/2 cDNA (*1′–4′*). The extract containing flotillin-1/2 greatly reduced or abolished the immune reaction of the serum on rat hippocampus (*1′*) and cerebellum (*2′*), primate cerebellum (*3′*), and HEK293-flotillin-1/2 (*4′*). The control extracts had no effect (*1–4*). Nuclei were counterstained by incubation with TO-PRO-3 iodide (*blue*). *Scale bar*: 50 μm. *PS* patient serum, *CS* control serum, *sg* stratum granulosum, *sm* stratum moleculare, *sp* stratum purkinjense

including 38 with anti-AQP4 (titers up to 1:3200), and from 444 healthy participants (blood donors of both sexes, 18–67 years) were analyzed as specificity controls. None of the sera reacted with HEK293-flotillin-1, HEK293-flotillin-2, and HEK293-flotillin-1/2.

Patient characteristics

In summary, 13 of the 14 anti-flotillin-1/2-positive patients for whom medical records could be evaluated had relapses, radiological signs of disseminated demyelination, and no evidence for a disorder other than MS, *ex post* fulfilling the revised diagnostic criteria of relapsing-remitting MS [24]. Providing direct evidence for the inflammatory nature of the disease, CSF analysis had revealed mild pleocytosis and/or CSF-specific oligoclonal band (OCB) in all patients. One patient had been diagnosed with secondary progressive MS. Thirteen (93%) patients were female. Nine (64%) patients had a history of optic neuritis. None of the patients displayed anti-AQP4 or anti-MOG antibodies. Where available (P1, P2, P3, and P5), CSF was found to harbor anti-flotillin-1/2. Specific antibody indices >4 indicative for intrathecal anti-flotillin-1/2 synthesis, as suggested by Reiber et al. for IFA analysis [25], were calculated for P1, P3, and P5. See Table 1 and Additional file 1 for more details.

Discussion

We report on IgG autoantibodies against the flotillin-1/2 complex. The autoantibodies were revealed during the serological work-up of patients referred for anti-AQP4 testing as an unexpected finding. The patients' sera and CSF reacted with cryosections of neural tissue but not with any of 30 previously established brain autoantigens in fixed recombinant cell-based IFA, including AQP4 and MOG. Histo-immunoprecipitation combined with mass spectrometry and recombinant expression identified the heterocomplex as the target antigen. All six index patients for whom medical records could be evaluated presented with a history of encephalomyelitis and/or inflammation of the optic nerve(s). *Ex post*, all patients fulfilled the revised diagnostic criteria for MS which prompted the search for anti-flotillin-1/2 in a cohort of 538 pre-diagnosed MS patients that revealed another 8 patients bearing the autoantibodies. Importantly, the antibodies were not detected in >500 controls.

Flotillin-1 and Flotillin-2 (synonyms: reggie-2 and reggie-1) were originally described to be upregulated in regenerating axons of goldfish retinal ganglion cells after traumatic injury of the optic nerve [22]. They are evolutionary well conserved in many eukaryotes including mammals [26, 27]. Human and rat flotillin-1 share 98% identity whereas the homology of human and rat/pig flotillin-2 is even 99%. In vertebrates, both proteins are ubiquitously expressed and abundant in striated muscle, adipose, lung tissue, and brain [15, 28]. On the cellular level, flotillins have been reported to be located in lipid rafts [28]. Functionally, flotillins have been shown to be involved in endocytosis, cell signaling, clustering of the amyloid precursor protein (APP) and amyloidogenic processing in neurons. Expression in glial cells has not been reported thus far. Moreover, artificial induction of flotillin expression in retinal ganglion cells in vivo leads to regeneration of subsequently crushed optic nerves in rats, thereby overcoming factors that inhibit this process in mammals under wild-type circumstances [27]. SiRNA-mediated downregulation of flotillin-2 affects neuronal differentiation and process formation in hippocampal neurons [29].

Despite of the abundant data on the individual flotillin proteins, information on expression, distribution, and function of flotillin-1 and flotillin-2 homo- and heterocomplexes is limited. Our own data indicate the presence of recombinant wild-type flotillin-1/2 on the surface of HEK293 cells whereas acylation-deficient but autoantibody-binding flotillin-1/2 is retained within the cells. Given that authentic flotillin-1/2 heterocomplexes were temporarily present on cell surfaces of neural cells in vivo or on signal-transducing exosomes [30], the autoantibodies could bear pathogenic potential. Furthermore, the antibodies univocally belong to the complement-activating IgG1 subclass, seem to be produced within the CNS, and remained detectable over the entire disease course in all three patients with long-term follow-up, and P5 favorably responded to plasma exchange. These facts are compatible with a role of anti-flotillin-1/2 in the inflammatory process. However, an involvement of anti-flotillin-1/2 and/or the flotillin proteins in MS pathogenesis is only speculative based on our data. The antibodies may as well be a result of an overshooting immune response during the inflammatory process and represent an immunological epiphenomenon.

In the six anti-flotillin-1/2-positive patients in whom the antibody was found prospectively and for whom we could evaluate medical records, testing for anti-AQP4 and anti-MOG was initially requested based on clinically assessed NMOSD core characteristics like myelitis and/or optic neuritis [10]. However, none met the latest international consensus criteria for NMOSD and all demonstrated "red flag" criteria according to that consensus, strongly suggesting another form of encephalomyelitis [10]. Neuroimaging; laboratory features, including the presence of typical MS lesions on brain MRI and of CSF-restricted oligoclonal bands; and fulfillment of the revised diagnostic criteria indicated MS in all patients [24]. Based on our prospective approach regarding the disease phenotype and the absence of anti-flotillin-1/2 in the controls, as well as based on the retrospective confirmation in a large cohort of pre-diagnosed MS patients, the flotillin-1/2 heterocomplex seems to be a B cell autoantigen in a subset of about 1–2% of MS patients.

Conclusions

Taken together, the compiled data indicate flotillin-1/2 heterocomplex as a target antigen of autoantibodies in a subset of patients with *bona fide* MS. More precise data regarding the time point at which anti-flotillin-1/2 is induced, and the phenotype relation and the prevalence have to be assembled in large cohorts of patients with inflammatory demyelinating CNS disorders including CIS; acute disseminated encephalomyelitis; NMOSD, each with and without ON; and isolated ON in order to discern the diagnostic, therapeutic, and prognostic value of these autoantibodies. Furthermore, these future data will help to elucidate the pathological relevance and functional relationship of flotillin antibodies.

Abbreviations

AQP4: Aquaporin-4; CIS: Clinically isolated syndrome; CSF: Cerebrospinal fluid; FITC: Fluorescein isothiocyanate; IFA: Indirect immunofluorescence assay; IP: Immunoprecipitation; MALDI-TOF: Matrix-assisted laser desorption/ionization-time of flight mass spectrometry; MRI: Magnetic resonance imaging; MS: Multiple sclerosis; OCB: Oligoclona bands; ON: Optic neuritis; PAGE: Polyacrylamide gel electrophoresis

Acknowledgements

We thank Laura Olejko, Susann Satow, Rita Komorowski, Sabrina Voigt, and Beatrice Witt for their excellent technical assistance and Johanna Fraune for critical reading of the manuscript.

Funding
The study was conducted without any third-party funding.

Authors' contributions
SH and MS were involved in immunoprecipitation and interpretation of data. SH, MS, RM, BT, SJ, and WS participated in antibody testing and microscopy. GT, KW, MB, AH, FS, MvD, TK, PE, HG, FP, SJ, and NM were involved in the clinical definition of the patients. YD performed mass spectrometric analysis. SB and CP performed molecular biology work. WS, GT, and LK were involved in the conception and organization of the research project and in the writing of the manuscript. All authors read and approved the final manuscript.

Competing interests
SH, MS, YD, SB, BT, CP, and LK are employees of the Euroimmun AG, a company that develops, produces, and manufactures immunoassays for the detection of disease-associated antibodies. WS is a member of the Board of the Euroimmun AG. WS and CP are shareholders of the Euroimmun AG. The Euroimmun has filed a patent application for the determination of autoantibodies against flotillin in patients with demyelinating disorders. The work of SJ was supported by a research grant from the Dietmar Hopp Foundation to the Department of Neurology, University of Heidelberg, Germany. NM has received honoraria for lecturing and travel expenses for attending meetings from Biogen Idec, GlaxoSmith Kline, Teva, Novartis Pharma, Bayer Healthcare, and Fresenius Medical Care and has received financial research support from Fresenius Medical Care and Diamed. The other authors have nothing to disclose.

Consent for publication
Not applicable.

Author details
[1]Institute of Experimental Immunology, Euroimmun AG, Seekamp 31, 23560 Lübeck, Germany. [2]Department of Neurology, University Medical Center Göttingen, Göttingen, Germany. [3]Clinical Immunological Laboratory Prof. Dr. med Stöcker, Lübeck, Germany. [4]Department of Neurology, University Medical Center Schleswig Holstein (UKSH), Lübeck, Germany. [5]Department of Neurology, University of Würzburg, Würzburg, Germany. [6]Department of Neurology, Caritas Hospital, Bad Mergentheim, Germany. [7]Medical Laboratory Osnabrück, Georgsmarienhütte, Germany. [8]Department of Neurology, Ammerland Klinik, Westerstede, Germany. [9]Institute of Clinical Neuroimmunology, Ludwig Maximilian University, Munich, Germany. [10]Institute of Clinical Chemistry, Ludwig Maximilian University, Munich, Germany. [11]Department of Neurology, Klinikum am Gesundbrunnen, Heilbronn, Germany. [12]NeuroCure Clinical Research Center and Clinical and Experimental Multiple Sclerosis Research Center, Department of Neurology, Charité Universitätsmedizin, Berlin, Germany. [13]Experimental and Clinical Research Center, Max Delbrück Center for Molecular Medicine and Charité Universitätsmedizin, Berlin, Germany. [14]Department of Neurology, University of Heidelberg, Heidelberg, Germany. [15]Department of Neurology, University of Münster, Münster, Germany.

References
1. Probst C, Saschenbrecker S, Stöcker W, Komorowski L. Anti-neuronal autoantibodies: current diagnostic challenges. Mult Scler Rel Dis. 2014;3:304–20.
2. Lennon VA, Kryzer TJ, Pittock SJ, Verkman AS, Hinson SR. IgG marker of optic-spinal multiple sclerosis binds to the aquaporin-4 water channel. J Exp Med. 2005;202:473–7.
3. Dalmau J, Gleichman AJ, Hughes EG, Rossi JE, Peng X, Lai M, Dessain SK, Rosenfeld MR, Balice-Gordon R, Lynch DR. Anti-NMDA-receptor encephalitis: case series and analysis of the effects of antibodies. Lancet Neurol. 2008.
4. Lancaster E, Lai M, Peng X, Hughes E, Constantinescu R, Raizer J, Friedman D, Skeen MB, Grisold W, Kimura A, Ohta K, Iizuka T, Guzman M, Graus F, Moss SJ, Balice-Gordon R, Dalmau J. Antibodies to the GABA(B) receptor in limbic encephalitis with seizures: case series and characterisation of the antigen. Lancet Neurol. 2010;9(1):67-76.
5. Irani SR, Alexander S, Waters P, Kleopa KA, Pettingill P, Zuliani L, Peles E, Buckley C, Lang B, Vincent A. Antibodies to Kv1 potassium channel-complex proteins leucine-rich, glioma inactivated 1 protein and contactin-associated protein-2 in limbic encephalitis, Morvan's syndrome and acquired neuromyotonia. Brain. 2010;133:2734–48.
6. Sabater L, Gaig C, Gelpi E, Bataller L, Lewerenz J, Torres-Vega E, Contreras A, Giometto B, Compta Y, Embid C, Vilaseca I, Iranzo A, Santamaria J, Dalmau J, Graus F. A novel non-rapid-eye movement and rapid-eye-movement parasomnia with sleep breathing disorder associated with antibodies to IgLON5: a case series, characterisation of the antigen, and post-mortem study. Lancet Neurol. 2014;13:575–86.
7. Hutchinson M, Waters P, McHugh J, Gorman G, O'Riordan S, Connolly S, Hager H, Yu P, Becker CM, Vincent A. Progressive encephalomyelitis, rigidity, and myoclonus: a novel glycine receptor antibody. Neurology. 2008;71: 1291–2.
8. Popescu BF, Guo Y, Jentoft ME, Parisi JE, Lennon VA, Pittock SJ, Weinshenker BG, Wingerchuk DM, Giannini C, Metz I, Bruck W, Shuster EA, Carter J, Boyd CD, Clardy SL, Cohen BA, Lucchinetti CF. Diagnostic utility of aquaporin-4 in the analysis of active demyelinating lesions. Neurology. 2015;84:148–58.
9. Wingerchuk DM, Lennon VA, Lucchinetti CF, Pittock SJ, Weinshenker BG. The spectrum of neuromyelitis optica. Lancet Neurol. 2007;6:805–15.
10. Wingerchuk DM, Banwell B, Bennett JL, Cabre P, Carroll W, Chitnis T, de SJ, Fujihara K, Greenberg B, Jacob A, Jarius S, Lana-Peixoto M, Levy M, Simon JH, Tenembaum S, Traboulsee AL, Waters P, Wellik KE, Weinshenker BG. International consensus diagnostic criteria for neuromyelitis optica spectrum disorders. Neurology. 2015;85:177–89.
11. Jarius S, Ruprecht K, Wildemann B, Kuempfel T, Ringelstein M, Geis C, Kleiter I, Kleinschnitz C, Berthele A, Brettschneider J, Hellwig K, Hemmer B, Linker RA, Lauda F, Mayer CA, Tumani H, Melms A, Trebst C, Stangel M, Marziniak M, Hoffmann F, Schippling S, Faiss JH, Neuhaus O, Ettrich B, Zentner C, Guthke K, Hofstadt-van OU, Reuss R, Pellkofer H, Ziemann U, Kern P, Wandinger KP, Bergh FT, Boettcher T, Langel S, Liebetrau M, Rommer PS, Niehaus S, Munch C, Winkelmann A, Zettl UU, Metz I, Veauthier C, Sieb JP, Wilke C, Hartung HP, Aktas O, Paul F. Contrasting disease patterns in seropositive and seronegative neuromyelitis optica: a multicentre study of 175 patients. J Neuroinflammation. 2012;9:14.
12. Balcer LJ, Miller DH, Reingold SC, Cohen JA. Vision and vision-related outcome measures in multiple sclerosis. Brain. 2015;138:11–27.
13. Brodsky M, Nazarian S, Orengo-Nania S, Hutton GJ, Buckley EG, Massey EW, Bhatti MT, Greer M, Goodwin J, Wall M, Savino PJ, Leist T, Miller NR, Irani D, Trobe JD, Cornblath W, Kaufman DI, Eggenberger E, Kupersmith MJ, Shults WT, McAllister L, Hamilton S, Beck RW, Dontchev M, Gal RL, Kollman C, Keltner JL, Smith CH, Optic Neuritis Study Group. Multiple sclerosis risk after optic neuritis: final optic neuritis treatment trial follow-up. Arch Neurol. 2008;65:727-32.
14. Heussinger N, Kontopantelis E, Gburek-Augustat J, Jenke A, Vollrath G, Korinthenberg R, Hofstetter P, Meyer S, Brecht I, Kornek B, Herkenrath P, Schimmel M, Wenner K, Hausler M, Lutz S, Karenfort M, Blaschek A, Smitka M, Karch S, Piepkorn M, Rostasy K, Lucke T, Weber P, Trollmann R, Klepper J, Haussler M, Hofmann R, Weissert R, Merkenschlager A, Buttmann M. Oligoclonal bands predict multiple sclerosis in children with optic neuritis. Ann Neurol. 2015;77:1076–82.
15. Zhao F, Zhang J, Liu YS, Li L, He YL. Research advances on flotillins. Virol J. 2011;8:479.
16. Bodin S, Planchon D, Rios ME, Comunale F, Gauthier-Rouviere C. Flotillins in intercellular adhesion—from cellular physiology to human diseases. J Cell Sci. 2014; 127:5139–47.
17. Malaga-Trillo E, Laessing U, Lang DM, Meyer A, Stuermer CA. Evolution of duplicated reggie genes in zebrafish and goldfish. J Mol Evol. 2002;54:235–45.

18. Morrow IC, Rea S, Martin S, Prior IA, Prohaska R, Hancock JF, James DE, Parton RG. Flotillin-1/reggie-2 traffics to surface raft domains via a novel golgi-independent pathway. Identification of a novel membrane targeting domain and a role for palmitoylation. J Biol Chem. 2002;277:48834–41.
19. Liu J, Deyoung SM, Zhang M, Dold LH, Saltiel AR. The stomatin/prohibitin/flotillin/HflK/C domain of flotillin-1 contains distinct sequences that direct plasma membrane localization and protein interactions in 3 T3-L1 adipocytes. J Biol Chem. 2005;280:16125–34.
20. Neumann-Giesen C, Falkenbach B, Beicht P, Claasen S, Luers G, Stuermer CA, Herzog V, Tikkanen R. Membrane and raft association of reggie-1/flotillin-2: role of myristoylation, palmitoylation and oligomerization and induction of filopodia by overexpression. Biochem J. 2004;378:509–18.
21. Li Y, Martin BR, Cravatt BF, Hofmann SL. DHHC5 protein palmitoylates flotillin-2 and is rapidly degraded on induction of neuronal differentiation in cultured cells. J Biol Chem. 2012;287:523–30.
22. Schulte T, Paschke KA, Laessing U, Lottspeich F, Stuermer CA. Reggie-1 and reggie-2, two cell surface proteins expressed by retinal ganglion cells during axon regeneration. Development. 1997;124:577–87.
23. Stöcker W, Otte M, Ulrich S, Normann D, Finkbeiner H, Stöcker K, Jantschek G, Scriba PC. Autoimmunity to pancreatic juice in Crohn's disease. Results of an autoantibody screening in patients with chronic inflammatory bowel disease. Scand J Gastroenterol Suppl. 1987;139:41–52.
24. Polman CH, Reingold SC, Banwell B, Clanet M, Cohen JA, Filippi M, Fujihara K, Havrdova E, Hutchinson M, Kappos L, Lublin FD, Montalban X, O'Connor P, Sandberg-Wollheim M, Thompson AJ, Waubant E, Weinshenker B, Wolinsky JS. Diagnostic criteria for multiple sclerosis: 2010 revisions to the McDonald criteria. Ann Neurol. 2011;69:292–302.
25. Reiber H, Lange P. Quantification of virus-specific antibodies in cerebrospinal fluid and serum: sensitive and specific detection of antibody synthesis in brain. Clin Chem. 1991;37:1153–60.
26. Hoehne M, de Couet HG, Stuermer CA, Fischbach KF. Loss- and gain-of-function analysis of the lipid raft proteins Reggie/Flotillin in Drosophila: they are posttranslationally regulated, and misexpression interferes with wing and eye development. Mol Cell Neurosci. 2005;30:326–38.
27. Koch JC, Solis GP, Bodrikov V, Michel U, Haralampieva D, Shypitsyna A, Tonges L, Bahr M, Lingor P, Stuermer CA. Upregulation of reggie-1/flotillin-2 promotes axon regeneration in the rat optic nerve in vivo and neurite growth in vitro. Neurobiol Dis. 2013;51:168–76.
28. Langhorst MF, Reuter A, Stuermer CA. Scaffolding microdomains and beyond: the function of reggie/flotillin proteins. Cell Mol Life Sci. 2005;62:2228–40.
29. Stuermer CA. How reggies regulate regeneration and axon growth. Cell Tissue Res. 2012;349:71–7.
30. Kowal J, Arras G, Colombo M, Jouve M, Morath JP, Primdal-Bengtson B, Dingli F, Loew D, Tkach M, Thery C. Proteomic comparison defines novel markers to characterize heterogeneous populations of extracellular vesicle subtypes. Proc Natl Acad Sci U S A. 2016;113:E968–77.

4

The contribution of the acute phase response to the pathogenesis of relapse in chronic-relapsing experimental autoimmune encephalitis models of multiple sclerosis

Silvy Mardiguian[1], Emma Ladds[1,2], Roberta Turner[1], Hazel Shepherd[1], Sandra J. Campbell[1] and Daniel C. Anthony[1*]

Abstract

Background: Increased relapse rates in multiple sclerosis (MS) as a consequence of peripheral immune system activation, owing to infection for example, have been widely reported, but the mechanism remains unclear. Acute brain injury models can be exacerbated by augmenting the hepatic acute phase response (APR). Here, we explored the contribution of the hepatic APR to relapse in two rodent models of MS.

Methods: Mice with MOG-CFA-induced chronic relapsing experimental autoimmune encephalitis (CR-EAE) were killed before, during and after the first phase of disease, and the brain and liver chemokine, cytokine and acute phase protein (APP) mRNA expression profile was determined. During remission, the APR was reactivated with an intraperitoneal lipopolysaccharide (LPS) and clinical score was monitored throughout. To explore the downstream mediators, CXCL-1, which is induced as part of the APR, was injected into animals with a focal, cytokine/MOG-induced EAE lesion (fEAE) and the cellularity of the lesions was assessed.

Results: Compared to CFA control, in a rodent CR-EAE model, an hepatic APR preceded clinical signs and central cytokine production in the initial phase of disease. Compared to administration in naïve animals, an LPS challenge during the asymptomatic remission phase of CR-EAE rodents provoked relapse and resulted in the increased and extended expression of specific peripheral hepatic chemokines. CXCL-1 and several other APPs were markedly elevated. A single intravenous administration of the highly induced chemokine, CXCL-1, was found to be sufficient to reactivate the lesions by increasing microglial activation and the recruitment of T cells in fEAE lesions.

Conclusions: The APR plays a contributing role to the pathology seen in models of chronic brain injury and in translating the effects of peripheral immune system stimulation secondary to trauma or infection into central pathology and behavioural signs. Further elucidation of the exact mechanisms in this process will inform development of more effective, selective therapies in MS that, by suppressing the hepatic chemokine response, may prevent relapse.

Keywords: Multiple sclerosis, Lipopolysaccharide, Acute phase response, VCAM-MPIO

* Correspondence: daniel.anthony@pharm.ox.ac.uk
[1]Department of Pharmacology, University of Oxford, Oxford OX1 4QT, UK

Background

The initial coordinated systemic response to physiological challenges such as infection or tissue injury is known as the acute phase response (APR). The APR mobilises the appropriate leukocyte populations to neutralise pathogens, whilst simultaneously initiating repair processes to restore normal function and limit secondary inflammatory damage [1, 2]. The APR occurs via a cascade of local vascular and systemic effects, facilitated by inflammatory mediators including chemokines, cytokines, pentraxins and serum amyloid proteins, which are largely produced by the liver and are often described as acute phase proteins (APP). Most commonly they are defined as a protein whose plasma concentration changes by 25% during an inflammatory response, and they may originate from both hepatic and extra-hepatic sites [2]. Although the APR evolved as a survival mechanism in the short term, prolonged or aberrant effects may be detrimental in chronic inflammation or autoimmune conditions [3].

The introduction of IL-1β into the basal ganglia rapidly induces APP expression by the liver and spleen including chemokine expression such as CXCL1 (the murine equivalent of IL-8) [4]. We have recently shown that astrocyte-shed extracellular vesicles regulate this peripheral APR to inflammatory brain lesions following acute CNS injuries [5] and that augmentation of the peripheral response can exacerbate acute CNS lesions [6]. This appears to be a direct consequence of enhanced mobilisation of leukocytes into the blood by the chemokines released by the liver [7]. Within the brain, multiple sclerosis (MS) lesions are known to be associated with local IL-1β production [8], and MS patients have higher IL-8 serum levels compared to controls [9]. However, it is unknown whether this local cytokine production is able to induce an APR and whether dysregulation of the APR in individuals with MS might impact on pathogenesis of MS. Infections have long been implicated in the pathogenesis in MS, and whilst no single pathogen has been consistently linked to aetiology or relapse, infection would be expected to generate an APR. Indeed, increased relapse rates have been demonstrated in patients with viral [10, 11] and bacterial [12] infections, but the pathway from infection to relapse has not been studied in a systematic manner. In a model of chronic relapsing experimental autoimmune encephalitis (CR-EAE) in SJL mice, Glabinski et al. reported coordinated chemokine upregulation in the brain and spinal cord during clinical relapse, but did not find evidence of CCL2 or CXCL10 expression in the liver [13]. However, in ABH mice with CR-EAE, we discovered that increased hepatic CXCL1 chemokine levels are associated with behavioural depression and the recruitment of neutrophils to the liver. This hepatic neutrophil recruitment was also found to be a histopathological feature in post-mortem liver from MS patients compared to controls [9]. The expression of hepatic CXCL1 in the ABH CR-EAE animals occurred well before the development of overt clinical signs and suggests that activation of the APR might precipitate clinical relapses experienced by MS patients [9]. In another acute EAE model, hepatic CCL2 and CXCL10 expression have been reported to precede the development of fulminant EAE disease, but it was unclear in this study whether this systemic inflammatory response was a 'primary determinant or a secondary reflection' of the occurrence of EAE in the affected animals [14].

As for MS, the disease course in EAE models can be affected by systemic cytokine production and infections. Direct intraperitoneal challenge with bacterial enterotoxins [15] or the cytokine IL-12 [16, 17], a critical component of innate resistance to bacterial infection, exacerbates CNS pathology and clinical signs, whilst intraperitoneal inoculation with *Chlamydia pneumonia* [18] or injection of live *Streptococcus pneumonia* [19] worsens disease. Such peripheral physiological challenges have been associated with increased levels of central pro-inflammatory cytokines [20, 21], but the contribution and temporal relationship between infection, the APR and relapse have not been investigated. Microbial recognition induces the production of pro-inflammatory chemokines, necessary for the recruitment of leukocytes to the diseased brain [22]. This has been shown to be important in the pathogenesis of MS and the acute model of EAE [23]. Systemic infection increases peripheral production of chemokines and, on the basis of our finding in acute CNS pathology, might be expected to modulate the pathogenesis of MS. Indeed, peripheral administration of interferon-beta (IFNβ), a mainstay therapy for MS, significantly inhibited hepatic CXCL-1 production and neutrophil recruitment induced by the microinjection of IL-1β into the brain [9].

Should the hepatic APR does play a role in mediating disease exacerbation in response to a peripheral stimulus, the process of recognition and initiation of changes in the chemokine expression profile would necessitate a time lag between the insult and the onset of worsening clinical symptoms. Thus, here we sought to investigate the temporal relationships between a peripheral inflammatory challenge, sufficient to stimulate an APR, and the central and hepatic production of chemokine and APP mRNA compared to the onset and duration of clinical symptoms in chronic models of MS.

Methods

Induction of EAE and LPS injection

Chronic relapsing EAE was induced in female Biozzi antibody-high (ABH) mice (6–8 weeks) by subcutaneous injection into both abdominal flanks of 150 μl of an emulsion consisting of 500 μg of mouse spinal cord homogenate in Freund's incomplete adjuvant (FIA) supplemented with mycobacteria (*Mycobacterium tuberculosis and Mycobacterium butyricum).* Animals were injected on days 0 and 7 and were weighed daily and assessed for clinical signs according to the following guidelines: 0—healthy, 1—limp tail, 2—incomplete hind limb paralysis, 3—complete hind limb paralysis and 4—forelimb paralysis. Animals (n = 6 per group) were killed on days 10, 14, 17 and 28 to examine the APR before, during and after the first phase of disease. A second cohort were established to determine the effect of a lipopolysaccharide (LPS) challenge during the remission period (1 mg/kg *Escherichia coli* 0111:B4; Sigma Chemical Co., St. Louis, MO, USA), when most APPs had returned to baseline. These animals (n = 5 or 6 per group) where killed on day 42. All experiments were performed with UK Home Office approval.

Behavioural testing

Hind limb muscle strength was evaluated using an inverted screen test as previously described [24]. The inverted screen was a square of wire mesh surrounded by a 4-cm-wide wooden edge. A mouse was placed on the screen, which was turned upside down and suspended above soft padding. After 2 min, it was rotated back and the mouse was removed. The time taken for the hind limbs to first drop from the screen, and the time (up to 120 s) that a mouse remained on the screen before falling were recorded. Testing was performed on days 1, 5, 6 and 7 following the lipopolysaccharide (LPS; 1 mg/kg) or vehicle challenge on days 30 and 31. The LPS-treated animals were killed 12 days after the first LPS injection on day 42.

Induction of focal EAE in Lewis rats

To examine the effect of chemokine administration on the histopathology of an MS-like lesion, focal, cytokine/MOG-induced EAE (fEAE) was generated in male Lewis rats (Charles River, UK) (80–120 g, n = 8). Animals were anaesthetized with 1.5–3% isoflurane in a mixture of nitrous oxide/oxygen (70%/30%) and injected subcutaneously at the base of the tail with 100 μl of MOG (35–55) peptide (25 μg diluted in saline) emulsified in IFA (1:1). Control animals were injected with the same volume of saline emulsified in IFA (1:1). To induce the targeted, focal EAE lesions, the immunised animals were anaesthetized with 2–3% isoflurane in a mixture of nitrous oxide/oxygen (70%/30%) and placed in a stereotaxic frame 21 days after the MOG injection (n = 8). A midline incision was made in the scalp, and a burr hole, drilled 1 mm anterior and 3 mm lateral to Bregma. Using a finely drawn glass microcapillary (< 50 μm) tip, 2 μl of a cytokine mixture containing 1.45 μg of recombinant rat tumour necrosis factor (TNF; PeproTech London, UK or NIBSC, Potters Bar, UK) and 1 μg of recombinant rat interferon gamma (IFN-γ; PeproTech London, UK) dissolved in sterile saline was injected stereotaxically into the corpus callosum over a 10-min period. After injection, the wound was closed and the animals were allowed to recover from anaesthesia; they displayed no overt clinical signs. A trace of monastral blue (Sigma-Aldrich) was added as a marker dye to enable easier lesion detection histologically. In the absence of an intracerebral cytokine challenge, no MOG-EAE lesions are detectable by MRI or by immunohistochemistry [25]. The focal lesions were allowed to develop and mature for 28 days. We have previously shown that there is no blood-brain barrier breakdown, but that the lesions continue to increase in size. At 28 days after lesion activation, the animals received a single intravenous dose (1 μg) of recombinant rat CXCL-1 (NIBSC, South Mimms) in 0.5 ml endotoxin-free saline or vehicle control.

EAE tissue collection and immunohistochemistry

The animals were deeply anaesthetised with sodium pentobarbital and transcardially perfused with 0.9% heparinised saline followed by 4% paraformaldehyde in 0.1 M phosphate buffer. Small pieces of fresh liver were removed and frozen immediately in dry ice for PCR analysis. Ten-micrometre-thick sections were cut from the liver and fixed for immunohistochemistry. We have previously shown that the site of the liver biopsy has no effect on the outcome; the expression of proteins is homogenous throughout [26].

Immunohistochemistry was carried out using standard three-step procedures [27] with appropriate biotinylated secondary reagents and standard avidin-biotin complex (ABC) amplification according to the manufacturer's instructions (Vector Laboratories, Peterborough UK). Neutrophils were identified using an anti-neutrophil serum as previously described [28]. To quantify the neutrophils, four representative, non-overlapping fields were chosen and the average number of positive cells were calculated and expressed per square millimetre.

fEAE tissue collection

To study the effect of increasing circulating levels of chemokine on the pathogenesis of MS-like disease, we chose to use a focal lesion model where direct histopathological comparison may be made that is not possible in disseminated disease models. Rats with the fEAE were killed 7 days after the injection of CXCL-1 or vehicle, which was the point at which maximum disease activity (clinical signs) was recorded following the LPS challenge in the CR-EAE experiment. Animals were perfusion-fixed with periodate-lysine-paraformaldehyde (PLP) as previously described. Immunohistochemistry was performed to quantify the number of T cells (anti-Phycoerythrin, OX22; Sigma-Aldrich) and activation of microglia (anti-iba1; Abcam, Cambridge, UK). As above, immunohistochemistry was carried out using standard three-step procedures [27] with appropriate biotinylated secondary reagents and standard ABC amplification according to the manufacturer's instructions (Vector Laboratories, Peterborough UK). The number of iba1 or OX22-postive cells was counted in three non-overlapping high-power (×400) fields in the injected striatum.

mRNA extraction and RT-PCR

RNA extraction from frozen liver and brain tissues was performed using the Qiagen RNeasy Extraction Kit ® (Qiagen Ltd. Crawley, UK) as per manufacturer's instructions quantitative real-time polymerase chain reaction (RT-PCR) assays were performed as previously described [29]. Results are expressed as number of copies of target per nanogram input RNA corrected to the housekeeping gene, glyceraldehyde 3-phosphate dehydrogenase (GAPDH).

Statistical analysis

Data is presented as mean ± SEM at each time point. Independent sample *t* tests were used to compare the behavioural outcomes and motor performance throughout the time course. One-way or two-way ANOVA (Prism 7.0, Graphpad software) was employed for all further analysis.

Results

Increased mRNA production of chemokines and APP proteins in the liver precedes clinical signs in EAE

Using quantitative RT-PCR, hepatic tissue collected from EAE and CFA control mice during the pre-symptomatic, symptomatic and remission phases of the disease (Fig. 1) was analysed for chemokine and APP expression. mRNA production of *CXCL1*, *SAA1*, *SAA2* and *SAP* was found to be significantly elevated ($p < 0.05$) in the liver in EAE mice at day 10 (before the onset of clinical signs) compared to levels in both CFA controls and EAE mice during the symptomatic (days 14 and 17) and remission phases of disease (day 28). mRNA *SAP* levels persisted in EAE animals during the symptomatic phase of the disease at day 14, whereas all other expression levels had declined to match those of the controls. By day 17, *SAP* levels had also returned to baseline.

Increased mRNA production of chemokines and APPs in the CNS in EAE during the acute phase of the disease

Quantitative RT-PCR was used to measure the mRNA production of representative APPs and chemokines in the CNS in tissue collected from EAE and CFA control animals at days 10, 14, 17 and 28 following the induction of EAE.

Whilst the production of chemokines and APPs in the periphery was highest at day 10 when the animals were asymptomatic (Fig. 1), in the brain, the highest expression was evident at day 14, during the acute disease phase. Compared to controls, significantly elevated *IL1B* (Fig. 2a) and *CCL5* ($p < 0.001$) (Fig. 2c) intracerebral levels were observed in EAE animals at days 14 and 17 alongside a significant elevation in the expression of *IL17*, *CXCL10* and *CCL2* ($p < 0.05$) at day 14 (Fig. 2).

Peripheral challenge with LPS exacerbates spontaneous relapse in EAE with a time delay before the onset of clinical symptoms

The first clinical signs were observed in the EAE models at day 13. The disease was most severe at day 17, followed by full or partial remission by day 28. Following the initial acute phase, 30 μg of LPS or saline was injected into EAE mice on days 31 and 32 when the animals were still in remission (Fig. 3a). LPS-treated animals suffered a relapse, with a significant increase in clinical scores from day 36 onwards ($p < 0.05$). There was therefore a time delay of 5 days before significant clinical effects were seen, although a non-significant decline was seen in the intervening period (Fig. 3a). LPS-treated mice also demonstrated a reduction in the period before falling off the inverted screen (Fig. 3b (i)), or before the first double hind limb foot-fault (Fig. 3b (ii)). These results were significant on days 37 and 38 ($p < 0.05$).

LPS treatment increases peripheral mRNA production of chemokines and APPs in EAE mice but does not affect levels in controls

The administration of a peripheral LPS challenge in EAE mice at days 31 and 32, i.e. during the disease remission phase, was associated with a significant increase in mRNA expression of the acute phase hepatic proteins *SAA1*, *SAA2*, *SAP* and *CXCL1* ($p < 0.05$) compared to the control mice who received a saline challenge (Fig. 4). LPS challenge was not associated with any altered mRNA expression in control CFA mice, suggesting that the increase was not attributable to the effects of LPS alone, but an interaction of the CR-EAE and the LPS administration. No significant differences were observed in the mRNA production of *CXCL10* or *CCL5*. Neither *IL17* nor tumour necrosis factor (*TNF*) expression was detected in the liver of these animals at this time point (data not shown).

LPS treatment is associated with increased central mRNA expression of chemokines and APPs in EAE mice compared to controls

Seven days after administration of peripheral LPS or saline, mRNA expression of the APPs *SAA1*, *SAA2* and *CCL5* in brain tissue was significantly increased ($p < 0.05$) in LPS-challenged EAE mice (Fig. 5). The expression

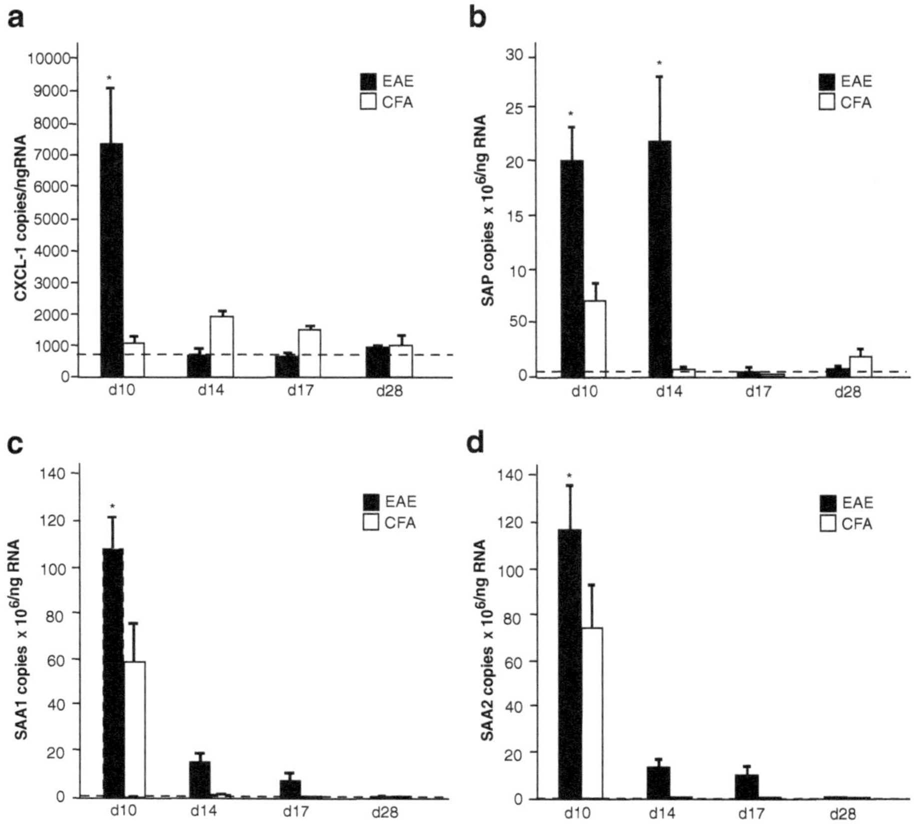

Fig. 1 Peripheral production of chemokines and APPs precedes clinical signs in EAE. Quantitative RT-PCR on hepatic tissue collected from EAE animals ($n = 6$) at days 10, 14, 17 and 28 revealed a significantly elevated mRNA expression of CXCL-10 (**a**), SAP (**b**), SAA1 (**c**) and SAA2 (**d**) at day 10, before the onset of clinical signs when compared to CFA mice at the same time point ($p < 0.05$). CXCL-10, SAA1 and SAA2 declined to control levels when the animals were symptomatic (days 14 and 17) and in remission (day 28). SAP levels persisted at day 14 and declined dramatically by day 17. The dotted line indicates the basal level of each marker in naive animals. *$p < 0.05$

profiles of *SAP, CXCL1, CXCL10, IL1B* and *IL17* were similar in both cohorts and CFA control mice also demonstrated no significant alterations.

The peripheral administration of CXCL-1 increases fEAE lesion activity

In order to assess the impact of increased circulating chemokine expression on MS lesions, CR-EAE animals were injected with CXCL-1 (10 μg) protein into the circulation (iv) and the status of inflammatory markers in the lesion tissue assessed using immunohistochemistry. Expression of both Iba-1 and OX-22 was higher 7 days after injection of the chemokine than after a saline injection ($p < 0.05$) (Fig. 6).

Discussion

Peripheral inflammatory insults, e.g. secondary to peripheral infection [30–32], acute medical illness [33, 34] or the chronic inflammation seen in metabolic syndrome [35] or autoimmune conditions [36], have been associated with an exacerbation of clinical symptoms in a wide range of CNS diseases [37]. Supportive evidence is emerging in many conditions for a mechanistic role played by systematic pro-inflammatory cytokines in this symptomatic deterioration [38–41].

Using the CR-EAE model of MS, in this study, we demonstrate hepatic production of APPs and chemokines prior to the onset of clinical signs. Production was also associated with clinical exacerbation following peripheral inflammatory stimulation during the relapse phase. These results are consistent with a feedforward model of peripheral-central cytokine interaction that underlies both stimulation and perpetuation of the hepatic APR and inflammatory-mediated production of neurological symptoms. Similar extensive cross-talk between peripheral and central insults and the production of central or peripheral cytokines has previously been demonstrated [42, 43]. Both acute and chronic non-immune-mediated injuries to the CNS result in a peripheral APR, which includes expression of hepatic APPs [4, 44]. In this study, acute and chronic non-immune-mediated damage within the CNS is associated with a similar peripheral response to CR-EAE.

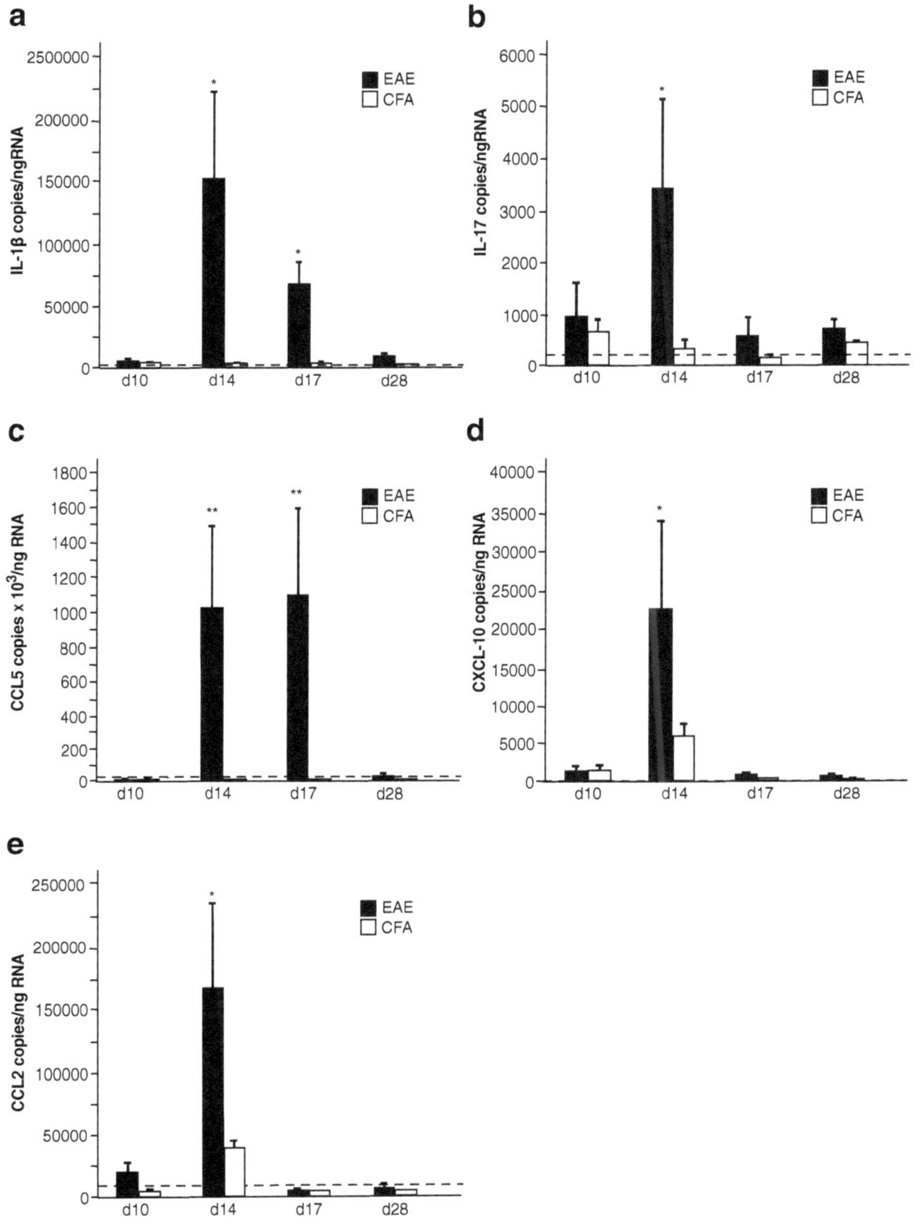

Fig. 2 Production of chemokines and APPs in the CNS is highest during the acute phase of EAE. Quantitative RT-PCR on brain tissue collected from EAE and CFA animals ($n = 6$) at days 10, 14, 17 and 28 revealed a significantly elevated mRNA expression of IL-1β (**a**), IL-17 (**b**), CCL5 (**c**) CXCL-10 (**d**) and CCL2 (**e**) at day 14, during the acute phase of the disease when compared to CFA mice ($p < 0.05$) and declined by day 17, with the exception of IL-1β and CCL5 which returned to control levels after day 17. The dotted line indicates the basal level of each marker in naive animals. *$p < 0.05$

Therefore, although MS and EAE are primarily considered CNS diseases, the production of peripheral chemokines and APPs may play an important role in the underlying disease process and clinical course.

The presence of a systemic component in MS is not a new idea. Most therapies for MS target processes occurring in the periphery rather than within the CNS. Natalizumab (Tysabri) suppresses peripheral leukocyte migration by both blocking the interaction of VLA4-positive lymphocytes with the brain endothelium and by controlling the localization of marginal zone B cells [45, 46]; fingolimod suppress microglial activation but its principal mode of action is to prevent lymphocyte migration from the lymph nodes [47] and by reducing peripheral secretion of IL-17 by CD8+ T cells [48], whilst glatiramer acetate is thought to compete with myelin

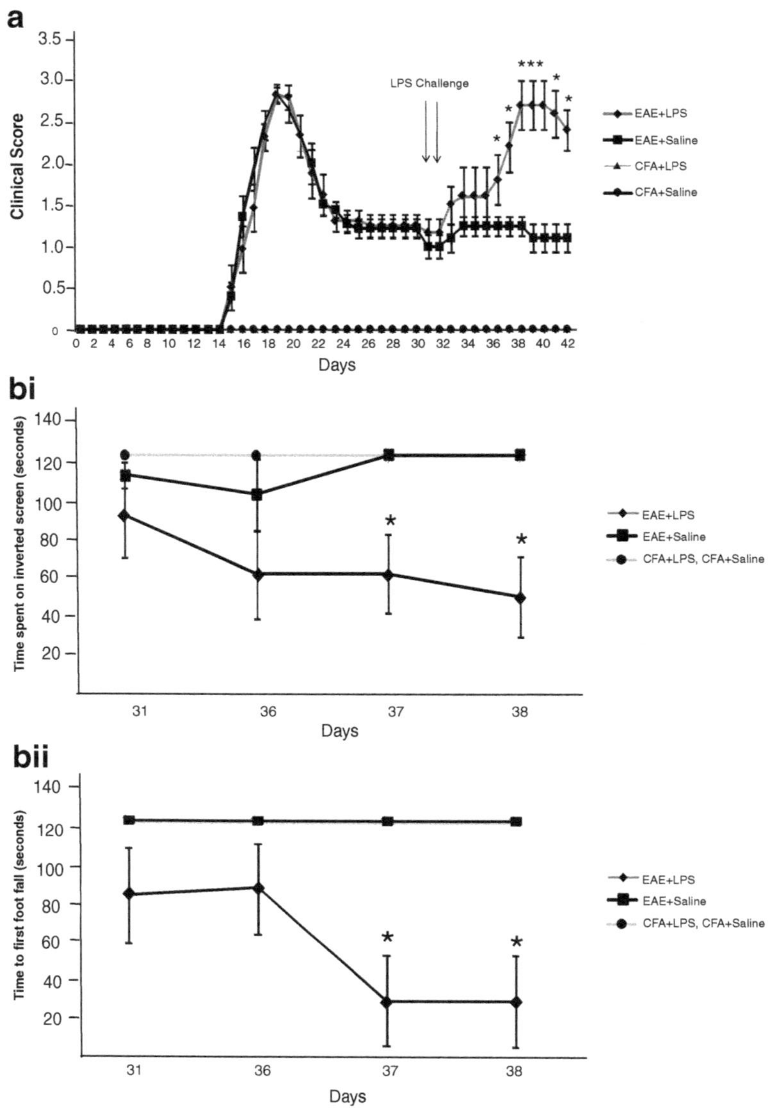

Fig. 3 Peripheral LPS administration in EAE exacerbates the relapse phase. EAE mice injected with LPS (n = 5) scored more than EAE mice injected with saline (n = 5) (**a**) There was a delay of 5 days from the administration of LPS until clinical signs were significantly greater than saline-treated mice. LPS-treated mice performed significantly worse in behavioural tests and spent less time on the inverted screen (**b** (i)) with a reduction in the time of the first foot-fall (**b** (ii)), which achieved significance on days 37 and 38

antigens within APCs in the periphery although there is very little evidence for this putative mode of action [49]. A more detailed characterisation of the exact processes underlying the peripheral contribution to disease pathology may contribute to the search for additional or more effective therapies.

In this study, expression of peripheral chemokines and APPs reached a peak prior to and then fell at the onset of clinical signs. By contrast, in the CNS, expression was highest during the acute disease phase. It is likely that the cellular source for the APP are astrocytes and microglia as both cell types have been reported to produce these chemokines and cytokines in previous studies [50–52]. Hepatic APP production has previously been shown to increase over a few hours following acute brain injury [4], which was thought to facilitate a concentration gradient firstly between the marrow and the blood and then between the blood and the CNS to encourage central leukocyte migration post-APR stimulation. However, the long-term expression of IL-1β in the brain gave rise to sustained high levels of hepatic cytokines expression [44], suggesting that the postulated role of the cytokines in immune cell recruitment is in fact more complex than the generation of simple gradients and that the continued

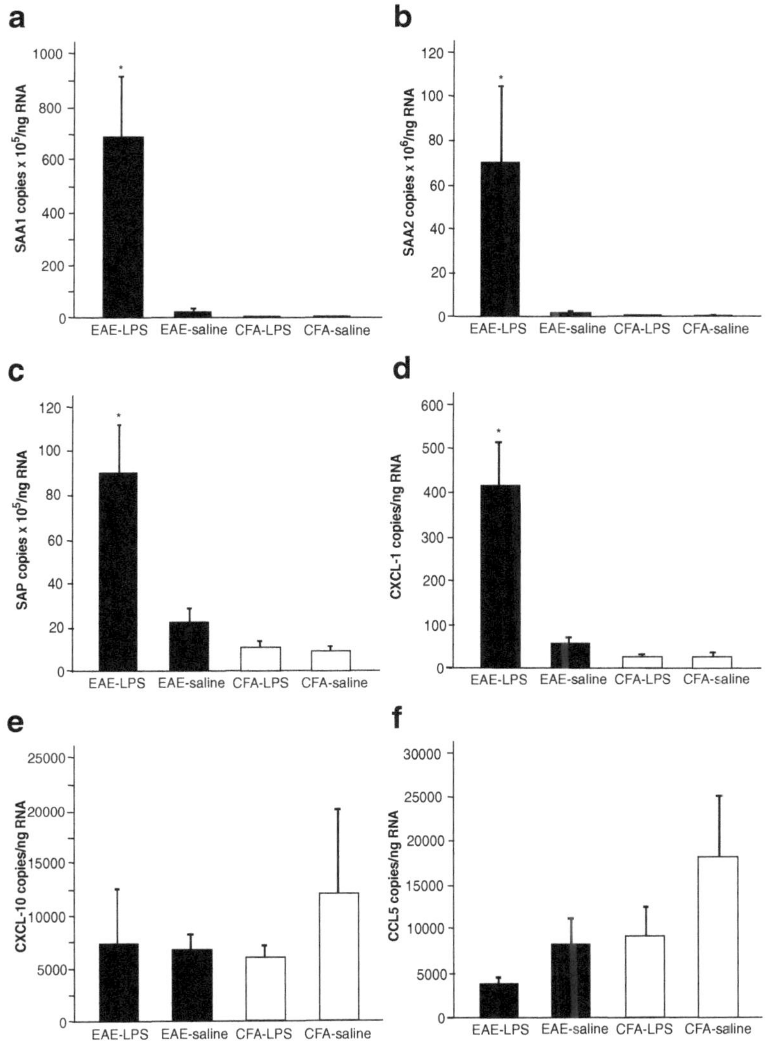

Fig. 4 Hepatic mRNA production of acute phase proteins and chemokines increases 8 days after LPS challenge in CR-EAE animals but not in CFA mice. Hepatic mRNA production of SAA1 (**a**), SAA2 (**b**), SAP (**c**) and CXCL-1 (**d**) was significantly higher in LPS-treated EAE mice (n = 5) when compared to that in saline-treated EAE mice (n = 5) ($p < 0.05$). No significant differences in CXCL-10 (**e**) and CCL5 (**f**) were found between the LPS-challenged mice and saline-treated animals. LPS administration in control CFA mice (n = 5) had no effect on the production of these acute phase proteins and chemokines when compared to saline-treated CFA mice (n = 4)

high level of induction of peripheral cytokines may play a role in more sustained responses.

Here we used LPS, a gram-negative bacterial endotoxin known to cause inflammation [53], to mimic a transient bacterial infection. The peripheral administration of LPS in CR-EAE mice brought forward and exacerbated the clinical signs seen in the disease relapse phase, in keeping with effects seen in other CNS diseases. Importantly, the APR remained elevated for days after the challenge compared the injection of LPS into naïve animals, which highlights the interaction between CNS and peripheral disease, and, once again, suggests that the gradient hypothesis is insufficient to explain the mobilisation and recruitment of leukocytes to the brain. Intraperitoneal LPS administration is also known to exacerbate brain damage and neurological deficits in stroke and prion disease models [38, 54] and is thought to mediate acute cognitive decline via production of pro-inflammatory cytokines [55]. The LPS-induced exacerbation of clinical signs in this study occurred after at least 5 days, longer than the time taken in previous work looking at peripheral LPS challenge [56]. However, this pattern resembles that seen in human MS patients following peripheral infection [11]. The lag may reflect the time needed for sufficient damage to occur to the blood-brain barrier, the destruction of myelin and generation of a conduction block [57].

Whilst MS is thought to largely be a macrophage and T cell-mediated disease, we have previously demonstrated

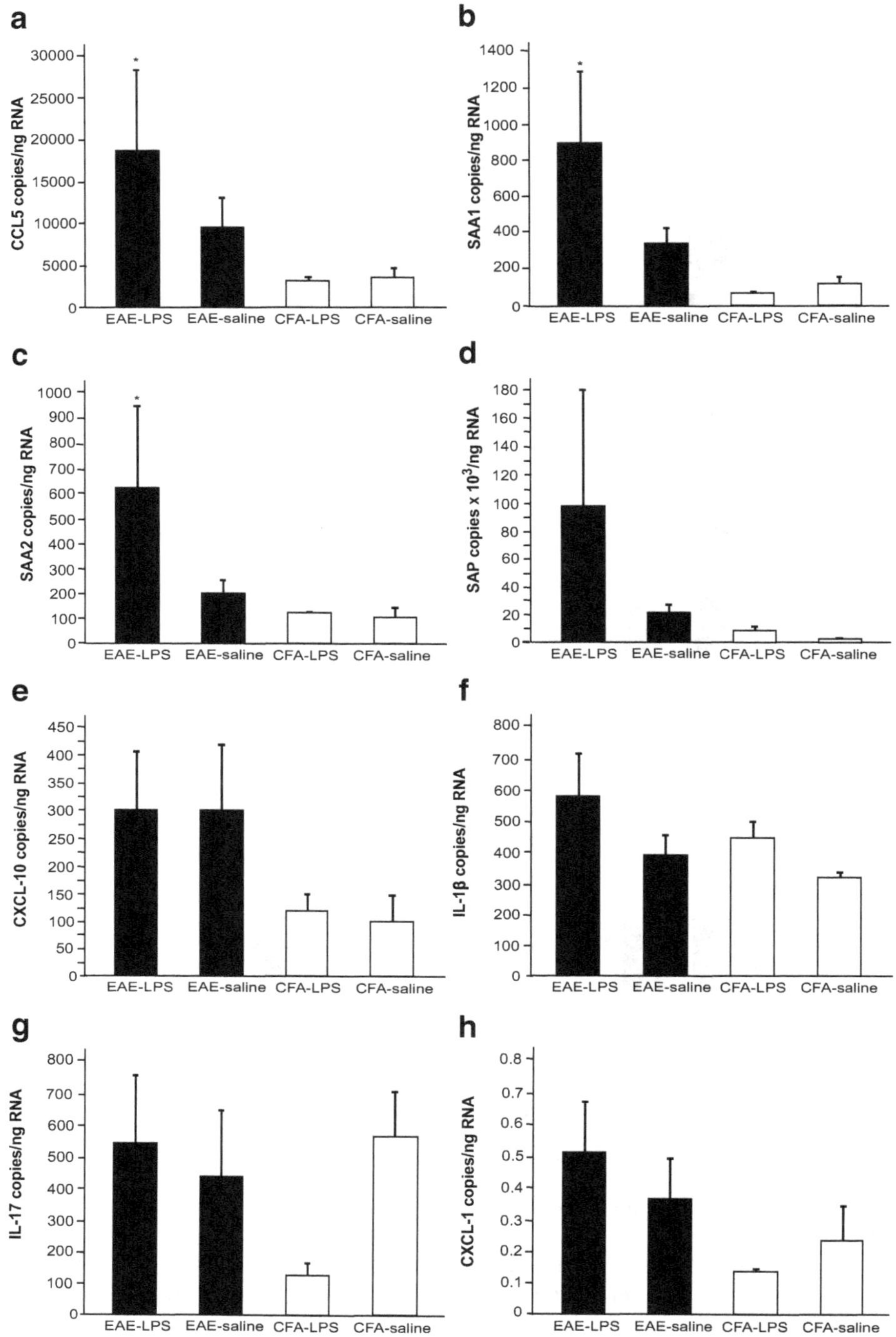

Fig. 5 In EAE acute phase, protein and chemokine expression increases in the brain 8 days after LPS challenge without having an effect in CFA mice. mRNA production of CCL5 (**a**), SAA1 (**b**) and SAA2 (**c**) in the brain was higher in LPS-treated EAE mice ($n = 5$) when compared to that in saline-treated EAE mice ($n = 5$) ($p < 0.05$). LPS administration in control CFA mice ($n = 5$) had no effect on the production of these acute phase proteins and expressed levels that were comparable to saline-treated CFA mice ($n = 4$). There were no significant changes in the levels of SAP (**d**), CXCL-10 (**e**), IL-1β (**f**), IL-17 (**g**) and CXCL-1 (**h**)

hepatic neutrophil recruitment as a feature of CR-EAE and MS, which appears to reduce during periods of clinical remission [9]. These findings would support an additional role for neutrophils and potentially associated cytokines such as IL-8 and CXCL-1 in the pathological process. As MS patients and CR-EAE models express

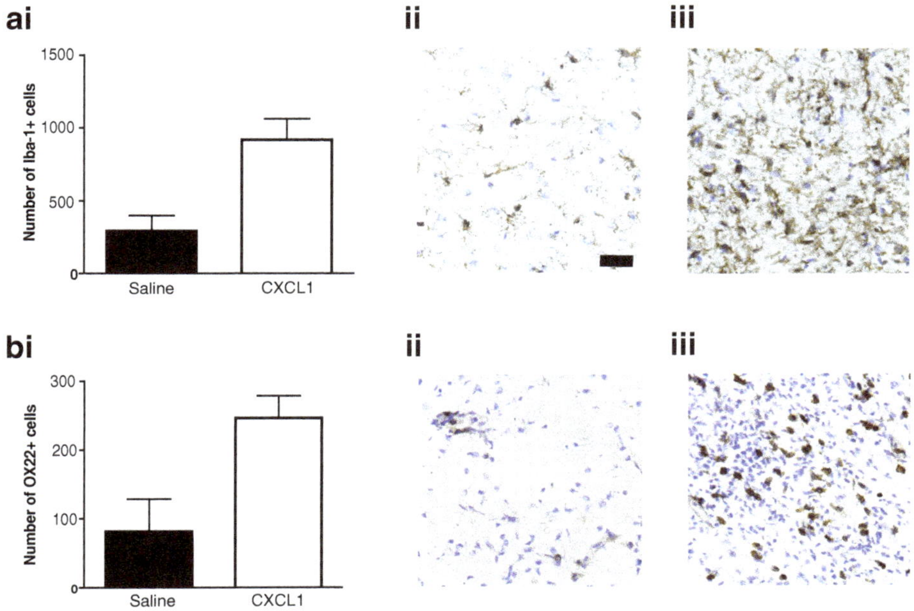

Fig. 6 CXCL-1 increases the lesion activity in the fEAE model. At 7 days, animals that received a peripheral injection of 1 μg CXCL-1 iv displayed more (**a**) Iba1 immunoreactive microglia/macrophages ($p < 0.05$) and **b** more T cells (OX-22-positive) were present within the lesions than in those animals that received saline vehicle. Photomicrographs of iba1 (Aii and Aiii) and OX22 (Bii and Biii) staining in the lesions of the control and CXCL-1-treated animals respectively. Scale bar = 20 μm

higher levels of circulating IL-8 and CXCL-1 [58, 59], the hepatic chemokine response may be involved in the control of leukocyte recruitment to chronic inflammatory lesions in the brain. Further support for the involvement of alterations in the peripheral cytokine profile in the pathology contributing to MS comes from studies of natalizumab, which not only inhibits the transmigration of leukocytes into the CNS but also decreases the plasma levels of GM-CSF, IL-6, IL-10 and TNF after 1 year—with IL-8 levels remaining unaltered [46].

In this study, the selective rise in the expression of hepatic chemokines and APPs in CR-EAE mice treated with LPS prior to clinical relapse suggests that LPS is able to induce and maintain the expression of peripheral immune markers. However, the mechanisms for this remain unclear. It has been shown that activation of the innate immune system in MS patients leads to the production of monocyte-derived dendritic cells that can modify autoreactive T cell populations and alter their cytokine secretion profile [60]. We have previously demonstrated that Kupffer cell-depleted CR-EAE rats experience a considerably reduced expression of selected chemokines following central IL-1ß microinjection, highlighting a role for Kupffer cells in the APR. However, this was not associated with decreased neutrophil mobilisation or CXCL-1 and MIP-1ß reduction, indicating that these processes may be Kupffer cell-independent [61]. The induction of high levels of CXCL-1 prompted us to examine the effect of CXCL-1 alone on the pathogenesis of a well-characterised focal model of pattern II MS, which is associated with the deposition of immunoglobulin and complement at sites of active myelin destruction [62]. The formation of stratified lesions in terms of spatial distribution and kinetics distinguishes these models from other types of EAE where lesion presentation is random and variable, and hence is not quantifiable. Here we showed that a single bolus injection of the downstream chemokine CXCL-1 was sufficient to increase microglial activation and increase the presence of T cells within the focal lesions over an extended period. Thus, whilst CXCL-1 is considered to be a neutrophil chemoattractant, it clearly has the potential to exacerbate an antibody-mediated MS-like disease in the CNS, which may be mediated via neutrophil activation or potentially by activating CXCR2 that is known to be expressed on endothelial cells in certain circumstances [63].

Conclusion

In this study, we demonstrated increased expression of hepatic chemokines and APPs in the CR-EAE model of chronic brain injury. This is consistent with previous findings in models of acute brain injury [4, 9, 44]. Peripheral expression of inflammatory markers was highest whilst the animals were asymptomatic, whereas central chemokine expression was greatest during the acute disease phase, suggesting that peripheral inflammatory mechanisms could contribute to the genesis of central inflammation and subsequent clinical signs. Peripheral LPS challenge results in exacerbation of spontaneous relapse 5 days after LPS administration, and this is associated with an increased expression of hepatic chemokines and APPs. Peripheral administration of CXCL-1 chemokine was sufficient to increase disease activity in focal MS-like lesions and thus chemokine signalling alone can account for the APR-induced exacerbation of central pathology. Therefore, we conclude that the hepatic APR may modulate the impact of the peripheral immune response on central pathology and relapse in MS patients.

Abbreviations

APPs: Acute phase proteins; CR-EAE: Chronic relapsing experimental autoimmune encephalomyelitis; LPS: Lipopolysaccharide; MRI: Magnetic resonance imaging; MS: Multiple sclerosis; VCAM-1: Vascular cell adhesion molecule-1

Acknowledgements

This work was supported by the University of Oxford.

Funding

This work was funded by a Raffy Manoukian scholarship to SM.

Authors' contributions

SM, RT and DA collected the data. SM, HS, SC and DA contributed to the analysis. SM, EL and DA prepared the figures and the manuscript for publication. All authors read and approved the final manuscript.

Consent for publication

Not applicable.

Competing interests

The authors declare that they have no conflict of interest.

Author details

[1]Department of Pharmacology, University of Oxford, Oxford OX1 4QT, UK.
[2]Department of Primary Care Health Sciences, University of Oxford, Oxford OX2 6GG, UK.

References

1. Baumann H, Gauldie J. The acute phase response. Immunol Today. 1994;15(2):74–80.
2. Morley JJ, Kushner I. Serum C-reactive protein levels in disease. Ann N Y Acad Sci. 1982;389:406–18.
3. Uhlar CM, Whitehead AS. Serum amyloid A, the major vertebrate acute-phase reactant. Eur J Biochem. 1999;265(2):501–23.
4. Campbell SJ, et al. CINC-1 is an acute-phase protein induced by focal brain injury causing leukocyte mobilization and liver injury. FASEB J. 2003;17(9):1168–70.
5. Dickens AM, et al. Astrocyte-shed extracellular vesicles regulate the peripheral leukocyte response to inflammatory brain lesions. Sci Signal. 2017;10(473):eaai7696.
6. Campbell S, et al. Central nervous system injury triggers hepatic CC and CXC chemokine expression that is associated with leukocyte mobilization and recruitment to both the central nervous system and the liver. Am J Pathol. 2005;166(5):1487–97.
7. Campbell SJ, et al. Hepatic nuclear factor kappa B regulates neutrophil recruitment to the injured brain. J Neuropathol Exp Neurol. 2008;67(3):223–30.
8. Rovaris M, et al. Patterns of disease activity in multiple sclerosis patients: a study with quantitative gadolinium-enhanced brain MRI and cytokine measurement in different clinical subgroups. J Neurol. 1996;243(7):536–42.
9. Campbell SJ, et al. Sickness behaviour is induced by a peripheral CXC-chemokine also expressed in multiple sclerosis and EAE. Brain Behav Immun. 2010;24(5):738–46.
10. Sibley WA, Bamford CR, Clark K. Clinical viral infections and multiple sclerosis. Lancet. 1985;1(8441):1313–5.
11. Buljevac D, et al. Prospective study on the relationship between infections and multiple sclerosis exacerbations. Brain. 2002;125(Pt 5):952–60.
12. Rapp NS, Gilroy J, Lerner AM. Role of bacterial infection in exacerbation of multiple sclerosis. Am J Phys Med Rehabil. 1995;74(6):415–8.
13. Glabinski AR, et al. Synchronous synthesis of alpha- and beta-chemokines by cells of diverse lineage in the central nervous system of mice with relapses of chronic experimental autoimmune encephalomyelitis. Am J Pathol. 1997;150(2):617–30.
14. Glabinski AR, et al. Central nervous system chemokine mRNA accumulation follows initial leukocyte entry at the onset of acute murine experimental autoimmune encephalomyelitis. Brain Behav Immun. 1995;9(4):315–30.
15. Brocke S, et al. Induction of relapsing paralysis in experimental autoimmune encephalomyelitis by bacterial superantigen. Nature. 1993;365(6447):642–4.
16. Smith T, et al. Interleukin-12 induces relapse in experimental allergic encephalomyelitis in the Lewis rat. Am J Pathol. 1997;150(6):1909–17.
17. Ahmed Z, et al. Myelin/axonal pathology in interleukin-12 induced serial relapses of experimental allergic encephalomyelitis in the Lewis rat. Am J Pathol. 2001;158(6):2127–38.
18. Du C, et al. Chlamydia pneumoniae infection of the central nervous system worsens experimental allergic encephalitis. J Exp Med. 2002;196(12):1639–44.
19. Herrmann I, et al. Streptococcus pneumoniae infection aggravates experimental autoimmune encephalomyelitis via Toll-like receptor 2. Infect Immun. 2006;74(8):4841–8.
20. Ban E, Haour F, Lenstra R. Brain interleukin 1 gene expression induced by peripheral lipopolysaccharide administration. Cytokine. 1992;4(1):48–54.
21. Gatti S, Bartfai T. Induction of tumor necrosis factor-alpha mRNA in the brain after peripheral endotoxin treatment: comparison with interleukin-1 family and interleukin-6. Brain Res. 1993;624(1–2):291–4.
22. Campbell SJ, et al. Immunomodulatory effects of etanercept in a model of brain injury act through attenuation of the acute-phase response. J Neurochem. 2007;103(6):2245–55.
23. Zhang GX, et al. Chemokines and chemokine receptors in the pathogenesis of multiple sclerosis. Mult Scler. 2000;6(1):3–13.
24. Jeyakumar M, et al. Delayed symptom onset and increased life expectancy in Sandhoff disease mice treated with N-butyldeoxynojirimycin. Proc Natl Acad Sci U S A. 1999;96(11):6388–93.
25. Serres S, et al. Comparison of MRI signatures in pattern I and II multiple sclerosis models. NMR Biomed. 2009;22(10):1014–24.
26. Campbell SJ, et al. Central nervous system injury triggers hepatic CC and CXC chemokine expression that is associated with leukocyte mobilization and recruitment to both the central nervous system and the liver. Am J Pathol. 2005;166(5):1487–97.
27. Hsu SM, Raine L, Fanger H. The use of antiavidin antibody and avidin-biotin-peroxidase complex in immunoperoxidase technics. Am J Clin Pathol. 1981;75(6):816–21.
28. Anthony DC, et al. Age-related effects of interleukin-1 beta on polymorphonuclear neutrophil-dependent increases in blood-brain barrier permeability in rats. Brain. 1997;120(Pt 3):435–44.
29. Campbell SJ, et al. Altered chemokine expression in the spinal cord and brain contributes to differential interleukin-1beta-induced neutrophil recruitment. J Neurochem. 2002;83(2):432–41.
30. Perry VH. The influence of systemic inflammation on inflammation in the brain: implications for chronic neurodegenerative disease. Brain Behav Immun. 2004;18(5):407–13.

31. Holmes C, et al. Systemic infection, interleukin 1beta, and cognitive decline in Alzheimer's disease. J Neurol Neurosurg Psychiatry. 2003;74(6):788–9.
32. Grau AJ, et al. Clinical and biochemical analysis in infection-associated stroke. Stroke. 1995;26(9):1520–6.
33. Witlox J, et al. Delirium in elderly patients and the risk of postdischarge mortality, institutionalization, and dementia: a meta-analysis. JAMA. 2010;304(4):443–51.
34. Pandharipande PP, et al. Long-term cognitive impairment after critical illness. N Engl J Med. 2013;369(14):1306–16.
35. Yaffe K, et al. The metabolic syndrome, inflammation, and risk of cognitive decline. JAMA. 2004;292(18):2237–42.
36. Wallin K, et al. Midlife rheumatoid arthritis increases the risk of cognitive impairment two decades later: a population-based study. J Alzheimers Dis. 2012;31(3):669–76.
37. Freeman LC, Ting JP. The pathogenic role of the inflammasome in neurodegenerative diseases. J Neurochem. 2016;136(Suppl 1):29–38.
38. McColl BW, Rothwell NJ, Allan SM. Systemic inflammatory stimulus potentiates the acute phase and CXC chemokine responses to experimental stroke and exacerbates brain damage via interleukin-1- and neutrophil-dependent mechanisms. J Neurosci. 2007;27(16):4403–12.
39. Terrando N, et al. Tumor necrosis factor-alpha triggers a cytokine cascade yielding postoperative cognitive decline. Proc Natl Acad Sci U S A. 2010;107(47):20518–22.
40. Mina F, et al. Il1-beta involvement in cognitive impairment after sepsis. Mol Neurobiol. 2014;49(2):1069–76.
41. Sun L, et al. Production of inflammatory cytokines, cortisol, and Abeta1-40 in elderly oral cancer patients with postoperative delirium. Neuropsychiatr Dis Treat. 2016;12:2789–95.
42. Vairetti M, et al. Impaired hepatic function and central dopaminergic denervation in a rodent model of Parkinson's disease: a self-perpetuating crosstalk? Biochim Biophys Acta. 2012;1822(2):176–84.
43. Strekalova T, et al. Tlr4 upregulation in the brain accompanies depression- and anxiety-like behaviors induced by a high-cholesterol diet. Brain Behav Immun. 2015;48:42–7.
44. Campbell SJ, et al. Overexpression of IL-1beta by adenoviral-mediated gene transfer in the rat brain causes a prolonged hepatic chemokine response, axonal injury and the suppression of spontaneous behaviour. Neurobiol Dis. 2007;27(2):151–63.
45. Lu TT, Cyster JG. Integrin-mediated long-term B cell retention in the splenic marginal zone. Science. 2002;297(5580):409–12.
46. Mellergard J, et al. Natalizumab treatment in multiple sclerosis: marked decline of chemokines and cytokines in cerebrospinal fluid. Mult Scler. 2010;16(2):208–17.
47. Massberg S, von Andrian UH. Fingolimod and sphingosine-1-phosphate—modifiers of lymphocyte migration. N Engl J Med. 2006;355(11):1088–91.
48. Serpero LD, et al. Fingolimod modulates peripheral effector and regulatory T cells in MS patients. J NeuroImmune Pharmacol. 2013;8(5):1106–13.
49. Sellner J, et al. Glatiramer acetate attenuates the pro-migratory profile of adhesion molecules on various immune cell subsets in multiple sclerosis. Clin Exp Immunol. 2013;173(3):381–9.
50. Hennessy E, Griffin EW, Cunningham C. Astrocytes are primed by chronic neurodegeneration to produce exaggerated chemokine and cell infiltration responses to acute stimulation with the cytokines IL-1beta and TNF-alpha. J Neurosci. 2015;35(22):8411–22.
51. Kang Z, et al. Astrocyte-restricted ablation of interleukin-17-induced Act1-mediated signaling ameliorates autoimmune encephalomyelitis. Immunity. 2010;32(3):414–25.
52. Simpson JE, et al. Expression of monocyte chemoattractant protein-1 and other beta-chemokines by resident glia and inflammatory cells in multiple sclerosis lesions. J Neuroimmunol. 1998;84(2):238–49.
53. Kohn FR, Kung AH. Role of endotoxin in acute inflammation induced by gram-negative bacteria: specific inhibition of lipopolysaccharide-mediated responses with an amino-terminal fragment of bactericidal/permeability-increasing protein. Infect Immun. 1995;63(1):333–9.
54. Combrinck MI, Perry VH, Cunningham C. Peripheral infection evokes exaggerated sickness behaviour in pre-clinical murine prion disease. Neuroscience. 2002;112(1):7–11.
55. Griffin EW, et al. Cyclooxygenase-1-dependent prostaglandins mediate susceptibility to systemic inflammation-induced acute cognitive dysfunction. J Neurosci. 2013;33(38):15248–58.
56. Doll DN, et al. Lipopolysaccharide exacerbates infarct size and results in worsened post-stroke behavioral outcomes. Behav Brain Funct. 2015;11(1):32.
57. Serres S, et al. Systemic inflammatory response reactivates immune-mediated lesions in rat brain. J Neurosci. 2009;29(15):4820–8.
58. Lund BT, et al. Increased CXCL8 (IL-8) expression in multiple sclerosis. J Neuroimmunol. 2004;155(1–2):161–71.
59. Rumble JM, et al. Neutrophil-related factors as biomarkers in EAE and MS. J Exp Med. 2015;212(1):23–35.
60. Correale J, Ysrraelit MC, Gaitan MI. Immunomodulatory effects of Vitamin D in multiple sclerosis. Brain. 2009;132(Pt 5):1146–60.
61. Campbell SJ, et al. Liver Kupffer cells control the magnitude of the inflammatory response in the injured brain and spinal cord. Neuropharmacology. 2008;55(5):780–7.
62. Anthony DC, et al. Anti-CD20 inhibits T cell-mediated pathology and microgliosis in the rat brain. Ann Clin Transl Neurol. 2014;1(9):659–69.
63. Heidemann J, et al. Angiogenic effects of interleukin 8 (CXCL8) in human intestinal microvascular endothelial cells are mediated by CXCR2. J Biol Chem. 2003;278(10):8508–15.

5

Monocyte-derived tissue transglutaminase in multiple sclerosis patients: reflecting an anti-inflammatory status and function of the cells?

Claudia Sestito[1,6], John J. P. Brevé[1], Marja C. J. A. van Eggermond[2], Joep Killestein[3], Charlotte E. Teunissen[4], Joram van Rossum[3], Micha M. M. Wilhelmus[1], Benjamin Drukarch[1], Peter J. van den Elsen[2,5] and Anne-Marie van Dam[1*]

Abstract

Background: Leukocyte infiltration into the central nervous system is an important feature of multiple sclerosis (MS) pathology. Among the infiltrating cells, monocytes comprise the largest population and are considered to play a dual role in the course of the disease. The enzyme tissue transglutaminase (TG2), produced by monocytes, plays a central role in monocyte adhesion/migration in animal models of MS. In the present study, we questioned whether TG2 expression is altered in monocytes from MS patients compared to healthy control (HC) subjects. Moreover, we determined the inflammatory status of these TG2-expressing monocytes, what inflammatory factor regulates TG2 expression, and whether TG2 can functionally contribute to their adhesion/migration processes.

Methods: Primary human monocytes from MS patients and HC subjects were collected, RNA isolated and subjected to qPCR analysis. Human THP-1 monocytes were lentivirally transduced with TG2 siRNA or control and treated with various cytokines. Subsequently, mRNA levels of inflammatory factors, adhesion properties, and activity of RhoA were analyzed in interleukin (IL)-4-treated monocytes.

Results: TG2 mRNA levels are significantly increased in monocytes derived from MS patients compared to HC subjects. In addition, correlation analyses indicated that TG2-expressing cells display a more anti-inflammatory, migratory profile in MS patients. Using THP-1 monocytes, we observed that IL-4 is a major trigger of TG2 expression in these cells. Furthermore, knockdown of TG2 expression leads to a pro-inflammatory profile and reduced adhesion/migration properties of IL-4-treated monocytes.

Conclusions: TG2-expressing monocytes in MS patients have a more anti-inflammatory profile. Furthermore, TG2 mediates IL-4-induced anti-inflammatory status in THP-1 monocytes, adhesion, and cytoskeletal rearrangement in vitro. We thus propose that IL-4 upregulates TG2 expression in monocytes of MS patients, driving them into an anti-inflammatory status.

Keywords: Multiple sclerosis, Tissue transglutaminase, Inflammation, Human monocytes, Cytokine, Adhesion/migration

* Correspondence: amw.vandam@vumc.nl
[1]Department of Anatomy and Neurosciences, Amsterdam Neuroscience, VU University Medical Center, Postbus 7057, 1007 MB Amsterdam, the Netherlands

Background

Multiple sclerosis (MS) is a chronic neurological disorder affecting mostly young adults that leads to, e.g., sensory, motor, and cognitive deficits [1]. Pathologically, it is characterized by inflammation, demyelination, and axonal loss in the central nervous system (CNS) [2]. Although the pathophysiology is not well understood, MS results in leukocyte infiltration into the CNS parenchyma which requires passage of the blood-brain barrier (BBB) [3]. This process is initiated by the secretion of cytokines and chemokines which induce leukocyte activation by stimulating conformational changes in the integrins, key regulators of the adhesion/migration cascade. These changes, together with cytoskeleton rearrangement and the secretion of matrix metalloproteinase (MMP) capable of cleaving components of the extracellular matrix (ECM), allow the arrest and finally the migration of the cells into the CNS [4, 5]. Monocytes and monocyte-derived macrophages constitute the major cell type in the perivascular infiltrates characteristic of several neuroinflammatory diseases including MS [6–9] and are considered to play a pivotal role in MS pathology. Indeed, depletion of monocytes and macrophages or inhibition of monocyte recruitment to the CNS leads to a reduction of clinical symptoms and pathology in animals suffering from experimental autoimmune encephalomyelitis (EAE), an animal model of MS [7, 10, 11]. Once migrated into the CNS, the recruited monocytes/macrophages, together with the locally activated microglia, release proteases, pro-inflammatory cytokines, and reactive oxygen species, contributing to myelin damage and, ultimately, axonal damage [12, 13]. Although monocytes/macrophages are thought to primarily have detrimental effects on MS pathogenesis and development, other studies point toward a dual role for these cells since it has been proven that they can also contribute to the clearance of tissue debris and promote tissue repair by secreting growth factors and anti-inflammatory cytokines, such as nerve growth factor (NGF) and interleukin (IL)-10 [14–16]. Furthermore, administration of anti-inflammatory-tuned monocytes to animals suffering from severe EAE ameliorates their clinical disease status [17–19].

Tissue transglutaminase, or transglutaminase 2 (TG2), is a calcium-dependent protein-crosslinking enzyme whose expression and activity can be increased by inflammatory mediators in various cell types, including monocytes [20–23]. A recent study from our group demonstrated TG2 immunoreactivity in human active MS lesions in infiltrating cells of which some express MHC-II. In addition, we observed in an animal experimental MS model that TG2 is present in infiltrating monocytes and contributes to pathology by promoting monocyte migration into the CNS [24]. Of interest is that TG2 has also been shown to be involved in the adhesion of monocytes onto ECM proteins in vitro (i.e., fibronectin, FN) as it serves as a β-integrin-associated co-receptor promoting binding to fibronectin [25].

Thus, we hypothesize that in monocytes of MS patients, TG2 expression is altered due to the inflammatory environment. Consequently, TG2 expressed by monocytes could contribute to adhesion and migration processes that are essential for cells entering the CNS, resulting in MS pathology. In the present study, we studied TG2 expression in monocytes from MS patients and healthy control (HC) subjects and we determined the inflammatory status of the TG2-expressing monocytes. In addition, using the human THP-1 monocyte cell line, we studied the regulation of TG2 expression by inflammatory mediators and its possible functional implication in monocyte adhesion/migration processes.

Methods

Isolation of primary human monocytes

Peripheral blood mononuclear cells (PBMCs) were obtained from 15 MS patients (13 relapsing-remitting and 3 primary progressive, RR-MS, and PP-MS respectively) diagnosed according to the Poser or McDonald criteria [26] and 10 HC subjects (Table 1). MS patients were recruited from the VU University Medical Center (VUmc) outpatient clinic while participating in different prospective cohort studies. Age and sex-matched control subjects were recruited from the Leiden University Medical Center (LUMC). All participants gave informed consent, and the study was approved by the Medical Research Ethics Committees of the VUmc and LUMC, respectively. At time of blood collection, the activity status of the disease was not measured. Peripheral blood was drawn by venipuncture and collected into sodium citrate tubes (Greiner, Kremsmünster, Austria). One part of blood was diluted with one part of buffer consisting of phosphate-buffered saline (PBS) + 10% *v*/*v* GPO (Sanquin, Amsterdam, The Netherlands) + 10% *v*/*v* sodium citrate. PBMCs were isolated by density centrifugation using Ficoll Isopaque PLUS (GE Healthcare Biosciences, Uppsala, Sweden). Monocytes were subsequently isolated from the PBMCs by anti-CD14 magnetic beads according to the manufacturer's instruction (MACS; Milteny Biotech, Bergisch Gladbach, Germany).

Cell culture and treatment

THP-1 cells (human monocytic cell line) were maintained in complete RPMI 1640 medium (Gibco, Waltham, Massachusetts, USA) containing 10% heat-inactivated fetal calf serum (PAA), penicillin (50 units/ml, Gibco), streptomycin (50 μg/ml, Gibco), and L-glutamine (2 mM, Gibco) at 37 °C in humidified air containing 5% CO_2.

Scramble control (SCR) and TG2-knockdown (TG2-KD) THP-1 cell lines were generated by double, subsequent

Table 1 Patient information

Subjects	Number	Female/male	Age (years) ± SD	Type MS	DMT
HC	Total 10	4/6	40 ± 12		
	1	Female	25	–	–
	2	Female	49	–	–
	3	Female	25	–	–
	4	Female	46	–	–
	5	Male	50	–	–
	6	Male	42	–	–
	7	Male	30	–	–
	8	Male	39	–	–
	9	Male	33	–	–
	10	Male	60	–	–
MS	Total 15	8/7	45 ± 16		
	11	Female	73	PP-MS	Untreated
	12	Male	51	PP-MS	Untreated
	13	Male	56	PP-MS	Untreated
	14	Female	25	RR-MS	Interferon beta-1a
	15	Female	71	RR-MS	Untreated
	16	Female	24	RR-MS	Glatiramer acetate
	17	Female	49	RR-MS	Glatiramer acetate
	18	Male	30	RR-MS	Interferon beta-1a
	19	Male	48	RR-MS	Natalizumab
	20	Female	30	RR-MS	Untreated
	21	Female	32	RR-MS	Untreated
	22	Female	46	RR-MS	Untreated
	23	Male	45	RR-MS	Untreated
	24	Male	58	RR-MS	Untreated
	25	Male	32	RR-MS	Untreated

HC healthy controls, *MS* multiple sclerosis, *PP-MS* primary progressive MS, *RR-MS* relapsing-remitting MS, *SD* standard deviation, *DMT* disease-modifying therapies

lentiviral transduction (MOI 1) with either a scramble or hTG2 specific short hairpin RNA (shRNA) (scramble: sc-108080, hTG2: sc-37514-V, Santa Cruz, Dallas, Texas, USA) for 24 h for each infection.

To create stable knockdown cell lines, cells were selected with 2 mg/ml puromycin (Sigma-Aldrich, Saint Louis, Missouri, USA). Subsequently, the cells were characterized by western blot analysis and semi-quantitative real-time PCR (qPCR) (see below) and used for functional assays. Stable cell lines were maintained in complete RPMI in presence of 2 mg/ml puromycin.

THP-1 cells were either untreated or treated with 50 ng/ml of the human recombinant IL-4, IL-10, IL-1β, or tumor necrosis factor (TNF)-α (BioLegend, San Diego, USA) for 24 h in culture medium. The dose of cytokine used was based on previous studies from our group [24, 27]. The incubation period was chosen based on the time-dependent TG2 expression in THP-1 cells showing that a 24-h treatment with cytokines resulted in the most increased TG2 expression (data not shown).

RNA isolation and cDNA synthesis from primary human monocytes

Primary human monocytes were centrifuged for 5 min at 500×*g*. Cells were lysed in RNAbee (Tel-Test, Friendswood, USA) according to the manufacturer's instructions. Lysates were stored at – 80 °C until further processing. Total RNA was extracted according to the manufacturer's instructions. The RNA concentration was determined by measuring the absorbance at 260 nm (NanoDrop ND-100 spectophotometer; Thermo Fisher scientific, Waltham, USA) and when approved, samples were included for cDNA synthesis. From 1 μg total RNA, cDNA was synthesized using Superscript III (Invitrogen, California, USA) with 250 ng random hexamers (Promega, Wisconsin, USA) and according to the manufacturer's instructions.

RNA isolation and cDNA synthesis from THP-1 cells

THP-1 cells were homogenized in Trizol reagent (Invitrogen) and total RNA was isolated as described by the manufacturer. RNA concentration was determined by measuring the absorbance at 260 nm (NanoDrop ND-1000 spectrophotometer) and when approved, samples were included for cDNA synthesis. Then, 1 µg of total RNA was reverse-transcribed into cDNA using the High-Capacity cDNA Reverse Transcription kit (Life Technologies, California, USA), using 0.5 µg oligo-dT primers and according to the manufacturer's instructions.

Semi-quantitative real-time PCR (qPCR)

For qPCR, the Power SYBR Green Master Mix (Life Technologies) was used. Primers were purchased from Eurogentec (Liège, Belgium) and qPCR was performed in MicroAmp Optical 96-well Reaction Plates (Applied Biosystems, California, USA) on a StepOnePlus Real-Time PCR system (Applied Biosystems). The reaction mixture (20 µl) was composed of 1× Power SYBR Green buffer (Applied Biosystems), 3.75 pmol of each primer (Table 2), and 100 ng cDNA. The thermal cycling conditions were an initial 10 min at 95 °C followed by 40 cycles of 15 s at 95 °C and 1 min at 60 °C. The specificity of the reaction was checked by melt curve analysis of the individual qPCR reaction. The relative expression level of the target genes was determined by the LinRegPCR software (http://www.hfrc.nl, downloads, applications, lin reg PCR, version 2017) using the following calculation $N0 = Nq/ECq$ ($N0$ = target quantity, Nq = fluorescence threshold value, E = mean PCR efficiency per amplicon, Cq = threshold cycle) [28], after which the value was normalized relative to the geometric mean of the mRNA levels of glyceraldehyde-3-phosphate-dehydrogenase (GAPDH) and polymerase (RNA) II polypeptide F (POLR2F). We chose GAPDH and POLR2F as reference genes based on the results of the GeNorm software analysis (version 3.5) in which the stability of six different human housekeeping genes (GAPDH, MRIP, POLR2F, HPRT1, PGK1, SDHA) was assessed in our primary human monocytes. Regarding the THP-1 cells, the value was normalized relative to the mRNA levels of GAPDH as previously described [29].

Western blotting (WB)

To determine TG2 protein expression, cells were homogenized in ice-cold RIPA buffer containing 150 mM NaCl, 20 mM Tris-HCl (pH 7.4), 1% NP-40, 1% sodium deoxycholate, 1 mM EDTA, 0.1% sodium dodecyl sulfate (SDS), 15 µM Pepstatin A, 100 µM phenylmethylsulfonyl fluoride (PMSF), 0.3 µM aprotinin, and 15 µM leupeptin. Cell lysates were cleared by centrifugation (14.000 rpm for 10 min at 4 °C). Protein concentration of the supernatant was determined by the bicinchoninic acid (BCA) method according to the instructions of the manufacturer (Pierce Biotechnology, Waltham, Massachusetts, USA).

Fifty micrograms of protein were denaturated by adding Laemmli buffer (0.012% bromophenol blue, 5% glycerol, 1.6% SDS, 125 mM Tris HCl pH 6.8) and 50 mM dithiothreitol (DTT). After boiling, the mixture was loaded on a 10% SDS-polyacrylamide gel and transferred onto a nitrocellulose membrane (Li-cor Biosciences, Lincoln, Nebraska, USA). Membranes were incubated overnight with the following primary antibodies: mouse anti-β-actin (1:10,000; Abcam, Cambridge, UK) and mouse anti-TG2 (Ab3, 1:2000; Thermo Scientific, Waltham, Massachusetts, USA) diluted in Li-cor buffer. For subsequent antigen detection, the membranes were incubated for 1 h at room temperature (RT) with corresponding IgG's labeled with IRDye 800CW or IRDye 680LT (1:10,000; Li-cor buffer) and subsequently scanned to detect fluorescence emission at 800 or 680 nm, respectively, using an Odyssey infrared imaging system (Li-Cor

Table 2 Primer sequences

Gene	Forward	Reverse
TG2	5'AGAGGAGCGGCAGGAGTATG 3'	5'AGGATCCCATCTTCAAACTGC 3'
GAPDH	5'TCAAGGGCATCCTGGGCTAC 3'	5'CGTCAAAGGTGGAGGAGTGG 3'
POLR2F	5'GAACTCAAGGCCCGAAAG 3'	5'TGATGATGAGCTCGTCCAC 3'
IL-1β	5'TACAGCTGGAGAGTGTAGATC 3'	5'CAAATTCCAGCTTGTTATTG 3'
TNF-α	5'CCCAGGCAGTCAGATCATCTTC 3'	5'CTCTCAGCTCCACGCCATTG 3'
IL-1ra	5'TCATCCGCTCAGACAGTGGC 3'	5'AGCTTCCATCGCTGTGCAGA 3'
TGF-β1	5'CTTTCCTGCTTCTCATGGCC 3'	5'CCGTGGAGCTGAAGCAATAG 3'
β1 integrin	5'TGTGGAGGAAATGGTGTTTGC 3'	5'TCTGTCCGTTGCTGGCTTCA 3'
β3 integrin	5'CAATGCCACCTGCCTCAACA 3'	5'GAGTCTTCATAGTACTGGAATC 3'
MMP-2	5'AAGGCCAAGTGGTCCGTGTG 3'	5'GTGCAGCTGTTGTACTCCTTGC 3'

TG2 Transglutaminase 2, *GAPDH* glyceraldehyde-3-phosphate-dehydrogenase, *POLR2F* polymerase (RNA) II polypeptide F, *IL-1β* interleukin-1β, *TNF-α* tumor necrosis factor-α, *IL-1ra* interleukin-1 receptor antagonist, *TGF-β* transforming growth factor-β1, *MMP-2* matrix metalloproteinase s2

Biosciences). The signal intensity was measured using the Odyssey Sa Infrared scanning software (version 1.1, Li-Cor Biosciences).

Adhesion assay

SCR or TG2-KD THP-1 monocytes were treated with 50 ng/ml IL-4. After 24 h treatment, cells were centrifuged and resuspended in adhesion medium (RPMI 1640 medium + 0.5% bovine serum albumin +25 mM HEPES). 5×10^4 of the treated cells were then added to a 96-well plate coated with 2 μg/cm^2 bovine FN (Sigma-Aldrich). Cells were allowed to adhere to the FN layer at 37° on an orbital shaker (Vibramax 100, Heidolph, Germany) at 300 rpm. After 1 h, the non-adherent cells were removed and the adherent cells were labeled with 0.5 μM calcein (Invitrogen) in the adhesion medium for 10 min at 37°. Then, excess of calcein was removed and cells were washed four times with PBS and lysed in 0.1 M NaOH. The fluorescence (emission 485 nm; extinction 520 nm) was then measured using a spectrophotometer (Fluostar Galaxy Microplate Reader, BMG Lab Technologies, Germany) and using FluoStar Software (BMG Lab Technologies).

RhoA GTPase activity assay

To determine the effect of TG2 on cytoskeletal reorganization, we measured RhoA GTPase activity. 2×10^6 SCR or TG2-KD THP-1 monocytes were treated with 50 ng/ml IL-4 for 24 h. Thereafter, cells were lysed with lysis buffer (50 mM Tris, pH 7.6, 150 mM NaCl, 1% Triton X-100, 20 mM MgCl2, 5 μg/ml Pepstatin A, 100 μM PMSF, 5 μg/ml aprotinin, and 5 μg/ml leupeptin). Of the cleared lysates, 30 μg was stored to determine the total amount of RhoA (total cell lysate). Remaining protein lysates were incubated with 60 μg bacterially produced GST-RBD (Rho Binding Domain of Rhotekin) bound to glutathione-agarose beads (Cytoskeleton, USA) for 30 min at 4°. Beads were washed four times with lysis buffer containing 50 mM Tris, pH 7.6, 150 mM NaCl, 1% Triton X-100, 10 mM $MgCl_2$. Bound proteins were eluted in 30 μl SDS Laemmli buffer and analyzed in parallel with the total cell lysate on a 12.5% SDS PAGE. The active form of RhoA and total RhoA were detected with a mouse monoclonal antibody (1:250, Santa Cruz Biotechnology) and were visualized as described under western blotting.

Statistical analysis

In the HC or MS patient-derived monocytes, the sample size varied between gene expression measurements due to availability of mRNA or cDNA or based on unreliable qPCR outcome (e.g., extreme values). Normal distribution of the data was tested using the Shapiro-Wilk procedure. When data from MS patients and HC were not normally distributed, either the logarithmic (for IL-1β and TNF-α) or the cubic root transformed parameter (for β3 Integrin) was used in order to normalize the variables. Subsequently, normally distributed data were analyzed by independent Student *t* test. Correlation analysis was assessed using Pearson correlation analysis. The data obtained with the THP-1 cells all met the criteria of normal distribution. Subsequently, one-way analysis of variance (ANOVA) followed by Bonferroni post hoc test was performed for multiple comparisons while for two group analysis, an independent Student *t* test was performed. Results were considered to be statistically significant if $p < 0.05$. All statistical analyses were performed using SPSS software, version 20.0 (IBM Corp, NY, USA).

Results

TG2 mRNA levels were increased in MS patient-derived monocytes compared to HC subject-derived monocytes

At first, we established that there was no significant difference in TG2 expression between untreated and drug-treated MS patients (see Additional file 1). Therefore, considering the relative low number of MS patients, all MS patient samples were further assessed as one group. When comparing TG2 mRNA levels between HC subjects and MS patients, there was a significant increase in TG2 expression in MS patient-derived monocytes compared to HC subject-derived monocytes ($p < 0.001$) (Fig. 1).

MS patient-derived monocytes showed a decrease in IL-1β mRNA and an increase in β3 integrin mRNA levels compared to HC subject-derived monocytes

Subsequently, we aimed to study the inflammatory phenotype of MS patient/HC subject-derived monocytes. We measured the expression of several pro- and anti-inflammatory mediators. Interestingly, MS patient-derived monocytes displayed a significant decrease in pro-inflammatory IL-1β expression compared to HC subject-derived monocytes ($p = 0.003$) (Fig. 2a), whereas pro-inflammatory TNF-α and anti-inflammatory IL-1 receptor antagonist (IL-1ra) and transforming growth factor (TGF)-β1 mRNA levels were not significantly different (Fig. 2b–d). In addition, we examined whether the expression of two relevant members of the β integrin family, β1 and β3, were also affected in monocytes derived from MS patients versus HC subjects. While β1 integrin mRNA levels were not significantly different between the two groups (Fig. 3a), we observed a significant increase in β3 integrin mRNA levels in MS patient-derived monocytes compared to HC subject-derived monocytes ($p = 0.01$) (Fig. 3b).

TG2 mRNA levels correlated with those of inflammatory mediators in MS patient-derived monocytes

Next, to determine the phenotype of TG2-expressing monocytes derived from MS patients and HC subjects,

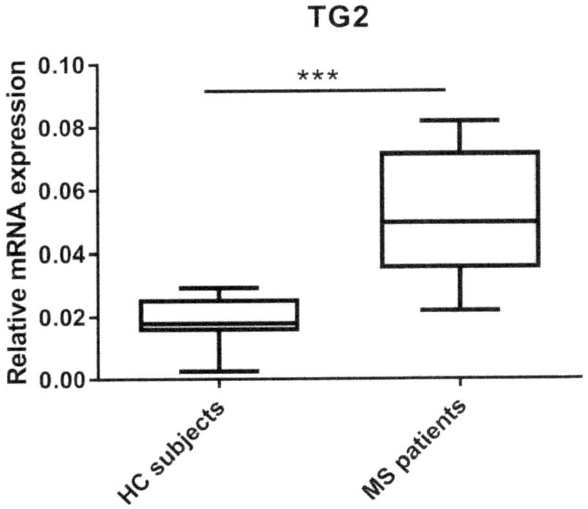

Fig. 1 TG2 expression in MS patient/HC subject-derived monocytes. qPCR analysis was performed to detect TG2 (HC $N = 8$/MS $N = 15$) mRNA levels in primary human monocytes isolated from MS patients and HC subjects. Data are shown in box-and-whiskers plots in which the median is represented by a horizontal line within the box and the lower and upper whiskers represent the 5 and 95 percentiles. ***$p < 0.001$. MS multiple sclerosis, HC healthy controls

we correlated TG2 mRNA levels with mRNA levels of pro- and anti-inflammatory mediators. In MS patient-derived monocytes (Fig. 4 black line), no significant correlation was observed between TG2 mRNA levels and either IL-1β mRNA levels ($r = 0.376$, $p = 0.168$) or TNFα mRNA levels ($r = 0.391$, $p = 0.186$) (Fig. 4a, b). However, TG2 mRNA levels correlated positively with the anti-inflammatory mediators IL-1ra ($r = 0.605$, $p = 0.02$) and TGF-β1 ($r = 0.532$, $p = 0.05$) (Fig. 4c, d). None of these correlations was observed in HC subject-derived monocytes (Fig. 4a–d, gray line).

TG2 expression was upregulated in IL-4-treated monocytes and sustained an anti-inflammatory phenotype

To determine which inflammatory stimulus modulates TG2 expression in monocytes, as might occur during MS, THP-1 monocytes were either untreated or treated with two pro-inflammatory stimuli, i.e., IL-1β or TNF-α or with two anti-inflammatory stimuli, i.e., IL-4 or IL-10. The qPCR analysis revealed that TG2 mRNA levels were highly upregulated by IL-4 treatment (Fig. 5a). WB analysis confirmed the upregulation of TG2 protein in IL-4-treated monocytes (Fig. 5b). Subsequently, we studied the relevance of TG2 in determining the phenotype of IL-4-treated monocytes, by using TG2-KD or SCR THP-1 cells. First, we showed that in TG2-KD cells, TG2 mRNA (Fig. 6a) and protein levels (Fig. 6b) were significantly decreased after IL-4 treatment compared to IL-4-treated SCR cells. In addition, IL-4-treated TG2-KD cells expressed significantly more of the pro-inflammatory cytokines IL-1β and TNFα (Fig. 6c, d, respectively). Moreover, we observed a significant reduction in the mRNA level of the anti-inflammatory cytokine IL-1ra (Fig. 6e) in IL-4-treated TG2-KD monocytes.

Effect of TG2-KD on adhesion and on cytoskeleton rearrangement in IL-4-treated THP-1 cells

To identify relevant functional aspects of TG2 in IL-4-treated THP-1 monocytes, we studied adhesion properties. We observed that knockdown of TG2 expression resulted in less cell adhesion onto FN in response to IL-4 (Fig. 7a). As β integrins can act in concert with TG2 to promote cell adhesion, it was of interest to observe that IL-4-treated TG2-KD cells expressed significantly less β1 integrin (Fig. 7b). In addition, we observed a reduction of almost 50% of active RhoA GTPase, indicative of reduced cytoskeletal rearrangement, in IL-4-treated TG2-KD monocytes compared to SCR monocytes (Fig. 7c). Furthermore, IL-4-treated TG2-KD monocytes expressed significantly less MMP-2 (Fig. 7d), a protein known to be involved in the cleavage of ECM proteins and therefore permissive for cell migration [30, 31].

Discussion

Alteration in TG2 expression and/or cross-linking activity has been extensively implicated in the pathogenesis of various human diseases, including neurodegenerative disorders [32], coeliac disease [33], and cancer [34]. Thus, based on our previous observations in rat and mouse models for MS, we here questioned whether monocyte-derived TG2 expression was altered in MS patients. Although a limited number of patients was included in the present study, we are the first to show that TG2 mRNA levels are significantly enhanced in monocytes derived from MS patients compared to HC subjects. The presence of low levels of TG2 in human monocytes is known for many years. Moreover, inflammatory factors have been shown to enhance TG2 levels in these cells [35–38]. Thus far, few studies have been performed to determine a physiological or pathological expression of TG2 in monocytes/macrophages in vivo. One of which is in a mouse model of atherosclerosis, showing increased TG2 immunoreactivity in infiltrated macrophages in the lesions, limiting lesion size [39].

As inflammation can alter TG2 expression, we characterized the inflammatory status of MS patient-derived monocytes and revealed that these cells expressed significantly lower mRNA levels of IL-1β. Interestingly, expression levels of either TNF-α or anti-inflammatory IL-1ra and TGF-β1 were unaffected.

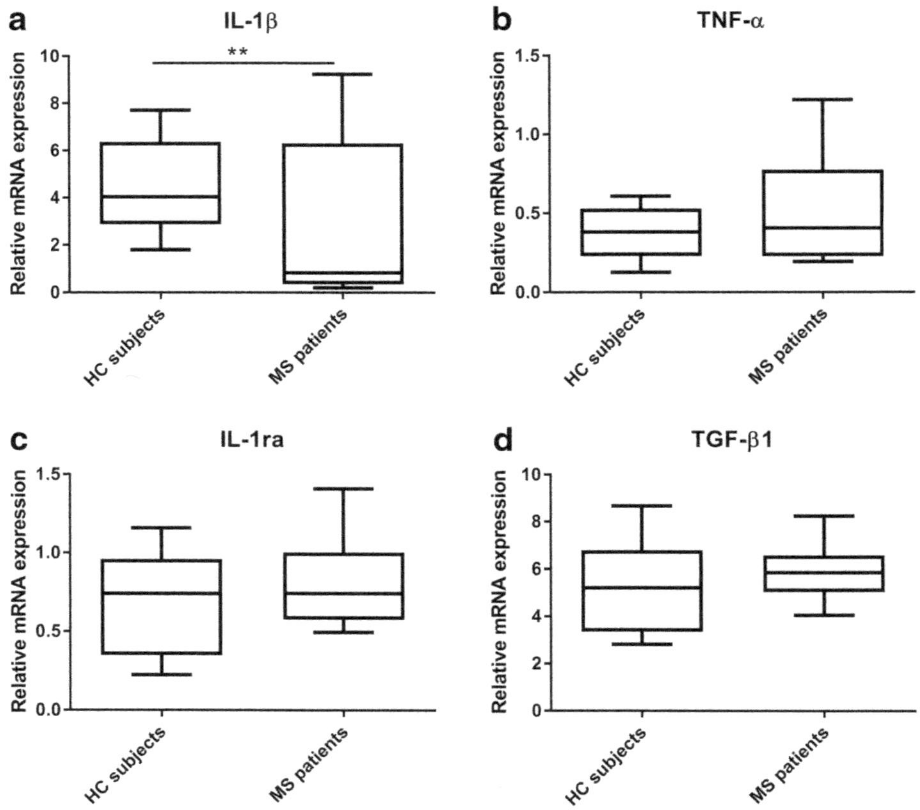

Fig. 2 IL-1β, TNF-α, IL-1ra, and TGF-β1 mRNA levels in MS patient/HC subject-derived monocytes. qPCR analysis was performed to detect **a** IL-1β (HC $N = 9$/MS $N = 15$), **b** TNF-α (HC $N = 10$/MS $N = 13$), **c** IL-1ra (HC $N = 8$/MS $N = 14$), and **d** TGF-β1 (HC $N = 8$/MS $N = 14$) mRNA levels in primary monocytes from MS patients and HC subjects. Data are shown in box-and-whiskers plots in which the median is represented by a horizontal line within the box, and the lower and upper whiskers represent the 5 and 95 percentiles. **$p < 0.01$. MS multiple sclerosis, HC healthy controls

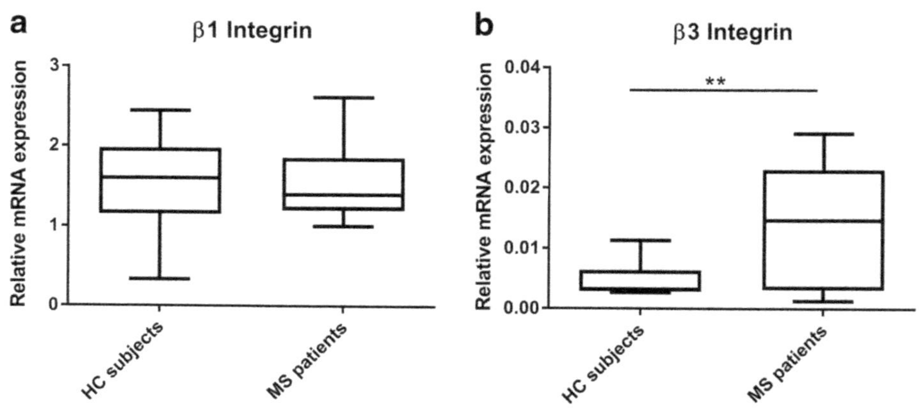

Fig. 3 β1 and β3 integrin mRNA levels in MS patient/HC subject-derived monocytes. qPCR analysis was performed to detect **a** β1 integrin (HC $N = 8$/MS $N = 14$) and **b** β3 integrin (HC $N = 7$/MS $N = 15$) mRNA levels in primary monocytes from MS patients and HC subjects. Data are shown in box-and-whiskers plots in which the median is represented by a horizontal line within the box, and the lower and upper whiskers represent the 5 and 95 percentiles. **$p < 0.01$. MS multiple sclerosis, HC healthy controls

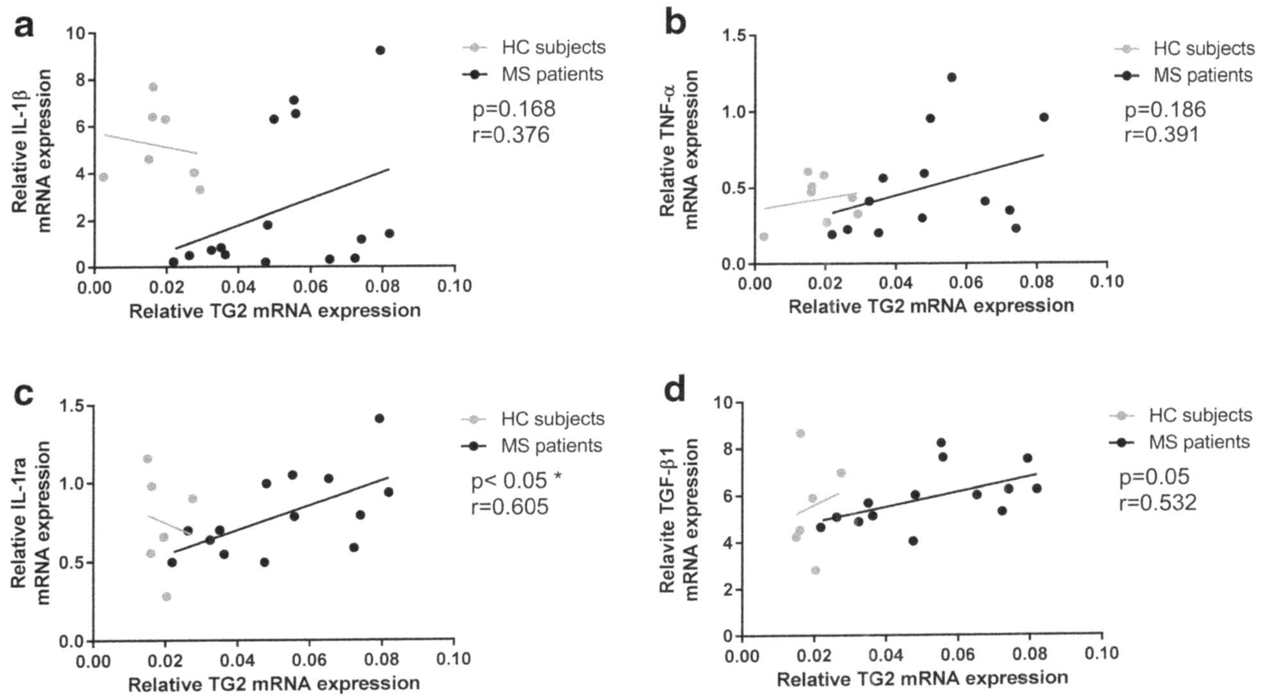

Fig. 4 Correlation of TG2 mRNA levels with pro/anti-inflammatory mediators. Pearson correlation analysis was performed to correlate TG2 mRNA levels with **a** IL-1β, **b** TNF-α, **c** IL-1ra, and **d** TGF-β1mRNA levels in MS patient-derived monocytes (*black line*) and HC subject-derived monocytes (*gray line*). $^{*}p < 0.05$. MS multiple sclerosis, HC healthy controls

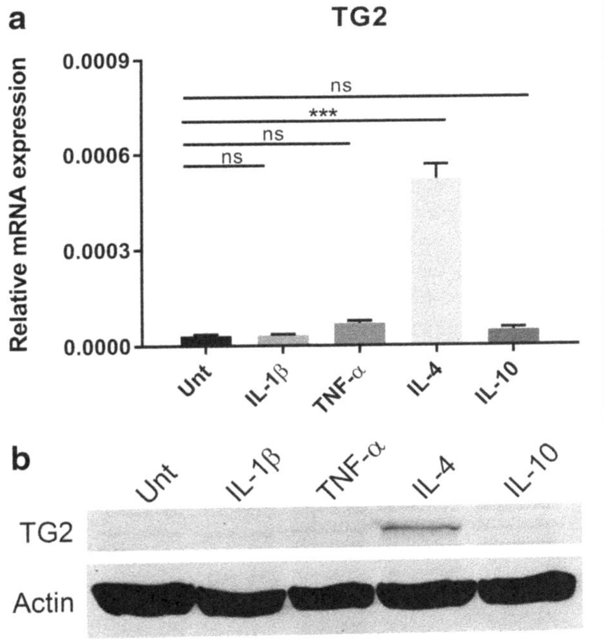

Fig. 5 TG2 expression under different inflammatory stimuli. THP-1 monocytes were either untreated or treated with 50 ng/ml of IL-1β, TNF-α, IL-4, or IL-10 for 24 h and TG2 expression was analyzed by **a** qPCR or **b** WB. Data presented are the mean values + SEM (standard error of the mean) of at least three independent experiments. $^{***}p < 0.001$. Unt untreated, ns not significant

Although, we cannot exclude the presence of separate cell populations with each specific pro- or anti-inflammatory phenotype, our data suggest that MS patient-derived monocytes have a mixed inflammatory phenotype, which is in agreement with the intermediate activation status displayed by monocyte-derived macrophages in active demyelinating MS lesions [40].

Noteworthy, elevated β3 integrin mRNA levels in MS patients indicate an increase migratory capacity of the cells [41, 42]. On the contrary, mRNA expression levels of the adhesion molecule β1 integrin were not affected.

In addition, our observation that TG2 does not correlate either with IL-1β or TNF-α expression but correlated positively with the expression of two anti-inflammatory markers, i.e., IL-1ra and TGF-β1 in MS monocytes, suggests that MS patient-derived monocytes expressing higher levels of TG2 have a more anti-inflammatory profile. We thus questioned what factor(s) could enhance monocyte-derived TG2, whose expression is known to be modulated by several inflammatory stimuli [27, 43, 44], due to the presence of various inflammatory factor-related response elements in the promotor region [45]. As inflammation occurs during MS pathogenesis, we determined the effect of inflammatory mediators on TG2 expression. In THP-1 cell, known to be responsive to inflammatory stimuli [46, 47], predominantly IL-4 induced TG2 mRNA and protein

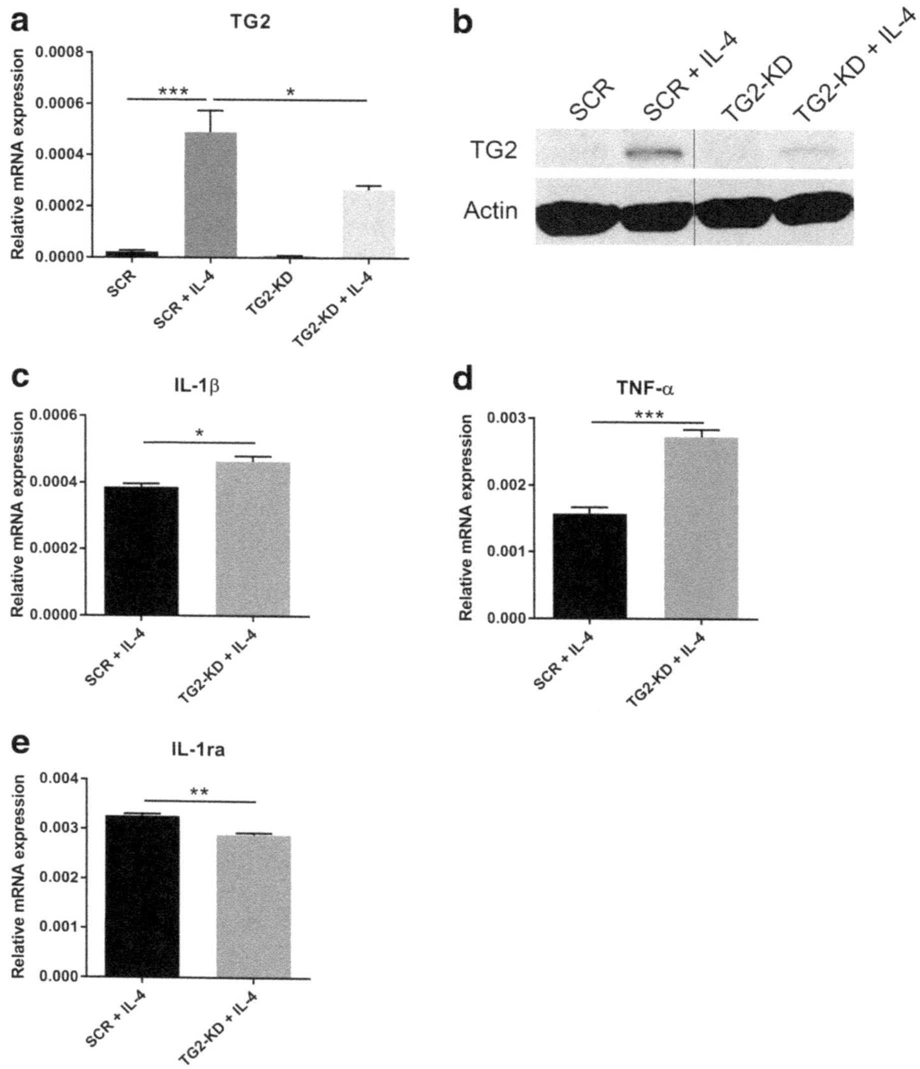

Fig. 6 Knockdown of TG2 expression drives IL-4-activated THP-1 monocytes into a pro-inflammatory phenotype. Lentiviral particles were used to efficiently knockdown TG2 expression in THP-1 monocytes as confirmed both by **a** qPCR or **b** WB. To study the phenotype of TG2-KD cells, mRNA expression levels of **c** IL-1β, **d** TNF-α, and **e** IL-1ra were measured by qPCR in SCR or TG2-KD THP-1 monocytes activated for 24 h with IL-4 (50 ng/ml). Data presented are the mean values + SEM (standard error of the mean) of at least three independent experiments. *$p < 0.05$, **$p < 0.01$, ***$p < 0.001$. SCR scramble control, TG2-KD TG2 knockdown

upregulation. These data suggest that the increased TG2 mRNA expression levels observed in MS patient-derived monocytes could, directly or indirectly, be mediated by circulating or autocrine IL-4, whose presence was described to be enhanced both in serum and in mononuclear cells of MS patients compared to HC subjects [48–51]. Subsequently, we found that knockdown of TG2 resulted in a pro-inflammatory phenotype of IL-4-treated THP-1 monocytes as indicated by the increased mRNA levels of IL-1β and TNF-α and by the reduced mRNA levels of the anti-inflammatory cytokine IL-1ra. These data suggest that the presence of TG2 drives an anti-inflammatory phenotype of monocytes. In agreement with this observation, TG2 was recently established as an anti-inflammatory marker of IL-4-treated human and mouse macrophages [52].

Furthermore, it is known that IL-4 affects adhesive/migratory properties of several cell types [53, 54]. Our findings regarding the attenuated adhesion, cytoskeleton rearrangement, and MMP-2 expression of IL-4-treated TG2-KD monocytes are the first to point out that these IL-4-mediated processes in human monocytes are, at least partly, regulated through TG2.

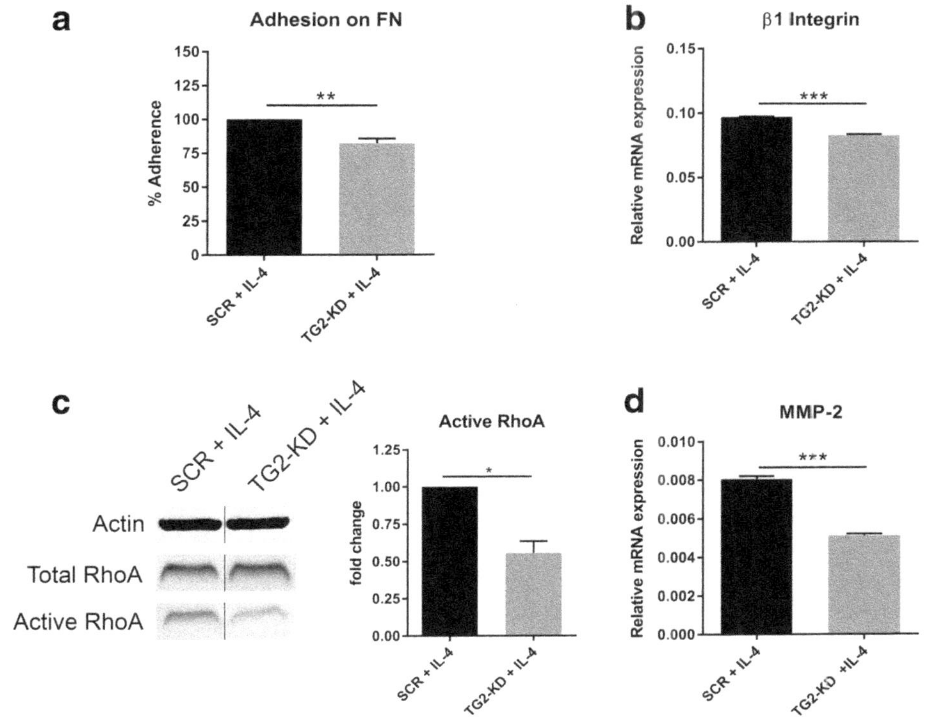

Fig. 7 Effect of TG2 knockdown on the adhesion/migration and cytoskeleton rearrangement in IL-4-activated THP-1 monocytes. SCR or TG2-KD monocytes were treated with IL-4 (50 ng/ml) for 24 h and then examined for **a** their ability to adhere onto a FN layer for 1 h, **b** mRNA expression of β1 integrin, **c** activation of the small GTPase protein RhoA, and **d** mRNA expression of MMP-2. Data presented are the mean values + SEM (standard error of the mean) of at least three independent experiments. *$p < 0.05$, **$p < 0.01$, ***$p < 0.001$. SCR scramble control, TG2-KD TG2 knockdown

Conclusion

In this study, we established that TG2 mRNA levels are increased in monocytes derived from MS patients and correlates with anti-inflammatory cytokine expression, proposing a more anti-inflammatory status of the TG2-expressing monocytes in MS. Furthermore, IL-4 is an important regulator of TG2 expression in THP1 monocytes and TG2 mediates IL-4-induced anti-inflammatory status of these cells as well as adhesion and cytoskeletal rearrangement in vitro. We thus propose that IL-4 upregulates TG2 expression in monocytes of MS patients, driving them into an anti-inflammatory status. This leads to the speculation that TG2 can mediate the enhanced adhesion of anti-inflammatory-tuned monocytes to the CNS endothelium of MS patients.

Abbreviations

ANOVA: One-way analysis of variance; BBB: Blood-brain barrier; BCA: Bicinchoninic acid; CNS: Central nervous system; DMT: Disease-modifying therapies; DTT: Dithiothreitol; EAE: Experimental autoimmune encephalomyelitis; ECM: Extracellular matrix; FN: Fibronectin; GAPDH: Glyceraldehyde-3-phosphate-dehydrogenase; HC: Healthy control; IL: Interleukin; IL-1ra: IL-1 receptor antagonist; MMP: Matrix metalloproteinase; MS: Multiple sclerosis; NGF: Nerve growth factor; PBMC: Peripheral blood mononuclear cells; PBS: Phosphate-buffered saline; PMSF: Phenylmethylsulfonyl fluoride; POLR2F: Polymerase II polypeptide F; PP-MS: Primary progressive; qPCR: Semi-quantitative real-time PCR; RR-MS: Relapsing-remitting MS; RT: Room temperature; SCR: Scramble control; SD: Standard deviation; SDS: Sodium dodecyl sulfate; SEM: Standard error of the mean; shRNA: Short hairpin RNA; TG2: Tissue transglutaminase or transglutaminase 2; TG2-KD: TG2-knockdown TGF: Transforming growth factor; TNF: Tumor necrosis factor; Unt: Untreated; WB: Western blotting

Acknowledgements

We thank all MS patients and HC subjects for giving their consent to contribute to this study.

Funding

This work was supported by European Union Framework Programme 7 Marie Curie TRANSPATH ITN (grant no. 289964) and by the Dutch MS Research Foundation (grant no. 14-865MS and no. 10-701MS).

Authors' contributions

CS conceived and carried out experiments, analyzed the data, and wrote the paper; JB, MvE, and JvR helped in data collection; JK, CT, MM, BD, and PvdE helped in the data interpretation and provided critical feedback on the paper; AvD designed the study, conceived the experiments, and helped in the data interpretation and in the writing of the paper. All authors read and approved the submitted manuscript.

Consent for publication

Not applicable

Competing interests

The authors declare that they have no competing interests.

Author details

[1]Department of Anatomy and Neurosciences, Amsterdam Neuroscience, VU University Medical Center, Postbus 7057, 1007 MB Amsterdam, the Netherlands. [2]Department of Immunohematology and Blood Transfusion, Leiden University Medical Center, Leiden, the Netherlands. [3]Department of Neurology, VU University Medical Center, Amsterdam, the Netherlands. [4]Department of Clinical Chemistry, VU University Medical Center, Amsterdam, the Netherlands. [5]Department of Pathology, VU University Medical Center, Amsterdam, the Netherlands. [6]Present Address: Brain Plasticity Group, Center for Neuroscience, Swammerdam Institute for Life Sciences, University of Amsterdam, Science Park 904, Amsterdam, the Netherlands.

References

1. Koch-Henriksen N, Sorensen PS. The changing demographic pattern of multiple sclerosis epidemiology. Lancet Neurol. 2010;9:520–32.
2. Noseworthy J, Lucchinetti C, Rodriguez M, Weinshenker B. Multiple sclerosis. N Engl J Med. 2000;343:938–52.
3. Lassmann H, van Horssen J. The molecular basis of neurodegeneration in multiple sclerosis. FEBS Lett. 2011;585:3715–23.
4. Chigaev A, Zwartz G, Graves SW, Dwyer DC, Tsuji H, Foutz TD, et al. alpha4beta1 integrin affinity changes govern cell adhesion. J Biol Chem. 2003;278:38174–82.
5. Shamri R, Grabovsky V, Gauguet JM, Feigelson S, Manevich E, Kolanus W, et al. Lymphocyte arrest requires instantaneous induction of an extended LFA-1 conformation mediated by endothelium-bound chemokines. Nat Immunol. 2005;6:497–506.
6. Adams CWM, Poston RN, Buk SJ. Pathology, histochemistry and immunocytochemistry of lesions in acute multiple sclerosis. J Neurol Sci. 1989;92:291–306.
7. Ajami B, Bennett JL, Krieger C, McNagny KM, Rossi FM. Infiltrating monocytes trigger EAE progression, but do not contribute to the resident microglia pool. Nat Neurosci. 2011;14:1142–9.
8. Brück W, Porada P, Poser S, Rieckmann P, Hanefeld F, Kretzschmarch HA, et al. Monocyte/macrophage differentiation in early multiple sclerosis lesions. Ann Neurol. 1995;38:788–96.
9. Hauser SL, Bhan AK, Gilles F, Kemp M, Kerr C, Weiner HL. Immunohistochemical analysis of the cellular infiltrate in multiple sclerosis lesions. Ann Neurol. 1986;19:578–87.
10. Huitinga I, Van Rooijen N, De Groot CJ, Uitdehaag BM, Dijkstra CD. Suppression of experimental allergic encephalomyelitis in Lewis rats after elimination of macrophages. J Exp Med. 1990;172:1025–33.
11. Tran EH, Hoekstra K, van Rooijen N, Dijkstra CD, Owens T. Immune invasion of the central nervous system parenchyma and experimental allergic encephalomyelitis, but not leukocyte extravasation from blood, are prevented in macrophage-depleted mice. J Immunol. 1998;161:3767–75.
12. McQualter JL, Bernard CC. Multiple sclerosis: a battle between destruction and repair. J Neurochem. 2007;100:295–306.
13. Miller E. Multiple Sclerosis. In: Ahmad S, editor. Neurodegenerative diseases. US: Springer; 2012. p. 222–38.
14. Boven LA, Van Meurs M, Van Zwam M, Wierenga-Wolf A, Hintzen RQ, Boot RG, et al. Myelin-laden macrophages are anti-inflammatory, consistent with foam cells in multiple sclerosis. Brain. 2006;129:517–26.
15. Elkabes S, DiCicco-Bloom EM, Black IB. Brain microglia/macrophages express neurotrophins that selectively regulate microglial proliferation and function. J Neurosci. 1996;16:2508–21.
16. Mosser DM, Edwards JP. Exploring the full spectrum of macrophage activation. Nat Rev Immunol. 2008;8:958–69.
17. Denney L, Kok WL, Cole SL, Sanderson S, McMichael AJ, Ho LP. Activation of invariant NKT cells in early phase of experimental autoimmune encephalomyelitis results in differentiation of Ly6Chi inflammatory monocyte to M2 macrophages and improved outcome. J Immunol. 2012;189:551–7.
18. Mikita J, Dubourdieu-Cassagno N, Deloire MS, Vekris A, Eiran M, Raffard G, et al. Altered M1/M2 activation patterns of monocytes in severe relapsing experimental rat model of multiple sclerosis. Amelioration of clinical status by M2 activated monocyte administration. Mult Scler. 2011;17:2–15.
19. Vaknin I, Kunis G, Miller O, Butovsky O, Bukshpan S, Beers DR, et al. Excess circulating alternatively activated myeloid (M2) cells accelerate ALS progression while inhibiting experimental autoimmune encephalomyelitis. PLoS One. 2011;6:e26921.
20. Bayardo M, Punzi F, Bondar C, Chopita N, Chirdo F. Transglutaminase 2 expression is enhanced synergistically by interferon-gamma and tumour necrosis factor-alpha in human small intestine. Clin Exp Immunol. 2012;168:95–104.
21. Kim SY, Jeong EJ, Steinert PM. IFN-gamma induces transglutaminase 2 expression in rat small intestinal cells. J Interf Cytok Res. 2002;22:677–82.
22. Shin DM, Jeon JH, Kim CW, Cho SY, Lee HJ, Jang GY, et al. TGF-beta mediates activation of transglutaminase 2 in response to oxidative stress that leads to protein aggregation. FASEB J. 2008;22:2498–507.
23. Yanagawa Y, Hiraide S, Matsumoto M, Shimamura K, Togashi H. Enhanced transglutaminase 2 expression in response to stress-related catecholamines in macrophages. Immunobiology. 2014;219:680–6.
24. van Strien ME, de Vries HE, Chrobok NL, Bol JG, Breve JJ, van der Pol SM, et al. Tissue transglutaminase contributes to experimental multiple sclerosis pathogenesis and clinical outcome by promoting macrophage migration. Brain Behav Immun. 2015;50:141–54.
25. Akimov SS, Belkin AM. Cell surface tissue transglutaminase is involved in adhesion and migration of monocytic cells on fibronectin. Blood. 2001;98:1567–76.
26. Polman CH, Reingold SC, Banwell B, Clanet M, Cohen JA, Filippi M, et al. Diagnostic criteria for multiple sclerosis: 2010 revisions to the McDonald criteria. Ann Neurol. 2011;69:292–302.
27. van Strien ME, Breve JJ, Fratantoni S, Schreurs MW, Bol JG, Jongenelen CA, et al. Astrocyte-derived tissue transglutaminase interacts with fibronectin: a role in astrocyte adhesion and migration? PLoS One. 2011;6:e25037.
28. Ruijter JM, Ramakers C, Hoogaars WM, Karlen Y, Bakker O, Van den Hoff MJB, et al. Amplification efficiency: linking baseline and bias in the analysis of quantitative PCR data. Nucleic Acids Res. 2009;36:e45.
29. Chanput W, Mes J, Vreeburg RA, Savelkoul HF, Wichers HJ. Transcription profiles of LPS-stimulated THP-1 monocytes and macrophages: a tool to study inflammation modulating effects of food-derived compounds. Food Funct. 2010;1:254–61.
30. Graesser D, Mahooti S, Haas T, Davis S, Clark RB, Madri JA. The interrelationship of alpha4 integrin and matrix metalloproteinase-2 in the pathogenesis of experimental autoimmune encephalomyelitis. Lab Investig. 1998;78:1445–58.
31. Yang L, Zheng Z, Zhou Q, Bai X, Fan L, Yang C, et al. miR-155 promotes cutaneous wound healing through enhanced keratinocytes migration by MMP-2. J Mol Histol. 2017;48:147–55.
32. Wilhelmus MM, de Jager M, Bakker EN, Drukarch B. Tissue transglutaminase in Alzheimer's disease: involvement in pathogenesis and its potential as a therapeutic target. J Alzheimers Dis. 2014;42(Suppl 3):S289–303.
33. Rauhavirta T, Hietikko M, Salmi T, Lindfors K. Transglutaminase 2 and transglutaminase 2 autoantibodies in celiac disease: a review. Clin Rev Allergy Immunol. 2016; doi:10.1007/s12016-016-8557-4.
34. Agnihotri N, Mehta K. Transglutaminase-2: evolution from pedestrian protein to a promising therapeutic target. Amino Acids. 2017;49:425–39.
35. Curro M, Ferlazzo N, Risitano R, Condello S, Vecchio M, Caccamo D, et al. Transglutaminase 2 and phospholipase A(2) interactions in the inflammatory response in human Thp-1 monocytes. Amino Acids. 2014;46:759–66.
36. Frisdal E, Lesnik P, Olivier M, Robillard P, Chapman MJ, Huby T, et al. Interleukin-6 protects human macrophages from cellular cholesterol accumulation and attenuates the proinflammatory response. J Biol Chem. 2011;286:30926–36.
37. Hodrea J, Demeny MA, Majai G, Sarang Z, Korponay-Szabo IR, Fesus L. Transglutaminase 2 is expressed and active on the surface of human monocyte-derived dendritic cells and macrophages. Immunol Lett. 2010;130:74–81.
38. Murtaugh MP, Arend WP, Davies PJ. Induction of tissue transglutaminase in human peripheral blood monocytes. J Exp Med. 1984;159:114–25.
39. Boisvert WA, Rose DM, Boullier A, Quehenberger O, Sydlaske A, Johnson KA, et al. Leukocyte transglutaminase 2 expression limits atherosclerotic lesion size. Arterioscler Thromb Vasc Biol. 2006;26:563–9.
40. Vogel DY, Vereyken EJ, Glim JE, Heijnen PD, Moeton M, van der Valk P, et al. Macrophages in inflammatory multiple sclerosis lesions have an intermediate activation status. J Neuroinflamm. 2013;10:35.
41. Brilha S, Wysoczanski R, Whittington AM, Friedland JS, Porter JC. Monocyte

adhesion, migration, and extracellular matrix breakdown is regulated by integrin alphaVbeta3 in mycobacterium tuberculosis infection. J Immunol. 2017;199:982–91.
42. Leavesley DI, Schwartz MA, Rosenfeld M, Cheresh DA. Integrin beta1-and beta3-mediated endothelial cell migration is triggered through distinct signaling mechanisms. J Cell Biol. 1993;121:163–70.
43. Kawabe K, Takano K, Moriyama M, Nakamura Y. Lipopolysaccharide-Stimulated Transglutaminase 2 Expression Enhances Endocytosis Activity in the Mouse Microglial Cell Line BV-2. Neuroimmunomodulation. 2015;22:243-9.
44. Johnson K, Hashimoto S, Lotz M, Pritzker K, Terkeltaub R. Interleukin-1 induces pro-mineralizing activity of cartilage tissue transglutaminase and factor XIIIa. Am J Pathol. 2001;159:149–63.
45. Gundemir S, Colak G, Tucholski J, Johnson GV. Transglutaminase 2: a molecular Swiss army knife. Biochim Biophys Acta. 2012;1823:406–19.
46. Krakauer T, Oppenheim JJ. IL-1 and tumor necrosis factor-alpha each up-regulate both the expression of IFN-gamma receptors and enhance IFN-gamma-induced HLA-DR expression on human monocytes and a human monocytic cell line (THP-1). J Immunol. 1993;150:1205–11.
47. Murthy PK, Dennis VA, Lasater BL, Philipp MT. Interleukin-10 modulates proinflammatory cytokines in the human monocytic cell line THP-1 stimulated with Borrelia burgdorferi lipoproteins. Infect Immunol. 2000;68:6663–9.
48. Hohnoki K, Inoue A, Koh CS. Elevated serum levels of IFN-gamma, IL-4 and TNF-alpha/unelevated serum levels of IL-10 in patients with demyelinating diseases during the acute stage. J Neuroimmunol. 1998;87:27–32.
49. Kallaur AP, Oliveira SR, Colado Simao AN, Delicato de Almeida ER, Kaminami Morimoto H, Lopes J, et al. Cytokine profile in relapsingremitting multiple sclerosis patients and the association between progression and activity of the disease. Mol Med Rep. 2013;7:1010–20.
50. CZ L, Jensen MA, Arnason BG. Interferon gamma- and interleukin-4-secreting cells in multiple sclerosis. J Neuroimmunol. 1993;46:123–8.
51. Soderstrom M, Hillert J, Link J, Navikas V, Fredrikson S, Link H. Expression of IFN-gamma, IL-4, and TGF-beta in multiple sclerosis in relation to HLA-Dw2 phenotype and stage of disease. Mult Scler. 1995;1:173–80.
52. Martinez FO, Helming L, Milde R, Varin A, Melgert BN, Draijer C, et al. Genetic programs expressed in resting and IL-4 alternatively activated mouse and human macrophages: similarities and differences. Blood. 2013;121:e57–69.
53. Chiba Y, Todoroki M, Misawa M. Interleukin-4 upregulates RhoA protein via an activation of STAT6 in cultured human bronchial smooth muscle cells. Pharmacol Res. 2010;61:188–92.
54. Elenstrom-Magnusson C, Chen W, Clinchy B, Obrink B, Severison E. IL-4-induced B cell migration involves transient interactions between beta 1 integrins and extracellular matrix components. Int Immunol. 1995;7:567–73.

6

Increased cortical lesion load and intrathecal inflammation is associated with oligoclonal bands in multiple sclerosis patients: a combined CSF and MRI study

Gabriele Farina[1,2†], Roberta Magliozzi[1,3†], Marco Pitteri[1], Richard Reynolds[3], Stefania Rossi[4,1], Alberto Gajofatto[1], Maria Donata Benedetti[1], Francesco Facchiano[4], Salvatore Monaco[1] and Massimiliano Calabrese[1*]

Abstract

Background: Although IgG oligoclonal bands (OCBs) in the cerebrospinal fluid (CSF) are a frequent phenomenon in multiple sclerosis (MS) patients, their relationship with grey matter lesions, intrathecal/meningeal inflammation and clinical evolution has not been clarified yet.

The aim of our study was to assess the relationship between the OCBs, the inflammatory/neurodegenerative CSF profile at diagnosis, the cortical lesion load and the clinical evolution after 10 years.

Methods: This is a 10-year observational, cross-sectional study based on a combined MRI, cognitive and CSF profiling of the examined patients.

Forty consecutive OCB-negative (OCB–) and 50 OCB-positive (OCB+) MS patients were included in this study. Both groups had mean disease duration of 10 years and were age and gender matched. Each patient underwent neurological and neuropsychological evaluation and 3-T MRI. Analysis of the presence and levels of 28 inflammatory mediators was performed in the CSF obtained from 10 OCB– MS, 11 OCB+ MS and 10 patients with other neurological conditions.

Results: Increased number of CLs was found in OCB+ compared to OCB– patients ($p < 0.0001$), whereas no difference was found in white matter lesion (WML) load ($p = 0.36$). The occurrence of OCB was also associated with increased levels of neurofilament light chains and of several inflammatory mediators linked to B lymphocyte activity and lymphoid-neogenesis (CXCL13, CXCL12, CXCL10, TNFSF13, TNFSF13B, IL6, IL10) and other pro-inflammatory molecules, such as IFN-γ, TNF, MMP2, GM-CSF, osteopontin and sCD163. Finally, the occurrence of OCB was found associated with poor prognosis, from both physical and cognitive points of view.

Conclusions: OCB at MS onset are associated with more severe GM pathology and with a more severe physical disability and cognitive impairment after 10 years. Increased levels of cytokines linked to B cell activation, lymphoid-neogenesis, and pro-inflammatory immune response in the CSF of OCB+ patients support the hypothesis of crucial role played by compartmentalized, intrathecal B cell response in the pathogenesis of CLs and OCB production.

Keywords: CSF, MRI, Oligoclonal bands, IgG, Multiple sclerosis, OCB, Cytokines, Grey matter, Neuroinflammation, Neurodegeneration

* Correspondence: massimiliano.calabrese@univr.it

†Equal contributors

[1]Neurology B, Department of Neurological, Biomedical and Movement Sciences, University of Verona, Policlinico "G.B. Rossi" Borgo Roma, Piazzale L.A. Scuro, 10, 37134 Verona, Italy

Background

Multiple sclerosis (MS) is a chronic immune-mediated disease of the central nervous system (CNS) characterized by demyelination, neurodegeneration and axonal/glial pathology. Persistent intrathecal inflammation, demonstrated by the presence of oligoclonal bands (OCBs) in the cerebrospinal fluid (CSF) [1, 2], is one of the main hallmarks of MS in about 87.7% of MS patients [3]. The early detection of OCB in the disease course, together with the deposition of antibody, activation of complement and demyelination [4, 5], supports the role for B cells in MS pathogenesis. Clonally expanded populations of memory B and plasma cells have been found in the perivascular spaces, in the meningeal infiltrates, and in the CSF of patients with MS, even at the disease onset.

B cells express a specific chemokine receptor profile dependent upon their state of differentiation and external microenvironment. Several chemokines have been shown to influence CNS B cell trafficking and activity: CCL2, CCL3, CCL20, CXCL10, CXCL12 and CXCL13 [6]. Among these factors, increased CSF levels of CXCL13, one of the most important chemokine regulating B cell migration and differentiation in MS patients and EAE models [7–9], corroborate the hypothesis that the abnormal B cell immune response persists and becomes compartmentalized in the CNS. Diffuse inflammation, sometimes accompanied by the formation of ectopic tertiary lymphoid tissues (TLT), and recently detected in the inflamed meninges of post-mortem secondary progressive MS cases [10–12], may represent the niches within cerebral sulci in which the B cell response persists and plays its role in disease exacerbation. Inflammation within the subarachnoid space is suggested to be involved in the creation of an intrathecal inflammatory milieu that, through circulating CSF, baths the external adjacent cortical grey matter (GM) and mediates neuronal and glia pathological alterations [10, 11, 13]. As shown by several studies, the consequent GM damage is strictly correlated with the accumulation of physical and cognitive disability, and with the evolution of the progressive phase of the disease [14–17]. In a previous preliminary, cross-sectional study [18], we observed an association between cortical lesions (CLs) and OCB but no formal hypotheses about the origin of such association were suggested.

The aim of the present study was to confirm the relationship between OCB expression, cortical damage and the unfavourable clinical evolution and to test the hypothesis that the presence of OCB and CLs might be related to the intrathecal inflammation and to the presence of subarachnoid tertiary B cell lymphoid-like structures.

Methods

Patients

All consecutive OCB− patients having a diagnosis of MS according to the most recent MS diagnostic criteria [19] and who consecutively underwent neurological examination at the MS Centre of Verona University Hospital, between January and December 2014, were asked to participate in this study. Among these 44 patients, 2 were excluded since their diagnosis was not confirmed, 2 did not agree to participate, and 40 were enrolled in this cohort study. The mean disease duration for these patients was 10.5 ± 7.3 years. Among the 815 OCB+ patients who underwent neurological examination in our MS centre in the same period, an MS population sex, age and disease duration matched with OCB− population was randomly pulled out by a homemade algorithm (flow chart in Additional file 1). Steroid therapy during the 2 months before the enrolment was an exclusion criterion. See Table 1 for demographic and clinical characteristics of the two populations studied. Furthermore, 10 age- and gender-matched control patients, with other neurological conditions, have also been recruited. The study was approved by the local ethic committee, and informed consent was obtained from all patients.

Clinical information

Each patient was assessed by means of the Expanded Disability Status Scale (EDSS) [20] at the time of inclusion in the study. Previous EDSS scores were retrospectively acquired from the clinical records of each patient. Data about previous and actual disease-modifying therapies were collected. Patients were classified into four categories, according to the type of drug administered (Table 1).

Neuropsychological assessment

Neuropsychological assessment was performed at the time of enrolment in the present study by means of the brief repeatable battery (BRB) of neuropsychological tests [21]—except the PASAT-2 subtest. The BRB is composed by tests of verbal learning and delayed memory recall (Selective Reminding Test, SRT), visuo-spatial learning and delayed memory recall (10/36 Spatial Recall Test, SPART), auditory information processing speed, working memory, attention, and calculation (Paced Auditory Serial Addition Test, PASAT), visual information processing speed and attention (Symbol Digit Modalities Test, SDMT), and semantic verbal fluency (Word List Generation, WLG). Test scores were considered failed according to the cut-off scores (5th percentile) derived from the Italian normative data [21]. Previous neuropsychological evaluations were excluded from the analysis since the types of tests administered were heterogeneous and then not comparable.

Table 1 Clinical and MRI parameters at diagnosis and at the enrolment (whole population)

	OCB+	OCB−	Whole group	*p* value
N (f/m)	50 (34/16)	40 (28/12)	90 (62/28)	0.511
Age (years)	42.5 ± 10.4 (19–67)	42.4 ± 11.2 (17–69)	42.5 ± 10.7 (17–69)	0.943
Years from onset to diagnosis	3.0 ± 5.1 (0–21)	2.6 ± 3.9 (0–17)	2.8 ± 4.6 (0–21)	0.356
Years from diagnosis to enrolment	7.8 ± 5.2 (0–20)	7.9 ± 6.4 (0–22)	7.9 ± 5.7 (0–22)	0.918
Years from onset to enrolment (disease duration)	10.8 ± 7.0 (1–31)	10.5 ± 7.3 (1–29)	10.7 ± 7.1 (1–31)	0.878
EDSS at diagnosis	1.5 (0–3.0)	1.0 (0–3.5)	1.5 (0–3.5)	0.645
EDSS at enrolment	2.8 (1.0–8.0)	1.5 (0–6.5)	2.0 (1.0–8.0)	<0.0001
RRMS/SPMS at enrolment	35/15	36/4	71/19	0.018
Time to SPMS transition in months	123 ± 23 (98–187)	183 ± 13 (165–198)	136 ± 33 (98–198)	<0.0001
Cognitive impairment CN/mCI/sCI	30/9/11	34/5/1	64/14/12	0.013
CL number at enrolment	6.1 ± 6.1 (0–24)	2.2 ± 2.8 (0–11)	4.4 ± 5.3 (0–24)	<0.0001
WMLV at enrolment (cm^3)	7.1 ± 3.6 (1.1–16.4)	6.5 ± 4.1 (1.3–18.1)	6.8 ± 4.0 (1.1–18.1)	0.258
Treatment until now				
None	0	5	5	0.033
Only 1° line[a]	34	28	62	
At least 2° line[a]	11	6	17	
At least 3° line[a]	5	1	6	

EDSS Expanded Disability Status Scale, *RRMS* relapsing-remitting multiple sclerosis, *SPMS* secondary progressive multiple sclerosis, *CN* cognitively normal, *mCI* mild cognitive impairment, *sCI* severe cognitive impairment, *CL* cortical lesion, *WML* white matter lesion
Data are reported as mean ± standard deviation (range). For the EDSS, median and (range) are provided
[a]1° line drugs: IFN-beta, GA, azathioprine; 2° line drugs: fingolimod, natalizumab; 3° line drug: cyclophosphamide, mitoxantrone

The presence of depression was assessed by means of the Beck Depression Inventory second edition (BDI-II) [22].

MS patients were classified into three groups: cognitively normal (CN = no failed test of the BRB), mild cognitive impairment (mCI = up to two failed tests), and severe cognitive impairment (sCI = three or more failed tests).

CSF analysis

The CSF, collected at the time of diagnosis from all the examined MS patients for diagnostic purposes, was then available for protein analysis from 21 (11 OCB+ and 10 OCB−, strictly representative of the two groups of examined MS patients) out of the 90 MS patients enrolled in the study and from 10 control patients (affected by other inflammatory neurological diseases, OIND). CSF sample collection and preparation were performed more than 2 months after the last relapse according to in-house guidelines (used since 1994 by the bio-bank at the MS Centre of Verona), which were in line with the Consensus Guidelines for CSF and Blood Biobanking [23]. CSF, obtained at the disease diagnosis, was centrifuged soon after collection, and both the supernatant fraction and the cell pellet were separately stored at −80 °C until use. The presence of OCBs was performed by using iso-electric focusing method and blindly assessed by two independent examiners [24]. When possible, the assessment of the OCB in OCB− MS patients was re-tested after second lumbar puncture showing confirmation of OCB absence.

The presence and levels of 28 inflammatory mediators, including either the major pro-inflammatory mediators or molecules mainly related to the B cell immune response (Table 2), were assessed using a combination of immune-assay multiplex techniques based on the Luminex technology (Table 2; Bio-Plex X200 System equipped with a magnetic workstation, BioRad, Hercules, CA, USA). The CSF analysis was optimized and performed by two independent investigators (RM and SR), blinded with respect to the presence/absence of OCB and to the clinical characteristics of the patient and according to previously published procedures [25, 26]. All samples were run in duplicate and a number of molecules have been measured in different immune-assay platform in order to verify the reproducibility and consistence of the results. The CSF level of each protein detected during the analysis was normalized to the protein concentration of each CSF sample (measured by Bradford protocol).

The levels of neurofilament light chain (NF-L) in CSF were measured using the Human NF-light ELISA kit (MyBioSource, San Diego, CA, USA) according to the manufacturer's instructions. The monoclonal antibody was allowed to bind to the antigen for 90 min at 37 °C and the unbound sample was washed away followed by addition of a biotinylated human NF-L

Table 2 Methodological details of the examined inflammatory proteins in the CSF of MS patients by Bio-Plex immunoassay System

		Detection limit (pg/ml)	Intra-assay variation (%)	Recovery percentage range (90–110%)
BCA1/CXCL13	Chemokine (C-X-C motif) ligand 13 (CXCL13) or B lymphocyte chemoattractant (BLC) or B cell-attracting chemokine 1 (BCA-1)	0.42–6694	6.0	100
SDF1αβ/CXCL12	C-X-C motif chemokine 12 (CXCL12) or stromal cell-derived factor 1 (SDF1)	12.73–160,858	5.4	104
6Ckine/CCL21	Chemokine (C-C motif) ligand 21	11.30–160,686	4.0	104
IP10/CXCL10	C-X-C motif chemokine 10 (CXCL10) or interferon gamma-induced protein 10 (IP-10)	1.04–14,668	1.5	95
BAFF/TNFSF13B	B cell activating factor (BAFF) or tumour necrosis factor ligand superfamily member 13B (TNFSF13B)	70.19–197,936	6.3	100
APRIL/TNFSF13	A proliferation-inducing ligand (APRIL), or tumour necrosis factor ligand superfamily member 13 (TNFSF13)	906.31–4,745,900	7.5	103
TWEAK/TNFSF12	TNF-related weak inducer of apoptosis (TWEAK) or tumour necrosis factor ligand superfamily member 12	3.59–6346	4.4	106
LIGTH/TNFSF14	Tumour necrosis factor superfamily member 14 (TNFSF14)	1.92–4647	5.8	98
TNFα	Tumour necrosis factor alpha	0.24–13,148	2.5	99
sTNFR1	Soluble- tumour necrosis factor-receptor 1	2.33–48,047	5.0	100
sTNFR2	Soluble- tumour necrosis factor-receptor 2	3.72–63,484	4.2	98
MIP3β/CCL19	Chemokine (C-C motif) ligand 19 (CCL19) or EBI1 ligand chemokine (ELC) or macrophage inflammatory protein-3-beta (MIP-3-beta)	3.08–49,150	2.8	103
MIG/CXCL9	Chemokine (C-X-C motif) ligand 9 (CXCL9) or monokine induced by gamma interferon (MIG)	1.19–23,643	5.4	97
sCD163	Soluble-CD163 (Cluster of Differentiation 163)	0.38–10,497	6.0	102
GM-CSF	Granulocyte-macrophage colony-stimulating factor (GM-CSF) or colony-stimulating factor 2 (CSF2)	2.32–34,028	5.2	104
INFα2	Interferon alpha-2	1.24–19,334	5.3	99
INFβ	Interferon beta	1.50–8727	6.0	100
INFγ	Interferon gamma	1.50–2326	3.0	99
IL1β	Interleukin-1 beta	0.15–2326	2.0	102
IL2	Interleukin-2	0.47–10,334	4.0	98
IL4	Interleukin-4	0.35–5258	6.0	100
IL6	Interleukin-6	0.68–57,162	3.0	99
IL8/CXCL8	Interleukin-8 (C-X-C motif) or chemokine ligand 8, CXCL8)	11.56–8523	1.0	103
IL10	Interleukin-10	0.84–2997	3.0	98
OPN	Osteopontin	123.64–286,066	7.3	100
MMP1	Matrix metallopeptidase 1	298.2–216,430	4.5	100
MMP2	Matrix metallopeptidase 2	90.63–2,109,030	3.3	104
MIF	Macrophage migration inhibitor factor	8.25–456,461	2.6	103

antibody at 37 °C for 1 h. The enzyme-conjugate liquid was added after plate washed for 30 min at 37 °C and plate was then washed. The plate was added with 3,3′,5,5′-tetrametilbenzidine (TMB) substrate according to the manufacturer's instructions and read at λ450 nm within 10 min and the quantification was carried out on VICTORTM X3 2030 Multilabel Plate Reader (Perkin Elmer, Walluf, Germany). Intra-assay variability (coefficients of variation) samples were below 10%. Data obtained were normalized for total protein concentration (mg/ml).

Image acquisition protocol

Each patient was scanned at enrolment using a 3.0-T Philips Achieva MRI (Philips Medical Systems, Best, The Netherlands), acquiring the following sequences:

- 3D fluid attenuated inversion recovery (FLAIR) TR/TE = 5500/292 ms, TI = 1650 ms, voxel dimension of 1 × 1 × 1 mm
- 3D double inversion recovery (DIR) TR/TE = 5500/292 ms, TI1/TI2 = 525 ms/2530 ms voxel dimension of 1 × 1 × 1 mm
- 3D T1 weighted fast field echo (FFE) TR/TE = 8.4/3.7 ms, voxel dimension of 1 × 1 × 1 mm

Previous MRI examinations acquired at the time of diagnosis (i.e. within 1 month from CSF collection) using a 1.5-T Philips Achieva MRI scanner, were available for 35 OCB− and 48 OCB+ patients.

The following sets of images were acquired at a 1.5-T scanner:

- 3D DIR: TR = 15,631 ms, TE = 25 ms, TI = 3400 ms, delay = 325 ms, ETL = 17, 50 contiguous axial slices with a thickness = 3 mm, matrix size = 130 × 256, and field of view (FOV) = 250 × 200 mm
- 3D FLAIR: TR = 10,000 ms, TE = 120 ms, TI = 2500 ms, ETL = 23, 50 contiguous axial slices with a thickness = 3.0 mm, matrix size = 172 × 288, and FOV = 250 × 200 mm
- 3D FFE: 120 contiguous axial slices with the off-centre positioned on zero, TR = 25 ms, TE = 4.6 ms, flip angle = 30°, slice thickness = 1.2 mm, matrix size = 256 × 256, and FOV = 250 × 250 mm

No major hardware upgrades were carried out on the MRI scanners during the study.

Image analysis

All DIR images were assessed by consensus of two experienced observers (MC and GF) blinded to patients' identities and clinical data. Each CL was identified according to the recent recommendations for CL scoring in patients with MS [27]. All FLAIR images were assessed by consensus of the same experienced observers, and the white matter lesion load was quantified. On FLAIR images, white matter lesion volume was quantified after lesion identification using a semi-automated local thresholding technique based on Fuzzy C-mean algorithm, part of the Medical Images Processing Analysis and Visualization (MIPAV) software (http://mipav.cit.nih.gov).

Statistics

Since EDSS scores were not normally distributed, the Wilcoxon or Mann-Whitney test was used to compare the two MS populations with respect to their EDSS score at diagnosis and at enrolment.

Pearson chi-square was used to test the difference between the two MS groups in terms of categorical data (i.e., female/male ratio; disease form: relapsing-remitting MS vs secondary progressive MS) and cognitive status (a ranked scale: CN vs mCI vs sCI). Univariate correlations among continuous variables were assessed using the Pearson correlation coefficient and those among discrete variables with the Spearman rank correlation coefficient. Differences among groups in continuous variables as age, time from diagnosis to enrolment, time from onset to diagnosis, and lesion load were assessed through analysis of variance (ANOVA). Mann-Whitney tests were also used to test differences in terms of CSF protein levels between OCB+ and OCB− MS patients. KEGG pathway analysis was also used to perform unsupervised pathway analysis on the CSF inflammatory mediators levels. The Bonferroni correction was applied. All statistical analyses were performed using SPSS v. 21 and R (http://www.r-project.org).

Results

Clinical parameters

Despite the same mean age, disease duration, and EDSS at the time of diagnosis (see Table 1), the OCB+ group showed more severe disease evolution. Ten years after the disease onset, the median EDSS score of OCB+ patients (2.8 [1.0–8.0]) was significantly higher than that of OCB− patients (1.5 [0–6.5], $p < 0.0001$). The proportion of patients who entered the SP phase was higher in OCB+ (15/50, 30.0%) than in OCB− (4/40, 10.0%, $p = 0.018$) and the time to reach the progressive phase was shorter in OCB+ (mean 123 ± 23 months; range 98–187 months) than in OCB− (mean 183 ± 13 months; range 165–198 months; $p < 0.0001$) patients. The greater severity of the pathological process in the OCB+ patients was also confirmed by the need of administering a higher rate of second- and third-line drug treatments compared to OCB− patients ($p = 0.033$).

Finally, a significant difference was also observed between OCB+ and OCB− patients according to their classification in the three groups considering the number of failed neuropsychological tests ($p = 0.013$): specifically, 30 OCB+ patients (60%) were classified as CN, 9 (18%) were classified as mCI, and 11 (22%) were classified as sCI; on the contrary, 34 OCB− patients (85%) were classified as CN, 5 (12.5%) were classified as mCI, and only 1 (2.5%) was classified as sCI (Table 1).

Imaging data

At the time of diagnosis, OCB+ patients showed 61.1% higher number of CLs (1.8 ± 2.0 [0–5]) compared to OCB− patients (1.1 ± 1.7 [0–6]; $p = 0.041$). CLs were detected in 25/48 (52%) OCB+ and in 11/35 (31%) OCB− patients ($p = 0.075$). No significant difference was observed in terms of WM lesion load ($p = 0.465$) between the OCB+ (mean = 2.0 ± 0.9 cm^3, range = 0.5–4.4 cm^3) and OCB− (mean = 1.6 ± 2.0 cm^3, range = 1.0–5.9 cm^3) patients.

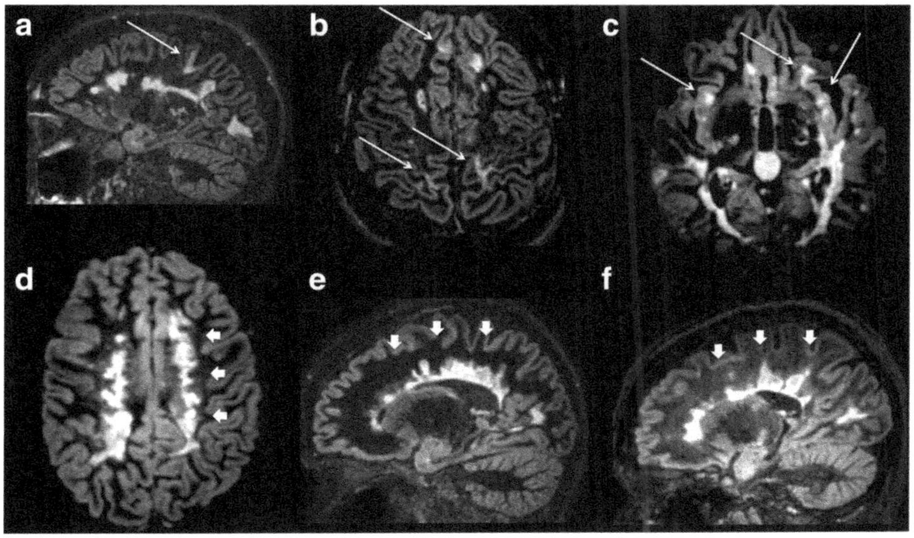

Fig. 1 3D double inversion recovery images of three RRMS OCB+ patients (**a**–**c**) and three RRMS OCB− patients (**d**–**f**). OCB+ patients show both white and grey matter demyelination (*arrows*) including insular lesions (*arrows*, **c**). OCB− patients do not show any grey matter lesion despite the severe white matter demyelination especially in the periventricular region (*arrowheads*, **d**–**f**)

After 10 years of disease, OCB+ patients showed 2.7 times higher number of CLs (6.1 ± 6.05 [0–24]) compared to OCB− patients (2.2 ± 2.8 [0–11]; $p < 0.0001$). CLs were detected in 46/50 (92%) of OCB+ and in 23/40 (57%) of OCB− patients ($p < 0.0001$) Fig. 1.

As detected at the time of diagnosis, after 10 years no significant difference was observed in terms of WM lesion load ($p = 0.258$) between the OCB+ (mean = 7.1 ± 3.6 cm^3, range = 1.1–16.4 cm^3) and OCB− (mean = 6.5 ± 4.1 cm^3, range = 1.3–18.1 cm^3) patients.

CSF analysis (at the time of diagnosis)

Among the clinical CSF parameters, significant increased in CSF cell count was found in OCB+ patients compared to controls ($p = 0.02$); furthermore, increased IgG index was detected in the CSF of OCB+ group compared to both controls ($p = 0.0075$) and to the OCB− group ($p = 0.039$).

Significantly higher levels of NF-L were detected in the CSF of OCB+ patients compared to both controls (fold change = 2.260; $p = 0.007$) and OCB− patients (fold change = 2.165; $p = 0.024$) (Fig. 2a). Among the 28 inflammatory molecules examined, 12 were significantly overexpressed ($p < 0.05$) in OCB+ compared to both controls and OCB− MS patients (Fig. 2b, c): IL6, IL8, IL10, CXCL13, CXCL12, TNF, APRIL, BAFF, IFNγ, MMP2, osteopontin (OPN), sCD163. No difference in the CSF levels of these molecules has been revealed in the OCB− group compared to controls. Although a trend towards an increase of few molecules was observed, such as MIF and CCL19, no significant overexpression was found in the CSF of OCB− patients. By using unsupervised pathway analysis, the occurrence of OCB in the CSF at MS onset was associated with the overexpression of molecules related to the B cell immune response, such as the lymphoid chemokines CXCL13 ($p < 0.001$), CXCL12 ($p < 0.001$), factors related to B cell activation and differentiation such as BAFF ($p = 0.019$), APRIL ($p = 0.015$), IL6 ($p = 0.0005$), and IL10 ($p = 0.035$) (Fig. 2b) or to those with a B cell regulatory role, such as OPN ($p = 0.019$). Concomitant overexpression of the major pro-inflammatory molecules, such as IFNγ ($p < 0.001$), TNF ($p = 0.012$), IL8 ($p = 0.042$), MMP2 ($p = 0.015$) and the marker of activated monocytes, sCD163 ($p = 0.003$), were found to be associated with the presence of OCB (Fig. 2b, c).

In the OCB+ MS patients, CL load significantly correlated with levels of several molecules linked to the B cell immune response, such as CXCL13 ($r = 0.922$; $p < 0.001$), CXCL12 ($r = 0.678$; $p = 0.022$), OPN ($r = 0.692$; $p = 0.018$), IL6 ($r = 0.628$; $p = 0.039$), TWEAK ($r = 0.629$; $p = 0.038$) (Fig. 3). EDSS scores positively correlated with the protein levels of CXCL12 ($r = 0.679$; $p = 0.022$), GM-CSF ($r = 0.626$; $p = 0.039$) and IL1beta ($r = 0.625$; $p = 0.040$) (Fig. 4).

Discussion

In this study we showed that a more inflammatory intrathecal profile and a more severe cortical demyelination are usually associated to the occurrence of OCB at MS diagnosis and to a more severe clinical evolution after 10 years of follow-up. To draw this conclusion, we evaluated the evolution of physical and cognitive disability, the time to progressive phase of the disease and the number of CLs in relapsing-remitting multiple sclerosis (RRMS) patients with and without OCB, at diagnosis and after about 10 years of disease duration. From the

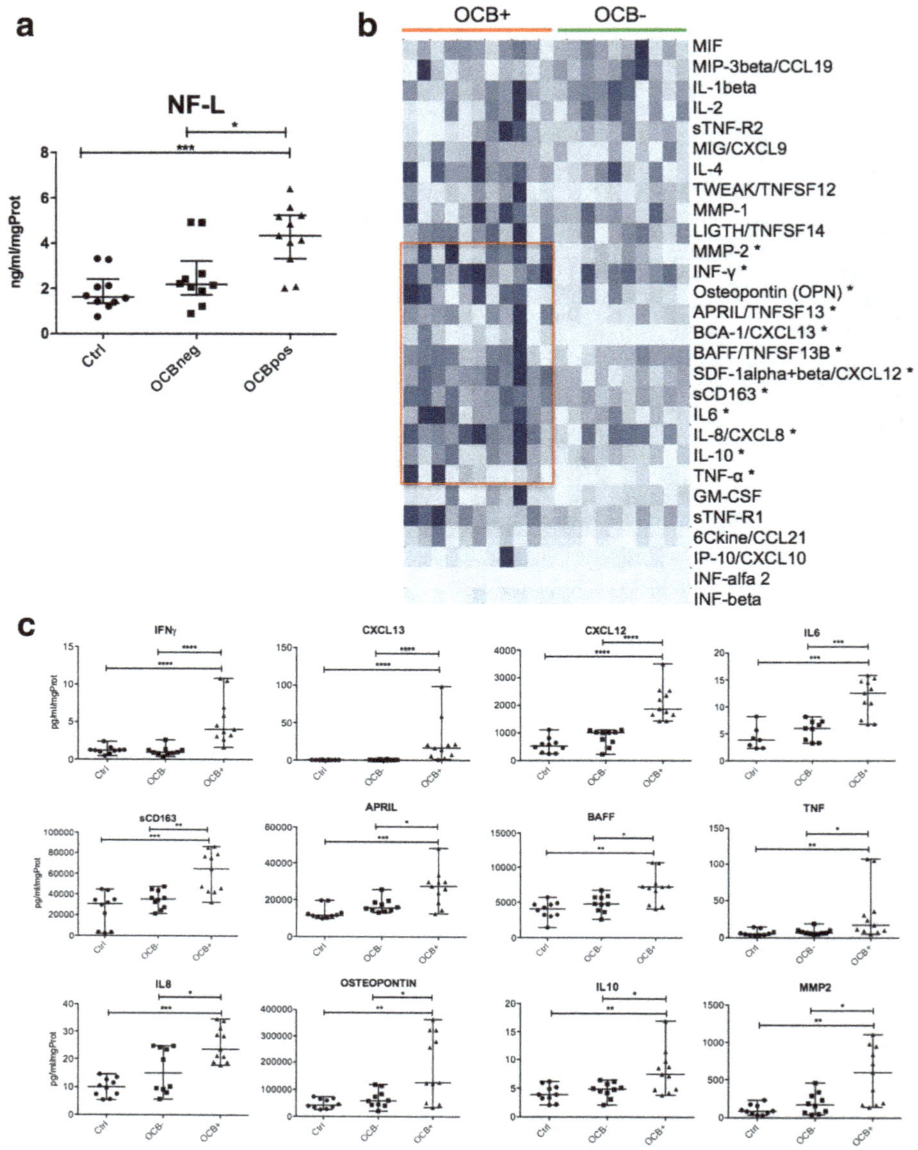

Fig. 2 Protein analysis of the presence and levels of neurofilament light chains (NF-L) and inflammatory mediators in CSF. **a** NF-L protein levels have been analysed in the CSF of controls, OCB– and OCB+ MS patients by using ELISA assessment, showing significant increased levels in OCB+ MS patients compared to both controls and OCB– MS patients. **b** Cluster analysis showing the level of expression of the 28 inflammatory mediators examined in OCB– and OCB+ MS patients: the red rectangle outlines a cluster of molecules significantly overexpressed only in OCB+ MS patients. **c** Statistical representation of the presence and levels of inflammatory mediators significantly overexpressed in OCB+ compared to controls and to OCB– MS patients. (Statistical analysis performed by using Mann-Whitney test; *p* value *<0.05; **<0.01; ***<0.001)

clinical point of view, physical and cognitive results suggest that the presence of OCB at diagnosis can be associated with a worse prognosis. In addition the presence of OCB in the CSF of MS patients is linked to increased CSF cell counts and IgG index, that could reflect the higher inflammatory condition of the CSF of the OCB+ group. In particular, while the cell count significantly differs in OCB + patients only compared to controls, the significant increase in IgG levels in OCB+ compared to both controls and OCB– may demonstrate the preponderance of the humoral response in OCB+ MS patients. In OCB+ group, the number of patients who entered the progressive phase of the disease was significantly higher, and the time to reach the progressive phase was significantly shorter than in OCB– patients group. Such differences of disease course could be explained by the presence of higher intrathecal inflammation and by the consequent higher cortical damage. Indeed, although the presence of CLs was not exclusive of patients with OCB, we showed that patients with OCB, despite the similar age, disease duration and

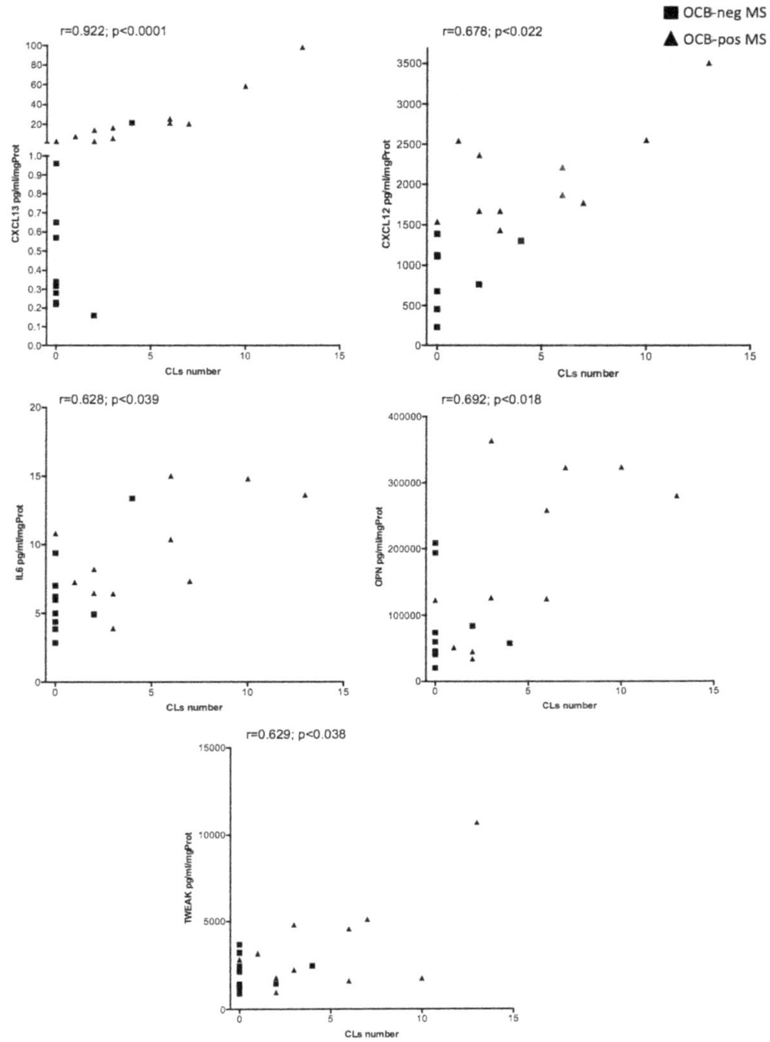

Fig. 3 Pearson correlation analysis between the CSF levels of overexpressed proteins and the number of cortical lesions detected by 3 T MRI in the subgroup of the 21 MS patients. All the represented correlations involve molecules related to B cell chemo-attraction (CXCL13, CXCL12) and activity (IL6, OPN, TWEAK). The *r* and *p* values are reported for each examined correlation in the correspondent graph

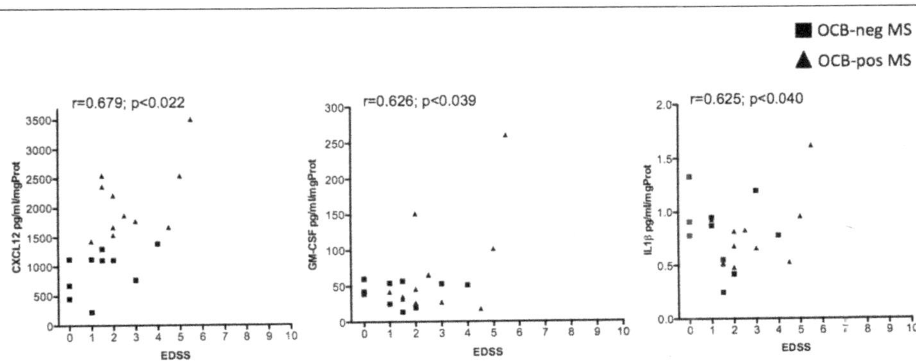

Fig 4 Pearson correlation analysis between the CSF levels of overexpressed proteins and the EDSS values of the subgroup of the 21 MS patients at the follow-up. The *r* and *p* values are reported for each examined correlation in the correspondent graph

WM lesion load, had a substantial increase of the CL load compared to patients without OCB, already at the time of diagnosis. Our hypothesis is that the presence of OCB might be an epiphenomenon of the compartmentalized intrathecal (meningeal) B cell response, which has been suggested to be associated with increased subpial demyelination and neuronal damage, both hallmarks of more rapidly progressive disease [12, 28–31]. While no difference in the levels of B cell-related CSF inflammatory mediators was found between controls and OCB– patients, it can be not excluded that differences in others CSF mediators may occur.

To provide more supporting evidence, we assessed the intrathecal CSF profile of a subgroup of patients with and without OCB. Our results confirmed that OCB+ patients have a greater intrathecal inflammatory activity already at the diagnosis. Such intrathecal inflammation was characterized by overexpression of molecules related to B cell differentiation/activity, inflammatory immune response and monocyte activation compared to both control and OCB– groups. Indeed, high levels of lymphoid chemokines CXCL13 and CXCL12, having a key role in the regulation of B cell migration and compartmentalization within secondary lymphoid organs [9], IL6 and IL10, involved in plasma blast differentiation/class switching as well as B cell regulatory immune activity, and BAFF, APRIL, and osteopontin, involved in the balance between activation, survival and apoptosis of B and T cells [30], were observed in OCB+ MS patients only. Our results confirm and extend previous observations of high levels of CXCL13 and increased numbers of naïve and memory B cells expressing its receptor, CXCR5, in the CSF of MS patients with intrathecal IgG synthesis and characterized by a more aggressive disease course [31–35]. Moreover, by stratifying patients on the basis of the OCB presence at diagnosis, we observed a direct correlation between high levels of CXCL13 (and other B cell-related molecules), CL load, and both long-term physical and cognitive disability. From the neurodegenerative point of view, the elevated level of CXCL12 detected in OCB+ MS patients, together with the high levels of NF-L discovered in the same MS patients, is in line with the high level of GM damage as suggested by the high number of CLs observed in OCB+ MS patients, suggesting a higher degree of neuronal and axonal damage in this subgroup of patients [36]. Indeed, in addition to its role in the immune system, CXCL12, which is produced by activated astrocytes, can induce neuronal apoptosis in certain conditions and promote survival of neurons in others [37]. Metalloproteinase (MMP)-2, that we also found overexpressed in the OCB+ MS patients, could have a direct role in cortical tissue damage by breakdown of extracellular matrix but could be also able to convert CXCL12 into a neurotoxic form [32].

The increased expression of several inflammatory molecules such as IFNγ, TNF, IL8, IL10, IL6, MMP2, and osteopontin found in OCB+ MS patients indicate higher levels of intrathecal inflammatory activity that may be directly involved in the cortical tissue damage, as well as indirectly by activation of resident glial cells. In particular, the high levels of IFNγ and TNF in the CSF of OCB+ MS patients with higher CL load is in agreement with the finding of increased IFNγ and TNF gene and protein expression in paired post-mortem meninges and CSF obtained from secondary progressive multiple sclerosis (SPMS) cases with increased meningeal inflammation, cortical damage and rapid disease progression [38]. Finally, the concurrent finding in OCB+ MS patients of increased levels of sCD163, that was proposed as possible informative marker of activated macrophages and disease activity [39–45], might suggest that an elevated intracerebral lymphocytic and macrophage activity is linked to more severe CL load and disease severity.

The intrathecal B cell activity and severe cortical pathology observed in OCB+ MS patients is also consistent with our previous studies demonstrating the presence of abnormal inflammation and tertiary lymphoid-like organs, rich in B-lymphocytes and plasma cells, in the meningeal infiltrates in the subarachnoid space in SPMS and primary progressive MS cases with a more rapid and severe disease progression [10, 12, 46]. Such a relationship would confirm our hypothesis that meningeal immune cell infiltrates may represent niches for the perpetuation of plasma cell activity and, therefore, together with the presence of long-lived plasma cells, of production sites of OCB immunoglobulins and of inflammatory factors. These inflammatory factors may diffuse across the glia-limitans and play a crucial role in the subpial damage, inducing demyelination, neurodegeneration, and glia alteration mediating a more severe and rapid progression [13, 38]. These events could occur since the early phases of the disease as suggested by the higher number of CLs observed in OCB+ patients since disease diagnosis and by other studies demonstrating the presence of increased meningeal inflammation [47] and meningeal enhancement [48] associated with increase subpial cortical demyelination in a subgroup of MS patients characterized by early and rapid disease progression.

We are aware that our study is not without limitations: first of all the limited number of the patients whose CSF was examined does not allow to drive any definitive conclusion; in addition, the limited number of patients does not allow further sub-analyses, stratifying the patients according to other clinical parameters (e.g., comparison between RRMS and SPMS forms of the OCB+ and OCB – groups, comparison of the same treatment lines, comparison of different MS forms in the same OCB group).

Moreover, although our MRI protocol was performed at a 3-T scanner and included a double inversion recovery sequence, a significant proportion of CLs could have escaped our detection. Finally, the retrospective nature of the study could be considered a limitation. However, it allowed us to choose patients whose diagnosis was confirmed by a very long clinical and radiological observation, and permitted us to correlate, for the first time, long-term clinical and radiological outcomes with the inflammatory features of the CSF obtained at the diagnosis.

Conclusions

The present study confirms and extends our previous observation [18] of strong relationship between OCB and CLs in MS and shows that after almost 10 years of disease duration the number of CLs was about threefold higher in OCB+ compared to OCB− patients, despite the same WM lesion load both at diagnosis and at follow-up. Intrathecal inflammation, in particular linked to B cell immune response, seems to be involved in the production of OCB and in the pathogenesis of cortical damage in MS. Although our data needs to be confirmed in different and larger MS cohorts and by longer perspective follow-up, we suggest that a well-defined pro-inflammatory CSF profile is associated with early occurrence of OCB in the CSF, with development of a more severe cortical pathology, and with a worse clinical (physical and cognitive) prognosis. These results indicate that the evaluation of intrathecal inflammation, combined with the assessment of GM lesion load at the time of diagnosis, might constitute a crucial prognostic tool, which could be helpful in selecting the most appropriate therapy.

Abbreviations

BRB: Brief repeatable battery; CL: Cortical lesion; CN: Cognitively normal; CNS: Central nervous system; CSF: Cerebrospinal fluid; DIR: Double inversion recovery; EDSS: Expanded Disability Status Scale; FLAIR: Fluid attenuated inversion recovery; GM: Grey matter; IgG: Immunoglobulin G; mCI: Mild cognitive impairment; MRI: Magnetic resonance imaging; MS: Multiple sclerosis; NF-L: Neurofilament light chains; OCB−: Oligoclonal bands negative; OCB +: Oligoclonal bands positive; OIND: Other inflammatory neurological diseases; PASAT: Paced Auditory Serial Addition Test; RRMS: Relapsing-remitting multiple sclerosis; sCI: Severe cognitive impairment; SPMS: Secondary progressive multiple sclerosis; WM: White matter; WML: White matter lesion

Acknowledgements

We would like to thank the technical assistance from the CPM Facility at Istituto Superiore di Sanità, Rome, Italy.

Dr Magliozzi was supported by the GR-2010-2313255 grant from Italian Ministry of Health and by the grant 2011/R/13 from Fondazione Italiana Sclerosi Multipla.

Prof Calabrese and Prof Reynolds were supported by Progressive Multiple Sclerosis Alliance grant (PA 0124).

Funding

R. Magliozzi was supported by the GR-2010-2313255 grant from Italian Ministry of Health.

M. Calabrese was supported by PMSA grant (PA 0124) and by GR-2013-02355322 from Italian Ministry of Health.

Authors' contributions

MC, RM and GF conceived and designed the study. MC, RM, GF, MP and SR acquired data. MC, RM, GF, SR and FF analysed and interpreted the data. MC, RM, GF and MP drafted the manuscript. MC, RM, GF, RR, AG, MDB, SM and FF made the critical revision of the manuscript. All authors read and approved the final manuscript.

Competing interests

The authors declare that they have no competing interests.

Consent for publication

Not applicable.

Author details

[1]Neurology B, Department of Neurological, Biomedical and Movement Sciences, University of Verona, Policlinico "G.B. Rossi" Borgo Roma, Piazzale L.A. Scuro, 10, 37134 Verona, Italy. [2]Unit of Neurology, Department of Clinical and Experimental Medicine, University of Sassari, Sassari, Italy. [3]Division of Brain Sciences, Faculty of Medicine, Imperial College London, London, UK. [4]Department EOMM, Istituto Superiore di Sanità, Rome, Italy.

References

1. Kabat EA, Moore DH, Landow H. An electrophoretic study of the protein components in cerebrospinal fluid and their relationship to the serum proteins. J Clin Invest. 1942;21:571–7.
2. Villar LM, Masterman T, Casanova B, Gómez-Rial J, Espiño M, Sádaba MC, et al. CSF oligoclonal band patterns reveal disease heterogeneity in multiple sclerosis. J Neuroimmunol. 2009;211:101–4. Elsevier B.V.
3. Dobson R, Ramagopalan S, Davis A, Giovannoni G. Cerebrospinal fluid oligoclonal bands in multiple sclerosis and clinically isolated syndromes: a meta-analysis of prevalence, prognosis and effect of latitude. J Neurol Neurosurg Psychiatry. 2013;84:909–14.
4. Meinl E, Krumbholz M, Hohlfeld R. B lineage cells in the inflammatory central nervous system environment: migration, maintenance, local antibody production, and therapeutic modulation. Ann Neurol. 2006;59:880–92.
5. Kanter JL, Narayana S, Ho PP, Catz I, Warren KG, Sobel RA, et al. Lipid microarrays identify key mediators of autoimmune brain inflammation. Nat Med. 2006;12:138–43.
6. Blauth K, Owens GP, Bennett JL. The Ins and outs of B cells in multiple sclerosis. Front Immunol. 2015;6:565.
7. Smith JR, Braziel RM, Paoletti S, Lipp M, Uguccioni M, Rosenbaum JT. Expression of B-cell-attracting chemokine 1 (CXCL13) by malignant lymphocytes and vascular endothelium in primary central nervous system lymphoma. Blood. 2003;101:815–21.
8. Magliozzi R, Columba-Cabezas S, Serafini B, Aloisi F. Intracerebral expression of CXCL13 and BAFF is accompanied by formation of lymphoid follicle-like structures in the meninges of mice with relapsing experimental autoimmune encephalomyelitis. J Neuroimmunol. 2004;148:11–23.
9. Cyster JG. Chemokines, sphingosine-1-phosphate, and cell migration in secondary lymphoid organs. Annu Rev Immunol. 2005;23:127–59.
10. Magliozzi R, Howell O, Vora A, Serafini B, Nicholas R, Puopolo M, et al. Meningeal B-cell follicles in secondary progressive multiple sclerosis associate with early onset of disease and severe cortical pathology. Brain. 2007;130:1089–104.
11. Magliozzi R, Howell OW, Reeves C, Roncaroli F, Nicholas R, Serafini B, et al. A gradient of neuronal loss and meningeal inflammation in multiple sclerosis. Ann Neurol. 2010;68:477–93.
12. Howell OW, Reeves CA, Nicholas R, Carassiti D, Radotra B, Gentleman SM, et al. Meningeal inflammation is widespread and linked to cortical pathology in multiple sclerosis. Brain. 2011;134:2755–71.
13. Calabrese M, Magliozzi R, Ciccarelli O, Geurts JJG, Reynolds R, Martin R. Exploring the origins of grey matter damage in multiple sclerosis. Nat Rev Neurosci. 2015;16:147–58. Nature Publishing Group.
14. Rovaris M, Filippi M. MRI correlates of cognitive dysfunction in multiple sclerosis patients. J Neurovirol. 2000;6 Suppl 2:S172–5.
15. Calabrese M, Poretto V, Favaretto A, Alessio S, Bernardi V, Romualdi C, et al.

Cortical lesion load associates with progression of disability in multiple sclerosis. Brain. 2012;135:2952–61.
16. Filippi M, Preziosa P, Copetti M, Riccitelli G, Horsfield MA, Martinelli V, et al. Gray matter damage predicts the accumulation of disability 13 years later in MS. Neurology. 2013;81:1759–67.
17. Zivadinov R, Uher T, Hagemeier J, Vaneckova M, Ramasamy DP, Tyblova M, et al. A serial 10-year follow-up study of brain atrophy and disability progression in RRMS patients. Mult Scler. 2016;22(13):1709–18.
18. Calabrese M, De Stefano N, Atzori M, Bernardi V, Mattisi I, Barachino L, et al. Detection of cortical inflammatory lesions by double inversion recovery magnetic resonance imaging in patients with multiple sclerosis. Arch Neurol. 2007;64:1416–22.
19. Polman CH, Reingold SC, Banwell B, Clanet M, Cohen JA, Filippi M, et al. Diagnostic criteria for multiple sclerosis: 2010 revisions to the McDonald criteria. Ann Neurol. 2011;69:292–302.
20. Kurtzke JF. Rating neurologic impairment in multiple sclerosis: an expanded disability status scale (EDSS). Neurology. 1983;33:1444–52.
21. Amato MP, Portaccio E, Goretti B, Zipoli V, Ricchiuti L, De Caro MF, et al. The Rao's Brief Repeatable Battery and Stroop Test: normative values with age, education and gender corrections in an Italian population. Mult Scler. 2006;12:787–93.
22. Beck AT, Steer RA, Brown GK. Manual for the Beck depression inventory-II. San Antonio: TX Psychol. Corp; 1996. p. 1–82.
23. Teunissen CE, Tumani H, Bennett JL, Berven FS, Brundin L, Comabella M, et al. Consensus guidelines for CSF and blood biobanking for CNS biomarker studies. Mult Scler Int. 2011;2011:246412.
24. Freedman MS, Thompson EJ, Deisenhammer F, Giovannoni G, Grimsley G, Keir G, et al. Recommended standard of cerebrospinal fluid analysis in the diagnosis of multiple sclerosis: a consensus statement. Arch Neurol. 2005;62:865–70.
25. Tanaka M, Matsushita T, Tateishi T, Ochi H, Kawano Y, Mei F-J, et al. Distinct CSF cytokine/chemokine profiles in atopic myelitis and other causes of myelitis. Neurology. 2008;71:974–81.
26. Studer V, Rossi S, Motta C, Buttari F, Centonze D. Peripheral B cell depletion and central proinflammatory cytokine reduction following repeated intrathecal administration of rituximab in progressive Multiple Sclerosis. J Neuroimmunol. 2014;276:229–31.
27. Geurts JJG, Roosendaal SD, Calabrese M, Ciccarelli O, Agosta F, Chard DT, et al. Consensus recommendations for MS cortical lesion scoring using double inversion recovery MRI. Neurology. 2011;76:418–24.
28. Haider L, Zrzavy T, Hametner S, Höftberger R, Bagnato F, Grabner G, et al. The topograpy of demyelination and neurodegeneration in the multiple sclerosis brain. Brain. 2016;139:807–15.
29. Serafini B, Rosicarelli B, Magliozzi R, Stigliano E, Aloisi F. Detection of ectopic B-cell follicles with germinal centers in the meninges of patients with secondary progressive multiple sclerosis. Brain Pathol. 2004;14:164–74.
30 Ma N, He Y, Xiao H, Han G, Chen G, Wang Y, et al. BAFF maintains T-cell survival by inducing OPN expression in B cells. Mol Immunol. 2014;57:129–37.
31 Krumbholz M, Theil D, Cepok S, Hemmer B, Kivisäkk P, Ransohoff RM, et al. Chemokines in multiple sclerosis: CXCL12 and CXCL13 up-regulation is differentially linked to CNS immune cell recruitment. Brain. 2006;129:200–11.
32 Sellebjerg F, Börnsen L, Khademi M, Krakauer M, Olsson T, Frederiksen JL, et al. Increased cerebrospinal fluid concentrations of the chemokine CXCL13 in active MS. Neurology. 2009;73:2003–10.
33 Haas J, Bekeredjian-Ding I, Milkova M, Balint B, Schwarz A, Korporal M, et al. B cells undergo unique compartmentalized redistribution in multiple sclerosis. J Autoimmun. 2011;37:289–99.
34 Ferraro D, Galli V, Vitetta F, Simone AM, Bedin R, Del Giovane C, et al. Cerebrospinal fluid CXCL13 in clinically isolated syndrome patients: association with oligoclonal IgM bands and prediction of multiple sclerosis diagnosis. J Neuroimmunol. 2015;283:64–9.
35 Corcione A, Casazza S, Ferretti E, Giunti D, Zappia E, Pistorio A, et al. Recapitulation of B cell differentiation in the central nervous system of patients with multiple sclerosis. Proc Natl Acad Sci U S A. 2004;101:11064–9.
36 Kornek B, Lassmann H. Axonal pathology in multiple sclerosis. A historical note. Brain Pathol. 1999;9:651–6.
37 Hesselgesser J, Taub D, Baskar P, Greenberg M, Hoxie J, Kolson DL, et al. Neuronal apoptosis induced by HIV-1 gp120 and the chemokine SDF-1 alpha is mediated by the chemokine receptor CXCR4. Curr Biol. 1998;8:595–8.
38 Gardner C, Magliozzi R, Durrenberger PF, Howell OW, Rundle J, Reynolds R. Cortical grey matter demyelination can be induced by elevated pro-inflammatory cytokines in the subarachnoid space of MOG-immunized rats. Brain. 2013;136:3596–608.
39 Vogel DYS, Vereyken EJF, Glim JE, Heijnen PDAM, Moeton M, van der Valk P, et al. Macrophages in inflammatory multiple sclerosis lesions have an intermediate activation status. J Neuroinflammation. 2013;10:35.
40 Zhang Z, Zhang Z-Y, Schittenhelm J, Wu Y, Meyermann R, Schluesener HJ. Parenchymal accumulation of CD163+ macrophages/microglia in multiple sclerosis brains. J Neuroimmunol. 2011;237:73–9.
41 Fabriek BO, Møller HJ, Vloet RPM, van Winsen LM, Hanemaaijer R, Teunissen CE, et al. Proteolytic shedding of the macrophage scavenger receptor CD163 in multiple sclerosis. J Neuroimmunol. 2007;187:179–86.
42 Boven LA, Van Meurs M, Van Zwam M, Wierenga-Wolf A, Hintzen RQ, Boot RG, et al. Myelin-laden macrophages are anti-inflammatory, consistent with foam cells in multiple sclerosis. Brain. 2005;129:517–26.
43 Stilund M, Reuschlein A-K, Christensen T, Møller HJ, Rasmussen PV, Petersen T. Soluble CD163 as a marker of macrophage activity in newly diagnosed patients with multiple sclerosis. PLoS One. 2014;9:e98588.
44 Stilund M, Gjelstrup MC, Petersen T, Møller HJ, Rasmussen PV, Christensen T. Biomarkers of inflammation and axonal degeneration/damage in patients with newly diagnosed multiple sclerosis: contributions of the soluble CD163 CSF/serum ratio to a biomarker panel. PLoS One. 2015;10:e0119681.
45 Komori M, Blake A, Greenwood M, Lin YC, Kosa P, Ghazali D, et al. Cerebrospinal fluid markers reveal intrathecal inflammation in progressive multiple sclerosis. Ann Neurol. 2015;78:3–20.
46 Choi SR, Howell OW, Carassiti D, Magliozzi R, Gveric D, Muraro PA, et al. Meningeal inflammation plays a role in the pathology of primary progressive multiple sclerosis. Brain. 2012;135:2925–37.
47 Lucchinetti CF, Popescu BFGG, Bunyan RF, Moll NM, Roemer SF, Lassmann H, et al. Inflammatory cortical demyelination in early multiple sclerosis. N Engl J Med. 2011;365:2188–97.
48 Absinta M, Vuolo L, Rao A, Nair G, Sati P, Cortese ICM, et al. Gadolinium-based MRI characterization of leptomeningeal inflammation in multiple sclerosis.Neurology. 2015;85(1):18–28.

7

Anti-CD52 antibody treatment depletes B cell aggregates in the central nervous system in a mouse model of multiple sclerosis

Micha Simon[1†], Rojda Ipek[1†], György A. Homola[2], Damiano M. Rovituso[1], Andrea Schampel[1], Christoph Kleinschnitz[3,4] and Stefanie Kuerten[1,5*]

Abstract

Background: Multiple sclerosis (MS) is a chronic autoimmune disease of the central nervous system (CNS) for which several new treatment options were recently introduced. Among them is the monoclonal anti-CD52 antibody alemtuzumab that depletes mainly B cells and T cells in the immune periphery. Considering the ongoing controversy about the involvement of B cells and in particular the formation of B cell aggregates in the brains of progressive MS patients, an in-depth understanding of the effects of anti-CD52 antibody treatment on the B cell compartment in the CNS itself is desirable.

Methods: We used myelin basic protein (MBP)-proteolipid protein (PLP)-induced experimental autoimmune encephalomyelitis (EAE) in C57BL/6 (B6) mice as B cell-dependent model of MS. Mice were treated intraperitoneally either at the peak of EAE or at 60 days after onset with 200 μg murine anti-CD52 vs. IgG2a isotype control antibody for five consecutive days. Disease was subsequently monitored for 10 days. The antigen-specific B cell/antibody response was measured by ELISPOT and ELISA. Effects on CNS infiltration and B cell aggregation were determined by immunohistochemistry. Neurodegeneration was evaluated by Luxol Fast Blue, SMI-32, and Olig2/APC staining as well as by electron microscopy and phosphorylated heavy neurofilament serum ELISA.

Results: Treatment with anti-CD52 antibody attenuated EAE only when administered at the peak of disease. While there was no effect on the production of MP4-specific IgG, the treatment almost completely depleted CNS infiltrates and B cell aggregates even when given as late as 60 days after onset. On the ultrastructural level, we observed significantly less axonal damage in the spinal cord and cerebellum in chronic EAE after anti-CD52 treatment.

Conclusion: Anti-CD52 treatment abrogated B cell infiltration and disrupted existing B cell aggregates in the CNS.

Keywords: Alemtuzumab, B cells, CD52, CNS, EAE, MS

* Correspondence: stefanie.kuerten@fau.de
†Micha Simon and Rojda Ipek contributed equally to this work.
[1]Department of Anatomy and Cell Biology, University of Würzburg, Würzburg, Germany
[5]Institute of Anatomy and Cell Biology, Friedrich Alexander University Erlangen-Nürnberg (FAU), Krankenhausstr. 9, 91054 Erlangen, Bavaria, Germany

Background

Multiple sclerosis (MS) is one of the most prevalent autoimmune disorders of the central nervous system (CNS) [1]. The disease is characterized by inflammation, demyelination, and axonal degeneration [2], eventually leading to severe and irreversible neurological deficits. The typical age of MS onset is between 20 and 40 years with a ratio of 2:1 female to male patients and a higher prevalence in the northern hemisphere. While the etiology of MS is not fully understood, a combination of genetic, environmental, and infectiological factors is assumed to be responsible for disease initiation and progression [1].

Traditionally, the autoimmune pathology of MS has been considered to be mainly T cell-driven [3], while more recent clinical observations as well as experimental data suggest a close interaction of T cells and B cells. Along these lines, depositions of immunoglobulins and of complement components have been found in active demyelinating brain lesions of MS patients [4], and oligoclonal bands (OCB) in the cerebrospinal fluid (CSF) of the majority of patients demonstrate local antibody production. Apart from antibody production, B cells function as highly potent antigen-presenting cells [5] particularly in the brain and are furthermore able to regulate ongoing inflammatory processes, e.g., by secreting pro- and/or anti-inflammatory cytokines. In addition, the overall clinical efficacy of B cell-depleting anti-CD20 antibody treatment and the therapeutic success of plasma exchange in a subset of MS patients with severe corticosteroid-resistant relapses further underlines the involvement of B cells in the immunopathology of MS [6, 7].

Alemtuzumab (Campath-1H) is a humanized anti-CD52 antibody [8], which was first approved for the treatment of patients with chronic lymphocytic leukemia. Alemtuzumab was later shown to be highly effective in patients with relapsing-remitting MS (RR-MS), lowering both the annual relapse rate and the sustained accumulation of disabilities in multiple clinical studies [9]. Improvement of pre-existing disabilities has also been reported. Cells of the acquired immune system, such as T cells and B cells, show high expression of CD52 molecules [10], hence being reduced drastically in numbers in the course of treatment, while cells of the innate system, such as natural killer cells and monocytes, are depleted to a lower extent due to lower CD52 expression. Plasma cells and hematopoietic stem cells lack CD52 and therefore remain unaffected. The absence of CD52 on hematological precursor cells enables maturation and repopulation after treatment, which appears to have a long-lasting tolerance-inducing effect in patients with MS, with more than 50% not requiring disease-modifying therapy 3 years after treatment [11]. This may be due to the slow repopulation of T cells with a relative expansion of $CD4^{+}CD25^{+}CD127^{low}$ regulatory T cells [12–14] as well as a rapid repopulation of mostly immature B cells transiently exceeding baseline levels [15, 16]. While there is no doubt about the value of alemtuzumab for the treatment of RR-MS, further studies are needed to determine if it is equally effective in the case of progressive MS and also to determine whether there are patient subgroups for which individualized treatment would be appropriate.

To further study the immunological mechanisms of action of alemtuzumab, a human CD52 transgenic mouse strain was established [17]. In this mouse strain, both the distribution of CD52 molecules on leukocytes and the depletory capacity of alemtuzumab are comparable to that in humans [18]. However, for the ease of experimentation, a murine anti-CD52 antibody was subsequently established and used in experimental autoimmune encephalomyelitis (EAE) [19], which is the most common animal model of MS. Studies of anti-CD52 treatment in EAE have so far involved the myelin oligodendrocyte glycoprotein (MOG) peptide 35-55 [19–21] and the rMOG:1-121 model in C57BL/6 (B6) mice, as well as the relapsing-remitting proteolipid protein (PLP) peptide 13-151 model in SJL mice [19]. In all of these models, mice were treated on five consecutive days in an early disease stage, which resulted in the depletion of T cells and B cells comparable to MS patients treated with alemtuzumab. Anti-CD52-mediated lymphocyte depletion significantly attenuated clinical EAE, altered peripheral cytokine production, and reduced CNS inflammation, demyelination, and axonal damage. In addition, elevated levels of $CD39^{+}$ regulatory T cells were observed in the gut-associated lymphatic tissue [20]. Since none of the aforementioned studies has used a B cell- and antibody-dependent model, the impact of anti-CD52 treatment on the peripheral vs. central B cell compartment in EAE still remains to be investigated. In addition, the antibody was previously given already with the onset of EAE when scores had not yet reached their maximal severity. Thus, it is unclear whether anti-CD52 antibody treatment is equally effective in more severe forms of EAE and in the chronic stage of the disease. To address these questions, we have employed the MP4-induced EAE model, in which mice are immunized with a fusion protein of myelin basic protein (MBP) and proteolipid protein (PLP) [22–24], and in which both pathogenic B cells and antibodies are induced. Our data demonstrate differential clinical effects of anti-CD52 treatment in acute and chronic EAE. In addition, this study is the first to show that treatment was highly effective in targeting both peripheral and central B cells, including those B cells that had already formed aggregates in the CNS. The disruption of these B cell aggregates was accompanied by a significant decrease in axonal pathology, even in late stages of the disease.

Methods

Mice

Six-week-old female B6 were purchased from Envigo (The Netherlands) and maintained under specific pathogen-free conditions at the animal facility of the Zentrum für Mund- und Kiefergesundheit at the University of Würzburg. The mice had free access to a standard rodent diet (Altromin Spezialfutter GmbH & Co. KG, Lage, Germany) and autoclaved water. Food was softened and kept at ground level for mice that displayed paralytic symptoms to ensure a sufficient diet. All animal experiments were performed according to protocols that were approved by the Regierung von Unterfranken (approval number 91/14) and complied with the German Law on the Protection of Animals and the "Principles of laboratory animal care" (NIH publication no. 86–23, revised 1985).

EAE induction and clinical score

For EAE induction, incomplete Freund's adjuvants was prepared by mixing paraffin oil (EM Science, Gibbstown, NJ, USA) and mannid monooleate (Sigma-Aldrich, St. Louis, USA) at a 9:1 ratio. To obtain complete Freund's adjuvants (CFA), 5 mg/ml *Mycobacterium tuberculosis* H37 Ra (Difco Laboratories, Franklin Lakes, NJ, USA) was added. Each mouse was immunized subcutaneously into both sides of the flank with a total dose of 200 μg MP4 (Alexion Pharmaceuticals, Cheshire, CT, USA), emulsified in a total volume of 200 μl CFA. In addition, mice received 200 ng pertussis toxin (List Biological Laboratories, Hornby, ONT, Canada) by intraperitoneal injection at the day of immunization and 48 h later. Mice were evaluated daily to record onset and progression of clinical symptoms based on the standard EAE scoring system: (0) no disease, (1) floppy tail, (2) hind limb weakness, (3) full hind limb paralysis, (4) quadriplegia, and (5) death. Increments of 0.5 were used to account for clinical deficits in between the defined hallmarks.

Treatment

Mice were treated either with a 200 μg (10 mg/kg body weight) anti-mCD52 antibody, obtained from Sanofi Genzyme (Cambridge, MA, USA), or with a murine IgG2a isotype control antibody (InVivo, Henningdorf, Germany) for five consecutive days. Treatment was given by intraperitoneal injection, and mice were subsequently monitored daily for at least 10 days to determine the treatment effect. Mice were treated either at the peak of EAE ("acute EAE") or at ~ 60 days after EAE onset ("chronic EAE"). For randomization purposes, each mouse in each cohort was assigned to one of the two treatment groups in an alternating fashion once the mouse had developed EAE. Yet, the extent of CNS inflammation was almost exclusively dependent on the EAE score, rather than on the disease duration after onset. Hence, slight variations of the initial randomization strategy occurred since the two groups were score-matched at the beginning of the treatment (Table 1).

Table 1 Clinical parameters of EAE in mice treated with IgG2a isotype control or anti-mCD52 antibody

	EAE onset (days after immunization)	Score at treatment onset	Disease duration before treatment	Final score	Score difference
Treatment at the peak of EAE					
Isotype					
n = 5	15.40 ± 1.40	2.75 ± 0.08	5.20 ± 1.83	2.15 ± 0.22	0.60 ± 0.15
Anti-mCD52					
n = 4	20.25 ± 1.11	2.94 ± 0.36	2.75 ± 1.11	1.50 ± 0.54	1.44 ± 0.21
p value	0.02	0.83	0.37	0.32	0.02
Treatment after ~ 60 days of EAE					
Isotype					
n = 14	16.29 ± 0.85	2.61 ± 0.09	61.57 ± 1.27	2.43 ± 0.15	0.18 ± 0.10
Anti-mCD52					
n = 18	15.28 ± 0.85	2.57 ± 0.11	61.72 ± 1.20	2.47 ± 0.13	0.10 ± 0.07
p value	0.29	0.59	0.95	0.85	0.47

All data are shown as mean values ± SEM. Mann-Whitney test was used to determine statistical significance

Tissue sampling and preparation

Blood samples for flow cytometry were taken from the tail vein 1 day before sacrifice. Mice were sacrificed with CO_2 before a non-perfused draining inguinal lymph node was collected for ELISPOT and blood was drawn from the inferior vena cava for ELISA analysis. Mice were then perfused with 4% paraformaldehyde (PFA) (Roth, Karlsruhe, Germany) in 0.01 M phosphate-buffered saline (PBS) (pH 7.4) for immunohistochemistry (IHC) or with 4% PFA/4% glutaraldehyde (GA) (Roth, Karlsruhe, Germany) in 0.01 M PBS (pH 7.4) for electron microscopy. The cerebellum, lumbar spinal cord, and the other draining inguinal lymph nodes were carefully dissected and post-fixed overnight at 4 °C under slight agitation. While samples for IHC were embedded in paraffin, samples for electron microscopy were embedded in Epon.

Flow cytometry

Blood was collected from the tail vein into heparinized tubes (Liquemin N25000, Roche, Basel, Switzerland). The blood was diluted 1:9 with PBS (total volume 1 ml), and red blood cells were lysed using an ammonium chloride-based lysis buffer. All samples were washed in PBS, transferred to cell culture plates (Greiner bio-one, Kremsmünster, Austria), and stained for 30 min with Fixable Viability Stain 450 (BD Biosciences, San Jose, CA, USA). Staining of T and B cells was performed with rat anti-mouse PerCP-Cy5.5-labeled CD4 (BD Biosciences) and APC-labeled rat anti-mouse CD19 antibody (BioLegend, San Diego, CA, USA) at 4 °C for 30 min. Samples were measured using a BD FACSCanto II (BD Biosciences) with BD FACS Diva software (version 6.1.3) at a flowrate of 1000–2000 events/min until at least 15,000 events were recorded. Further analysis was performed with FlowJo® (version 10.0.6, Tree Star Inc., Ashland, USA). Only viable single cells were included in the analysis. A lymphocyte gate on the FSC-H (forward scatter height)/FSC-A (forward scatter area) profile was set. B cells were characterized as $CD19^{+}CD4^{-}$ and T cells as $CD19^{-}CD4^{+}$ applying a CD4/CD19 bivariate gate. Gates were first set identically for all samples and adjusted individually according to unstained samples. The overall gating strategy is demonstrated in Additional file 1.

ELISPOT analysis

MultiScreen HTS 96-well 0.45-μm ELISPOT plates (Merck-Millipore, Darmstadt, Germany) were coated overnight at 4 °C with 100 μl per well of either 10 μg/ml MP4 (Alexion Pharmaceuticals) or 15 μg/ml anti-mouse IgG (MabTech, Nacka Strand, Sweden) in sterile PBS (Sigma-Aldrich) or with sterile PBS only for negative controls. Plates were blocked with 10% fetal bovine serum (FBS; Gibco, Thermo Fisher Scientific, Waltham, MA, USA) in sterile PBS at room temperature for 2 h. Non-perfused inguinal lymph nodes were dissected, and the suspension was passed through a 70-μm cell strainer (Falcon, Corning, NY, USA). Cells were washed in RPMI-1640 medium before counting them with 0.2% trypan blue (Roth). Samples were resuspended in HL-1 (Lonza, Basel, Switzerland) containing 1% L-glutamine (Sigma-Aldrich) and 1% penicillin/streptomycin (Sigma-Aldrich) and plated at a concentration of 10^6 cells/well. Plates were incubated at 37 °C and 7% CO_2 for 24 h. Goat anti-mouse IgG served as secondary antibody (Dako, Glostrop, Denmark) diluted 1:2000 in 0.5% FBS/PBS and was incubated overnight at 4 °C. Afterwards, streptavidin-alkaline phosphatase (1:800) in 0.5% FBS/PBS was incubated at room temperature for 2 h before Vector Blue substrate kit (Vector Laboratories, Burlingame, CA, USA) was applied according to the manufacturer's instructions. Scanning and image analysis of the plates was performed using an ImmunoSpot Series 6 UV Analyzer (CTL-Europe, Bonn, Germany).

MP4-specific antibody ELISA

ELISA plates (Nunclon™ Delta Surface™ 96 MicroWell, Nalge Nunc International, Rochester, NY, USA) were coated overnight at 4 °C with 100 μl of 3 μg/ml MP4 in PBS. The plates were blocked with 1% milk powder (MP; Herler Bio Magermilchpulver, Heirler-Cenovis GmBH) in PBS/0.05% Tween (Biochemica, Billingham, UK) at room temperature for 2 h. The serum samples were diluted 1:1000 in 1% MP/0.05% Tween in PBS and incubated at 4 °C overnight. Negative control wells contained 1%MP/0.05% Tween in PBS. Biotinylated anti-mouse IgG (eBioscience, Waltham, MA, USA) was diluted 1:800 in 0.1% MP/PBS and incubated overnight at 4 °C. Strepavidin-horseradish peroxidase (BD Biosciences) was diluted 1:1000 in 0.1% MP/PBS and added for 2 h before 100 μl tetrametyhylbenzidin substrate (eBioscience) was used for development. The reaction was stopped with 0.16 M sulfuric acid and analyzed at 450 nm using a Perkin Elmer (Waltham, MA, USA) Victor^3 1420 Multilabel Counter with Wallac 1420 software version 3.00 revision 5.

IHC for $CD3^{+}$ T cells and $B220^{+}$ B cells

In MP4-induced EAE, a focus of B cell infiltration is observed in the cerebellum [25]. To this end, paraffin-embedded cerebella were cut into 4–5-μm-thick serial sections covering the entire tissue. Every seventh (acute treatment group) or ninth (chronic treatment group) section was stained with hematoxylin/eosin in order to screen for the presence of inflammatory infiltrates. To this end, $n = 12$ sections were analyzed per mouse. In case of infiltration, the adjacent section was stained for $CD3^{+}$ T cells and $B220^{+}$ B cells by IHC. The diaminobenzidine (DAB)/Vector Blue staining protocol consisted of the following steps: paraffin-embedded sections were rehydrated and endogenous peroxidase was blocked. After citrate buffer-mediated epitope retrieval and protein blocking, the primary antibodies rabbit anti-mouse CD3 (1:200; Abcam, Cambridge, UK) and rat anti-mouse B220 (1:500; eBioscience) were incubated in 1% normal goat serum (NGS; Sigma-Aldrich)/PBS at 4 °C overnight. Inguinal lymph node sections (5 μm thick) served as positive controls. Biotinylated anti-rabbit and anti-rat antibodies (both Vector Laboratories; diluted 1:250 in PBS) were used as secondary antibodies and incubated at room temperature for 1 h. For CD3 detection, the sections were incubated with rabbit-peroxidase-anti-peroxidase complex (diluted 1:250 in PBS) for 30 min in the dark. The sections were developed with a horseradish peroxidase-based VECTASTAIN ABC kit (Vector Laboratories) and monitored under microscopic control in a solution containing nickel sulfate, glucose, ammonium chloride, DAB, and glucose oxidase. For B220 staining, alkaline phosphatase-conjugated streptavidin and Vector Blue substrate kit (Vector Laboratories) were used. The sections were examined with a Leica DM 2000 LED microscope equipped with a Leica MC150HD digital camera and Leica Application Suite 4.40 Build 454 software (Leica, Wetzlar, Germany). Hematoxylin/eosin-stained sections were used to determine the parenchymal area of the cerebella by ImageJ 2.0.0.-rc-54/1.51b software (National Institutes of Health, USA). All infiltrates were further categorized into non-B cell infiltrates, diffuse B cell infiltrates, and B cell aggregates. Since anti-CD52 treatment completely abrogated the formation of B cell aggregates or disrupted these structures during chronic EAE, staining for lymphoid neogenesis was not performed.

Assessment of demyelination and axonal damage by Luxol Fast Blue (LFB) and SMI-32 IHC staining

The spinal cords and cerebella of the chronic EAE cohort were cut into serial sections of 4 μm. Tissue was stained with LFB to detect demyelination ($n = 12$ sections per mouse) and with anti-SMI-32 antibody to detect axonal damage ($n = 4$ sections per mouse). The DAB staining protocol for SMI-32 consisted of the following steps: paraffin-embedded sections were rehydrated and endogenous peroxidase was blocked. After citrate buffer-mediated epitope retrieval and protein blocking, staining was performed with the M.O.M kit according to the manufacturer's instructions (Vector Laboratories). The primary antibody was used at 1:500 dilution (Covance, Princton, NJ, USA). The sections were developed with a horseradish peroxidase-based VECTASTAIN ABC kit (Vector Laboratories) and monitored under microscopic control in a solution containing nickel sulfate, glucose, ammonium chloride, DAB, and glucose oxidase. For LFB staining, slides were also deparaffinized and subsequently stained with a 0.2% solution of Solvent Blue 38 (Sigma-Aldrich) in 96% ethanol at 60 °C overnight. The process was stopped in 50% ethanol, followed by distilled water. To distinguish between myelinated and non-myelinated areas, the slides were stored in 0.05% lithium carbonate solution for 30 s before removing the dye for 30 s in 75% ethanol and stopping the reaction in distilled water. Differentiation was repeated until gray and white matter were clearly distinguishable. All sections were examined with a Leica DM 2000 LED microscope. Analysis and quantification were done with ImageJ 2.0.0.-rc-54/1.51b (National Institutes of Health). Total white matter area and the demyelinated regions within the white matter were measured, and SMI-32$^+$ axons were counted.

Olig2$^+$APC$^+$ IHC

In the chronic EAE cohort, 4-μm-thick paraffin-embedded sections of $n = 3$ lumbar spinal cords and cerebella were deparaffinized and rehydrated before citrate buffer-based antigen retrieval was performed. Sections were permeabilized for 10 min in 0.25 Triton X/PBS before blocking in 5% NGS/PBS at room temperature for 1 h. Rabbit anti-mouse Olig2 antibody (1:500; Merck Milipore) was incubated at 4 °C overnight. The following day, sections were incubated with biotinylated goat anti-rabbit antibody (1:250; Vector Laboratories) in PBS and with DAPI (1:5000; Roche) at room temperature for 30 min. To perform double staining, the sections were again blocked in 5% NGS/PBS at room temperature for 1 h before incubation with APC primary antibody (Calbiochem, USA) diluted 1:100 in 1% NGS/PBS at room temperature for 2 h. Biotinylated goat anti-mouse IgG (Vector Laboratories) was subsequently applied at a dilution of 1:250 in 1% NGS/PBS at room temperature for 30 min before incubation with NeutrAvidin DyLight 550 (Thermo Scientific). Sections were coverslipped with Mowiol 4-88 (Roth). For analysis, six to eight images of each segment were acquired using a Keyence BZ-9000 fluorescence microscope (Osaka, Japan). Olig2$^+$APC$^+$ cells were counted and white matter area measurements were performed using ImageJ 2.0.0.-rc-54/1.51b software (National Institutes of Health).

Phosphorylated neurofilament heavy (pNF-H) ELISA

pNF-H ELISA was performed with the sera of the same mice that were used for histological analysis. We used a commercially available ELISA kit from Merck according to the manufacturer's instructions.

Electron microscopy

For EM analysis, we obtained a standardized tissue block from the lumbar spinal cord of each mouse. We carefully prepared the whole spine and isolated the part that contained the spinal cord between thorax and the beginning of the cauda equina. Ultra-thin sections were then obtained from the top of each tissue block. For EM analysis of the cerebellum, the tissue of each mouse was cut into six similar blocks. These blocks corresponded to those areas that most likely contained B cell aggregates and thus neurodegeneration according to our previous experience. All six blocks were screened, and images were acquired from those blocks that were affected by neuroinflammation.

For embedding, samples were first washed with PBS and subsequently with 0.1 M cacodylate buffer (CACO, sodium dimethyl arsenate in aqua dest) (EMS, München, Germany) (pH 7.35) three times for 10 min each. Afterwards, samples were stored in 0.1 M CACO buffer at 4 °C under slight agitation. For epon embedding, samples were washed again with 0.1 M CACO buffer three times on a rotating wheel for 10 min each. Then, they were placed into 0.1 M CACO buffer containing 1% osmium tetroxide (OsO_4) (EMS, München, Germany) at room temperature for 4 h. During that time, the tissue was protected from light and deposited on a rotator. The tissue was then washed with aqua bidest twice for 15 min and then for 15 min each in 30%, 50%, 70%, 80%, 90%, and 96% ethanol. After washing twice in 100% ethanol for 15 min each, the tissue was incubated in propylene oxide (EMS, München, Germany) twice for 30 min. The samples were then transferred into a 1:1 mixture of propylene oxide and epon at room temperature overnight and afterwards incubated with pure fresh epon for 2 h. Epon was changed again, and embedded tissue samples were polymerized at 60 °C for 48 h. Epon was prepared by mixing 26 g glycid ether (Serva, Heidelberg, Germany), 11 g dodecenyl succinic-acid anhydride (DDSA) (Serva, Heidelberg, Germany), 15 g methylacid anhydride (MNA) (Serva, Heidelberg, Germany), and 0.25 g 2-,4-,6-tris(dimethylaminomethyl)phenole (DMP) (Serva, Heidelberg, Germany). Embedded tissue was cut transversely at 1 μm on an ultra-microtome (Leica, Wetzlar, Germany, serial number 365952) for semi-thin analysis. Sections were dried at 60 °C for at least 20 min and rinsed in methylene blue (Merck, Darmstadt, Germany) for approximately 45 s. After sections had been washed and dried on a heating plate, they were covered in DEPEX (Serva, Heidelberg, Germany). Digital images were acquired using a Leica DM LB2 microscope, equipped with a Zeiss camera (AxioCam MRc) and Zeiss software (AxioVision 40 4.7). For EM analysis, tissue was cut into 65–85-nm-thick sections. Sections were stretched with chloroform (Roth, Karlsruhe, Germany) while floating in the water tub of the diamond knife (EMS, München, Germany). Afterwards they were carefully put on 100 mesh formvar-coated nickel grids (EMS, München, Germany). For contrast enhancement, the sections were stained with 2% uranyl acetate (Serva, Heidelberg, Germany) in 70% ethanol for 20 min and Reynold's lead citrate solution (Plano, Wetzlar, Germany) for 7 min. The tissue was analyzed using a Zeiss AB912 LEO transmission electron microscope at 80-kV acceleration voltage. Digital images were acquired with an EM digital camera system (Tröndle sharp eye camera, Moorenweis, Germany) equipped with Zeiss software (Image SP × 64) at × 6300 magnification. At least 10 images per mouse and tissue were analyzed, which covered the areas of the spinal cord and cerebellar lesions.

Statistical analysis

Mann-Whitney and one-way ANOVA tests were used for statistical analysis and computed using GraphPad Prism 6 (La Jolla, CA, USA). Statistical significance was set at $p \leq 0.05$. Mean values and standard errors of the mean (SEM) are shown in the graphs.

Results

Anti-mCD52 antibody treatment attenuates acute but not chronic MP4-induced EAE

MP4-immunized B6 mice received 200 μg of anti-mCD52 antibody or IgG2a isotype control by intraperitoneal injection on five consecutive days either at the peak of acute EAE or at ~ 60 days after EAE onset. The mean EAE onset of all treated mice was 16.12 ± 0.55 days after immunization. There was no significant difference in disease severity in anti-mCD52- and isotype control-treated mice at the beginning of treatment in both acute ($p = 0.83$) and chronic ($p = 0.59$) EAE (Fig. 1a–d, Additional file 2, Table 1). In acute EAE, anti-mCD52-treated mice displayed a significant decrease in disease severity 11.56 ± 0.18 days post-treatment, while the scores of isotype control-treated mice remained unaffected (Fig. 1a, Table 1; $p = 0.02$). In chronic EAE, anti-mCD52 treatment did not have any effect on the difference between pre- and post-treatment scores (Fig. 1b; Table 1; $p = 0.47$). In order to determine the extent of depletion of circulating lymphocytes after anti-mCD52 treatment, we performed flow cytometry on tail vein blood obtained 10.37 ± 0.18 days post-treatment and we determined the percentages of viable $CD4^+$ T cells and $CD19^+$ B cells. In the chronic cohort, $CD4^+$ T cells showed a significant reduction from 24.02 ± 1.71% to 3.39 ± 0.52% ($p < 0.001$; Fig. 1e). The percentage of $CD19^+$ B cells was significantly reduced to 6.70 ± 1.23% in anti-mCD52-treated mice compared to 38.28 ± 2.82% in the isotype control group ($p < 0.001$; Fig. 1f). In the acute EAE cohort, comparable results were observed for both T cells (compare 33.82 ± 3.68% to 0.92 ± 0.19%; $p = 0.016$) and B cells (compare 21.51 ± 4.41% to 3.22 ± 1.34%; $p = 0.016$).

Anti-mCD52 treatment does not affect MP4-specific B cells and autoantibodies

In order to determine the effect of anti-mCD52 treatment on peripheral MP4-specific B cells, we performed ELISPOT on draining lymph node cells (Fig. 2a, b) of both anti-mCD52- and isotype control-treated mice in the acute and chronic EAE cohort. Samples were collected 11.37 ± 0.18 days after treatment onset. As shown in Fig. 2, there was no difference between the numbers of MP4-specific antibody secreting B cells expressed as anti-MP4 IgG/total IgG ratio in anti-mCD52- vs. isotype control-treated animals ($p_{acute} = 0.51$; $p_{chronic} = 0.81$). There was also no difference between anti-MP4-specific IgG titers in the sera of both groups ($p_{acute} = 0.73$; $p_{chronic} = 0.75$) (Fig. 2c, d).

Anti-mCD52 treatment significantly decreases immune cell infiltration in the cerebella of acute and chronic MP4-immunized mice

Since our results showed a reduction in blood lymphocyte counts in FACS analysis, we set out to further determine the impact of this lymphocyte depletion on immune infiltration in the CNS. To this end, we screened the cerebella of mice treated at the peak of

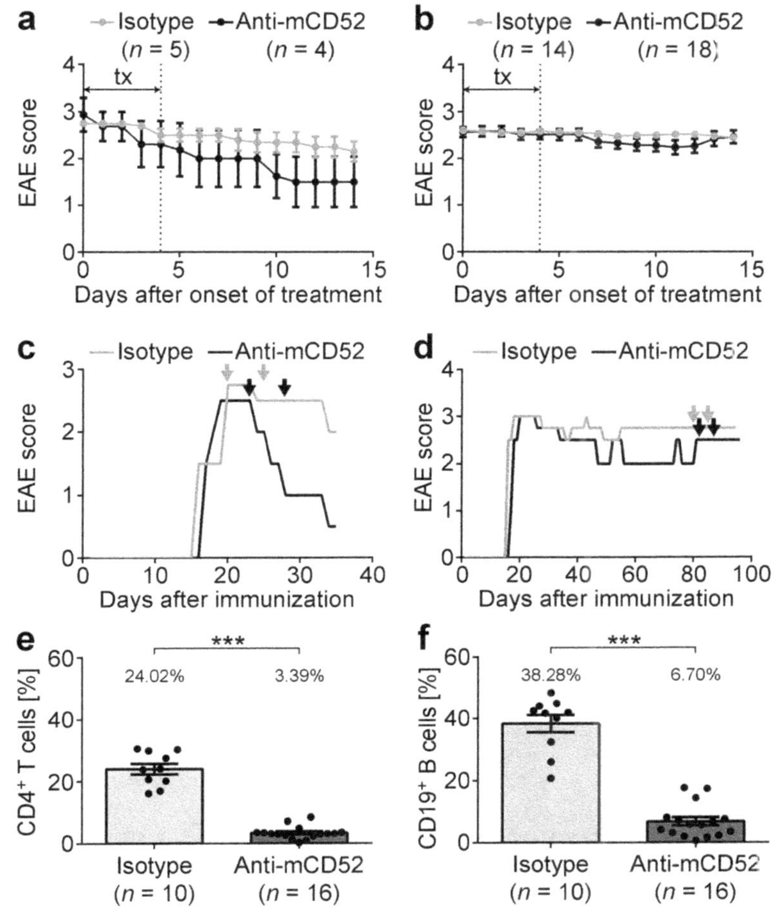

Fig. 1 Disease course in mice treated with anti-mCD52 antibody in the acute or chronic stage of EAE. MP4-immunized mice were treated with 200 μg anti-mCD52 antibody or IgG2a isotype control for five consecutive days (tx) either **a** at the peak of the disease or **b** at ~ 60 days after EAE onset. **c**, **d** Representative disease course of individual animals treated during **c** acute or **d** chronic EAE. Arrows indicate the treatment period. **e**, **f** Flow cytometry of $CD4^+$ T cells and $CD19^+$ B cells in the blood after treatment with anti-mCD52 compared to vehicle. $^{***}p < 0.001$, Mann-Whitney test. Mean values ± SEM are shown. For EAE scores, statistics were calculated based on differences on a daily basis

EAE and ~ 60 days after EAE onset for $CD3^+$ T cell and $B220^+$ B cell infiltration by IHC. The tissue was collected 11.37 ± 0.18 days after treatment. To further differentiate infiltrate categories in the CNS, we defined three different types of lymphocyte infiltration (Fig. 3a–c). Loose perivascular infiltrates of $CD3^+$ T cells in the absence of $B220^+$ B cells were defined as non-B cell infiltrates, while the simultaneous presence of individual $CD3^+$ T cells and $B220^+$ B cells was characteristic of diffuse B cell infiltrates. B cell aggregates were defined as highly compact perivascular aggregation of stained lymphocytes containing at least one-third $B220^+$ B cells. The percentage of perivascular infiltration per parenchymal area was determined for each category in acute and chronic EAE. As shown in Fig. 3, there was a significant overall reduction in immune cell infiltration in the cerebella of anti-mCD52-treated animals in the acute ($p = 0.03$) (Fig. 3d–f) and chronic EAE cohort ($p = 0.002$) (Fig. 3g–i). Strikingly, B cell aggregates were entirely absent in all of the $n = 14$ anti-mCD52-treated animals, while only $n = 4$ of 15 isotype control-treated mice were aggregate-free. Because of this complete depletion of B cell aggregates in the anti-CD52-treated group, we did not perform any further analysis on potential lymphoid neogenesis resulting from B cell aggregation in this study.

Anti-mCD52 therapy does not have neuroprotective effects in MP4-induced EAE

We have demonstrated that anti-mCD52 treatment significantly reduced both peripheral lymphocyte counts and CNS infiltration in MP4-induced EAE. Yet, there was no impact on clinical disease severity in the chronic stage of the disease. This lack of effect on late-stage EAE may be explained by the absence of primarily neuroprotective properties of the drug. We stained sections of the

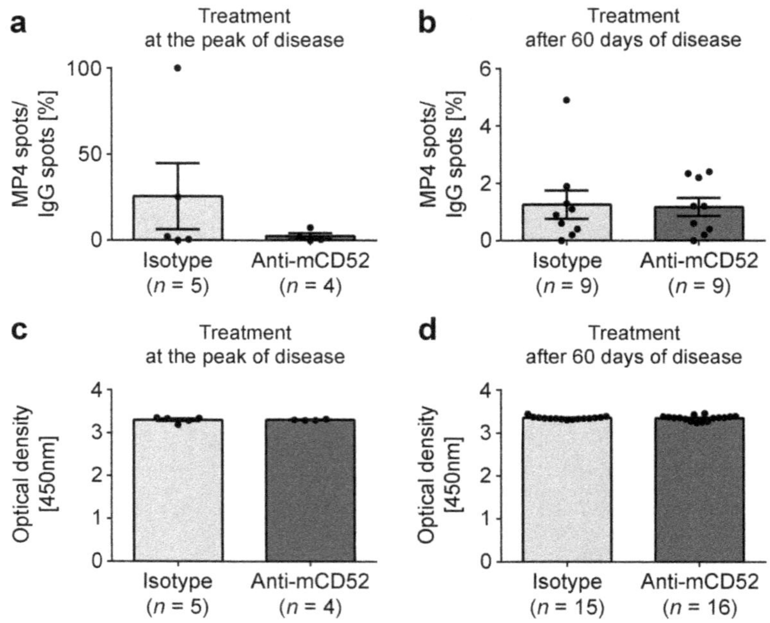

Fig. 2 Measurements of MP4-specific B cells and antibodies. B cell ELISPOT was performed on draining inguinal lymph nodes of MP4-immunized mice to detect the number of MP4-specific B cell spots in relation to the number of total IgG spots during **a** acute or **b** chronic EAE. MP4-specific serum antibodies were measured by ELISA during **c** acute or **d** chronic treatment. Mice were treated with either 200 μg anti-mCD52 antibody or IgG2a isotype control for five consecutive days. Means ± SEM are shown

lumbar spinal cord of anti-mCD52- and isotype control-treated B6 mice of the chronic treatment cohort for demyelination using LFB (Fig. 4a) and for SMI-32$^+$ damaged axons (Fig. 4b). Both the demyelinated area and the number of SMI-32$^+$ axons were set in relation to the total white matter (WM) spinal cord area that was analyzed. We also determined the cell densities of Olig2$^+$APC$^+$ oligodendrocytes (Fig. 4c). The data show that the extent of demyelination ($p = 0.74$) and axonal damage ($p = 0.97$) as well as the cell densities of Olig2$^+$APC$^+$ oligodendrocytes ($p = 0.07$) were comparable between anti-mCD52- and isotype control-treated mice. Similar results were obtained when the cerebellum was analyzed (Additional file 3). To further corroborate these results, we performed pNF-H ELISA on serum samples from the same mice that were used for histology (Fig. 5). It has previously been proposed that the detection of pNF-H in CSF and blood of patients with neurodegenerative diseases provides information about the degree of axonal injury [26]. Indeed, pNF-H has been reported to be present in large amounts in CSF and blood following experimental spinal cord and brain injury in rats [27]. In addition, the detection of pNF-H has been associated with amyotrophic lateral sclerosis [28, 29], optic neuritis [30], and also with MS [31]. In our study, elevated levels of pNF-H were detectable in the sera of MP4-immunized compared to non-immunized control mice. However, there was no difference between anti-CD52- and isotype control-treated mice (Fig. 5).

While light microscopic and serum analyses provide a first impression on neurodegeneration, ultrastructural analysis is needed for detailed quantification. To this end, we used electron microscopy to assess myelin pathology as well as beginning and irreversible axonal damage in both anti-mCD52- and isotype control-treated mice in the spinal cord (Fig. 6) and cerebellum (Fig. 7). In order to distinguish between de- and remyelinating nerve fibers, the g-ratio was used. This ratio describes the relationship of the myelin sheath to its respective nerve fiber. Analysis of $n = 8$ naïve mice allowed us to determine the physiological range of the g-ratio in both the spinal cord (0.40–0.86) and cerebellum (0.48–0.82). While beginning axonal damage can be assessed by the so-called nearest neighbor neurofilament distance (NNND) with a decreased NNND indicating pathology, irreversible axonal damage is reflected by axolysis and axonal loss. Figures 6 and 7 demonstrate that both anti-mCD52- and isotype control-treated mice displayed a significantly increased number of pathological nerve fibers both in terms of demyelination and axonal damage, which pertained both to the spinal cord and the cerebellum. Along these lines, the number of axons was significantly reduced in both EAE groups. While there was no difference in the extent of de- and remyelination comparing anti-mCD52- and isotype

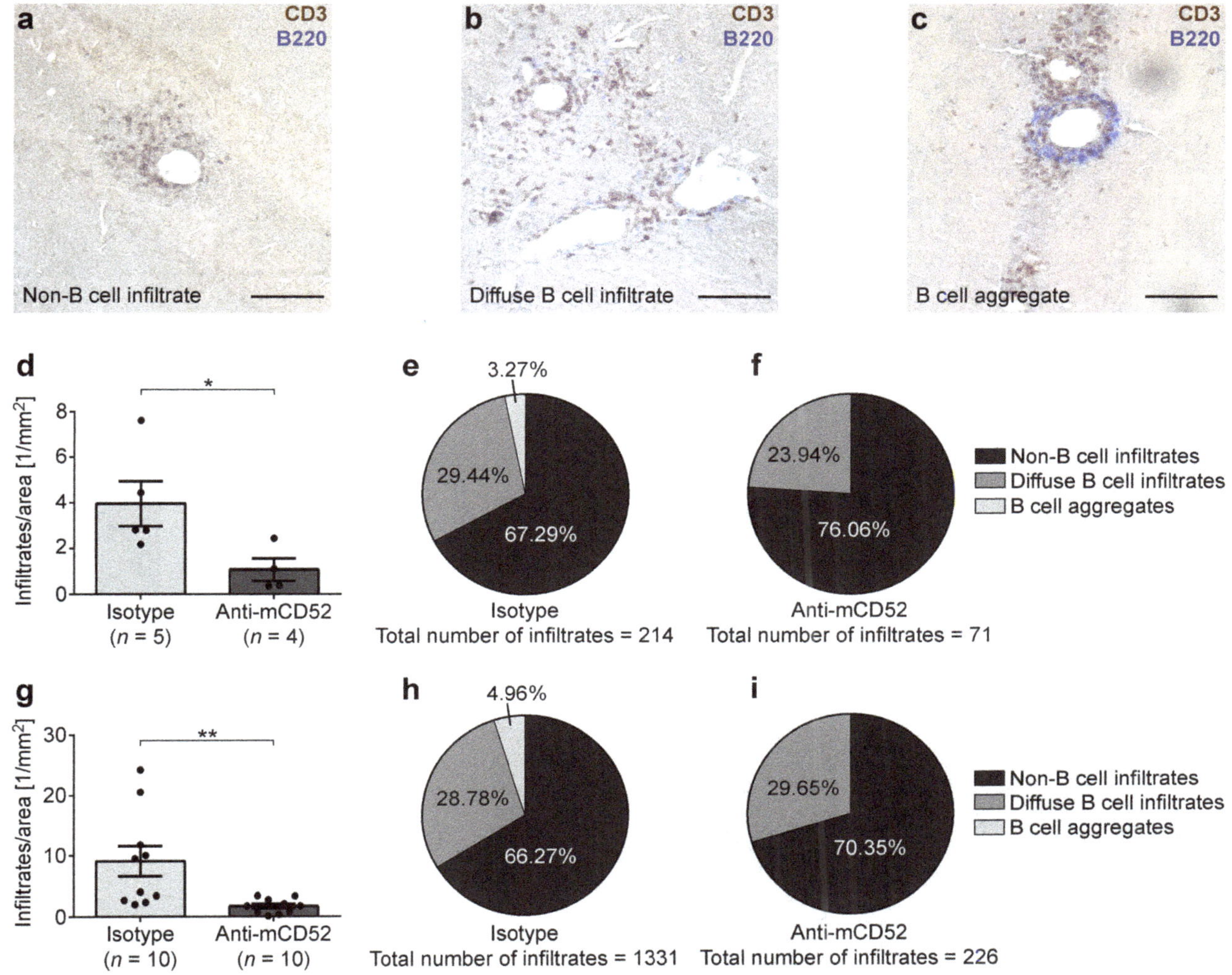

Fig. 3 Histological analysis of B cell aggregates in the cerebella of MP4-immunized mice. **a**–**c** CD3/B220 double staining of representative cerebellar sections of a mouse treated with isotype control at the peak of disease. The panels demonstrate the different infiltrate categories. Scale bars represent 100 μm. **d**–**f** Quantification of the number of infiltrates per parenchymal area and distribution of infiltrate categories in mice treated either with anti-mCD52 antibody or isotype control at the peak of disease. **g**–**i** Quantification of the number of infiltrates per parenchymal area and distribution of infiltrate categories in mice treated ~ 60 days after disease onset. Graphs show means ± SEM. $^{*}p < 0.05$, $^{**}p < 0.01$, Mann-Whitney test

control-treated mice (Figs. 6b and 7b), anti-mCD52-treated displayed significantly decreased axonal pathology and axonal loss (Figs. 6c and 7c).

Discussion

Alemtuzumab, a humanized anti-CD52 antibody, is a relatively new approved treatment option for MS with promising results in multiple clinical trials [32–35]. Yet, the mechanistic effects of the drug on different aspects of MS pathogenesis have remained subject to further research, including the impact of alemtuzumab on the B cell component of the disease. The most recent reports of treatment failure in individual patients with subsequent severe and possibly B cell-mediated relapses underline the importance of further research along these lines [36]. While longitudinal studies on the impact of alemtuzumab on peripheral and CNS B cells are difficult to perform in MS patients themselves, the EAE model offers the possibility of investigating long-term effects of anti-CD52 antibody treatment on both the autoimmune response and also on neurodegeneration and nueroregeneration.

In our model, anti-CD52 antibody treatment drastically reduced the numbers of circulating $CD4^{+}$ T cells and $B220^{+}$ B cells, while the titers of MP4-specific serum antibodies and the numbers of the corresponding plasmablast population in the blood remained unaffected. This was expected and well in line with previous studies in EAE [19–21] and in humans [12, 13, 15, 37] and could be explained

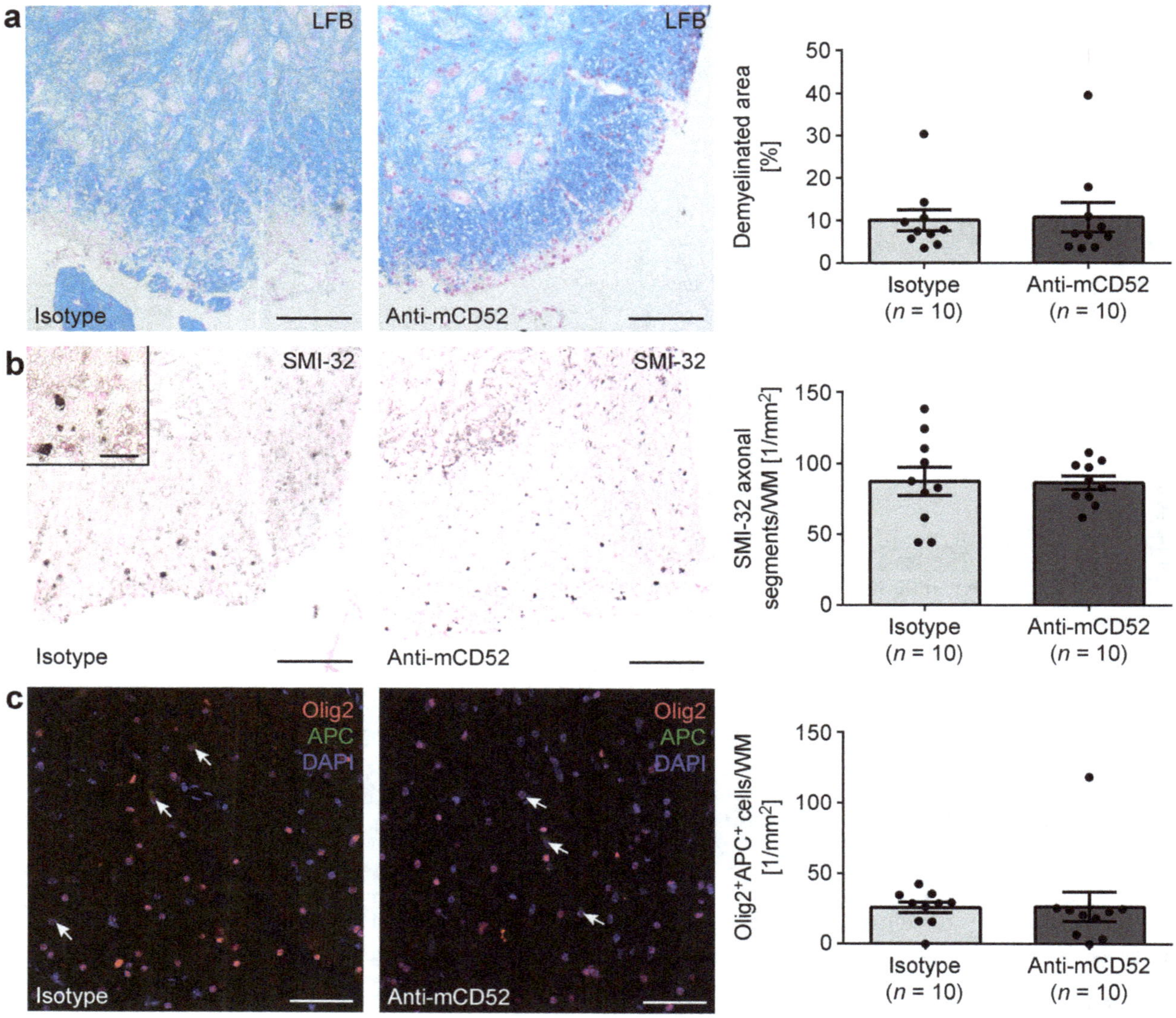

Fig. 4 Detection of spinal cord demyelination, axonal damage, and remyelination in MP4-immunized mice. **a** Luxol Fast Blue staining for the detection of demyelination in spinal cord white matter. **b** IHC for SMI-32 for the detection of axonal damage in spinal cord white matter. **c** IHC for $Olig2^+APC^+$ oligodendrocytes in spinal cord white matter. Analysis was performed in mice that had received treatment in the chronic stage of EAE. Scale bars denote 100 μm. Graphs show means ± SEM

by differences in the expression of CD52 on different lymphocyte subsets. In particular, low levels of CD52 on plasmablasts have been noted before [37].

Unlike previous studies that all relied on T cell-dependent EAE, we immunized mice with the MP4 molecule that induces both encephalitogenic T cells and B cells/antibodies. Using this model, we were able to show that anti-CD52 treatment did not only deplete circulating B cells, but also B cells that had formed aggregates in the CNS. Interestingly, treatment not only prevented the formation of aggregates, but also disrupted already existing aggregates in MP4-induced EAE. The clinical relevance of B cell aggregates in the brains of MS patients is still subject to debate, but an association with an earlier disease onset, progression, and death and with more severe cortical pathology is assumed [38, 39]. These results may support recently published data that found alemtuzumab to reduce the relapse rate in MS patients more efficiently than fingolimod, while being comparable to natalizumab [40]. Mechanistically, it is unclear whether the disruption of B cell aggregates in the brain after anti-CD52 antibody treatment is the result of direct B cell depletion or rather due to a lack of replenishment from circulating peripheral B cells. Natalizumab is a potent anti-VLA4-antibody that blocks the migration of lymphocytes through the blood-brain barrier (BBB) by inhibiting their binding to the cell adhesion molecules

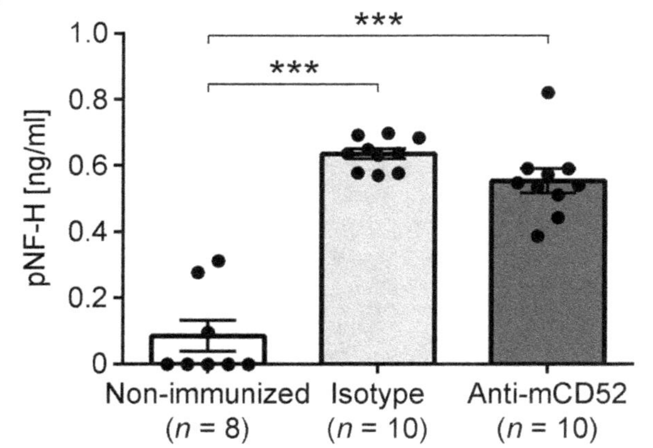

Fig. 5 ELISA detection of pNF-H in MP4-immunized mice. The assay was performed on serum samples from non-immunized control mice as well as from isotype control- and anti-mCD52-treated MP4-immunized EAE mice that had received treatment ~ 60 days after EAE onset. Graphs show means ± SEM. ***$p < 0.001$, ANOVA

VCAM-1 and MAdCAM-1 on the endothelium. The resulting complete or partial disappearance of OCBs in the CSF of a group of RRMS patients treated with natalizumab [41, 42] indicates that constant supply from the periphery is necessary to maintain B cell aggregates if they are considered at least partially responsible for OCB development. We have previously shown that treatment with the $S1P_1$ receptor agonist fingolimod, which inhibits lymphocyte egress from secondary lymphoid organs, prevented the development of B cell aggregates in the CNS in acute MP4-induced EAE, while it did not affect existing infiltrates in the chronic stage of the disease [43]. This rather suggests the independence of B cell aggregates, at least partially, from peripheral support. Yet, our data have also shown that the effect of fingolimod on B cells was much less pronounced than on T cells. Therefore, it is conceivable that there is still ongoing migration of autoreactive B cells into the CNS in the setting of fingolimod treatment, while natalizumab blocks B cell migration more effectively and alemtuzumab depletes the majority of migrating lymphocytes.

Any efficient depletion of lymphocytes in the CNS relies on the penetration of the antibody through the BBB, on sufficient binding to the target cell, and on the activation of antibody-dependent cellular and/or complement-dependent cytotoxicity (ADCC/CDC) in case of the currently available type I antibodies. This has been confirmed for alemtuzumab in vitro [44] and in vivo [17]. While in gadolinium-enhanced magnetic resonance imaging (MRI) studies of lesions in RR-MS patients the BBB has been described to be permeable for antibodies, and complement levels have been reported to be elevated in the CNS, the BBB in secondary progressive (SP-MS) and primary progressive (PP-MS) patients exhibits lower permeability. Indeed, a clinical trial comparing a combination of intrathecal and intravenous application of the anti-CD20 antibody rituximab to placebo in patients with low-inflammatory SP-MS was terminated early since it failed to reach the expected efficiency in the depletion of intrathecal B cells and axonal damage markers in the CSF [45]. Decreased CDC, lack of natural killer cells, and lower CSF flow were made responsible for the failure of the trial. These arguments may also apply to alemtuzumab treatment.

In order to prevent further or even reverse pre-existing neurological disabilities, the search for new treatment options for MS patients focuses not only on immune modulation, but also on neuroprotection [46, 47]. A post hoc subgroup analysis of patients in the CAMMS223 cohort with no clinical evidence of immunological disease activity before treatment and no clinical and radiological disease activity on-trial displayed an overall reduction of clinical disabilities [48]. This could not be explained by the suppression of inflammation due to the depletion of lymphocytes since ongoing neuroinflammation was not detectable in this subgroup. These findings raised hope that alemtuzumab may create an environment of "neuroprotective autoimmunity," with reported higher levels of neurotrophins and oligotrophins resulting in disability reduction. Along these lines, Turner et al. [19] described the reversal of EAE scores in the MOG_{35-55}, MOG_{1-121}, and $PLP_{139-151}$ model early after disease onset after anti-CD52 antibody treatment. Furthermore, they demonstrated neuroprotective effects of the drug in the spinal cord of MOG_{35-55}-immunized mice during acute EAE, reporting a significant reduction in demyelinated white matter, axonal damage, as well as the preservation of axonal conductance. When we applied the anti-CD52 antibody at the peak of MP4-induced EAE, we observed a similar attenuation of clinical EAE. However, there was no effect on EAE scores when treatment was initiated in the chronic stage of the disease ~ 60 days after EAE onset, which had not been evaluated in the other EAE models before [19–21]. Further analysis revealed differential effects of the treatment on CNS degeneration in chronic MP4-immunized mice. In contrast to the results of Turner et al., we did not observe any difference between isotype- and anti-CD52 antibody-treated mice in the light microscopic analysis of demyelination and SMI-32$^+$ axons, indicating axonal damage in the lumbar spinal cord and cerebellum of MP4-immunized mice. These results were underlined by similar levels of pNF-H in the sera obtained from the two mouse groups. Furthermore, we did not observe ongoing remyelination when staining for Olig2$^+$APC$^+$ oligodendrocytes or when performing ultrastructural electron microscopic analysis. Yet, on the ultrastructural level, the numbers of damaged axons were significantly decreased after anti-CD52 treatment. Indeed, electron microscopy allows the precise evaluation of CNS pathology on the level of individual nerve fibers and

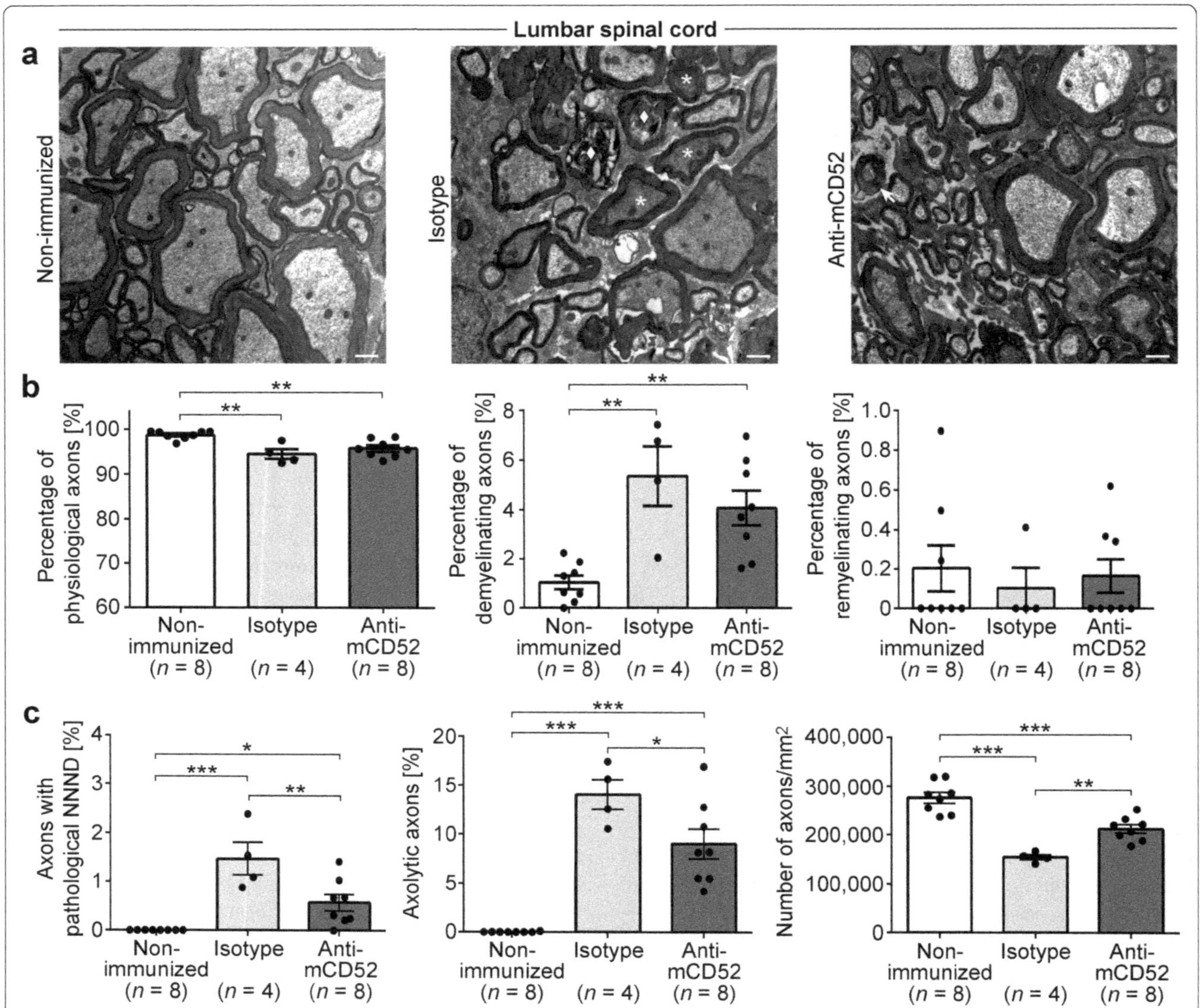

Fig. 6 Electron microscopic analysis of demyelination and axonal damage in the spinal cord of MP4-immunized mice. **a–c** Representative electron microscopic images of the spinal cord of non-immunized control and in MP4-immunized mice that had received treatment with either isotype control or anti-mCD52 antibody ~ 60 days after EAE onset. Scale bars denote 1 μm. The arrow indicates a demyelinating axon. The asterisks represent axons with a decreased NNND, and the diamond shows an axolytic axon. **b** Quantification of the percentage of physiological and of de- and remyelinating nerve fibers in non-immunized control vs. MP4-immunized mice of the two treatment cohorts. **c** Quantification of axonal damage and loss in non-immunized control vs. MP4-immunized mice of the two treatment cohorts. Graphs show means ± SEM. *$p < 0.05$, **$p < 0.01$, ***$p < 0.001$, ANOVA

is therefore much more sensitive than the light microscopic techniques. These beneficial effects on CNS histopathology are likely to the result of reduced CNS inflammation and potentially the disruption of B cell aggregates, which have been described to secrete soluble toxic molecules into the adjacent tissue inducing CNS pathology [39]. This assumption is supported by a 6-year follow-up clinical trial that displayed sustained reduction of the relapse rate, however without improvement of clinical disabilities in a more selective group of alemtuzumab-treated patients with poor prognostic indicators such as high relapse rate, active disease on cMRI scans, and rapidly accumulating disability [34].

Conclusion

This study underlines the potency of anti-CD52 antibody treatment to deplete T cells and B cells in the context of EAE. The novel aspect of this study is the demonstration of a treatment effect on B cell aggregates in the CNS. It will be subject to future studies to determine whether alemtuzumab is equally effective in depleting B cell aggregates in MS patients and whether such depletion is actually associated with clinical benefit. On the one hand,

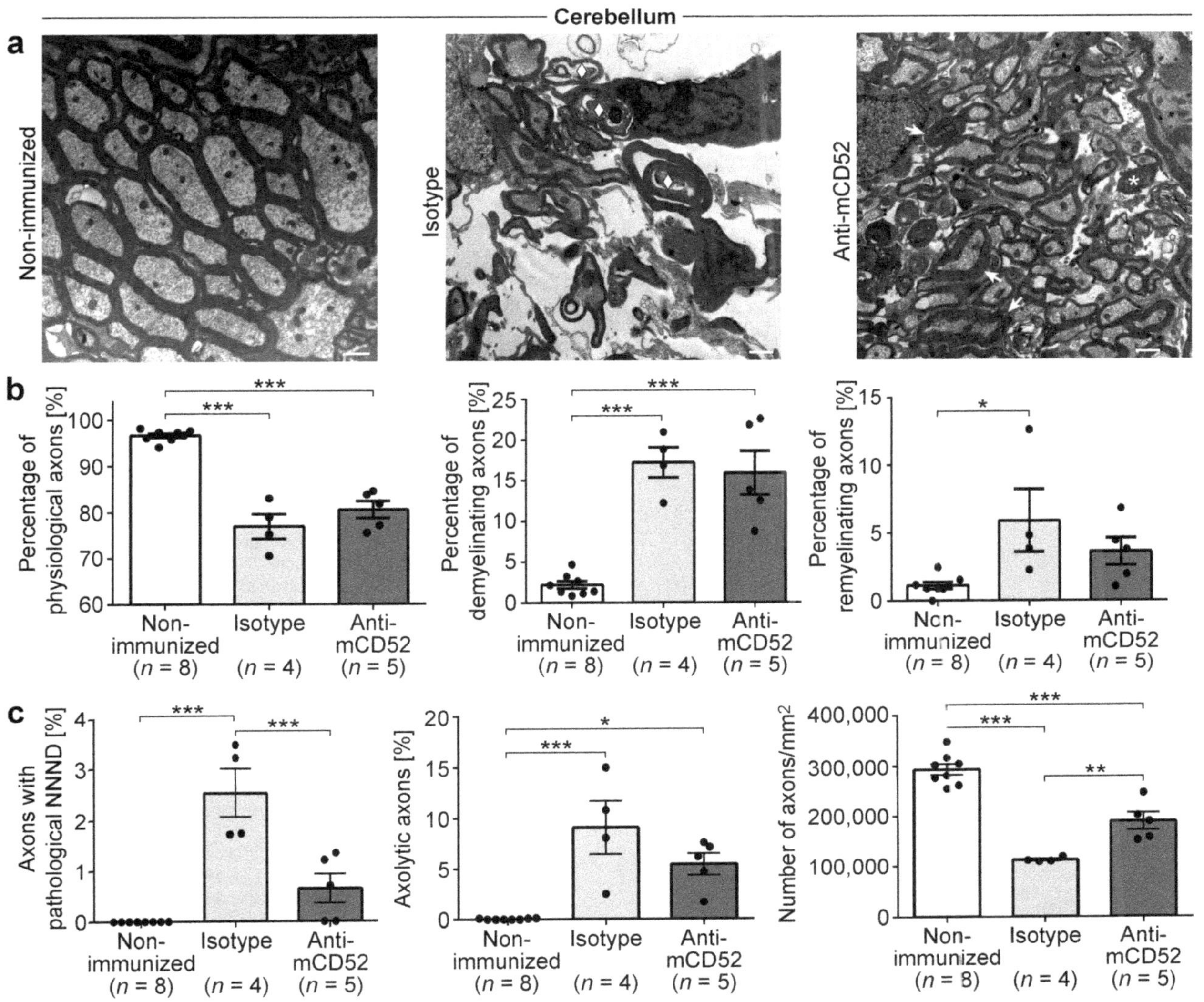

Fig. 7 Electron microscopic analysis of demyelination and axonal damage in the cerebellum of MP4-immunized mice. **a–c** Representative electron microscopic images of the cerebellum of non-immunized control and MP4-immunized mice that had received treatment with either isotype control or anti-mCD52 antibody ~ 60 days after EAE onset. Scale bars denote 1 µm. The arrow indicates a demyelinating axon. The asterisk represents an axon with a decreased NNND, and the diamond shows an axolytic axon. **b** Quantification of the percentage of physiological and of de- and remyelinating nerve fibers in non-immunized control vs. MP4-immunized mice of the two treatment cohorts. **c** Quantification of axonal damage and loss in non-immunized control vs. MP4-immunized mice of the two treatment cohorts. Graphs show means ± SEM. $^{*}p < 0.05$, $^{**}p < 0.01$, $^{***}p < 0.001$, ANOVA

suitable imaging tools to detect B cell aggregate formation in the brains of MS patients would help to address this question. Until such tools may eventually be available, the development of blood- and/or CSF-based biomarkers to measure autoantigen-specific B cell activity may be useful to predict and monitor the effect of alemtuzumab on the B cell compartment in patients and to correlate such an effect with clinical outcomes. On the other hand, while B cell aggregate formation is a characteristic feature of the MP4 model, the actual existence and relevance of these structures in the MS brain is still heavily debated.

Eventually, the permeability of alemtuzumab through the BBB and its mode of action in the CNS itself needs to be further investigated. It may also be worthwhile to consider a type II anti-CD52 antibody, which is supposed to be less dependent on CDC and ADCC by inducing apoptosis directly.

Additional files

Additional file 1: Gating strategy for flow cytometric analysis of viable $CD19^+$ B cells and $CD4^+$ T cells in the blood.

Additional file 2: Comprehensive disease course of mice treated with anti-mCD52 antibody in the acute or chronic stage of EAE, respectively.

Additional file 3: Detection of cerebellar demyelination, axonal damage, and remyelination in MP4-immunized mice. (a) Luxol Fast Blue staining for the detection of demyelination in the cerebellum. (b) IHC for SMI-32 for the detection of axonal damage in the cerebellum. (c) IHC for Olig2$^+$APC$^+$ oligodendrocytes in the cerebellum. Analysis was performed in mice that had received treatment in the chronic stage of EAE. The scale bar denotes 50 µm in (a) and (b) and 100 µm in (c).

Abbreviations

ADCC: Antibody-dependent cellular cytotoxicity; B6: C57BL/6; BBB: Blood-brain barrier; CACO: Cacodylate; CDC: Complement-dependent cytotoxicity; CFA: Complete Freund's adjuvant; CNS: Central nervous system; CSF: Cerebrospinal fluid; DAB: Diaminobenzidine; EAE: Experimental autoimmune encephalomyelitis; GA: Glutaraldehyde; IHC: Immunohistochemistry; IL-4: Interleukin-4; LFB: Luxol Fast Blue; MBP: Myelin basic protein; MOG: Myelin oligodendrocyte glycoprotein; MP: Milk powder; MP4: MBP-PLP fusion protein; MRI: Magnetic resonance imaging; MS: Multiple sclerosis; NGS: Normal goat serum; NNND: Nearest neighbor neurofilament distance; OCB: Oligoclonal bands; PBS: Phosphate-buffered saline; PFA: Paraformaldehyde; PLP: Proteolipid protein; pNF-H: Phosphorylated neurofilament heavy; PP-MS: Primary progressive MS; RR-MS: Relapsing-remitting MS; SEM: Standard error of the mean; SP-MS: Secondary progressive MS; WM: White matter

Acknowledgements

We would like to thank Alla Ganscher, Brigitte Treffny, Karin Reinfurt, and Sieglinde Schenk for the excellent technical support and Michael Christof for the graphical procession of the figures.

Funding

This study was funded by a research grant from Sanofi Genzyme.

Authors' contributions

MS and RI conducted ELISA experiments and statistical analyses. MS conducted the ELISPOT experiments, immunohistochemistry, and drafted the manuscript. RI was responsible for electron microscopy. DRM, MS, and RI conducted the flow cytometry experiments. AS scored the mice. CK, GH, and SK were responsible for the design of the study. SK immunized and treated the mice, conducted ELISA experiments, supervised the study, interpreted the data, and drafted the manuscript. All authors read and approved the final manuscript.

Consent for publication

Not applicable.

Competing interests

The authors declare that they have no competing interests.

Author details

[1]Department of Anatomy and Cell Biology, University of Würzburg, Würzburg, Germany. [2]Department of Diagnostic and Interventional Neuroradiology, University Hospital Würzburg, Würzburg, Germany. [3]Department of Neurology, University Hospital Würzburg, Würzburg, Germany. [4]Department of Neurology, University Hospital Essen, Essen, Germany. [5]Institute of Anatomy and Cell Biology, Friedrich Alexander University Erlangen-Nürnberg (FAU), Krankenhausstr. 9, 91054 Erlangen, Bavaria, Germany.

References

1. Compston A, Coles A. Multiple sclerosis. Lancet. 2008;372:1502–17.
2. Popescu BF, Pirko I, Lucchinetti CF. Pathology of multiple sclerosis: where do we stand? Continuum (Minneap Minn). 2013;19:901–21.
3. Disanto G, Morahan JM, Barnett MH, Giovannoni G, Ramagopalan SV. The evidence for a role of B cells in multiple sclerosis. Neurology. 2012; 78:823–32.
4. Lucchinetti C, Bruck W, Parisi J, Scheithauer B, Rodriguez M, Lassmann H. Heterogeneity of multiple sclerosis lesions: implications for the pathogenesis of demyelination. Ann Neurol. 2000;47:707–17.
5. Meinl E, Krumbholz M, Hohlfeld R. B lineage cells in the inflammatory central nervous system environment: migration, maintenance, local antibody production, and therapeutic modulation. Ann Neurol. 2006;59: 880–92.
6. Hauser SL, Bar-Or A, Comi G, Giovannoni G, Hartung HP, Hemmer B, Lublin F, Montalban X, Rammohan KW, Selmaj K, Traboulsee A, Wolinsky JS, Arnold DL, Klingelschmitt G, Masterman D, Fontoura P, Belachew S, Chin P, Mairon N, Garren H, Kappos L, OPERA I, OPERA II Clinical Investigators. Ocrelizumab versus inteferon Beta-1a in relapsing multiple sclerosis. N Engl J Med. 2017; 376:221–34.
7. Cortese I, Chaudhry V, So YT, Cantor F, Cornblath DR, Rae-Grant A. Evidence-based guideline update: Plasmapheresis in neurologic disorders: report of the Therapeutics and Technology Assessment Subcommittee of the American Academy of Neurology. Neurology. 2011;3:294–300.
8. Hale G, Xia MQ, Tighe HP, Dyer MJ, Waldmann H. The CAMPATH-1 antigen (CDw52). Tissue Antigens. 1990;35:118–27.
9. Willis MD, Robertson NP. Alemtuzumab for multiple sclerosis. Curr Neurol Neurosci Rep. 2016;16:84.
10. Rao SP, Sancho J, Campos-Rivera J, et al. Human peripheral blood mononuclear cells exhibit heterogeneous CD52 expression levels and show differential sensitivity to alemtuzumab mediated cytolysis. PLoS One. 2012;7: e39416.
11. Wiendl H, Bourdette D, Ciccarelli O. Can immune reprogramming with alemtuzumab induce permanent remission in multiple sclerosis? Neurology. 2017;89:1098–100.
12. Cox AL, Thompson SA, Jones JL, et al. Lymphocyte homeostasis following therapeutic lymphocyte depletion in multiple sclerosis. Eur J Immunol. 2005; 35:3332–42.
13. Zhang X, Tao Y, Chopra M, et al. Differential reconstitution of T cell subsets following immunodepleting treatment with alemtuzumab (anti-CD52 monoclonal antibody) in patients with relapsing-remitting multiple sclerosis. J Immunol. 2013;191:5867–74.
14. Havari E, Turner MJ, Campos-Rivera J, et al. Impact of alemtuzumab treatment on the survival and function of human regulatory T cells in vitro. Immunology. 2014;141:123–31.
15. Thompson SA, Jones JL, Cox AL, Compston DA, Coles AJ. B-cell reconstitution and BAFF after alemtuzumab (Campath-1H) treatment of multiple sclerosis. J Clin Immunol. 2010;30:99–105.
16. Heidt S, Hester J, Shankar S, Friend PJ, Wood KJ. B cell repopulation after alemtuzumab induction-transient increase in transitional B cells and long-term dominance of naive B cells. Am J Transplant. 2012;12:1784–92.
17. Hu Y, Turner MJ, Shields J, et al. Investigation of the mechanism of action of alemtuzumab in a human CD52 transgenic mouse model. Immunology. 2009;128:260–70.
18. Turner MJ, Lamorte MJ, Chretien N, et al. Immune status following alemtuzumab treatment in human CD52 transgenic mice. J Neuroimmunol. 2013;261:29–36.
19. Turner MJ, Pang PT, Chretien N, et al. Reduction of inflammation and preservation of neurological function by anti-CD52 therapy in murine experimental autoimmune encephalomyelitis. J Neuroimmunol. 2015; 285:4–12.
20. Pant AB, Wang Y, Mielcarz DW, Kasper EJ, Telesford KM, Mishra M, Haque A, Channon JY, Kasper LH, Begum-Haque S. Alteration of CD39+Foxp3+ CD4 T cell and cytokine levels in EAE/MS following anti-CD52 treatment. J Neuroimmunol. 2017;303:22–30.
21. Barbour M, Wood R, Hridi SU, Wilson C, McKay G, Bushell TJ, Jiang HR. The therapeutic effect of anti-CD52 treatment in murine experimental autoimmune encephalomyelitis is associated with altered IL-33 and ST2 expression levels. J Neuroimmunol. 2018;318:87–96.
22. Kuerten S, Lichtenegger FS, Faas S, Angelov DN, Tary-Lehmann M, Lehmann PV. MBP-PLP fusion protein-induced EAE in C57BL/6 mice. J Neuroimmunol. 2006;177:99–111.

23. Kuerten S, Schickel A, Kerkloh C, et al. Tertiary lymphoid organ development coincides with determinant spreading of the myelin-specific T cell response. Acta Neuropathol. 2012;124:861–73.
24. Kuerten S, Gruppe TL, Laurentius LM, et al. Differential patterns of spinal cord pathology induced by MP4, MOG peptide 35-55, and PLP peptide 178-191 in C57BL/6 mice. APMIS. 2011;119:336–46.
25. Kuerten S, Kostova-Bales DA, Frenzel LP, Tigno JT, Tary-Lehmann M, Angelov DN, Lehmann PV. MP4- and MOG:35-55-induced EAE in C57BL/6 mice differentially targets brain, spinal cord and cerebellum. J Neuroimmunol. 2007;189:31–40.
26. Shaw G. Brain neurotrauma: molecular, neuropsychological, and rehabilitation aspects. In: Kobeissy FH, editor. Chapter 21. Frontiers in Neuroengineering. Boca Raton: CRC Press/Taylor & Francis; 2015.
27. Shaw G, Yang C, Ellis R, et al. Hyperphosphorylated neurofilament NF-H is a serum biomarker of axonal injury. Biochem Biophys Res Commun. 2005;336: 1268–77.
28. Lu CH, Macdonald-Wallis C, Gray E, et al. Neurofilament light chain: a prognostic biomarker in amyotrophic lateral sclerosis. Neurology. 2015;84: 2247–57.
29. Li Y, Zhang L, Kallakuri S, Cohen A, Cavanaugh JM. Correlation of mechanical impact responses and biomarker levels: a new model for biomarker evaluation in TBI. J Neurol Sci. 2015;359:280–6.
30. Petzold A, Rejdak K, Plant GT. Axonal degeneration and inflammation in acute optic neuritis. J Neurol Neurosurg Psychiatry. 2004;75:1178–80.
31. Gresle MM, Liu Y, Dagley LF, et al. Serum phosphorylated neurofilament-heavy chain levels in multiple sclerosis patients. J Neurol Neurosurg Psychiatry. 2014;85:1209–13.
32. Cohen JA, Coles AJ, Arnold DL, et al. Alemtuzumab versus interferon beta 1a as first-line treatment for patients with relapsing-remitting multiple sclerosis: a randomised controlled phase 3 trial. Lancet. 2012;380:1819–28.
33. Investigators CT, Coles AJ, Compston DA, et al. Alemtuzumab vs. interferon beta-1a in early multiple sclerosis. N Engl J Med. 2008;359:1786–801.
34. Willis MD, Harding KE, Pickersgill TP, et al. Alemtuzumab for multiple sclerosis: long term follow-up in a multi-centre cohort. Mult Scler. 2016;22:1215–23.
35. Havrdova E, Arnold DL, Cohen JA, et al. Alemtuzumab CARE-MS I 5-year follow-up: durable efficacy in the absence of continuous MS therapy. Neurology. 2017;89:1107–16.
36. Haghikia A, Dendrou CA, Schneider R, et al. Severe B-cell-mediated CNS disease secondary to alemtuzumab therapy. Lancet Neurol. 2017;16:104–6.
37. Ellebedy AH, Jackson KJ, Kissick HT, Nakaya HI, Davis CW, Roskin KM, McElroy AK, Oshansky CM, Elbein R, Thomas S, Lyon GM, Spiropoulou CF, Mehta AK, Thomas PG, Boyd SD, Ahmed R. Defining antigen-specific plasmablast and memory B cell subsets in human blood after viral infection or vaccination. Nat Immunol. 2016;17:1226–34.
38. Serafini B, Rosicarelli B, Magliozzi R, Stigliano E, Aloisi F. Detection of ectopic B-cell follicles with germinal centers in the meninges of patients with secondary progressive multiple sclerosis. Brain Pathol. 2004;14:164–74.
39. Magliozzi R, Howell O, Vora A, et al. Meningeal B-cell follicles in secondary progressive multiple sclerosis associate with early onset of disease and severe cortical pathology. Brain. 2007;130:1089–104.
40. Kalincik T, Brown JWL, Robertson N, et al. Treatment effectiveness of alemtuzumab compared with natalizumab, fingolimod, and interferon beta in relapsing-remitting multiple sclerosis: a cohort study. Lancet Neurol. 2017;16:271–81.
41. Harrer A, Tumani H, Niendorf S, et al. Cerebrospinal fluid parameters of B cell-related activity in patients with active disease during natalizumab therapy. Mult Scler. 2013;19:1209–12.
42. von Glehn F, Farias AS, de Oliveira AC, et al. Disappearance of cerebrospinal fluid oligoclonal bands after natalizumab treatment of multiple sclerosis patients. Mult Scler. 2012;18:1038–41.
43. Bail K, Notz Q, Rovituso DM, et al. Differential effects of FTY720 on the B cell compartment in a mouse model of multiple sclerosis. J Neuroinflammation. 2017;14:148.
44. Lowenstein H, Shah A, Chant A, Khan A. Different mechanisms of Campath-1H-mediated depletion for CD4 and CD8 T cells in peripheral blood. Transpl Int. 2006;19:927–36.
45. Komori M, Lin YC, Cortese I, et al. nsufficient disease inhibition by intrathecal rituximab in progressive multiple sclerosis. Ann Clin Transl Neurol. 2016;3:166–79.
46. Stys PK, Zamponi GW, van Minnen J, Geurts JJ. Will the real multiple sclerosis please stand up? Nat Rev Neurosci. 2012;13:507–14.
47. Ransohoff RM, Hafler DA, Lucchinetti CF. Multiple sclerosis—a quiet revolution. Nat Rev Neurol. 2015;11 134–42.
48. Jones JL, Anderson JM, Phuah CL, et al. Improvement in disability after alemtuzumab treatment of multiple sclerosis is associated with neuroprotective autoimmunity. Brain. 2010;133:2232–47.

8

Purinergic receptors P2Y12R and P2X7R: potential targets for PET imaging of microglia phenotypes in multiple sclerosis

Wissam Beaino[1*], Bieneke Janssen[1], Gijs Kooij[2], Susanne M. A. van der Pol[2], B. van Het Hof[2], Jack van Horssen[2], Albert D. Windhorst[1] and Helga E. de Vries[2]

Abstract

Background: Microglia are major players in the pathogenesis of multiple sclerosis (MS) and may play a dual role in disease progression. The activation status of microglia in vivo is highly dynamic and occurs as a continuum, with the pro-inflammatory and anti-inflammatory phenotypes on either end of this spectrum. Little is known about in vivo dynamics of microglia phenotypes in MS due to the lack of diagnostic tools. Positron emission tomography (PET) imaging is a powerful non-invasive technique that allows real-time imaging of microglia activation phenotypes in the central nervous system, depending on the availability of selective PET tracers. Our objective is to investigate and characterize the expression of the purinergic receptors P2Y12R and P2X7R as potential targets for PET tracer development and subsequent PET imaging in order to evaluate the dynamics of microglia status in vivo.

Methods: We used immunohistochemical analysis to explore the expression of P2Y12R and P2X7R in experimental autoimmune encephalomyelitis (EAE) post-mortem tissues and different stages of well-characterized MS lesions. We evaluated by quantitative real-time polymerase chain reaction the expression of P2Y12R and P2X7R in human polarized microglia, and we performed autoradiography binding assay with radiolabeled P2Y12R and P2X7R antagonists using MS and rat EAE tissues.

Results: Here, we demonstrate that P2X7R is associated with a pro-inflammatory phenotype of human microglia in vitro, and is highly expressed in microglia in MS lesions as well as during the peak of EAE. In contrast, P2Y12R was associated with an anti-inflammatory phenotype in human microglia in vitro and was expressed at lower levels in active inflammatory MS lesions compared to normal-appearing white matter (NAWM) and similarly in EAE, while its expression increased in the remission phase of EAE. Binding of radiolabeled tracers specific for P2Y12R and P2X7R on ex vivo tissues validated the value of these receptors as PET imaging targets for microglia phenotypes in vivo.

Conclusion: Our results suggest that P2Y12R and P2X7R are excellent targets for PET imaging to discriminate distinct microglia phenotypes in MS. Ultimately, this may provide insight into the role of microglia in disease progression and monitor novel treatment strategies to alter microglia phenotype.

Keywords: Multiple sclerosis, P2Y12R, P2X7R, PET imaging, Neuroinflammation, Microglia

* Correspondence: w.beaino@vumc.nl
[1]Department of Radiology and Nuclear Medicine, VU University Medical Center, Amsterdam, The Netherlands

Background

Multiple sclerosis (MS) is an inflammatory autoimmune disease of the central nervous system (CNS) characterized by massive immune cell infiltration, glia activation, severe demyelination, and neurodegeneration [1]. In the disease progression, microglia play a profound role through the secretion of pro-inflammatory mediators, myelin phagocytosis, and antigen presentation. However, recent insights indicate that in MS, microglia also exert protective and anti-inflammatory effects by the production of neuroprotective factors, thereby playing a role in disease resolution [2–4]. Microglia are highly dynamic cells that are constantly sensing their microenvironment [5, 6]. The activation status of microglia in vivo is highly dynamic and occurs as a continuum, with pro-inflammatory cytotoxic microglia on one end of the spectrum and anti-inflammatory, repair promoting microglia on the other side [7, 8]. In the experimental autoimmune encephalomyelitis (EAE) model, the well-established animal model for MS, it has been shown that pro-inflammatory microglia and macrophages contribute to disease development by secreting inflammatory cytokines and recruitment of cytotoxic T cells into the CNS [9, 10]. On the other hand, anti-inflammatory microglia and macrophages are predominant in the recovery phase where they contribute to phagocytosis of myelin debris and associated axonal regeneration [11, 12]. This protective role was corroborated by several studies showing that injection of macrophages polarized towards a more anti-inflammatory phenotype inhibited or ameliorated EAE associated clinical signs in mice [13, 14].

The role of microglia in MS pathology and its contribution to disease progression remains unclear. The development of new treatments for MS relies heavily on improved understanding of neuroinflammation and the role of activated microglia in the disease evolution. Many questions are still pending concerning the role of pro- and anti-inflammatory microglia in MS and how immunomodulatory therapy affects the state of microglia activation. Getting insights into the molecular dynamics and polarization of activated microglia in vivo is only possible through a highly sensitive and non-invasive imaging technique as positron emission tomography (PET). Current developments in PET imaging of activated microglia are centered around targeting translocator protein (TSPO), a mitochondrial protein overexpressed in activated microglia [15]. TSPO imaging provided valuable information in detecting the presence of active neuroinflammation, but failed to discriminate between pro- and anti-inflammatory states of microglia and was subjected to significant level of polymorphism between different subjects which limited its utility [16]. Hence, there is an urgent need for new PET imaging tools and new target receptors for imaging activated microglia in neuroinflammation.

Ionotropic and metabotropic receptors P2X7R and P2Y12R, respectively, are expressed on microglia and are involved in microglia response to brain tissue damage and neurodegeneration [9]. P2X7R is a purinergic, ATP binding, receptor expressed on immune cells such as monocytes, macrophages, and microglia [17]. In addition, P2X7R plays an important role in activating the inflammasome and subsequent release of IL-1β [18–20]. P2Y12R belong to the family of G protein-coupled receptor, and studies have shown that P2Y12R is only expressed on microglia and not peripheral or infiltrated macrophages in the brain [21, 22].

In this study, we investigated P2X7R and P2Y12R receptors as potential targets for PET imaging of pro- and anti-inflammatory microglia in well-characterized MS tissue samples and the EAE model.

Our data indicate that P2X7R and P2Y12R are promising selective targets for PET imaging of microglia phenotypes in vivo. Visualization of microglia activation and the dynamics of their activation status will provide valuable insights into the status and role of microglia during MS disease progression. Furthermore, it may contribute to a better understanding of the relation between microglia activation status and neurodegeneration, and in the development and evaluation of new immunomodulatory and disease-modifying therapies.

Methods

Reagents

Chemicals were obtained from commercial sources and used without further purification. Solvents were purchased from Sigma-Aldrich (Zwijndrecht, The Netherlands), MERCK (Darmstadt, Germany) and Biosolve (Valkenswaard, The Netherlands) and used as received unless stated otherwise. Tetrahydrofuran (THF) was first distilled from $LiAlH_4$ and then stored on 3 Å molecular sieves. [^{3}H]methyl nosylate stock solution (717 MBq/mL in toluene, molar radioactivity of 3.08 GBq.μmol^{-1}) was obtained from Novandi Chemistry AB (Södertälje, Sweden) and dried at 60 °C under an argon flow prior to use.

Radioligand synthesis

[^{3}H]A-740003

[^{3}H]A-740003 was synthesized in a similar manner as previously described for [^{11}C]A-740003 [23]. Briefly, desmethyl precursor was reacted with [^{3}H]methyl nosylate in the presence of tetrabutylammonium hydroxide for 16 h at room temperature. HPLC purification was performed on a Reprospher 100 C18-DE (50 × 8 mm, 5 μm) column (Dr. Maisch GmbH, Ammerbuch, Germany) using MeCN/H_2O/diisopropylamine (22:78:0.1, *v/v/v*) as eluent at a flow rate of 3 mL.min^{-1}. Fractions containing product (t_R = 16 min) were collected and formulated in

1.5 mL 96% EtOH. Radioactivity concentration (10.9 kBq.μL^{-1}) was determined by liquid scintillation counting (LSC) (LKB/Wallac 1219 Rackbeta, Mount Waverley, Australia) using 5 mL of Optiphase "Highsafe 3" scintillation liquid (PerkinElmer, Waltham, MA, USA). The identity of the product was confirmed with analytical HPLC by coinjection of the product and non-labeled A-740003 ($t_R = 10$ min), and the (radiochemical) purity was > 99%. Analytical isocratic HPLC was performed on an Xbridge C18 5 μm (100 × 4.6 mm) column (Waters, Milford, MA, USA) using $MeCN/H_2O$ (30:70, *v/v*) as eluent at a flow rate of 1 mL.min^{-1}.

[^{11}C]P2Y12R antagonist

Ethyl 6-(3-(3-((5-chlorothiophen-2-yl)sulphonyl)[^{11}C]ureido)azetidin-1-yl)-5-cyano-2-methylnicotinate, as well as precursors ethyl 6-(3-aminoazetidin-1-yl)-5-cyano-2-methylnicotinate and 5-chlorothiophene-2-sulphonyl azide were synthesized as previously described [24]. Hereafter, we will refer to this antagonist as [^{11}C]P2Y12R-ant. Briefly, [^{11}C]CO was transferred to a vial containing a solution of the precursors, chloro(1,5-cyclooctadiene)rhodium(I) dimer and triphenylphosphine in dry THF. The reaction mixture was heated at 100 °C for 5 min, and subsequently, the excess of the azide precursor was quenched, simultaneously evaporating most of THF. After semi-preparative HPLC purification on an Altima C18 5 μm (250 × 10 mm) column (Grace, Columbia, MD, USA) using $MeCN/H_2O$/TFA (55:45:0.1, *v/v/v*) as eluent at a flow rate of 4 mL.min-1, ethyl 6-(3-(3-((5-chlorothiophen-2-yl)sulphonyl)[^{11}C]ureido)azetidin-1-yl)-5-cyano-2-methylnicotinate ($t_R = 16$ min) was formulated in 1 mL of EtOH and diluted with 5 mL of 7.09 mM NaH_2PO_4 in saline. The tracer was obtained in a decay-corrected radiochemical yield (RCY) of 6 ± 2% ($n = 2$; calculated from [^{11}C]CO_2 at end of bombardment) with a radiochemical purity > 99%, a molar radioactivity of 37 ± 4 GBq.μmol^{-1} ($n = 2$). The identity of the product was confirmed with analytical HPLC on a Platinum C18 5 μm (250 × 4.6 mm) column (Grace, Columbia, MD, USA) using $MeCN/H_2O$/trifluoroacetic acid (TFA) (45:55:0.1, *v/v/v*) as eluent at a flow rate of 1 mL.min^{-1} by coinjection of the product and non-labeled reference compound ($t_R = 12$ min).

Human brain tissue

Brain tissue from three controls and eight MS patients were used in this study. Patient details are presented in Additional file 1: Table S1. Brain tissue samples were obtained from the Netherlands Brain Bank (coordinator Dr. Huitinga, Amsterdam, The Netherlands). The Netherlands Brain Bank received permission to perform autopsies for the use of tissue and for access to medical records for research purposes from the Ethical Committee of the VU University Medical Center, Amsterdam, The Netherlands. All patients and controls, or their next of kin, had given informed consent for autopsy and use of brain tissue for research purposes.

EAE model

We used EAE tissues acquired from an independent study performed in our laboratory and the acute experimental autoimmune encephalomyelitis (EAE) was induced as follows. Eight- to 11-week-old male Lewis rats (200 g) obtained from Harlan (Zeist, The Netherlands), as described before [25]. Rats were injected s.c. with 20 μg synthetic myelin basic protein 63–88 peptide, 500 μg Mycobacterium tuberculosis type 37HRa (Difco, Detroit, MI, USA), and 50 μl complete Freund's adjuvant (CFA) (Difco) supplemented with PBS to reach a volume of 100 μl. Rats were examined daily (weight and clinical disease) and graded on a scale from 1 to 5 for neurological signs. Clinical disease in EAE animals was apparent around day 10 post-immunization with a maximum clinical score between days 14 and 15. Animals were housed under standard laboratory conditions with water and food ad libitum. CFA-immunized animals were used as a control. Animals were sacrificed at day 14 dpi (peak of the disease) and day 20 dpi (recovery phase, end of clinical signs).

Immunohistochemistry

For human tissue staining, air-dried frozen sections (5 μm) were fixed with acetone (10 min at RT). For single immunohistochemistry staining of proteolipid protein (PLP), MHC-II, purinergic receptor P2X7R, and P2Y12R, we used the protocol described previously by Vogel et al. [4] using Envision-HRP (Dako) and 3,3′-diaminobenzidine (Dako) as detection method.

For immunofluorescence staining on human tissue, sections were fixed with acetone then blocked for non-specific binding with goat serum (10%) for 20 min at RT. Sections were then incubated with the primary antibody (anti-P2Y12R or anti-P2X7R) in PBS/1% serum overnight at 4 °C. Sections were then washed with PBS three times for 5 min and incubated with fluorescence-labeled secondary antibody (1/400) in PBS/1% serum or for 1 h at RT. Sections were then washed three times for 5 min with PBS and blocked with mouse serum (10%) for 20 min at RT followed by incubation with anti-MHC-II or anti-CD31 or anti-GFAP antibody in PBS/1% BSA for 1 h at RT. After three times of washes for 5 min, a fluorescently labeled secondary antibody was added in PBS/1% BSA for 1 h at room temperature. Nuclei were stained with Hoechst (1/1000) for 1 min in the dark. After a final wash for three times for 5 min with PBS, sections were mounted with coverslips using aqueous mounting media Mowiol.

For rat tissue immunofluorescence double staining, air-dried frozen sections (7 μm) were used. Tissues from three different EAE animals at day 14 post-immunization and three different EAE animals at day 20 post-immunization, and three CFA control rat brains were used. Sections were fixed with acetone for 10 min at RT and blocked for non-specific binding using BSA 2%. Sections were then incubated with a mix of both primary antibodies overnight at 4 °C or 1 h at room temperature. Sections were then washed three times in PBS/0.05% Tween-20 and then incubated with fluorescently labeled secondary antibodies and DAPI (1/1000) for nuclear staining for 1 h at RT. Sections were then washed three times for 5 min with PBS/0.05% Tween-20. Sections were mounted with coverslips using aqueous mounting media Mowiol.

Fluorescence images were acquired using Leica DM6000 microscope equipped with a motorized stage. Whole-slide low-zoom images were acquired using ×10 objective and merged by tile stitching to get the final image. For fluorescence quantification and comparison, sections were stained in a single run and images were collected in a single session with the same exposure time between different areas and different slides. Bright field images were acquired on a Zeiss bright field microscope equipped with a colored camera. Images were analyzed using Leica LAS AF or Zen 2012 software. The list of antibodies used for immunohistochemistry and immunofluorescence are described in Additional file 1: Table S3.

Human microglia isolation

Human microglia isolation and preparation was performed as described elsewhere [3]. In brief, 5 to 10 g of brain white matter was obtained at autopsy, and microglia isolation procedure was performed within 4 to 24 h. Single-cell suspension was prepared using 0.05% trypsin (Sigma, St Louis, MO). Cells were then filtered through a 100-μm nylon mesh (BD Bioscience, Durham, NC) and centrifuged, and the pellet is resuspended in a gradient buffer (3.56 g/L $Na_2HPO_4{\cdot}2H_2O$, 0.78 g/L $NaH_2PO_4{\cdot}H_2O$, 8 g/L NaCl, 4 g/L KCl, 2 g/L d-(+)-glucose, and 2 g/L BSA, pH 7.4) and centrifuged for 35 min at 1200×*g*. The cell debri-myelin layer was removed. The cell pellet was treated with red blood cell lysis buffer (8.3 g/L NH_4CL and 1 g/L $KHCO_3$, pH 7.4) for 10 min at 4 °C. Cells were then suspended and cultured in DMEM/Ham nutrient mixture F10 (1:1), 1% penicillin-streptomycin-glutamine, and 25 ng/mL granulocyte-macrophage colony-stimulating factor (GM-CSF is only added for the first 2 days). After 7 days, microglia were polarized into a pro-inflammatory status by priming with recombinant IFN-γ (1 × 103 U/mL) (U-Cytech, Utrecht, The Netherlands) for 24 h, followed by addition of *Escherichia coli* LPS (10 ng/mL) (LPS-EB ultrapure; Invitrogen, San Diego, CA) to the medium for 24 h. To induce anti-inflammatory microglia, cells were stimulated with IL-4 (10 ng/mL) (Immunotools, Friesoythe, Germany) for 48 h. Untreated cells were referred to as M0.

RNA isolation and real-time quantitative polymerase chain reaction

All oligonucleotides were synthesized by Ocimum Biosolutions (Ocimum Biosolutions, Ijsselstein, The Netherlands). RNA was isolated using triazol. cDNA was synthesized with the Reverse Transcription System kit (Promega, Madison, WI, USA) following manufacturer's guidelines as described previously [26]. QPCR reactions were performed on an Applied Biosystems ViiA 7 machine with the SYBR Green method (Applied Biosystems, Carlsbad, CA, USA). Obtained expression levels of transcripts were normalized to GAPDH and PolRF2 expression levels. Here, we report only the results normalized to GAPDH as we did not observe any difference of normalized data between GAPDH and PolRF2. All primer sequences are listed in Additional file 1: Table S2.

Western blot

Cells were lysed with RIPA lysis buffer containing protease inhibitors for 1 h on ice. The cells were then centrifuged at 14,500 rpm for 15 min, the pellet was discarded, and the supernatant was collected. Electrophoresis was performed under denaturating conditions on 10% SDS polyacrylamide gel. The proteins were transferred to a nitrocellulose membrane. Blots were saturated in Odyssey buffer/PBS (1:1) for 1 h at RT. The blots were incubated with primary antibodies Rabbit anti-human P2X7R (Alomone, Jerusalem BioPark (JBP), Israel), or Rabbit anti-human P2Y12R (Ananspec, LIEGE Science Park, Belgium) in Odyssey buffer/PBS (1:1) + Tween-20 (0.1%) overnight at 4 °C followed by fluorescently labeled secondary antibody (Odyssey) in Odyssey buffer/PBS (1:1) + Tween-20 (0.1%) for 1 h at room temperature. Blots were imaged using Odyssey imager. Blot were then washed and stained with goat anti-human β-actin (Santa Cruz, Heidelberg, Germany) antibody following the same procedure as above. Western blot relative quantification was realized by calculating the ratio of the integrated intensity of the band of the protein of interest over the integrated intensity of the band of β-actin.

Autoradiography

For autoradiography tissues from three non-neurological controls, three active, two chronic active, and three chronic inactive MS lesions, and from three different EAE animals at day 14 post-immunization and three different EAE animals at day 20 post-immunization, and three CFA control rat brains were used. Tissue cryosections (20 μm) of acute EAE and human MS were mounted on glass slides, air dried and stored at −80 °C until use. Sections were washed in assay buffer (50 mM Tris-HCl, pH 7.4) for three times 5 min and then dried under an air flow. Sections were incubated with [^{11}C]P2Y12R-ant (10 nM) for 30 min at room temperature, or incubated with [^{3}H]A740003 for 1 h and 30 min at room temperature. Sections were then washed three times for 90 s with Tris-HCl (50 mM, pH 7.4) and dipped twice in deionized water. Sections were dried under an air flow and exposed to phosphor screen BAS-IP TR 2025 (for tritum-labeled tracer) or phosphor screen BAS-IP SR 2025 (for carbon-11-labeled tracer) (General Electric, Eindhoven The Netherlands) for 1 h for [^{11}C]P2Y12R or 48 h for [^{3}H]A740003. Phosphor screen were then imaged using Typhoon FLA 7000 imager (General Electric, Eindhoven, The Netherlands). The intensity of the signal was quantified using image Quant software (General Electric, Eindhoven, The Netherlands). Three independent experiments were performed.

Statistical analysis

All data are presented as mean ± SD. Groups were compared using the two-tailed Student t test (normal), and Mann-Whitney (non-normal) and analysis were done with Graphpad prism 5 (San Diego, CA, USA). p values of less than 0.05 were considered statistically significant.

Results

Dynamic of expression of P2Y12R and P2X7R in human polarized microglia

To investigate the regulation of P2Y12R and P2X7R expression, human microglia were freshly isolated from 10 different adult post-mortem brains, cultured for 7 days and then polarized into an inflammatory phenotype with IFN-γ/LPS or anti-inflammatory phenotype with IL-4 as described previously [3] (Additional file 1: Figure S1). Expression levels of P2Y12R, P2X7R, and TSPO were measured using quantitative PCR. P2Y12R was significantly downregulated in inflammatory polarized microglia compared to non-stimulated microglia (fourfolds lower, $p < 0.001$). In anti-inflammatory polarized microglia, the expression of P2Y12R was strongly increased compared to non-stimulated microglia (threefolds higher, $p < 0.01$) and pro-inflammatory polarized microglia (12-folds higher, $p < 0.001$) (Fig. 1a).

P2X7R expression revealed an opposite expression pattern with a significant increase in pro-inflammatory microglia (fivefolds higher, $p < 0.01$) compared to non-stimulated microglia and anti-inflammatory stimulated microglia (fivefolds higher, $p < 0.01$). No significant change was observed in anti-inflammatory microglia, which indicates a strong association of P2X7R with a pro-inflammatory microglia phenotype (Fig. 1b). The increased expression of P2X7R in pro-inflammatory microglia and P2Y12R in anti-inflammatory microglia was also observed at the protein level as shown by western blot from the same donors (Fig. 1d, e). Protein level was only evaluated in two donors due to the low amount of microglia cells obtained from the isolations which makes it challenging to have enough protein for western blot analysis. We next investigated the expression of TSPO as this marker is considered to be the state of art for PET imaging of activated microglia. TSPO was highly expressed in pro-inflammatory microglia (1.5-folds higher, $p < 0.05$), albeit less pronounced compared to P2X7R (1.5-folds vs fivefolds, respectively). In anti-inflammatory microglia, no significant change of TSPO expression was observed compared to non-stimulated microglia (Fig. 1c).

Expression of P2Y12R and P2X7R in multiple sclerosis lesions

In order to investigate P2Y12R and P2X7R as targets for imaging microglia phenotype in MS, we analyzed their expression in white matter samples from three non-neurological controls, three active, two chronic active, and three chronic inactive MS lesions (control, Fig. 2a–d; active, Fig. 2e–l; chronic active, Fig. 2m–p, chronic inactive, Fig. 2q–t; Additional file 1: Figure S2-5). P2X7R and P2Y12R were expressed on ramified cells in control brain and normal-appearing white matter (NAWM) that were identified as microglia by their colocalization with MHC-II (Fig. 3). In inflamed MS lesions, P2X7R and P2Y12R are expressed on activated microglia characterized by their round shape and high MHC-II expression (Figs. 2 and 3; Additional file 1: Figure S2-S5). GFAP-(marking activated astrocytes) and CD31- (marking endothelial cells) positive cells in MS lesion, NAWM, or control tissue did not express P2X7R or P2Y12R (Additional file 1: Figure S7-10).

P2X7R and P2Y12R expression on microglia is affected by their activated state. To compare the change of expression of P2X7R and P2Y12R between ramified and activated microglia, we performed colocalization studies with MHC-II in active and chronic active MS lesions. P2X7R was more robustly expressed on activated microglia in active lesions and on microglia in the active rim of the chronic active lesions compared to microglia in the NAWM (Fig. 3m–x; Additional file 1: Figure S11). In contrast, P2Y12R immunolabeling showed a gradual decrease of expression on microglia from the NAWM towards the center of the active lesion (Fig. 3a–l). Interestingly, at the border of the active lesion, we observe a mixed population of activated microglia expressing either high or low levels of P2Y12R; the same pattern was also observed in activated microglia in the

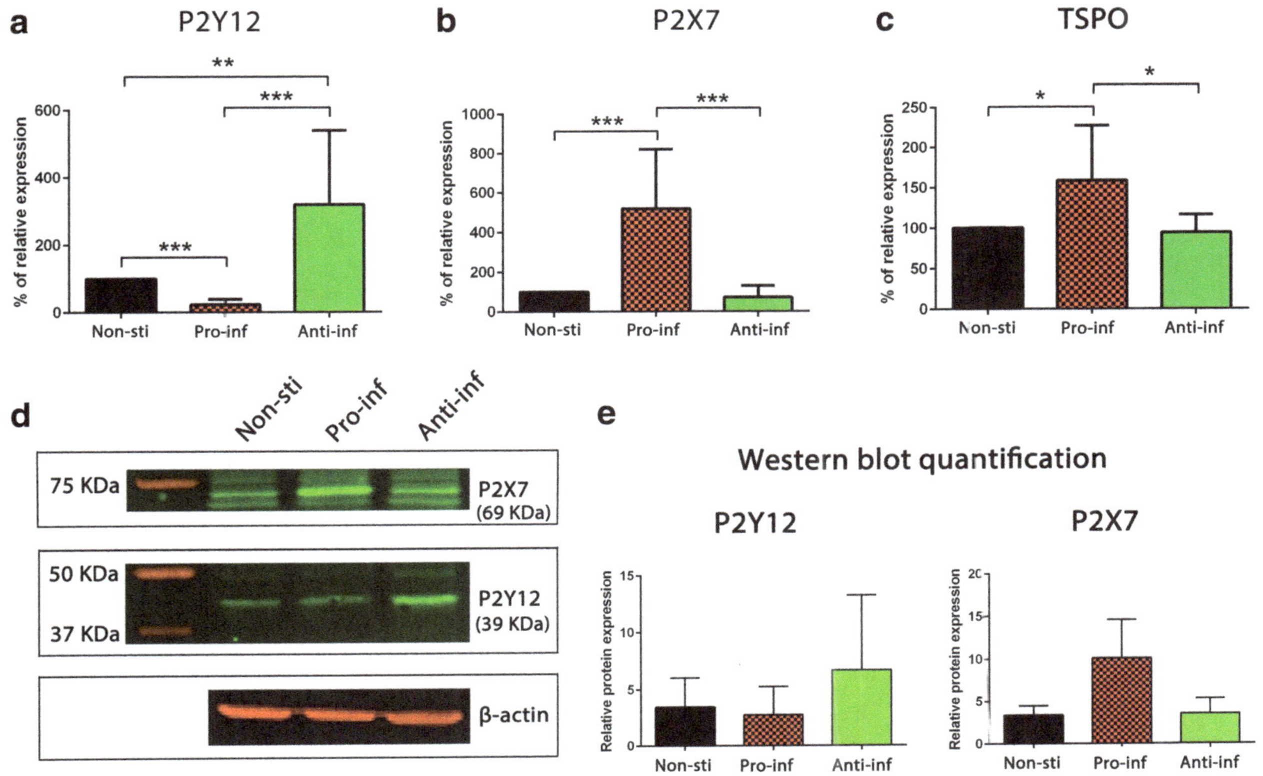

Fig. 1 P2Y12R, P2X7R, and TSPO expression in non-stimulated (non-sti), pro-inflammatory (pro-inf), and anti-inflammatory (anti-inf) polarized human adult microglia. Quantitative PCR analysis and western blot were performed on mRNA and cell lysate collected from non-stimulated, LPS-stimulated pro-inflammatory, and IL-4-stimulated anti-inflammatory human cultured microglia. Expression level of P2Y12R (**a**), P2X7R (**b**), and TSPO (**c**) was evaluated. P2X7R and TSPO were significantly upregulated in pro-inflammatory microglia, and P2Y12R was significantly upregulated in anti-inflammatory microglia ($n = 10$ donors; each sample is done in duplicate). Representative western blot (**d**) and quantification (**e**) of P2Y12R and P2X7R protein expression in non-stimulated, pro-inflammatory, and anti-inflammatory human microglia ($n = 2$ donors). Error bars represent SD. Each sample was done in duplicate. (one asterisk) $p < 0.05$, (two asterisks) $p < 0.01$, (three asterisks) $p < 0.001$

rim of the chronic active lesions (Additional file 1: Figure S12).

P2Y12R and P2X7R expression on microglia in human MS lesions

We observe that P2X7R and P2Y12R are differentially expressed within MS active lesions. In order to investigate the dynamic of expression of P2X7R and P2Y12R, we compared their respective change of expression on ramified microglia in the NAWM and activated microglia in MS lesions. Enhanced expression of P2X7R on activated microglia in the MS lesion is accompanied by a decrease in microglial P2Y12R expression on the same cells (Fig. 4a, b). To further evaluate the relation between the expression of P2Y12R and P2X7R, we quantified their expression by drawing regions of interest (ROIs) around microglia in the NAWM and MS lesion. When comparing the microglia at the ramified less activated state to the highly activated state, we detected that in the majority of microglia an increase of expression of P2X7R coincides with a decrease of P2Y12R expression (Fig. 4c, d). We also observed a small population of activated microglia that shows an increase of P2X7R expression and no decrease in P2Y12R expression; these cells were mostly located at the border of the lesion.

Expression of P2Y12R and P2X7R in acute EAE lesions

To investigate whether the change of expression of P2Y12R and P2X7R that we observed in post-mortem human MS tissue also occurs in EAE, a well-established animal model of MS, we performed immunohistochemistry on tissues from acute EAE induced in Lewis rats. We used cerebellum and brain stem tissue sections where the majority of neuroinflammation and immune cell infiltration occurs in this particular model. Tissues were collected from EAE animals at the peak of the disease (day 14 post-immunization) and in the recovery phase (day 20 post-immunization). Tissues from animals immunized with complete Freund's adjuvant (CFA) were used as control. Microglia were stained with anti-CD11b, and sections were analyzed by differentiating a highly inflamed and a less inflamed area based on the CD11b staining.

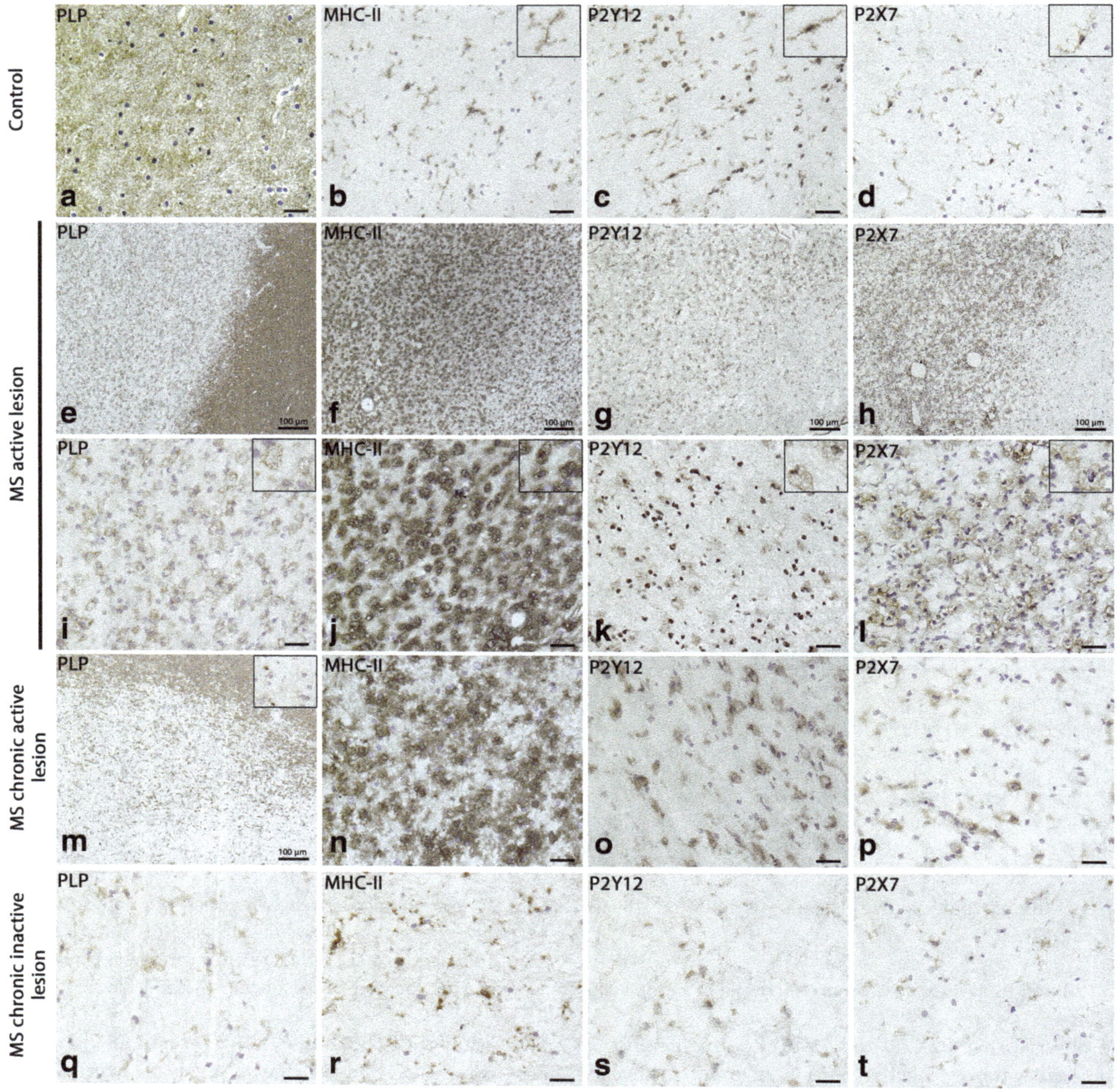

Fig. 2 Expression of P2Y12R and P2X7R in controls, MS active, chronic active, and inactive lesions. PLP and MHC-II staining in different MS lesions and control (**a**, **b**, **e**, **f**, **i**, **j**, **m**, **n**, **q**, **r**). P2Y12R and P2X7R expression on ramified microglia in control human brain tissue (**c**, **d**). P2Y12R expression in MS active lesion (**g**, **k**), chronic active lesion (**o**), and chronic inactive lesion (**s**). P2X7R expression in MS active lesion (**h**, **l**), chronic active lesion (**p**), and chronic inactive lesion (**t**). The images were taken at the middle of the lesion for active sections and at the rim of the lesion for chronic active sections. Scale bar is 20 μm when not specified

We first investigated the expression of P2X7R and P2Y12R in control animals. P2Y12R immunoreactivity localized with CD11b-positive microglia in control brain tissue (Additional file 1: Figure S13). No P2X7R expression was detected in control brain tissue, which may be due to the low expression of P2X7R and/or the low sensitivity of the antibody (Additional file 1: Figure S16).

At the peak of the disease, we observed a marked decrease of P2Y12R on CD11b-positive cells in the highly inflamed area. Quantification of the P2Y12R fluorescence signal revealed a significant reduction of the staining in the inflamed area compared to the less inflamed area (Fig. 5a–d). In EAE, at the end of the recovery phase, P2Y12R is markedly expressed on CD11b-positive microglia compared to microglia in the less inflamed

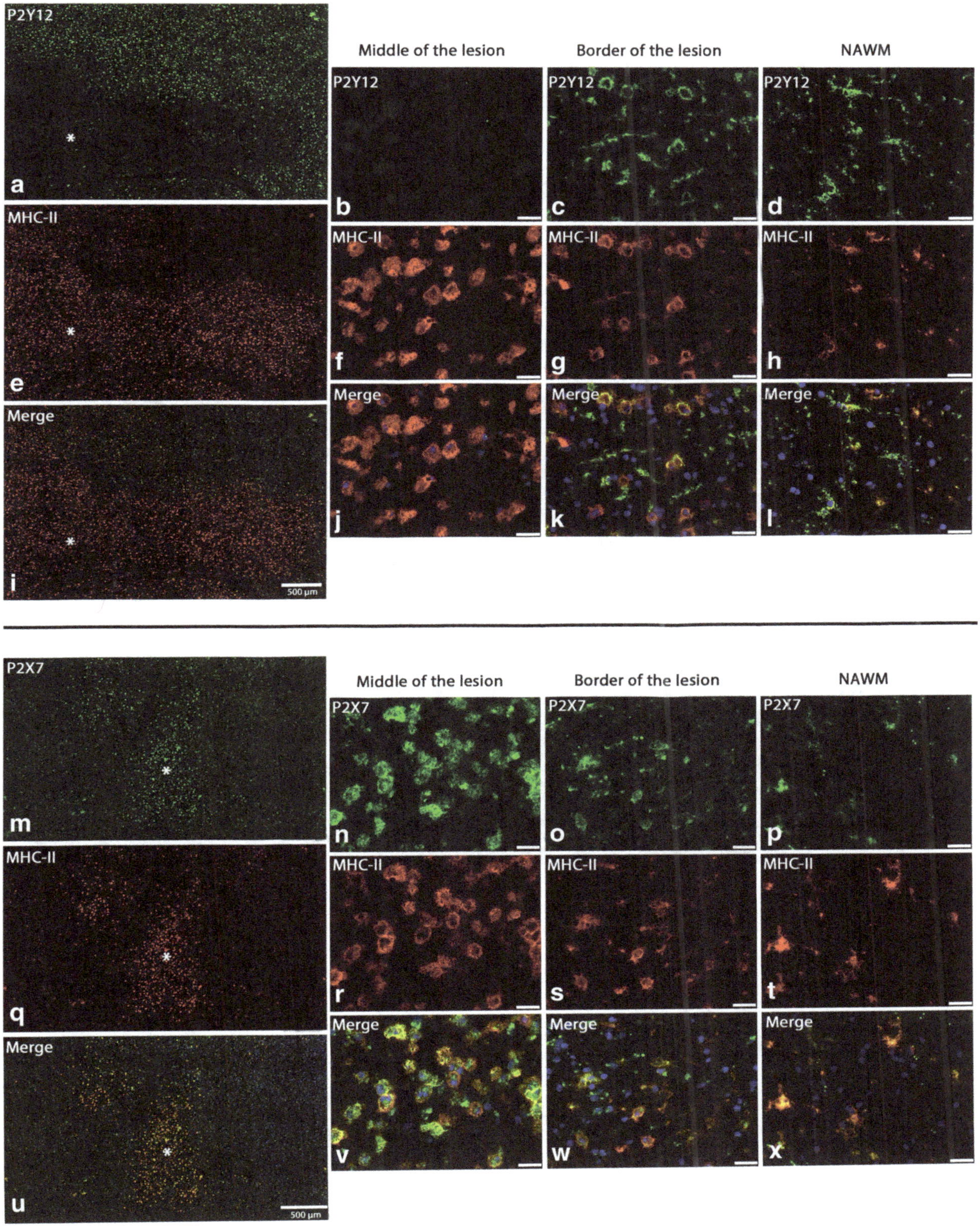

Fig. 3 (See legend on next page.)

(See figure on previous page.)
Fig. 3 Expression of P2Y12R and P2X7R on MHC-II-positive cells in MS active lesion. Low-zoom images showing P2Y12R and MHC-II double staining in MS active lesion (**a**, **e**, **i**); asterisk indicates the center of the lesion. High-magnification images of P2Y12R and MHC-II double staining taken at the center of the lesion (**b**, **f**, **j**), the border of the lesion (**c**, **g**, **k**), and the NAWM (**d**, **h**, **l**). Low-zoom images showing P2X7R and MHC-II double staining in MS active lesion (**m**, **q**, **u**). High-magnification images of P2X7R and MHC-II double staining taken at the center of the lesion (**n**, **r**, **v**), the border of the lesion (**o**, **s**, **w**), and the NAWM (**p**, **t**, **x**). All images were acquired in the same session using same exposure time between different areas to allow comparison. Blue is nuclear staining with Hoechst. Scale bar is 25 μm when not specified

area (Fig. 6a, b). The quantification of the P2Y12R expression showed a significant increase of the P2Y12R expression in the inflamed area compared to the less inflamed area (Fig. 6c, d). Infiltrating monocyte-derived macrophages (ED1-positive) in the perivascular area did not express P2Y12R (Additional file 1: Figure S14).

P2X7R was highly expressed on CD11b-positive cells in the EAE tissue at the peak of the disease and at the end of the recovery phase. The expression of P2X7R on activated microglia in the inflamed area was higher compared to the ramified microglia in the less inflamed area (Fig. 7a, b).

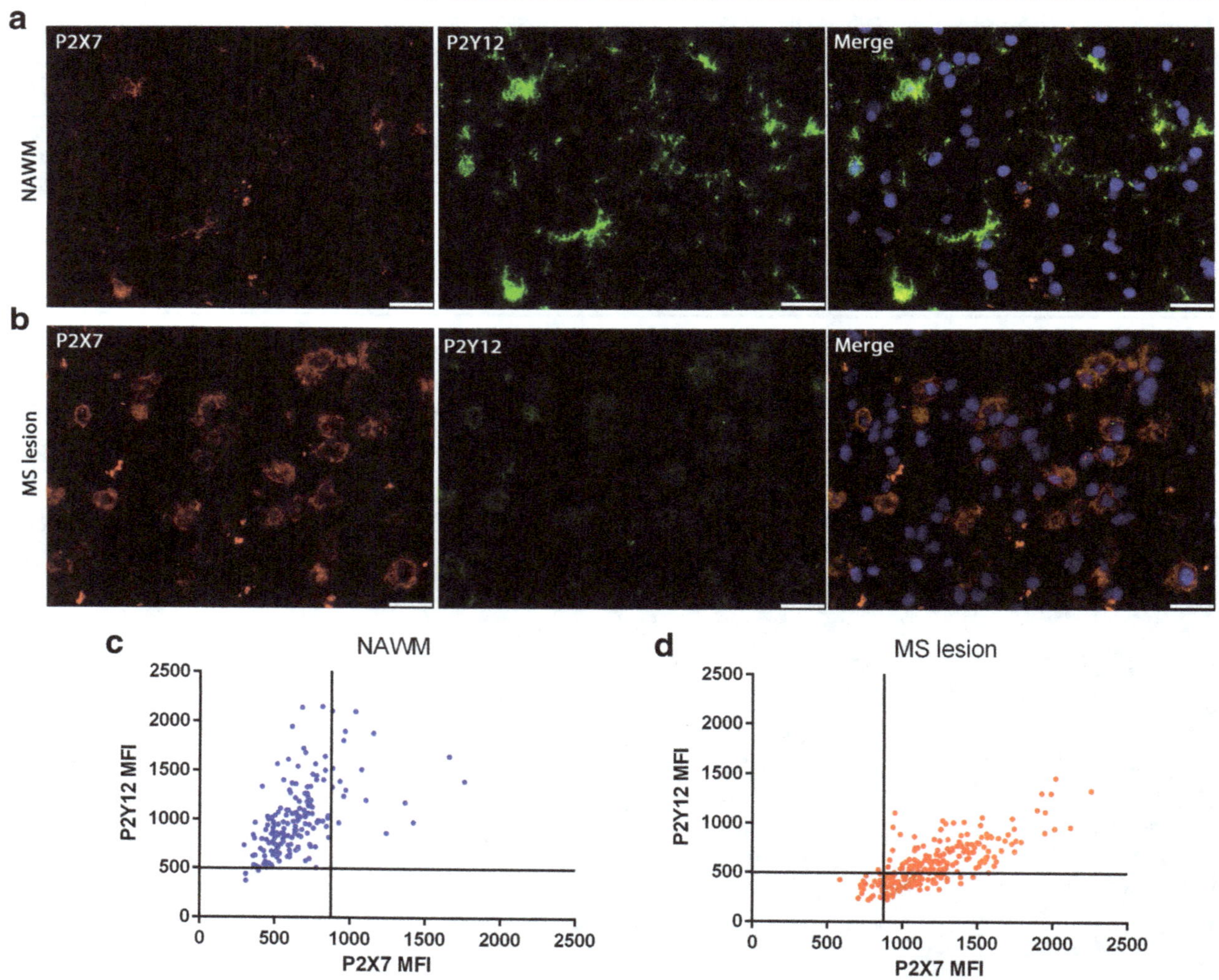

Fig. 4 Expression of P2Y12R and P2X7R on microglia in NAWM and human MS active lesion. Double staining showing the expression of P2Y12R and P2X7R in NAWM (**a**) and MS active lesion (**b**). Images were collected from the same section with the same exposure time between different areas to allow comparison. Scatter plot showing quantification of P2Y12R and P2X7R fluorescence mean intensity (MFI) on microglia in NAWM (179 cells quantified) (**c**), and active MS lesion (241 cells quantified) (**d**). Each dot represents a single cell. All images for quantification were collected from a single section and were acquired in a single imaging session with the same exposure time. Regions of interest (ROIs) were drawn manually delineating each cell using Leica LAS AF software

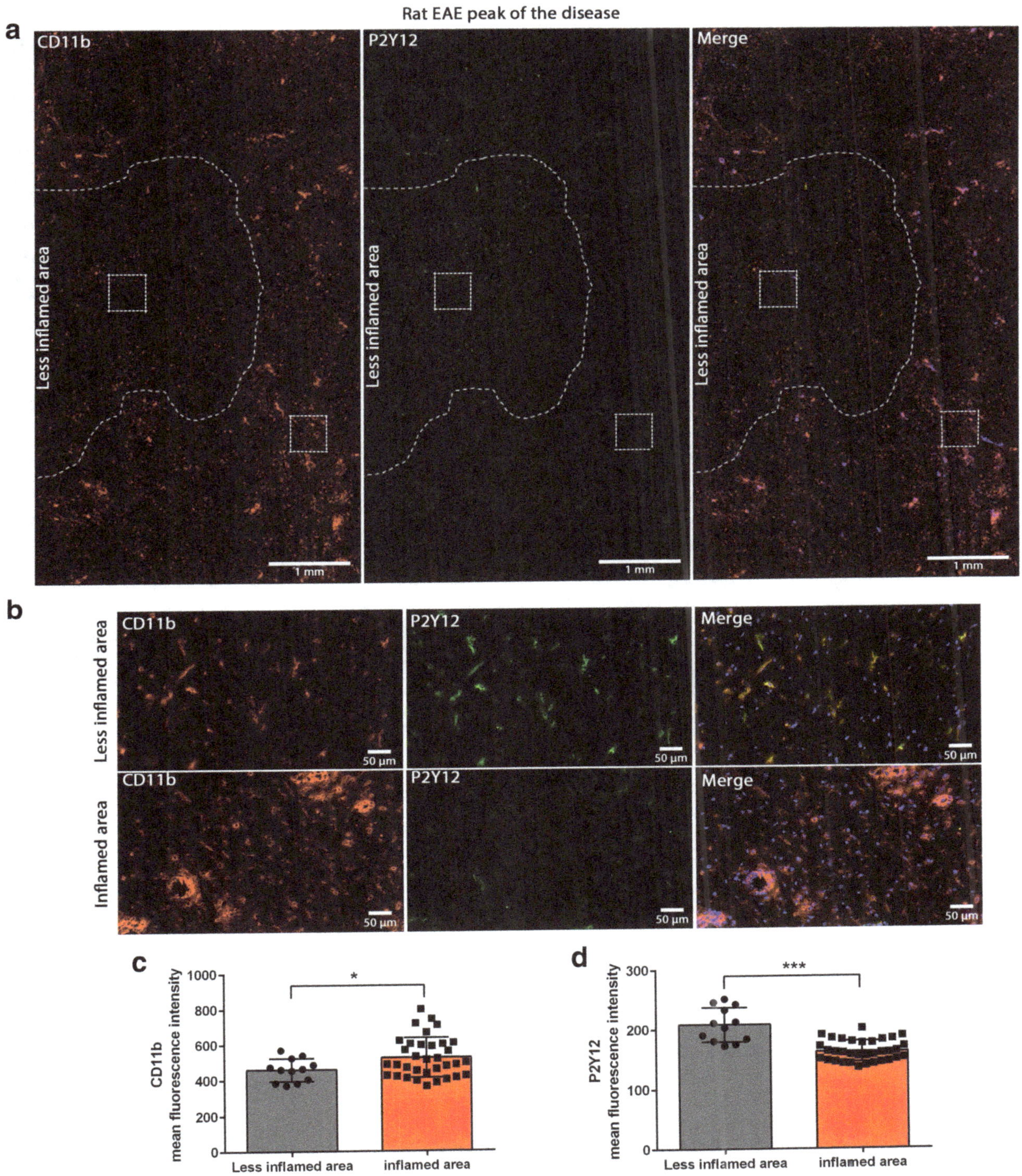

Fig. 5 P2Y12R expression is downregulated on activated microglia in EAE at the peak of the disease. P2Y12R and CD11b double staining on EAE tissues from the peak of the disease showing a highly infiltrated and inflamed area, and a less inflamed area (**a**). Higher magnification images of P2Y12R and CD11b staining showing a reduction of P2Y12R expression on microglia in the high inflamed area comparec the less inflamed area (**b**). Fluorescence quantification of CD11b (**c**) and P2Y12R (**d**) showing a significant increase in CD11b expression and a significant decrease of P2Y12R expression in the highly inflamed area compared to the less inflamed area. Each circle and square represents one drawn region of interest (ROI) and represents tissues from two different rats. Different groups were compared using the Student *t* test, (one asterisk) $p < 0.05$, (three asterisks) $p < 0.0001$. Blue is nuclear staining with DAPI

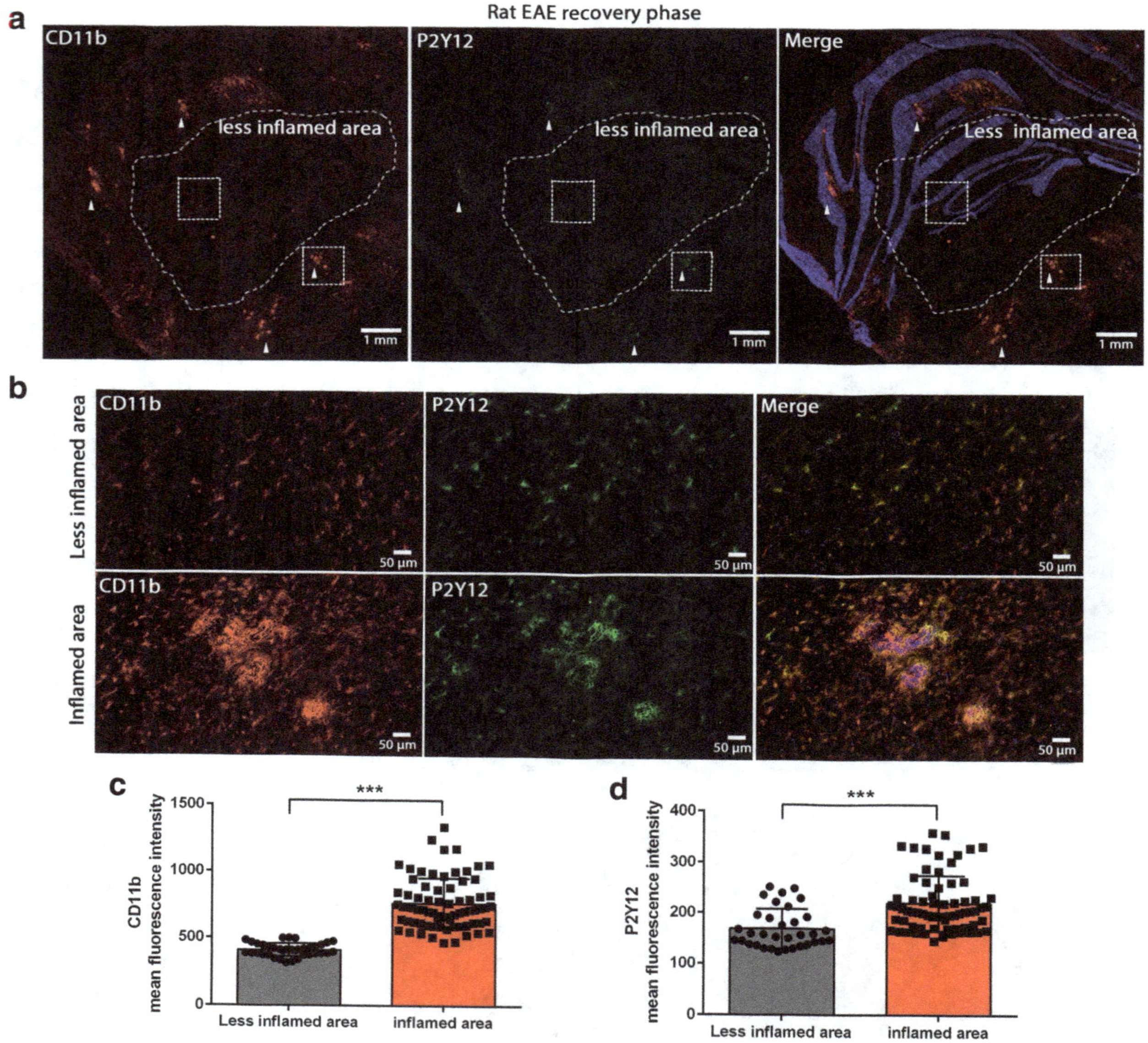

Fig. 6 P2Y12R expression is upregulated on activated microglia in EAE in the recovery phase. P2Y12R and CD11b double staining on EAE tissues from the recovery phase showing a highly infiltrated and inflamed area, and a less inflamed area. Arrow head shows high P2Y12R staining on CD11b positive cells (**a**). Higher magnification images of P2Y12R and CD11b staining showing an increase of P2Y12R expression on microglia in the high inflamed area compared the less inflamed area (**b**). Fluorescence quantification of CD11b (**c**) and P2Y12R (**d**) showing a significant increase in CD11b and P2Y12R expression in the highly inflamed area compared to the less inflamed area. Each circle and square represents one drawn region of interest (ROI) and represents tissues from three different rats. Different groups were compared using student t-test, (one asterisk) $p < 0.05$, (three asterisks) $p < 0.0001$. Blue is nuclear staining with DAPI

Binding of P2Y12R and P2X7R radiolabeled tracers on MS and acute EAE tissue

To investigate the binding of PET tracers and their ability to predict and follow the change of P2Y12R and P2X7R expression, we performed autoradiography binding experiment using a carbon-11-labeled specific P2Y12R tracer ([^{11}C]P2Y12R-ant) and tritium-labeled P2X7R-specific tracer ([^{3}H]A-740003) for binding to EAE and human MS post-mortem tissues. For these binding experiments, we used sections from the same human MS and EAE tissues blocks as for the immunostaining experiments. In tissue from acute EAE animals, we observed a significant decrease of binding of the [^{11}C]P2Y12R-ant tracer at the peak of the disease compared to the control that increases back in the recovery phase. P2X7R tracer, [^{3}H]A-740003, showed a significant increase of binding to EAE tissues from the peak of the disease compared to control. The binding of [^{3}H]A-

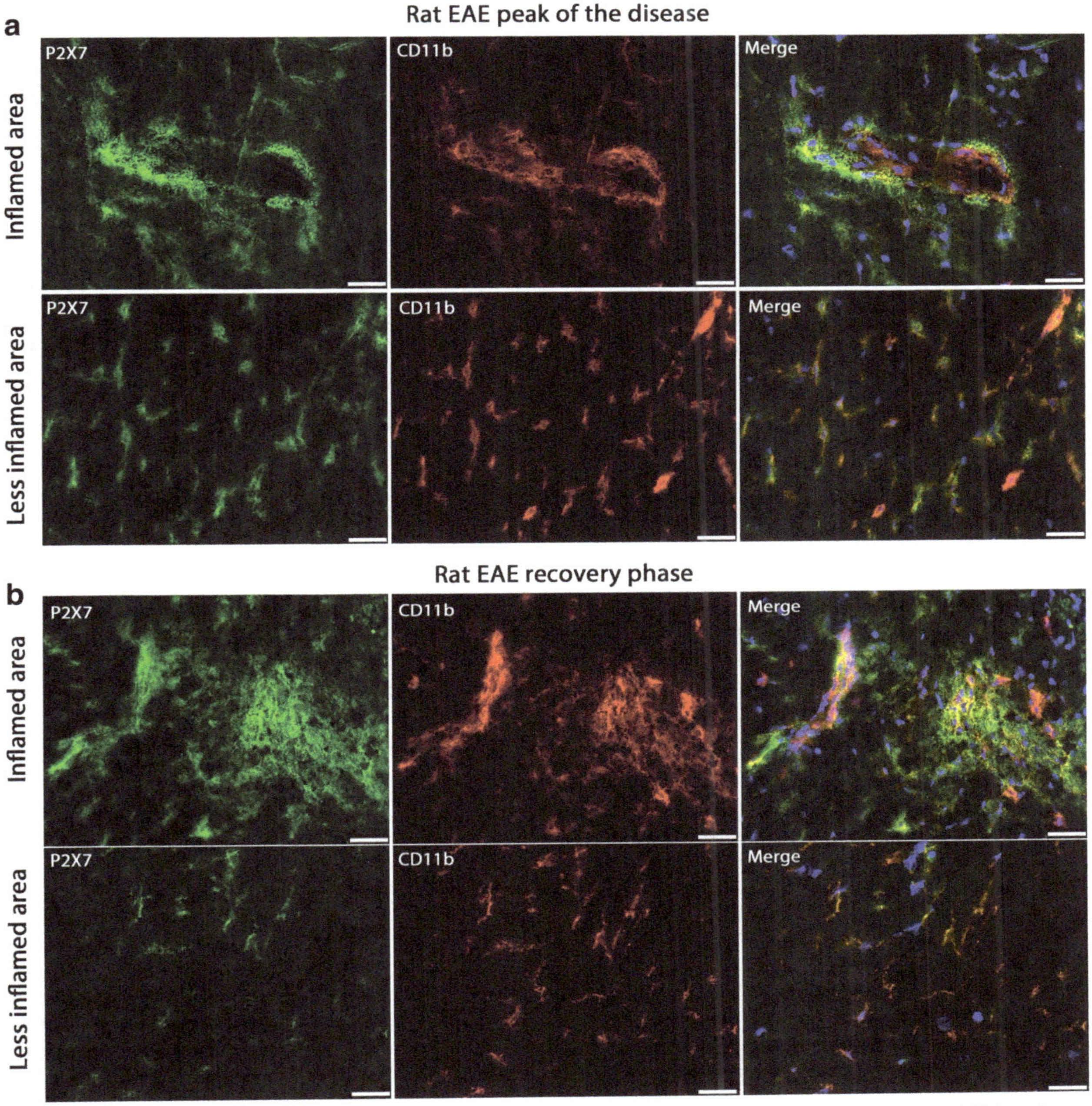

Fig. 7 P2X7R expression in rat EAE at the peak of the disease and in the recovery phase. P2X7R and CD11b double staining on EAE tissue from the peak of the disease (**a**) and the recovery phase (**b**). Blue is nuclear staining with DAPI. Scale bar is 25 μm

740003 slightly decreased in the recovery phase (Fig. 8a–c). In human MS tissues, the binding of [^{11}C]P2Y12R-ant tracer was significantly decreased in all types of MS lesions (active, chronic active, and chronic inactive) compared to control (Fig. 8d, f). The binding of P2X7R tracer [^{3}H]A-740003 was significantly increased only in the MS active lesion while there was a slight non-significant increase in chronic active lesions and a decrease in the chronic inactive lesions compared to control (Fig. 8e, f). We also performed blocking studies and post-autoradiography immunostaining; our data showed that the binding of both tracers is specific and matches the antibody staining (Additional file 1: Figure S17-19). The binding of the P2X7R and P2Y12R tracers correlated with our immunohistochemistry results which further validate these receptors as potential targets for use in PET imaging of activated microglia.

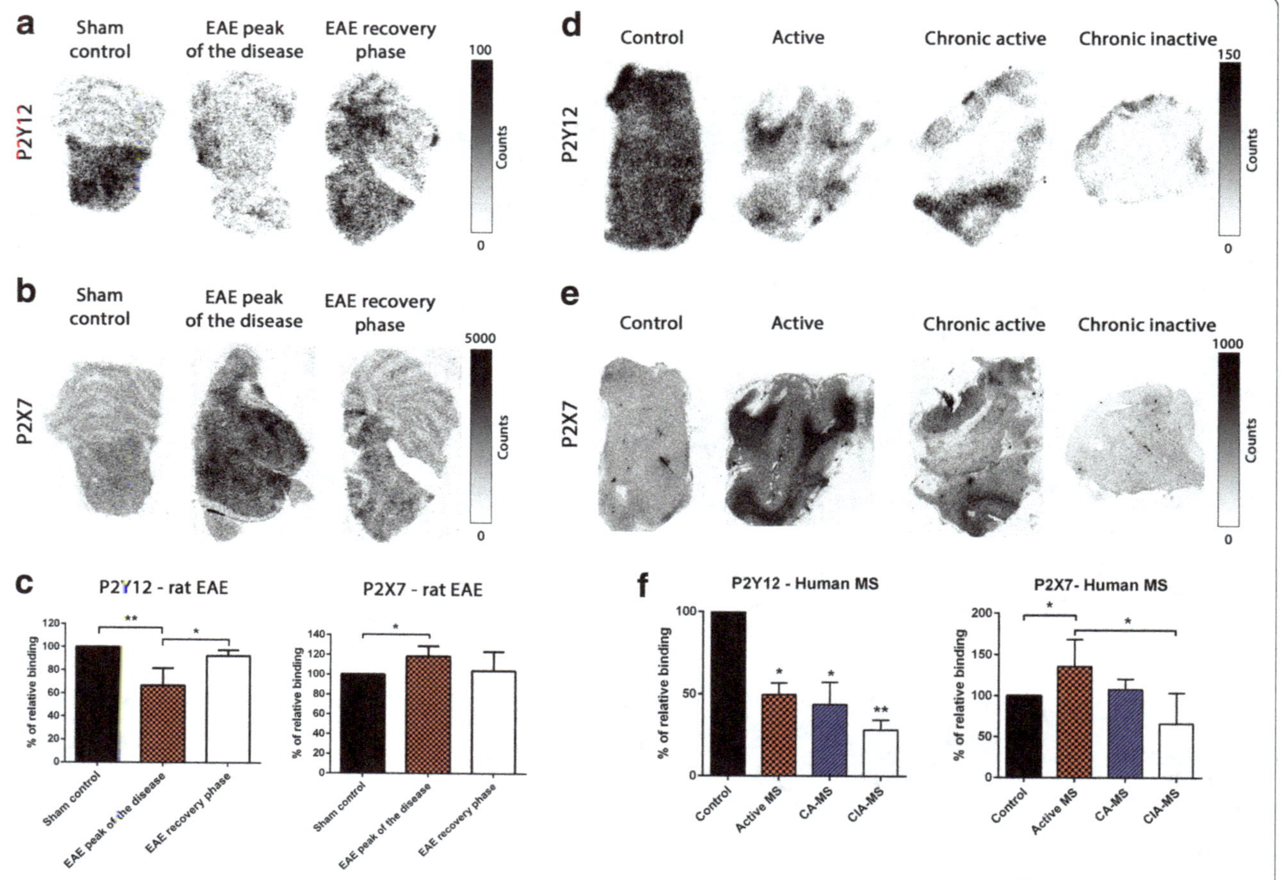

Fig. 8 Autoradiography on acute rat EAE tissue and human MS tissue using P2Y12R and P2X7R radiotracers. Representative autoradiograms of carbon-11-labeled P2Y12R-ant on rat control and EAE tissues (**a**). Representative autoradiograms of tritium-labeled A-740003 (P2X7R specific antagonist) on rat control and EAE tissues (**b**). Quantification of binding of [^{11}C]P2Y12R-ant and [^{3}H]A-740003 on rat control and EAE tissues (data presented is the summary of $n = 3$ animals per time point and three independent experiments) (**c**). Representative autoradiograms of [^{11}C]P2Y12R-ant on different human MS lesion types (**d**). Representative autoradiograms of tritium-labeled A-740003 (P2X7R specific antagonist) on different human MS lesion types (**e**). Quantification of binding of [^{11}C]P2Y12R and [^{3}H]A-740003 on different human MS lesions (data presented is a summary of three independent experiments using three non-neurological controls, three active, two chronic active, and three chronic inactive MS lesions) (**f**)

Discussion

Our data show that P2X7R and P2Y12R can be used for PET tracer development and have the potential to discriminate between pro- and anti-inflammatory microglia in vivo by PET imaging upon successful development of a PET tracer. This may help in obtaining insights into the role of microglia in disease progression and enabling the development of novel treatment strategies aimed at altering microglial phenotype in order to promote neuro-protection. The pathogenesis of MS is complex, and the role of microglia in the development and resolving of the disease is still poorly understood mainly due to the lack of tools to visualize such dynamics. In vitro, microglia can be polarized into pro-inflammatory or anti-inflammatory phenotype depending on stimulus, but in vivo, it has been hypothesized that the microglia activation is very dynamic and show rather a spectrum of activation phenotypes with pro- and anti-inflammatory characteristics on either end of this spectrum. PET imaging is a non-invasive technique and the method of choice for imaging neuroinflammation due to its high sensitivity and quantifiable images. Our data suggests that purinergic receptors P2X7R and P2Y12R could be of high value as PET imaging targets in order to identify a pro- or anti-inflammatory-balanced microglia environment that may suggests new insights into disease progression towards worsening or more resolving state.

P2X7R is markedly expressed on activated microglia and infiltrated macrophages in inflamed MS tissue compared to microglia in the NAWM. P2X7R might be activated by increased levels of ATP that are released during the inflammatory process and cellular damage that is prominent in MS active lesions [27]. P2X7R signaling is also involved in the activation of the inflammasome and the release of IL-1β by activated microglia that is a main inflammatory cytokine potentially playing a role in the MS pathogenesis [28]. The increase in P2X7R receptor in MS and EAE were reported previously using western blot analysis on whole brain homogenate [17, 29] and on microglia/macrophages cells in spinal cord of MS lesion [30]. Our data suggests that microglial P2X7R immunoreactivity correlated with a pro-inflammatory environment and ongoing neuroinflammation. We also observed an increase in P2X7R expression on activated microglia and macrophages at the peak of EAE when the level of inflammation is at the highest. Surprisingly, P2X7R is not reduced on activated microglia in the recovery phase of the EAE. Inflammatory cytokines, i.e., IL-17, IFN-γ, TNF-α, are still present in the recovery phase, but are counter balanced by enhanced levels of anti-inflammatory cytokines, i.e., IL-4 and IL-10 [31]. This implies that P2X7R expression on microglia is less regulated by anti-inflammatory stimuli that occur in the recovery phase in EAE and more responsive to inflammatory cytokines.

P2Y12R expression behaved in opposite direction to P2X7R where the expression was significantly downregulated on activated microglia in MS lesion compared to the microglia in the NAWM. In the EAE model at the peak of the disease, we observe a downregulation of P2Y12R expression on activated microglia in line with earlier reports [13, 22, 32]. However, in the recovery phase of EAE, P2Y12R expression was robustly increased on activated microglia suggesting that P2Y12R expression is more regulated by anti-inflammatory cytokines. In a recent study, Zrzavy et al. reported that a loss of P2Y12R expression on microglia was observed in both active MS lesions and the surrounding normal-appearing white matter (NAWM), suggesting that the chronic inflammatory environment in MS may contribute to the P2Y12R downregulation [32]. Moreover, a higher expression of P2Y12R was detected on microglia in inactive lesions where inflammation was subsided which support our observations about P2Y12R dynamic expression and sensitivity to cytokine environment.

It is apparent that P2X7R and P2Y12R are differentially expressed when comparing ramified microglia to activated microglia in MS lesions; an upregulation of P2X7R is associated with a downregulation of P2Y12R. Our in vitro data using human microglia polarized into pro- or anti-inflammatory phenotypes showed similar responses of P2X7R and P2Y12R expression and correlates with our observation in MS and EAE tissues. P2Y12R response to pro- or anti-inflammatory stimuli in isolated microglia was also in accordance with previous report by Moore et al. [33]. An upregulation of P2Y12R could occur in the remission phase of MS as it happened in the recovery phase of the EAE, but the limitation of post-mortem tissue make it challenging to investigate, which emphasize the importance of PET imaging for non-invasive evaluation of such molecular processes. In addition, the use of M1 and M2 markers to define pro-inflammatory vs anti-inflammatory microglia phenotypes has drawbacks as most of the microglia in the MS lesions adopt an intermediate M1/M2 phenotype [4]. This further stress the need of specific PET imaging markers for the visualization of pro- and anti-inflammatory microglia status in vivo.

Thorough examination of the immunostainings revealed a profound microglial staining pattern of P2Y12R expression. No staining was observed in other cell types, including astrocytes and endothelial cells. These results are in accordance with other studies showing that the expression of P2Y12R is restricted to microglia [21, 22, 32]. However, the specificity of P2X7R to microglia is more controversial. Our results show that P2X7R expression is restricted to microglia and macrophages in MS lesion and NAWM which is not fully in line with other studies showing its expression on other cells in the brain [34]. We cannot exclude the expression of P2X7R on other brain cells; however, the expression level may be lower compared to microglia and the differences in antibody used or tissue treatment could be the reasons of the discrepancy.

It is crucial that PET tracers are able to reflect the changes of expression for these two receptors that we observe in MS and EAE. Our autoradiography data on EAE and human MS tissues show that the binding of the radiolabeled P2X7R and P2Y12R antagonists are in strong accordance with the antibody staining strengthening the rationale of using PET imaging for evaluating the expression of these two receptors. Our autoradiography results give further support to P2X7R and P2Y12R as valuable targets for PET imaging of pro- and anti-inflammatory microglia and that the overall change of expression is significant enough to be detected by in vivo imaging. Combining PET imaging of these two receptors may also provide some insight into the pathological type of lesions in MS as we observe differential tracers binding in different types of MS lesions.

Altogether, our data shows that P2X7R and P2Y12R are PET targetable receptors that have the potential of discriminating between a pro- or anti-inflammatory microglia environment which may help in predicting a worsening or more resolving neuroinflammation in MS and EAE. A possible scenario is that an increase uptake of P2X7R tracer that is accompanied by a decrease uptake of P2Y12R may indicate a progressing MS lesion, while upon immunomodulatory treatment if an increase of P2Y12R uptake is observed, this may indicate that the lesion is shifting to more anti-inflammatory environment and thus indicating a possible resolution of neuroinflammation and treatment efficiency. To that end, we are currently finalizing the characterization of specific P2X7R and P2Y12R PET tracers for the next step of in vivo evaluation of microglia and/or macrophage dynamics in the EAE model. Moreover, a new P2X7R PET tracer was recently reported and showed promising results in an in vivo model in which the human P2X7 was overexpressed through an AAV vector [35]. In addition, the change of P2X7R and P2Y12R expression on activated microglia is not restricted to MS and EAE and has been also described in other neuroinflammatory disease.

Conclusion

The data we present in this study is the first step in the process that may lead to better understanding of the role of microglia in MS and other neuroinflammatory diseases. Furthermore, it may contribute to a better understanding of the relation between microglia activation status and neurodegeneration, and in the development of new immunomodulatory and disease-modifying therapies.

Abbreviations

CFA: Complete Freund's adjuvant; CNS: Central nervous system; EAE: Experimental autoimmune encephalomyelitis; GM-CSF: Granulocyte-macrophage colony-stimulating factor; LSC: Liquid scintillation counting; MS: Multiple sclerosis; NAWM: Normal-appearing white matter; PET: Positron emission tomography; PLP: Proteolipid protein; QPCR: Quantitative real-time polymerase chain reaction; RCY: Radiochemical yield; ROIs: Regions of interest; TSPO: Translocator protein

Acknowledgements

We would like to acknowledge the AO|2M core facility (www.ao2m.amsterdam) for their technical support and expertise.

Funding

This study was financed by an unrestricted Global Multiple Sclerosis Innovation (GMSI) research grant, provided by Merck KGaA (Darmstadt, Germany), and received funding from the European Union's Seventh Framework Programme (FP7/2007-2013) under grant agreement no. HEALTH-F2-2011-278850 (INMiND).

Authors' contributions

WB designed and coordinated the study, carried the in vitro work on human microglia, the immunostaining on rat tissue, autoradiography experiments, and drafted the manuscript. BJ performed the synthesis of the radiotracers. GK assisted in the isolation and preparation of the human microglia. SvP performed the immunostaining on human MS tissues. BvHH carried out the QPCR and western blot experiments. JvH, AD, and HV participated in the study design and coordination and helped to draft the manuscript. All authors read and approved the final manuscript.

Consent for publication

Not applicable

Competing interests

The authors declare that they have no competing interests.

Author details

[1]Department of Radiology and Nuclear Medicine, VU University Medical Center, Amsterdam, The Netherlands. [2]Department of Molecular Cell Biology and Immunology, VUmc MS Center Amsterdam, Amsterdam Neuroscience, VU University Medical Center, Amsterdam, The Netherlands.

References

1. Garg N, Smith TW. An update on immunopathogenesis, diagnosis, and treatment of multiple sclerosis. Brain Behav. 2015;5:e00362. https://doi.org/10.1002/brb3.362 .
2. Prinz M, Tay TL, Wolf Y, Jung S. Microglia: unique and common features with other tissue macrophages. Acta Neuropathol. 2014;128:319–31. https://doi.org/10.1007/s00401-014-1267-1 .
3. Peferoen LAN, Vogel DYS, Ummenthum K, Breur M, Heijnen, Priscilla DAM, Gerritsen WH, et al. Activation status of human microglia is dependent on lesion formation stage and remyelination in multiple sclerosis. J Neuropathol Exp Neurol. 2015;74:48–63. https://doi.org/10.1097/NEN.0000000000000149 .
4. Vogel DYS, Vereyken EJF, Glim JE, Heijnen PDAM, Moeton M, van der Valk P, et al. Macrophages in inflammatory multiple sclerosis lesions have an intermediate activation status. J Neuroinflammation. 2013;10:35. https://doi.org/10.1186/1742-2094-10-35 .
5. Gomez-Nicola D, Perry VH. Microglial dynamics and role in the healthy and diseased brain: a paradigm of functional plasticity. Neuroscientist. 2015;21:169–84. https://doi.org/10.1177/1073858414530512 .
6. Parkhurst CN, Gan W. Microglia dynamics and function in the CNS. Curr Opin Neurobiol. 2010;20:595–600. https://doi.org/10.1016/j.conb.2010.07.002.
7. Correale J. The role of microglial activation in disease progression. Mult Scler. 2014;20:1288–95. https://doi.org/10.1177/1352458514533230 .
8. Giunti D, Parodi B, Cordano C, Uccelli A, Kerlero de Rosbo N. Can we switch microglia's phenotype to foster neuroprotection? Focus on multiple sclerosis. Immunology. 2014;141:328–39. https://doi.org/10.1111/imm.12177 .
9. Kettenmann H, Hanisch U, Noda M, Verkhratsky A. Physiology of microglia. Physiol Rev. 2011;91:461–553. https://doi.org/10.1152/physrev.00011.2010 .
10. Heppner FL, Greter M, Marino D, Falsig J, Raivich G, Hovelmeyer N, et al. Experimental autoimmune encephalomyelitis repressed by microglial paralysis. Nat Med. 2005;11:146–52. https://doi.org/10.1038/nm1177 .
11. Kotter MR, Li W, Zhao C, Franklin RJM. Myelin impairs CNS remyelination by inhibiting oligodendrocyte precursor cell differentiation. J Neurosci. 2006;26:328–32. https://doi.org/10.1523/JNEUROSCI.2615-05.2006 .
12. Filbin MT. Myelin-associated inhibitors of axonal regeneration in the adult mammalian CNS. Nat Rev Neurosci. 2003;4:703–13. https://doi.org/10.1038/nrn1195 .
13. Butovsky O, Ziv Y, Schwartz A, Landa G, Talpalar AE, Pluchino S, et al. Microglia activated by IL-4 or IFN-gamma differentially induce neurogenesis and oligodendrogenesis from adult stem/progenitor cells. Mol Cell Neurosci. 2006;31:149–60. https://doi.org/10.1016/j.mcn.2005.10.006 .
14. Tierney JB, Kharkrang M, La Flamme AC. Type II-activated macrophages suppress the development of experimental autoimmune encephalomyelitis. Immunol Cell Biol. 2009;87:235–40. https://doi.org/10.1038/icb.2008.99 .
15. Airas L, Rissanen E, Rinne JO. Imaging neuroinflammation in multiple sclerosis using TSPO-PET. Clin Transl Imaging. 2015;3:461–73. https://doi.org/10.1007/s40336-015-0147-6 .
16. Vivash L, O'Brien TJ. Imaging microglial activation with TSPO PET: lighting up neurologic diseases? J Nucl Med. 2016;57:165–8. https://doi.org/10.2967/jnumed.114.141713 .
17. Yu Y, Ugawa S, Ueda T, Ishida Y, Inoue K, Kyaw Nyunt A, et al. Cellular localization of P2X7 receptor mRNA in the rat brain. Brain. 2008;1194:45–55. https://doi.org/10.1016/j.brainres.2007.11.064 .
18. Clark AK, Staniland AA, Marchand F, Kaan TKY, McMahon SB, Malcangio M. P2X7-dependent release of interleukin-1 beta and nociception in the spinal cord following lipopolysaccharide. J Neurosci. 2010;30:573–82. https://doi.org/10.1523/JNEUROSCI.3295-09.2010 .
19. Monif M, Burnstock G, Williams DA. Microglia: proliferation and activation driven by the P2X7 receptor. Int J Biochem Cell Biol. 2010;42:1753–6. https://doi.org/10.1016/j.biocel.2010.06.021 .
20. Bhattacharya A, Biber K. The microglial ATP-gated ion channel P2X7 as a CNS drug target. Glia. 2016;64:1772–87. https://doi.org/10.1002/glia.23001.

21. Butovsky O, Jedrychowski MP, Moore CS, Cialic R, Lanser AJ, Gabriely G, et al. Identification of a unique TGF-beta-dependent molecular and functional signature in microglia. Nat Neurosci. 2014;17:131–43. https://doi.org/10.1038/nn.3599 .
22. Mildner A, Huang H, Radke J, Stenzel W, Priller J. P2Y12 receptor is expressed on human microglia under physiological conditions throughout development and is sensitive to neuroinflammatory diseases. Glia. 2017;65:375–87. https://doi.org/10.1002/glia.23097 .
23. Janssen B, Vugts DJ, Funke U, Spaans A, Schuit RC, Kooijman E, et al. Synthesis and initial preclinical evaluation of the P2X7 receptor antagonist [^{11}C]A-740003 as a novel tracer of neuroinflammation. J Label Compd Radiopharm. 2014;57:509–16. https://doi.org/10.1002/jlcr.3206 .
24. Janssen B, Vugts DJ, Funke U, Perry S, Kruijer, Dolle F, Bormans G, et al. Synthesis of the first carbon-11 labelled P2Y12 receptor antagonist for PET imaging of microglial activation in neuroinflammation. J Label Compd Radiopharm. 2015;58:S1–S74. https://doi.org/10.1002/jlcr.3302_1 .
25. de Vries HE, JJA H, Honing H, de Lavalette CR, SMA v d P, Hooijberg E, et al. Signal-regulatory protein -CD47 interactions are required for the transmigration of monocytes across cerebral endothelium. J Immunol. 2002;168:5832–9. https://doi.org/10.4049/jimmunol.168.11.5832 .
26. Garcia-Vallejo JJ, van Dijk W, van Het Hof B, van Die I, Engelse MA, Hinsbergh V, Victor WM, Gringhuis SI. Activation of human endothelial cells by tumor necrosis factor-alpha results in profound changes in the expression of glycosylation-related genes. J Cell Physiol. 2006;206:203–10. https://doi.org/10.1002/jcp.20458 .
27. Rodrigues RJ, Tomé AR, Cunha RA. ATP as a multi-target danger signal in the brain. Front Neurosci. 2015;9:148. https://doi.org/10.3389/fnins.2015.00148 .
28. Lin C, Edelson BT. New insights into the role of IL-1β in experimental autoimmune encephalomyelitis and multiple sclerosis. J Immunol. 2017;198:4553–60. https://doi.org/10.4049/jimmunol.1700263 .
29. Matute C, Torre I, Perez-Cerda F, Perez-Samartin A, Alberdi E, Etxebarria E, et al. P2X(7) receptor blockade prevents ATP excitotoxicity in oligodendrocytes and ameliorates experimental autoimmune encephalomyelitis. J Neurosci. 2007;27:9525–33. https://doi.org/10.1523/JNEUROSCI.0579-07.2007 .
30. Yiangou Y, Facer P, Durrenberger P, Chessell IP, Naylor A, Bountra C, et al. COX-2, CB2 and P2X7-immunoreactivities are increased in activated microglial cells/macrophages of multiple sclerosis and amyotrophic lateral sclerosis spinal cord. BMC Neurol. 2006;6:12. https://doi.org/10.1186/1471-2377-6-12.
31. Ruuls SR, Sedgwick JD. Cytokine-directed therapies in multiple sclerosis and experimental autoimmune encephalomyelitis. Immunol Cell Biol. 1998;76:65–73. https://doi.org/10.1046/j.1440-1711.1998.00715.x .
32. Zrzavy T, Hametner S, Wimmer I, Butovsky O, Weiner HL, Lassmann H. Loss of 'homeostatic' microglia and patterns of their activation in active multiple sclerosis. Brain. 2017;140:1900–13. https://doi.org/10.1093/brain/awx113 .
33. Moore CS, Ase AR, Kinsara A, Rao VTS, Michell-Robinson M, Leong SY, et al. P2Y12 expression and function in alternatively activated human microglia. Neurol Neuroimmunol Neuroinflamm. 2015;2:e80. https://doi.org/10.1212/NXI.0000000000000080.
34. Bartlett R, Stokes L, Sluyter R. The P2X7 receptor channel: recent developments and the use of P2X7 antagonists in models of disease. Pharmacol Rev. 2014;66:638–75. https://doi.org/10.1124/pr.113.008003 .
35. Ory D, Celen S, Gijsbers R, van den Haute C, Postnov A, Koole M, et al. Preclinical evaluation of a P2X7 receptor-selective radiotracer: PET studies in a rat model with local overexpression of the human P2X7 receptor and in nonhuman primates. J Nucl Med. 2016;57:1436–41. https://doi.org/10.2967/jnumed.115.169995 .

Expression of the neuroprotective protein aryl hydrocarbon receptor nuclear translocator 2 correlates with neuronal stress and disability in models of multiple sclerosis

Tissa Rahim†, Pierre Becquart†, Maria-Elizabeth Baeva and Jacqueline Quandt*

Abstract

Background: Axonal degeneration and neuronal loss have been described as the major causes of irreversible clinical disability in multiple sclerosis (MS). The aryl-hydrocarbon receptor nuclear translocator 2 (ARNT2) protein has been associated with neuroprotection in models of ischemia and neuronal responses to stressors.

Methods: To characterize its potential to influence inflammatory neurodegeneration, we examined ARNT2 expression in the experimental autoimmune encephalomyelitis (EAE) model of MS and characterized mediators that influence ARNT2 expression as well as plausible partners and targets.

Results: *Arnt2* message and protein levels dropped significantly in EAE spinal cords as disease developed and were lowest at peak disability. ARNT2 expression is prominent in neuronal cell bodies within the gray matter with some staining in glial fibrillary acidic protein (GFAP)$^+$ astrocytes in healthy animals. At peak disease, ARNT2 expression is reduced by 20–50% in gray matter neurons compared to healthy controls. ARNT2 intensity in neurons throughout the EAE spinal cord correlated inversely with the degree of immune cell infiltration ($r = -0.5085$, $p < 0.01$) and axonal damage identified with SMI32 staining ($r = -0.376$, $p = 0.032$). To understand the relationship between ARNT2 expression and neuronal health, we exposed enriched cortical cultures of neurons to hydrogen peroxide (H_2O_2) to mimic oxidative stress. H_2O_2 at lower doses rapidly increased ARNT2 protein levels which returned to baseline within 3–4 h. Exposure to higher doses of H_2O_2) dropped ARNT2 levels below baseline, preceding cytotoxicity measured by morphological changes and lactate dehydrogenase release from cells. Decreases in ARNT2 secondary to staurosporine and H_2O_2 preceded increases in cleaved caspase 3 and associated apoptosis. We also examined expression of neuronal pas 4 (*Npas4*), whose heterodimerization with ARNT2 drives expression of the neurotrophic factor brain-derived neurotrophic factor (*Bdnf*). Like ARNT2, *Npas4* levels also decline at the onset of EAE and are linked to decreases in *Bdnf*. In vitro, H_2O_2 exposure drives *Npas4* expression that is tied to increases in *Bdnf*.

Conclusion: Our data support ARNT2 as a neuronal transcription factor whose sustained expression is linked to neuronal and axonal health, protection that may primarily be driven through its partnering with Npas4 to influence BDNF expression.

Keywords: Multiple sclerosis, Aryl hydrocarbon receptor nuclear translocator 2, Neuroprotection, Experimental autoimmune encephalomyelitis

* Correspondence: jquandt@pathology.ubc.ca
†Tissa Rahim and Pierre Becquart contributed equally to this work.
Department of Pathology and Laboratory Medicine, University of British Columbia, G227-2211 Wesbrook Mall, Vancouver, BC V6T 2B5, Canada

Background

The aryl-hydrocarbon receptor nuclear translocator 2 (ARNT2) is a member of the basic-helix-loop-helix period-ARNT-single-minded protein (bHLH/PAS) transcription factor family [1]. ARNT2 heterodimerizes with other bHLH/PAS members to direct transcription of target genes in response to various environmental and physiological stimuli. These include hypoxia (hypoxia-inducible factor 1α (HIF-1α)), early cell determination/differentiation (single-minded homolog 1 (SIM1)) and environmental toxins (aryl hydrocarbon receptor (AhR)) [2]. Notably, AhR has been implicated in regulating pathogenic responses in an animal model of multiple sclerosis (experimental autoimmune encephalitis, EAE), mediating environmental influence on astrocytes and as a key component in the postulated mechanism of action for laquinimod (an MS disease-modulating therapy currently in clinical trials) [3–6].

ARNT2 is a nuclear transcription factor found almost exclusively in the central nervous system (CNS), but also localized to kidneys, the urinary tract, and the thymus [7–10]. ARNT2 was first described as an isoform of the aryl hydrocarbon receptor nuclear translocator (ARNT), named after its purported role in the nuclear translocation of the aryl hydrocarbon receptor (AhR). ARNT2 has been associated with neuroprotective properties in ischemic insults and cells undergoing oxidative damage. *Arnt2* gene transcript levels declined significantly following 2 h of recirculation post-ischemic injury, preceding neuronal death at 24 h of recirculation [10]. ARNT2 acts as an anti-apoptotic factor in PC12 cells (a cell line derived from a pheochromocytoma of the rat adrenal medulla), as downregulation of ARNT2 by RNA interference resulted in apoptosis of these cells, and oxidative stress-induced PC12 cell death was preceded by rapid and strong downregulation of ARNT2 [10]. *Arnt2* homozygous knockout mice and rats die perinatally (within the first day to 2 weeks after birth) secondary to a lack of hypothalamic neuroendocrine lineage formation, impaired regulation of HIF-1 target genes and thymic defects [11–14]. The importance of *Arnt2* has also been demonstrated in a case study of a family with a nonsense mutation in *Arnt2*, where children exhibited microcephaly and delayed or loss of myelination [15].

Physiological levels of synaptic activity result in a rapid and transient rise in calcium, which can activate a program of gene expression that promotes dendritic growth, synapse development, and neuronal plasticity, including but not limited to neuronal PAS domain protein 4 (NPAS4), a CNS-specific bHLH transcription factor that is the primary partner for ARNT2 in the CNS [16, 17]. Under excitatory conditions, a rapid and enhanced influx of calcium into the cell induces NPAS4 transcription, followed by heterodimerization with ARNT2, binding the PER-ARNT-SIM response element (PASRe) and guiding transcription of brain-derived neurotrophic factor (BDNF) at BDNF promoters I and IV of a total of nine promoters [18, 19]. This ARNT2:NPAS4 guidance of BDNF [20] transcription has been described under excitatory and neurodegenerative conditions [18, 19]. Notably, lack of NPAS4 and/or BDNF expression has been linked to neurodegenerative diseases and worsened disease stroke/ischemia models [21–23] and reductions of both *Npas4* and *Arnt2* mRNA have been observed in a rat model of depression [19].

Multiple sclerosis (MS) is a chronic inflammatory and demyelinating neurodegenerative disorder confined to the central nervous system (CNS) and characterized pathologically by alterations in the vasculature, inflammatory infiltrates, demyelination, glial scarring, oligodendrocyte loss, and axonal damage and loss [24]; the irreversible axonal loss and neurodegeneration is thought to be the major correlate of chronic disability in MS [25]. Recent investigations highlight that axonal injury starts early in the disease course [26, 27], and these pathological changes are confirmed by in vivo magnetic resonance imaging (MRI) studies showing early brain volume loss [28, 29].

Lymphocytes contribute to damage directly via cell-cell death or indirectly via soluble mediators including cytokines, antibodies, or proteases. The resident antigen-presenting cells, microglia, become activated, and recruited monocytes generate macrophages, the primary mediators of tissue injury and the most abundant inflammatory cells found in MS lesions [30, 31]. Oxidative stress, glutamate excitotoxicity, and inflammatory mediators, typically driven by surrounding glia/microglia, macrophages and lymphocytes, can all contribute to mitochondrial dysfunction [26, 32] and may contribute to disease progression [33, 34].

These disease mediators can induce rapid influx or release of calcium into the cell, which leads to activation of proteolytic enzymes, cleaved caspase processing initiating apoptosis, and damage to the mitochondrial membrane [35]. While many attribute demyelination and subsequent axonal loss as secondary to inflammatory cells and mediators in MS [26], this explains neither the neurodegeneration seen prior to inflammatory cell infiltration in animal models nor the progressive loss of function after the inflammatory phase has subsided [36, 37], or axonal loss despite intact myelin [37]. There is considerable interest in characterizing both gray matter disease and disease progression, where disability progresses despite suppression of new inflammatory activity [38]. Recent findings implicate mitochondrial dysfunction secondary to energy imbalance and increases in ROS as sources of oxidative damage not directly attributable to inflammation [39, 40] and suggest inflammation is secondary to more primary degenerative processes.

While the importance of ARNT2 in cell survival has been shown in models of ischemic injury, its expression patterns or role in chronic inflammatory and neurodegenerative disease of the CNS have not been characterized. We hypothesized that alterations in ARNT2 expression in vitro or in vivo in models of MS are associated with changes in cell viability and clinical disease, through processes relevant to pathogenesis in a model of MS. We report that *Arnt2* levels are significantly altered over the preclinical and acute phases of EAE compared to baseline and are lowest at times of peak disability. We found that ARNT2 expression in neuronal cells within the gray matter of EAE mice is lower at peak disease than observed in controls and propose that a loss in ARNT2 in EAE that is also tied to the loss of its primary CNS partner *Npas4* and downstream regulation of *Bdnf*, may be a primary driver for the neurodegeneration and disability seen in chronic inflammatory demyelinating disease. Decreases in neuronal ARNT2 correlate with the degree of inflammation and axonal damage. Furthermore, inflammatory and apoptotic mediators can influence neuronal expression of ARNT2 in vitro: ARNT2 protein increases in response to stressors, yet high doses or prolonged exposure is associated with decreases in ARNT2 that precede cell death and cleaved caspase 3 expression. This is the first report implicating ARNT2 in neurodegenerative processes relevant to inflammatory neurodegenerative disorders such as MS, and provides data to warrant its consideration as a primary contributor to disease development and progression.

Methods

EAE induction

All animal work was in compliance with our protocol approved by the University of British Columbia Animal Care Committee (certificate #A130281) and per the Canadian Council on Animal Care guidelines. Eight-week-old female C57BL/6 (Jackson Laboratories, Bar Harbor, ME) mice were immunized for chronic progressive EAE as previously described [41, 42] with 200 μg of MOG35-55 peptide (MEVGWYRSPFSRVVH LYRNGK; Stanford Pan Facility, Stanford, CA) in 4 mg/mL *Mycobacterium tuberculosis* (H37Ra) in incomplete Freund's adjuvant (IFA) (Difco Laboratories, Detroit, MI). Pertussis toxin (200 ng, List Biologicals, Campell, CA) was delivered intraperitoneally that day and 2 days later. Mice were scored daily on a scale from 0 to 5 for severity of clinical symptoms: 0–0.5 indicated no disease/distal limp tail, 1.0 limp tail, 2.0 weakness in one or 2.5 in both hind limbs/slipping on bars, 3.0 paralysis in one or 3.5 both hind limbs, 4.0 hind limb paralysis plus weakness in one or in 4.5 both forelimbs, and 5 for moribund animals.

Processing of EAE tissues

For qPCR and western blotting analyses, C57BL/6 mice spinal columns and brains were isolated from healthy mice and EAE mice immediately following CO_2 exposure and decapitation at the following intervals: day 7, day 10 (pre-onset), day 14 (onset), day 18 (peak disease), day 25 (recovery), and days 32 and 45 which reflect some degree of worsening. Controls included healthy animals or sham/CFA-immunized (no MOG) animals that also received pertussis toxin harvested at days 7, 14, 25, and 45. For immunohistochemistry, animals were anesthetized with a ketamine/xylazine formulation, with subsequent transcardial perfusion with PBS followed by buffered formalin. Tissues were fixed for 3–5 days, and spinal cords removed before cryoprotection in 30% sucrose solution for at least 5 days. Spinal cords were cut into 5 mm pieces representing five to seven different levels and embedded in optimal cutting temperature compound (OCT) (VWR, Radnor, PA) and frozen until sectioning at 5 μM on a cryostat.

Tissue staining and image acquisition

Sectioned tissues were permeabilized with 0.05% triton and blocked with 10% normal goat or donkey serum. Tissues were incubated with antibodies to NeuN, microtubule-associated protein 2 (MAP2), a neuronal marker) and glial fibrillary acidic protein (GFAP, a marker of astrocytes, all from EMD Millipore, Etobicoke, ON), myelin basic protein (MBP, Santa Cruz Biotechnology, Dallas, TX), SMI-32 (Biolegend, San Diego, CA) or ARNT2 (Santa Cruz) overnight. After incubation, tissues were washed with TBST followed by incubation with secondary antibody at room temperature. Normal goat, chicken, rat, mouse, and rabbit IgG (Santa Cruz) served as isotype controls.

Tissue sections and cells were visualized on a Zeiss Axio Vert 200 Inverted Fluorescence Microscope (Oberkochen, DE), and images acquired with an Axiocam 506 monochrome camera. Analysis was performed with Zeiss software Zen (Version 2.3). To quantify immunostaining results, sections from five to seven spinal levels spanning the entire cord (C4/5, T1/2, T5/6, T12/13, L5/6, S3/4) were examined from seven healthy/CFA control-immunized mice and five EAE mice at day 18 for a total of 26–40 sections per treatment group. Disease scores ranged from 2.5 to 4.0 with an average score of 3.25 ± 0.67, and all animals showed evidence of inflammatory infiltration of the spinal cord. Images were captured at × 20 with identical light intensity and exposure times applied to all images from each experimental set. ARNT2 expression in neurons was quantified by measuring the average intensity per pixel for ARNT2 over the area of NeuN-positive nuclei. First, a binary mask was created to select only the gray matter (based on regions of

NeuN staining positivity) and then another one to select all nuclei of the section using the DAPI staining. Nuclei with a high fluorescence intensity (set at greater than 1500 mean intensity per pixel for NeuN) were selected, and the average fluorescence intensity per pixel for ARNT2 over the area of the DAPI-positive nucleus was measured. Neuronal cells were quantified by counting the NeuN/DAPI$^+$ cells per square millimeter in the whole gray matter region, and ARNT2 intensity was quantified in cells in this larger region as well as those in the dorsal horn at each level based on anatomical outlines in the © 2008 Allen Institute for Brain Science Allen Spinal Cord Atlas available from http://mousespinal.brain-map.org. The values of all of the cells within one side of the spinal cord were first normalized to the average value for ARNT2 mean intensity measured in central canal ependymal cells (negative for ARNT2 expression) to account for any background staining between sections. The values for each spinal cord section within this region from each mouse were then pooled and averaged for analysis. The number of astrocytes in the gray matter was assessed using the same gray matter mask to select all the nuclei in the gray matter with DAPI staining. The nuclei with a high fluorescence intensity (greater than 1600 mean intensity per pixel) for GFAP were selected as GFAP$^+$ cells and normalized to the surface area of the gray matter mask to obtain cell number per square millimeter.

Assessment of inflammatory infiltrates, demyelination, and axonal damage

Immunostained sections from five levels of each EAE mouse spinal cord ($n = 5$, total of 25 levels) were assessed for the degree of inflammatory infiltration according to the criteria in Additional file 1: Table S1. MBP-negative regions of the white matter were outlined in Zen, and demyelinated areas (in μm^2) were summed from each level and divided by the area of the entire white matter with the same binary mask approach used for gray matter to get a % area of demyelination for each level. SMI32-positive regions of interest, or spheroids, were selected as those regions with a staining intensity above the threshold set by averaging regions of white matter in healthy animals; the number of SMI32+ spheroids was evaluated per square millimeter of white matter at each of five levels from five EAE mice as for infiltrates. The relative sum of inflammation, % demyelination, and SMI32$^+$ staining per level of the spinal cord was compared to the relative intensity of ARNT2 in neurons at that level.

Primary cortical neuron-enriched cultures

Embryonic day 18 (E18) rat cortices were graciously provided by Dr. Shernaz Bamji (University of British Columbia) and were cultured as previously described [43]. Cortices were washed with 37 °C Hank's Balanced Salt Solution (HBSS, Gibco, Carlsbad, CA), incubated in 0.25% Trypsin-EDTA (Sigma-Aldrich®, St. Louis, MO), DNase (Sigma-Aldrich) and HBSS, and dissociated and seeded at 50,000 cells/cm^2 for western blotting/qPCR and 35,000 cells/cm^2 for immunocytochemistry on poly-L-lysine-coated plates in Neurobasal® media (Thermo Fisher Scientific, Waltham, US) supplemented with B-27 (Gibco, Thermo Fisher Scientific). Cells were maintained at 5% CO_2 and 37 °C until experiments at 7–16 days in vitro (DIV). Hydrogen peroxide (H_2O_2, Fisher, Waltham, MA) was used to mimic oxidative damage, and staurosporine (Sigma-Aldrich), a non-selective protein kinase inhibitor, was used to induce apoptosis, modeling pathological processes associated with degeneration in MS [44, 45].

Cell lysis, protein quantification, and western blotting

Cells were lysed in radioimmunoprecipitation assay buffer (RIPA, tris-hydrochloric acid (MP Biomedicals, Santa Ana, CA), sodium chloride (Fisher), sodium deoxycholate (Fisher), NP-40 (Thermo Fisher Scientific, sodium dodecyl sulfate (SDS, MP Biomedicals), and EDTA (MP Biomedicals)) with 5% protease inhibitor (Roche, Basel, CH) and lysate stored at − 20 °C. Samples run on 12% tris/glycine gels (Bio-Rad, Hercules, USA) were transferred to nitrocellulose membranes, blocked with 2% skim milk, and incubated with primary antibodies overnight at 4 °C. Membranes were washed and incubated with secondary antibody at room temperature with Clarity™ Western ECL Blotting Substrate (Bio-Rad) added before imaging on a Bio-Rad ChemiDoc™ MP System. Blots were analyzed using quantitative densitometry on Image Lab™ (Bio-Rad 5.2) and normalized to tubulin as a loading control following normalization of data on different blots to a positive control spinal cord lysate that was loaded on each blot run; this enabled blot to blot comparisons when run in an identical manner and using the same exposure times.

Reverse transcription and quantitative polymerase chain reaction

Tissues were processed with the AllPrep kit (Qiagen, Hilden, DE) per manufacturer guidelines and RNA stored until use. In vitro cell culture RNA was isolated using the Qiagen RNeasy Mini Kit, and protein was precipitated using buffer APP (Qiagen) per manufacturer's guidelines). RNA was measured using a NanoDrop™ spectrophotometer (Wilmington, USA). Reverse transcription was performed using the QuantiTect® Reverse Transcription Kit (Qiagen) with Fast Start Essential DNA Green Master (Roche). cDNA, SYBR Green and ultrapure dH_2O were combined and loaded on to LightCycler® 480 Multiwell plates (Roche) and run on a LightCycler® 480 Instrument II (Roche); qPCR primers are included in Additional file 1: Table S2. Data was subsequently analyzed using the

LightCycler® 480 software (Version 1.5, Roche). Standard curves (*Arnt2*, *Npas4*, *Bdnf*, and *β-actin* cDNA generated from mouse brain, diluted in 10-fold successions) were included on each run for absolute quantification. Precipitated proteins from spinal cord were quantified and analyzed by western blotting as outlined above for cell cultures.

Lactate dehydrogenase assay

Cell viability measurements were performed using a lactate dehydrogenase (LDH) cytotoxicity assay kit (Thermo Fisher Scientific™ Pierce™) per protocol guidelines. Controls included samples from dead cells (killed with lysis buffer provided for maximum LDH release) against which % cytotoxicity of treatments could be measured. Absorbance was measured using a Spectra Max plate reader (Molecular Devices, Sunnyvale, USA).

Immunocytochemistry

Cells in culture were fixed with 10% phosphate-buffered formalin (Fisher), permeabilized with 0.1% Triton-X 100 (Fisher), and blocked with 10% normal goat serum (Gibco). Cells were washed with PBS, and incubated with primary antibodies for ARNT2, NeuN, MAP-2, GFAP, or cleaved caspase 3 (R&D Systems, Minneapolis, MN) in 2% normal goat serum overnight at 4 °C and secondary antibodies at RT (Additional file 1: Table S2). After counterstaining with 4′,6-diamidino-2-phenylindole (DAPI), images were acquired and analysis was performed with Zeiss software Zen (Version 2.3). ARNT2 staining was examined in NeuN-, GFAP-, or MAP-2-positive cells and cleaved caspase 3 in neuronal cells.

Statistical analysis

All statistical analysis was performed using GraphPad Prism (version 5, La Jolla, CA). A repeated measures one-way ANOVA was performed, and if the data was not normally distributed, a repeated measures ANOVA on ranks (Friedman test) was performed when comparing multiple treatments. Both were followed with a Tukey multiple comparisons post-test. All data are reported as mean ± standard deviation unless otherwise indicated. For comparison of immunohistochemical evaluations in EAE to healthy/CFA-immunized mice, a Mann-Whitney comparison test was performed and significance reported at $p < 0.05$. The correlation of inflammation, MBP, and SMI32 staining to ARNT2 intensity was examined using a Pearson correlation.

Results

Arnt2 expression is altered over the course of EAE

We began our investigation by characterizing *ARNT2* levels in the spinal cord where inflammation and degeneration are most prevalent in the MOG-induced model of MS. This is also the region where tissue changes are thought to contribute to disability in this model. qPCR analysis of chronic EAE spinal cord samples was performed with tissues from pre-onset, onset, peak, recovery/stabilization, and worsening stages of the disease compared to sham-immunized controls or healthy non-immunized littermates (Fig. 1a). Compared to CFA-immunized littermates, *Arnt2* levels in the spinal cord are decreased by onset (day 14) and are lowest at peak disease (Fig. 1b). Notably, *Arnt2* message levels have begun to increase again by day 25 where the animals have shown some recovery. By day 45 however, the RNA levels are still significantly below levels observed in healthy or sham-immunized animals. We also examined expression of the primary CNS partner for ARNT2, *Npas4*, and one of their downstream targets, *Bdnf*, over the course of EAE (Additional file 2). While *Arnt2* message tended to show increases prior to disease onset, both *Npas4* message and *Bdnf* message were elevated compared to sham-immunized animals prior to disease onset (at days 7 and 10 post EAE induction respectively). Like ARNT2, expression of *Npas4* and *Bdnf* decreased significantly over the course of EAE, with levels at their lowest at peak disability and recovering as animals recovered. Notably, ARNT2 protein was also lowest at peak clinical disease on day 18 (Fig. 1c) and was the only time point where ARNT2 protein levels were significantly different than healthy or sham CFA-immunized control mice.

ARNT2 expression is altered during acute EAE

We next examined the expression of ARNT2 in the spinal cord of EAE animals at peak disease compared to controls, localizing ARNT2 to distinct cell populations and regions. In the spinal cords of sham-immunized animals, ARNT2 was localized to regions of both the gray as well as the myelin-rich white matter. In gray matter, ARNT2 staining was frequently associated with the nuclei of $NeuN^+$ cells, either larger motor neurons in the ventral horns (arrows) or smaller cells of the dorsal horns or intermediate regions (arrowheads, Fig. 2a). While ependymal cells lining the central canal were negative for ARNT2 expression (Fig. 2b), ARNT2 was commonly associated with the nuclei of $GFAP^+$ cells lining the midline and surrounding the central canal (insets, Fig. 2b, c respectively). ARNT2 positivity was also detected in several $GFAP^+$ astrocytes lining the meninges.

Compared to the gray matter of healthy animals which typically showed numerous $ARNT2^+/NeuN^+$ cells, ARNT2 expression was detected at lower levels in the $NeuN^+$ cells in EAE mice (Fig. 3). In the gray matter of an EAE spinal cord with moderate disability but at a higher level of the spinal cord (C4/5) with few infiltrates (Fig. 3a, b), there were far fewer double-staining $NeuN^+$ cells in the EAE mouse than in the healthy mouse; this

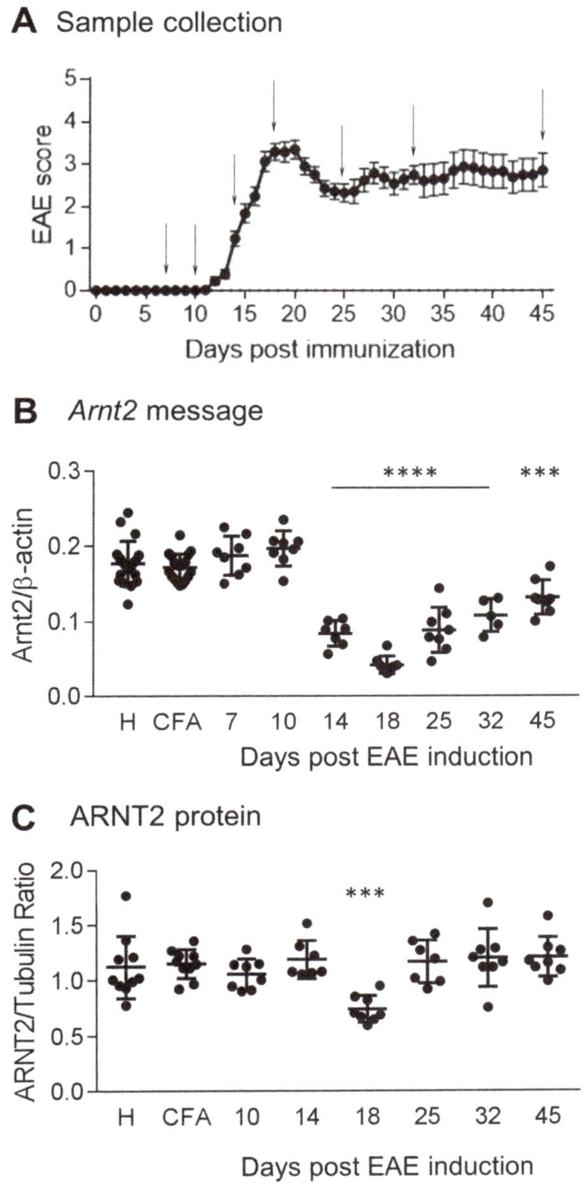

Fig. 1 qPCR analyses of ARNT2 expression over the course of MOG-induced chronic EAE. **a** A cohort of 95 mice were induced for EAE or received only CFA and pertussis as sham-immunized healthy controls; healthy non-immunized mice also served as controls. Mice were scored as outlined in the Materials & Methods and points represent the mean score ± SEM of all mice with clinical symptoms. Tissues from 5 to 8 mice with similar disease scores were harvested at times indicated by arrows (days 7, 10, 14, 18, 25, 32, and 45) representing preclinical, onset, peak, recovery and times with some degree of worsening over time and analyzed by qPCR to obtain ARNT2 message levels normalized to β-actin (**b**) or analyzed by western blotting to quantify ARNT2 protein compared to tubulin (**c**). Each point represents the value obtained from one mouse; bars represent the mean ± SD. One way ANOVA followed by Dunnett's multiple comparison test against CFA/sham immunized mice, $^{***}p < 0.001$, $^{****}p < 0.0001$

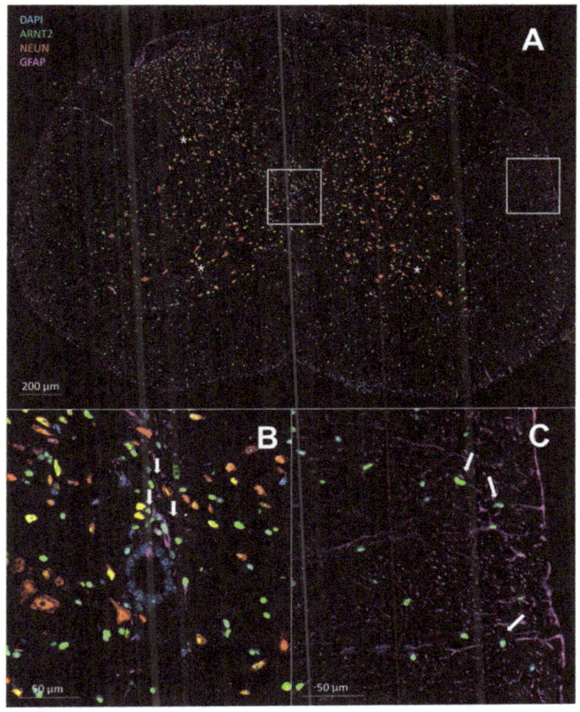

Fig. 2 ARNT2 is localized to neurons and glia in the healthy mouse spinal cord. **a** A cross section of the mouse spinal cord at approximately C5 shows numerous ARNT2 (green) expressing cells throughout the gray and white matter of the cord. ARNT2 positivity colocalizing with NeuN$^+$ (red) cells is observed frequently as yellow cells in the dorsal and ventral horns (asterisk) as well as throughout the intermediate zones. **b** An inset of the central canal from A shows ependymal cells of the central canal are negative for ARNT2, but indeed many GFAP$^+$ cells in the area show positivity for ARNT2 (arrows). **c** In the white matter, ARNT2 positivity is often associated with GFAP$^+$ astrocytes (arrows) with a fibrous phenotype in arrangements that extend away from the meninges

pattern was prominent in the ventral horn and intermediate zones of the gray matter though it seemed most pronounced in many levels within the dorsal horns (Fig. 3b, c insets). Notably, there was also a significant reduction in the number of NeuN$^+$ cells/mm^2 of gray matter in EAE animals compared to healthy controls (Fig. 4a). The reduction observed when samples were pooled from all levels of the cord (cervical, thoracic, and lumbar) was 535.9 ± 23.3 in healthy vs 281.7 ± 26.3 in EAE animals ($p < 0.001$); the greatest differences were observed in the thoracic and lumbar levels while differences in the cervical regions were not significant (430.7 ± 34.8 vs 389.9 ± 36.3, data not shown). Using a threshold for negative staining set by ARNT2 staining of the ependymal cells in each section, we measured the mean fluorescence intensity per pixel of each NeuN$^+$ nucleus to compare healthy animals to EAE animals. We analyzed the entire gray matter and also performed a separate analysis of cells in the dorsal

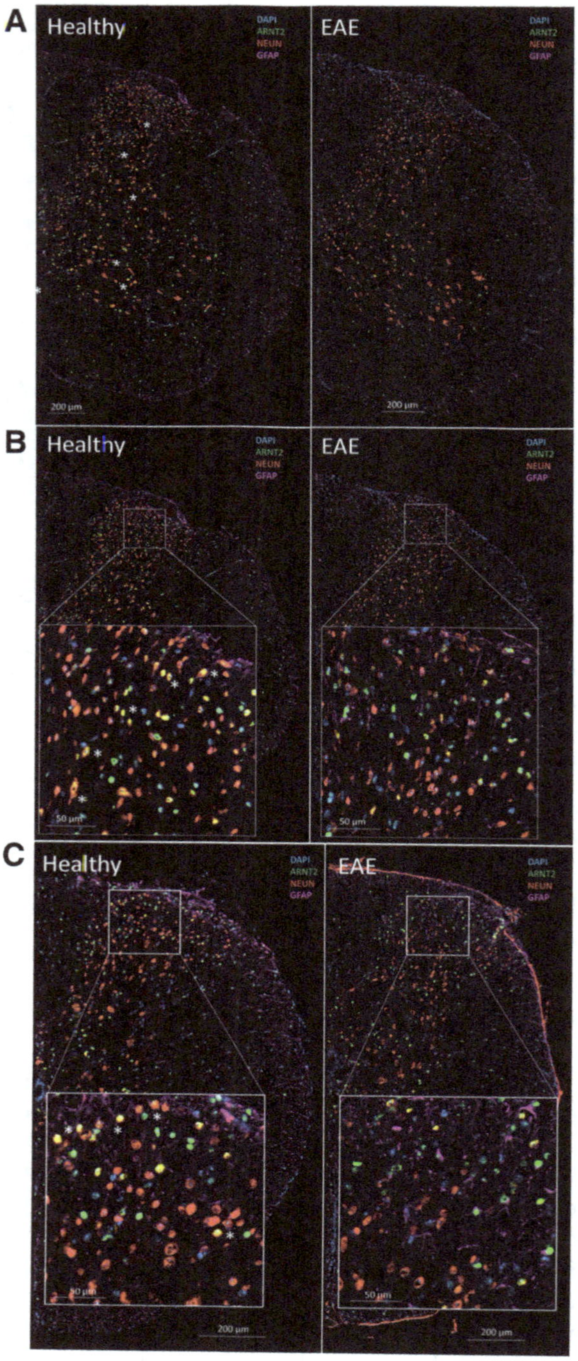

Fig. 3 ARNT2 is expressed differentially between healthy immunized and EAE mice. Staining for ARNT2 in neuronal (NeuN$^+$) or astrocytic (GFAP$^+$) populations was localized predominantly to gray matter neurons and some astrocytes in the gray and white matter of healthy mice. **a** Compared to healthy mice, less NeuN+ cells stain for ARNT2 as well, giving rise to fewer yellow co-labeled cells (asterisk) in this C5 level image of EAE mice than observed in the healthy mice. With a focus on the dorsal horn (**b**), this loss in ARNT2 staining in NeuN$^+$ cells seems even more pronounced; the same is true in **c** where images of the dorsal horn of EAE mice at T5/T6 show lower ARNT2 positivity in NeuN$^+$ cells than observed in the dorsal horn of healthy mice (asterisk)

horn only. Separate from the determination of positive cells, we also distinguished the percent of moderate (> 1.5× negligible intensity threshold) versus highly staining cells (> 2× negligible intensity threshold) as illustrated in Fig. 4b. We did not detect a significant difference in the % of NeuN$^+$ cells which were positive for ARNT2 between the two groups, 65.8 ± 3.1 versus 66.6 ± 3.4% in healthy vs EAE animals respectively over the entire gray matter region; numbers were also similar when only the dorsal horns were compared in the healthy (66.6 ± 3.4%) vs. EAE animals (63.0 ± 4.1%). However, the relative intensities of the stained cells were significantly lower in EAE animals than healthy mice (Fig. 4c). Over the entire gray matter region, the percentage of NeuN$^+$ cells staining moderate to high was significantly lower in EAE animals (33.7 ± 2.6% of cells vs 22.6 ± 2.7%, $p = 0.0065$). This decrease was particularly marked in highly staining ARNT2 cells which dropped from 11.0 ± 1.4% of NeuN$^+$ cells in healthy animals to 5.1 ± .9% of NeuN$^+$ cells in EAE animals ($p = 0.0024$). Decreases in ARNT2 expression were even more pronounced within the dorsal horns; the proportion of moderate to highly stained NeuN$^+$ cells dropped by 50% (36.0 ± 3.0% in healthy vs 18.2 ± 3.0% in EAE mice) whereas the proportion of highly expressing ARNT2 cells dropped by more than 80% (10.1 ± 1.7% in healthy vs 1.9 ± .9% in EAE mice). The number of GFAP$^+$ cells in the gray matter of EAE mice was also significantly increased compared to healthy sham-immunized mice (Fig. 4d, e; 419.2 ± 40.4 vs 161.7 ± 14.1 cells/mm^2, $p < 0.0001$). In Fig. 4f, notably, the intensity of ARNT2 expression in NeuN$^+$ cells correlated inversely with the degree of immune cell infiltration. Declines in neuronal ARNT2 intensity were correlated with increased infiltrates ($r = -0.508$, $R^2 = 0.259$, $p = 0.0047$). In this EAE model, regions of immune cell infiltration often correlated with areas of demyelination (reduced staining for myelin basic protein, MBP) and also axonal damage which is apparent as axonal spheroids detectable by staining for non-phosphorylated neurofilaments with the SMI32 antibody [26, 46]. As expected, demyelination was not detected in our sham

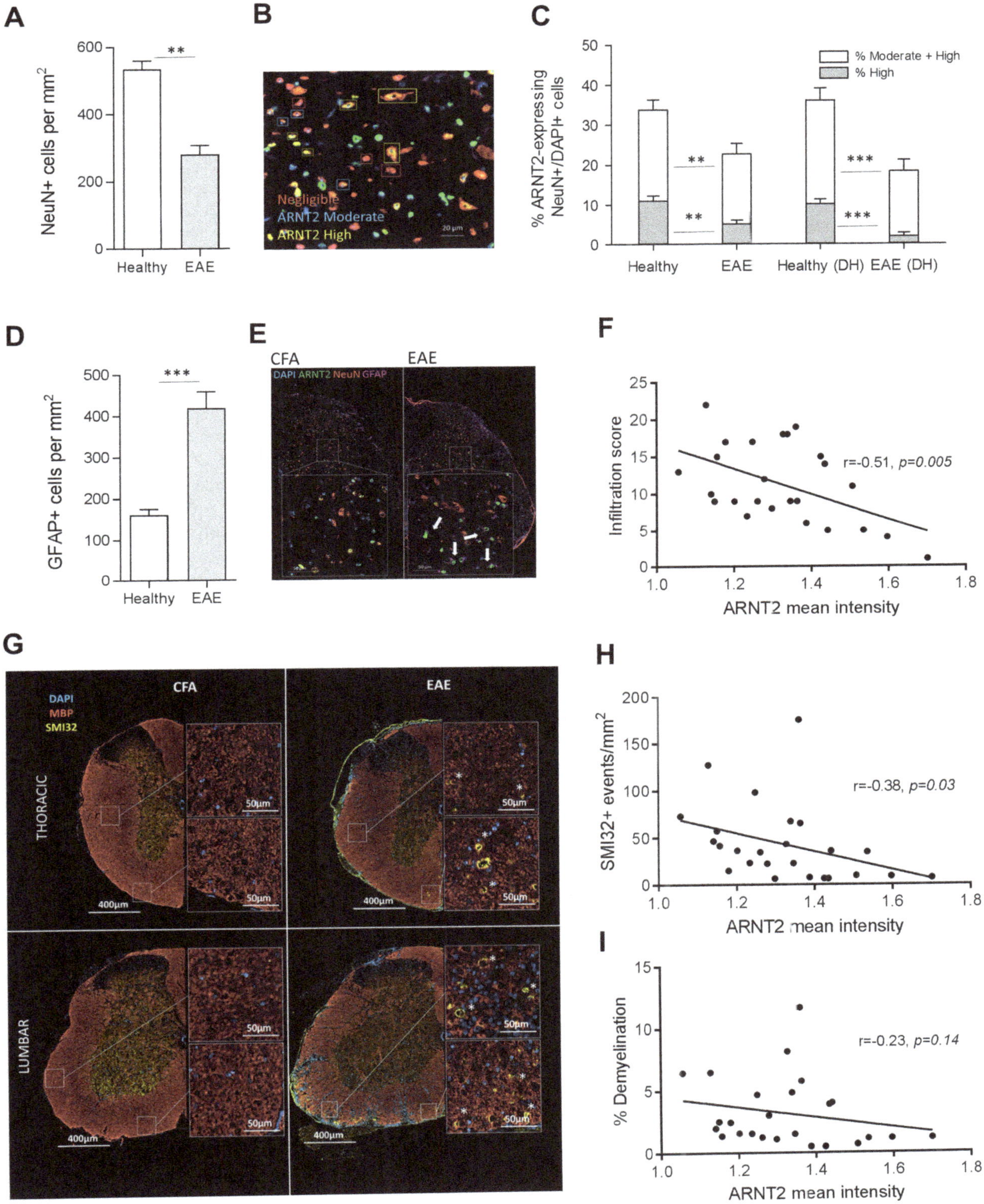

Fig. 4 (See legend on next page.)

(See figure on previous page.)
Fig. 4 ARNT2 expression is decreased during peak disease in neuronal populations. **a** A relative loss of NeuN$^+$ cells is observed in EAE mice compared to healthy sham-immunized controls examined in five to seven levels from three to four mice each. **b** Expression levels of ARNT2 were normalized to the staining of ependymal cells and categorized as high (mean intensities greater than 2× the background) or moderate (greater than 1.5× the background) as shown in representative images. **c** The % of NeuN$^+$ cells expressing moderate or greater ARNT2 intensity was reduced by almost 30% in animals at peak disease. These differences were even greater in analyses of the dorsal horn (DH) regions in each section. Bars represent the mean intensity of 4–6 levels pooled from 7 healthy/CFA immunized animals ($n = 39$) compared to levels pooled from 5 EAE animals ($n = 29$) where whiskers indicate the SEM. $p \leq 0.05$*, $p \leq 0.01$**, $p \leq 0.001$***, Mann-Whitney *T* test. **d** GFAP$^+$ astrocytes were enumerated per mm^2 of gray matter in each of the same levels analyzed in **c**. **e** A comparison of healthy to EAE animals at the L5/L6 level showed a marked increase in the frequency of GFAP$^+$ cells in the gray matter of EAE mice; notably, these cells are largely positive for ARNT2 (arrows). **f** Each infiltrate was scored and pooled per each of 5 levels from 5 EAE mice. This infiltration score from 25 levels of EAE cord was compared to the mean intensity of ARNT2 in NeuN$^+$ cells in the GM. **g** Serial sections from the same levels examined in C were stained for MBP and SMI-32. SMI32 positivity was not detected in sham-immunized animals, nor was a decrease in MBP staining. Associated with regions of infiltrates in EAE animals (inset), SMI32$^+$ axons and spheroids were more frequent and in the lower areas of cord tended to be associated with regions of demyelination. In higher thoracic areas of the cord, SMI32 positivity was still present but demyelination was less prevalent. **h** The no. of SMI32+ events/mm2 and **i** % demyelination as calculated by masking regions devoid of MBP staining were correlated with ARNT2 mean intensity as outlined in **f**

immunized animals (Fig. 4g). In contrast, all levels of EAE mice examined exhibited some degree of demyelination, typically associated with areas of inflammatory infiltration; the degree of demyelination ranged from 1.4 to 21.5% of the white matter area in a single level with an average of 4.7 ± 0.9% demyelination over all levels examined from EAE mice. Similarly, few SMI32$^+$ axons were detected in sham-immunized animals at any level. In contrast, SMI32$^+$ spheroids were detected in all levels of EAE animals examined, with an average of 62.7 ± 13.3 (range 6 to 300) spheroids per square millimeter. In EAE animals, we found a direct correlation between the frequency of SMI32$^+$ spheroids and the degree of demyelination ($r = 0.878$, $R^2 = 0.772$, $p < 0.0001$ (data not shown). Notably, the frequency of SMI32$^+$ spheroids or axon “rings” stained with SMI32 (as in insets) per square millimeter correlated inversely with the ARNT2 intensity of NeuN$^+$ cells at each level of the EAE mice examined (Fig. 4h; $r = -0.376$, $R^2 = 0.141$, $p = 0.032$). The degree of demyelination did not correlate with the ARNT2 intensity as closely throughout all levels examined (Fig. 4i; $r = -0.229$, $R^2 = 0.052$, $p = 0.136$). Examination of different levels of the spinal cord showed that SMI32$^+$ were frequent in areas of extensive demyelination yet were also detected in areas where demyelination was less apparent, such as those in higher/thoracic levels of the cord (Fig. 4f, insets).

Cell stressors alter ARNT2 protein levels

After establishing the relationship between inflammation and ARNT2 expression in vivo, we set out to examine factors which alter ARNT2 expression as well as the outcome of decreasing ARNT2 expression in vitro. Cultures routinely consist of 92.6 ± 6.9% MAP2$^+$ neuronal cells ($n = 3$) by DIV10-14 (Additional file 3: Table S3) with some GFAP$^+$ astrocytes (7.4 ± 6.9%). Healthy neurons, characterized by large cell bodies with complex axonal and dendritic processes, ranged in nuclear area from 50 to 200 μm^2. Occasional astrocytes exhibited a reactive morphology with extensive ramifications in comparison to non-reactive astrocytes that are more flat and polygonal [47].

Staurosporine potently induces apoptosis by preventing ATP binding to kinases, preventing protein kinase activity and resulting in growth factor withdrawal [48]. Reduced growth factor activity is linked to caspase-3 and cytochrome c activity, resulting in activation of the apoptotic pathway [49]. We tested staurosporine at a range of doses from 5 to 1000 nM for 24 h, where previous studies showed neuronal apoptosis in vitro with 500–1000 nM [48, 49]. Ten nanomolars of staurosporine increased ARNT2 levels by greater than 50% compared to vehicle-treated cells at 24 h (Fig. 5a, $n = 3$, $p \leq 0.05$). At 500 to 1000 nM, cell death became evident by phase microscopy showing numerous cell bodies and cellular debris (Fig. 5b), which was not observed with ARNT2 levels nearer to vehicle controls. We next examined ARNT2 and cleaved caspase 3 intensities in enriched neuronal cultures and found that 6 or 12 h of exposure to 1 μM staurosporine significantly decreased ARNT2 expression and these decreases in ARNT2 were accompanied by increases in cleaved caspase 3 (Fig. 5c–e). In staurosporine-treated wells, cells staining brightly for cleaved caspase 3 typically showed negligible levels of ARNT2 compared to vehicle-treated controls.

Oxidative stress significantly alters ARNT2 protein expression

To model mild to severe oxidative stress in primary cortical-enriched neuronal cultures, we applied 25, 50, 100, and 300 μM H_2O_2 (Fig. 6). Twenty-five micromolars of H_2O_2 was associated with a significant increase in ARNT2 tested over 0.5 to 3 h compared to untreated controls (Fig. 6a, $n = 6$, $p \leq 0.01$). Notably, phase microscopy showed no changes in cell morphology or signs of blebbing and LDH release was also negligible over the

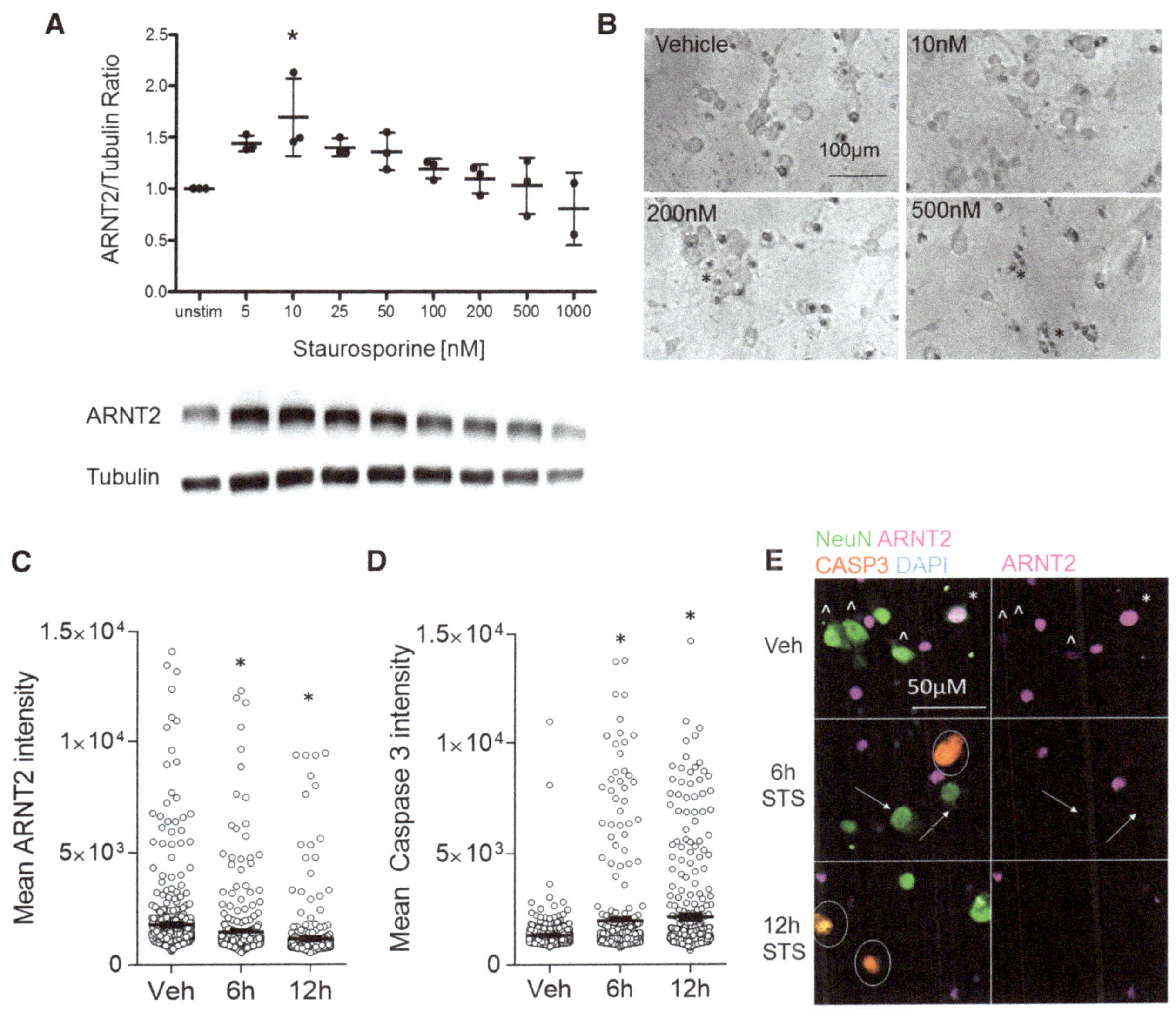

Fig. 5 Staurosporine significantly increases ARNT2 protein levels. **a** Enriched neuronal cultures were treated with staurosporine at different doses for 24 h prior to analysis. Lines and whiskers indicate mean and standard deviation from results in three experiments with representative blots. *$p \leq 0.05$ repeated measures ANOVA on ranks with Tukey's multiple comparison test to vehicle (0.1% DMSO)-treated cells. **b** Phase microscopy images show dead/dying neurons following exposure to 500–1000 nM staurosporine. No change in % cytotoxicity as measured by LDH release was observed (data not shown). Enriched neuronal cortical cultures were treated with 1 μM staurosporine for 6 or 12 h and stained for NeuN to distinguish neurons for **c** ARNT2 and **d** cleaved caspase 3 intensity. Data points represent cells pooled from 11 random regions from wells treated in duplicate. *$p \leq 0.05$ ANOVA followed by Bonferroni's multiple comparisons test to vehicle-treated cells; bars represent the average mean intensity and whiskers the SEM. **e** Representative images from the wells analyzed in **c** and **d** reveal NeuN$^+$ cells in vehicle-treated wells that stain brightly (asterisk) or faintly (circumflex accent) for ARNT2; cleaved caspase-3 staining (red) is negligible. With 6 or 12 h exposure to staurosporine (STS), ARNT2 intensity is significantly lowered in neurons (arrows) whereas Caspase3$^+$ intensity increases in NeuN$^+$ cells (circled)

24 h treatment period (Fig. 6a). There were no changes in ARNT2 from 10 to 24 h in longer term experiments (data not shown).

Similar to 25 μM, 50 μM H_2O_2 increased ARNT2 protein levels with peak levels measured at 2 h after addition (Fig. 6b, $n = 6$, $p \leq 0.05$); ARNT2 levels then returned to baseline by 3–4 h and ultimately dropped below baseline. The dropping of ARNT2 levels below baseline was not associated with morphological alterations within the first 5 to 10 h (Fig. 6e). Cell cytotoxicity measured by LDH release, while not apparent at 6 h, was significantly increased to 15–17% cytotoxicity by 12 and 18 h of cell exposure.

Exposure to a higher dose of H_2O_2 (100 μM) increased detectable ARNT2 protein at 0.5 and 1 h compared to controls (Fig. 6c, $n = 7$, $p \leq 0.05$). By 3–4 h exposure, ARNT2 levels dropped below baseline in most experiments, but cells maintained their complex morphology

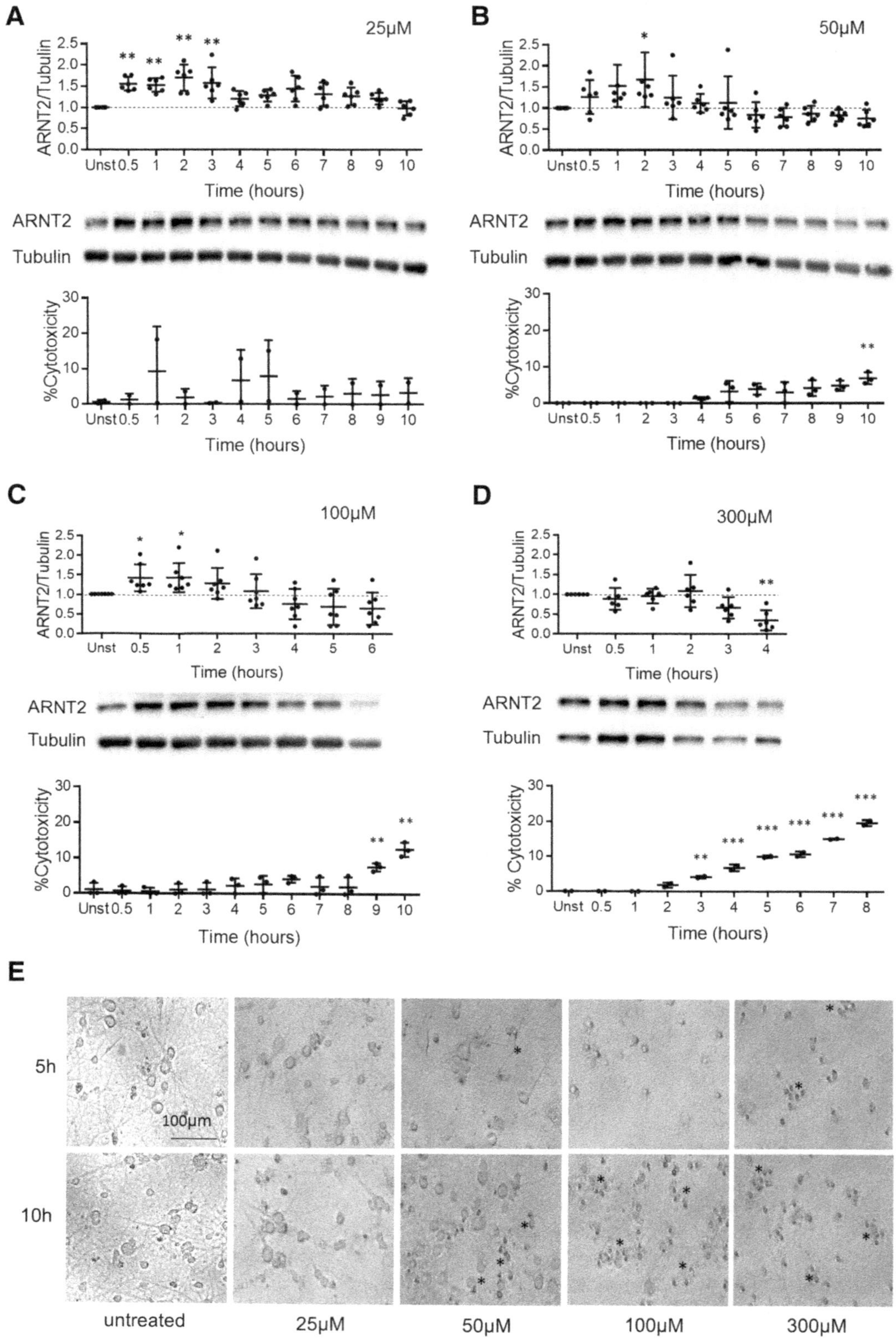

Fig. 6 (See legend on next page.)

(See figure on previous page.)
Fig. 6 Hydrogen peroxide significantly alters ARNT2 protein expression. Four doses were applied: **a–d** 25, 50, 100, and 300 μM H_2O_2. Graphs represent the ARNT2/β-actin ratios of protein expression from western blotting. Points represent six biological replicates, with two technical replicates each, where lines and whiskers indicate mean and standard deviation, with representative blots. Cytotoxicity measured by lactic dehydrogenase (LDH) release is reported as the % cytotoxicity or % of total death relative to wells lysed with lysis buffer. Supernatants were collected at intervals following H_2O_2 treatment and compared to spontaneous LDH release in untreated controls. $p \leq 0.05$*, $p \leq 0.01$**, $p \leq 0.001$***, repeated measures ANOVA on ranks with Tukey's multiple comparison test to unstimulated. **e** Representative phase contrast photomicrographs show neuronal bodies with numerous complex dendrites and processes throughout the culture in untreated cultures. Addition of increasing doses of H_2O_2 over time leads to a loss in cell viability evidenced by decreasing processes and complexity of neurons with increasing amounts of cellular debris and condensed nuclei (asterisk)

through 5 h of treatment. Increases in LDH release became significant by 6 h ($p \leq 0.05$) and were followed by a relative loss of dendrites and increased neuronal blebbing, nuclear condensation, and cell death apparent by 10 h (Fig. 6e). Notably, exposure to the highest tested dose H_2O_2 at 300 μM did not significantly increase ARNT2 levels and instead was associated with significant declines in ARNT2 expression beginning at 3–4 h which preceded blebbing of many cells by 5 h and loss of all dendritic morphology by 10 h (Fig. 6e).

We analyzed mRNA for *Arnt2, Npas4,* and *Bdnf* in H_2O_2-treated neuronal-enriched cultures compared to PBS-treated cells. Notably, *Arnt2* mRNA was not influenced by oxidative stress in primary cortical neuron-enriched cultures, indicating no relative change in transcript levels (Additional file 4). Over the time intervals where ARNT2 protein changed (0.5 to 2 h in response to H_2O_2), we saw no change in ARNT2 message. However, *Npas4* mRNA increased rapidly and specifically in response to oxidative stress and was followed closely by increases in *Bdnf* mRNA.

We next examined the relationship between declines in ARNT2 intensity and expression of cleaved caspase 3. Using early DIV7 neuronal cultures, we minimized the likelihood of glial contamination with the potential for MAP2 losses by neurons following exposure to stressors or undergoing cell death or apoptosis. Exposure to 25 μm H_2O_2 for 1 h had no effect on ARNT2 expression but 50 μM significantly reduced the mean ARNT2 intensity in neurons (Fig. 7a, $p < 0.05$). In this 1 h of exposure, there were no increases in cleaved caspase 3 expression in either group (Fig. 7b). In contrast, 3 h exposure to both 25 and 50 μM of H_2O_2 both significantly reduced ARNT2 intensity in neurons (Fig. 7c). Only exposure to the greater dose of H_2O_2 was associated with increases in cleaved caspase 3, although the majority of these cells also showed condensed nuclei (Fig. 7b, c) indicative of reduced cell viability that was also apparent in our earlier phase micrographs (Fig. 6e).

We also examined ARNT2 expression at the individual cell level in our enriched neuronal cultures; 15–20% of the cells in the culture stained negligibly for ARNT2 (Fig. 8a). The majority of cells (60–70%) were low to moderate in their expression of ARNT2 while 10–15% had more intense ARNT2 staining. Notably, the few contaminating astrocytes were also positive for ARNT2. We tested the same doses of H_2O_2 (25 μM and 100 μM) previously used, focusing on earlier time points (0.5, 1, 2, 4, and 6 h). Total DAPI$^+$ cells, MAP2$^+$ cells, and GFAP$^+$ cells were analyzed (Fig. 8b). With 100 μM H_2O_2, there was a significant increase in ARNT2 protein detected at 1 h exposure compared to untreated controls ($n = 3$, $p \leq 0.05$ for DAPI$^+$, 0.001 for MAP2$^+$, and 0.01 for GFAP$^+$ cells); this matched the increases in ARNT2 observed by western blotting (Fig. 6c). The staining intensity of ARNT2 was at or below baseline in neurons and astrocytes treated for 2–4 h and reached levels significantly lower than baseline (i.e., all three data groups, $n = 3$ for each; at 2 h: $p \leq 0.01$ for GFAP$^+$; at 4 h: $p \leq 0.05$ for DAPI$^+$, $p \leq 0.01$ for GFAP$^+$; at 6 h: $p \leq 0.001$ for all three) which preceded changes in cell viability. Using this cell-specific analysis, we report a significant early upregulation of ARNT2 by 100 μM H_2O_2 in both neurons and astrocytes, which after extended exposure results in similar decreases in ARNT2 expression that precede cytotoxicity as in Fig. 6a–d.

Discussion

ARNT2 has been characterized for its expression patterns and functional roles in vivo throughout development and under conditions of hypoxia, ischemic injury, and neuroprotection, as well as in in vitro models, including in primary cells and cell lines [10]. In this study, we set out to characterize changes in the amount and cellular localization of ARNT2 during inflammatory demyelinating disease of the CNS and to examine the ability of specific factors and stressors to alter ARNT2 protein expression in primary cortical neuron-enriched cultures.

We examined ARNT2 expression in both healthy and EAE animals in what is to our knowledge the first description of ARNT2 in the healthy spinal cord and in chronic inflammatory CNS disease. ARNT2 localization to NeuN$^+$ neuronal cell bodies throughout gray matter in the healthy spinal cord was expected, with moderate to high expression observed throughout the gray matter in both the dorsal and ventral horns as well as in the intermediate zones. At peak disease, we observed a significant drop in ARNT2 expression in NeuN$^+$ cells, associated with a loss of these cells throughout the gray

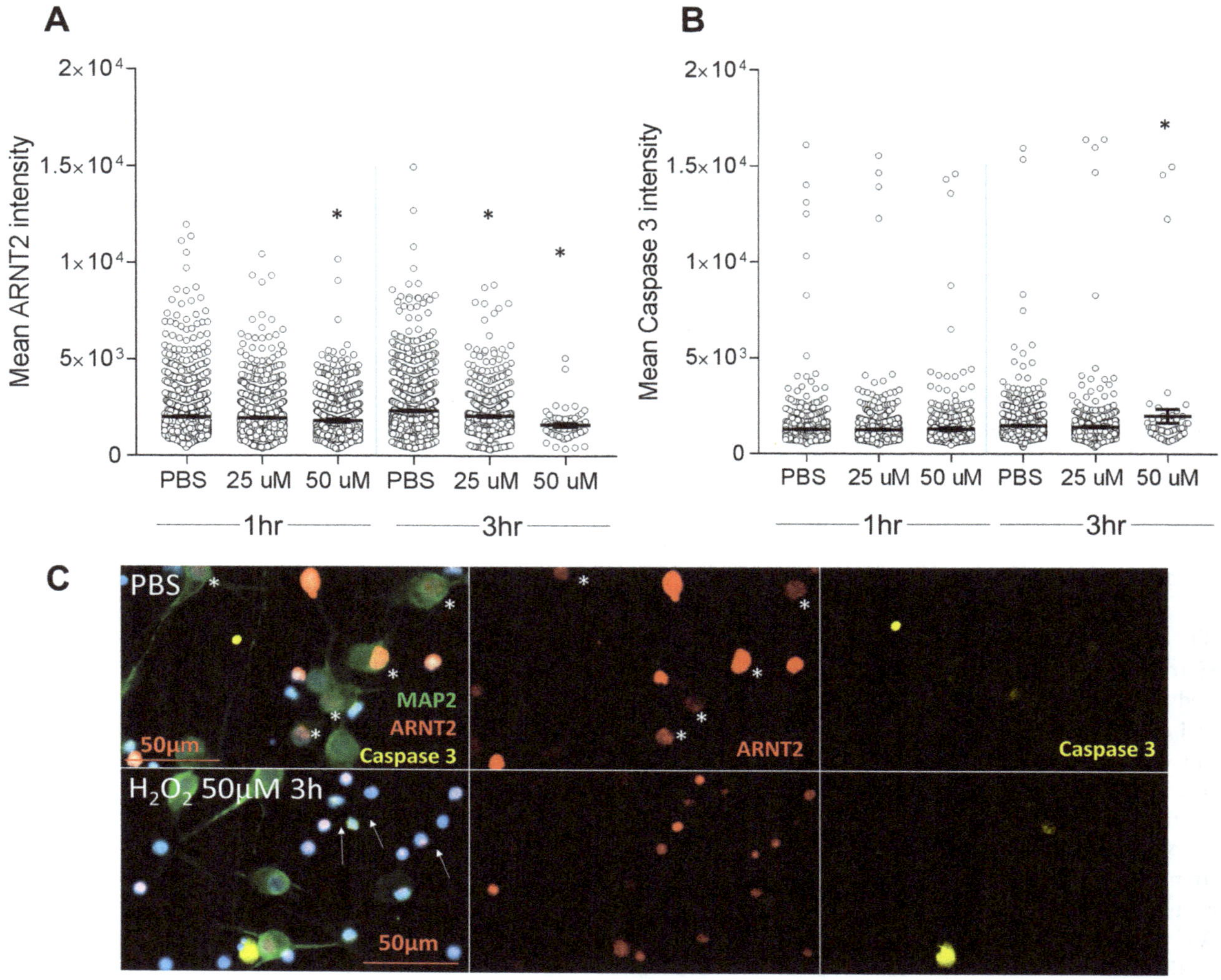

Fig. 7 H_2O_2-treated neurons display decreased ARNT2 which precedes increases in cleaved-caspase 3 staining/apoptotic cell death. DIV7 neurons were treated with 25 or 50 μM H_2O_2 for 1 and 3 h and stained to examine ARNT2 and cleaved caspase-3 intensity. Data points represent cells pooled from 11 random regions from wells treated in duplicate. *$p \leq 0.05$ ANOVA followed by Bonferroni's multiple comparisons test to PBS-treated cells for the same treatment time; bars represent the average mean intensity and whiskers the SEM; 1 of 2 representative experiments with similar results is shown. **c** Representative images from **a** to **b** are shown. PBS-treated wells show numerous MAP2$^+$ cells staining brightly or moderately for ARNT2 (asterisk); staining for cleaved caspase-3 is negligible. In contrast, exposure to 25uM H_2O_2 significantly reduced ARNT2, without associated increases in cleaved caspase-3 that are not detected until exposure to 50 μM H_2O_2 for 3 h. Fifty micromolars of H_2O_2 also increased the number of condensed nuclei and reductions in MAP2$^+$ dendrites (arrow)

matter. A loss of NeuN$^+$ cells in the spinal cord during acute EAE has been described previously [50], but is not typically examined in most studies. Notably, decreases in ARNT2 expression correlated with increased numbers of inflammatory infiltrates. Given the regulation of ARNT2 in response to stressors and a role in neuroprotection, concurrent loss of ARNT2 expression and neuronal integrity and axonal damage evidenced by increased SMI32 positivity at peak disease highlights a potential role for ARNT2 in neuronal health and survival. In the chronic progressive model of EAE, we found a significant downregulation of *Arnt2* mRNA at peak disease in the spinal cord. Our histological data showed that loss of ARNT2 expression in spinal cord neuronal populations correlates with the drop in *Arnt2* message and protein that we observed in whole spinal cord lysates from preclinical to peak stages in our model.

Somewhat unexpectedly, we found ARNT2$^+$/GFAP$^+$ astrocytes lining the meninges, midline, and central canal of healthy animals with some scattering through the white matter. This is the first description of ARNT2 in astrocytes at brain interfaces in healthy animals, and increases in their number through the gray matter may implicate ARNT2$^+$ astrocytes in processes mitigating damage with the potential to aid in repair that require further characterization. Astrocytes are a key source of

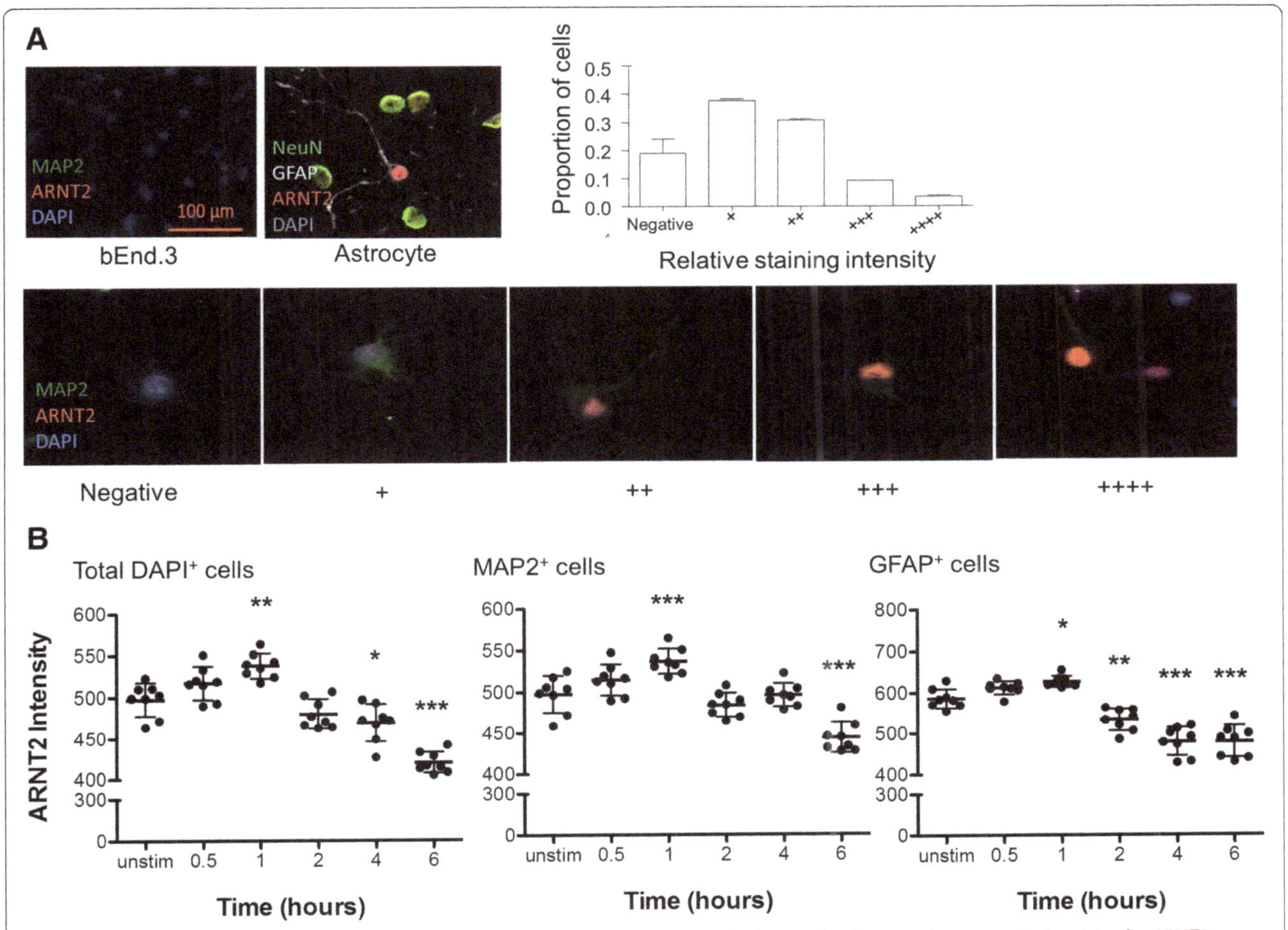

Fig. 8 ARNT2 protein is localized to both neurons and astrocytes in neuronal-enriched cortical cultures. **a** Immunocytochemistry for ARNT2 reveals negligible ARNT2 staining in the Bend3 mouse immortalized brain microvascular endothelial cell line. Using threshold sets by the staining intensity in negative cells as described in the "Methods" section and Additional file 3, cells were divided according to staining intensity: negligible to ++++. The majority of MAP2$^+$ neurons in the culture showed low to moderate staining for ARNT2; staining was also detected in the few contaminating GFAP$^+$ astrocytes which demonstrated a reactive phenotype. One of three representative experiments is shown where eight regions from each of two duplicate wells were analyzed. **b** Following exposure to 100 μM H_2O_2, the entire enriched population as well as MAP2$^+$ neurons and GFAP$^+$ astrocytes examined individually demonstrated increases in ARNT2 staining intensity at 1 h; the same decreases after longer exposure observed with western blotting to baseline levels and below were replicated by immunocytochemistry. Points represent eight biological replicates, with two technical replicates each, where lines and whiskers indicate mean and standard deviation. $p \leq 0.05$*, $p \leq 0.01$**, $p \leq 0.001$***, repeated measures ANOVA on ranks with Tukey's multiple comparison test to unstimulated

neurotrophins throughout neuronal development and afford neuroprotection in response to trauma or insult; indeed, astrocytes express BDNF and this expression is upregulated under conditions of CNS injury [1]. ARNT2 expression by these cells in proximity to the meninges and proximal to the cerebrospinal fluid may define the ability to respond to stressors locally as well as those produced remotely. Expression of ARNT2 in astrocytes in vivo may not have been previously reported either because it was not detected in the specific brain regions examined, or a lower likelihood of detection may exist in healthy tissues. In our analyses, astrocytic ARNT2 expression in the white matter of the healthy spinal cord was relatively sparse and largely overshadowed by neuronal ARNT2 expression. During acute disease, ARNT2$^+$ astrocytes morphologically resembled reactive astrocytes found in vivo in EAE as well as MS post-mortem tissue, with increased ramifications and high GFAP expression [51]. These cells are thought to play a role in the disease process through astrogliosis or expansion of astrocyte numbers due to nearby damage, causing scar formation and potential inhibition of axonal regeneration [51]. Preliminary stains to characterize GFAP$^-$/ARNT2$^+$ cells showed that ARNT2 was apparent in Olig2$^+$ cells (a marker of oligodendrocytes but also present on reactive astrocytes [42] which warrants further investigation). In contrast, we could not detect ARNT2 in Iba-1+ microglia in healthy spinal cords nor in Iba-1+ cells in EAE spinal cords in preliminary analyses.

We report for the first time the effect of stressors involved in inflammatory and neurodegenerative processes on ARNT2 expression in primary enriched cultures of cortical neurons. We have shown that ARNT2 expression is increased under certain stress-initiating stimuli, including mild and more concentrated exposure to H_2O_2 and staurosporine. While ARNT2 protein is significantly increased by 25 to 100 μM H_2O_2 within a couple of hours, there is no change at the mRNA level in *Arnt2* over these doses or time points. This suggests early increases in ARNT2 protein are not secondary to enhanced mRNA transcription and subsequent translation. It may instead result from post-transcriptional/post-translational modifications or epigenetics, as described for other bHLH factors under developmental conditions [52, 53]. Indeed, epigenetic regulation of ARNT2 has previously been described in the context of neuronal differentiation of P19 cells, in which expression of ARNT2 was dependent upon downregulation of the expression of a repressor gene [2].

The upregulation of ARNT2 protein in primary cortical neurons in response to oxidative stress and apoptotic stimuli is a novel finding. Overall, ARNT2 protein levels in neurons appeared to follow two patterns when exposed to different levels of oxidative stress: an early upregulation with 25, 50, and 100 μM H_2O_2 and a return to constitutive levels versus exposure to higher doses (300 μM H_2O_2) where declining ARNT2 expression precedes losses in cell integrity as well as increases in cleaved caspase3 expression. A previous study has shown that pre-treatment of mouse hippocampal neurons with bicuculline reduced the percentage of cells undergoing apoptosis following staurosporine treatment which was abolished with knockdown of NPAS4 [54]. As the primary binding partner of NPAS4 in the CNS is ARNT2 and given the previous implication of ARNT2 as an anti-apoptotic factor in PC12 cells, it is plausible that their heterodimerization may play a role in protection of cells against apoptotic cell death [1, 10].

A neuroprotective role for ARNT2 is supported by both our in vitro and in vivo findings of changes in *Bdnf* that coincide with changes in *Npas4*. BDNF is a major mediator of physiological functions including activity-dependent functions, axonal growth, and a key molecule in neuronal and axonal survival with impact on memory, learning, and neurogenesis [55–59]. Npas4 controls activity-dependent Bdnf mRNA levels. BDNF expression is reduced by almost twofold in cultures expressing Npas4-RNA interference [17], and overexpressing dominant/negative forms of ARNT2 and Npas4 protein prevent BDNF induction [18]. BDNF has garnered particular interest in MS pathogenesis as one of only a handful of "protective" pathways described in MS models. In vitro, de novo expression of otherwise negligible *Npas4* in cortical neurons is driven rapidly by oxidative stress in our studies, a response which has not previously been described. This is closely associated with increases in *Bdnf* message, also an immediate early gene. Similarly, in vivo analyses of animals developing clinical disease secondary to autoimmune inflammatory neurodegeneration show that the presence of *Arnt2* RNA and protein prior to the onset of disease has the potential to partner with significant increases in *Npas4* RNA at day 7 to yield the observed increases in *Bdnf* RNA by day 10. As both ARNT2 message and protein decrease, similar decreases are seem with *Npas4* that are closely mirrored by reductions in *Bdnf*. Together, these findings demonstrate that the presence of ARNT2 can be closely linked to neurotrophic support via BDNF increases associated with the induction of Npas4.

Conclusions

This study has uniquely characterized the expression of ARNT2 in an inflammatory neurodegenerative disease model of MS. We link changes in ARNT2 to inflammatory processes and mediators, where decreases are associated with losses in neuronal integrity in vitro and immune infiltration and axonal damage and disability in vivo. Our data support ARNT2 as a neuronal transcription factor whose sustained expression is linked to neuronal and axonal health, protection that may primarily be driven through its partnering with Npas4 to influence BDNF expression. This characterization of ARNT2 expression and regulation points to ARNT2 and its partner Npas4 as potential targets to effect neuroprotection and warrants further examination in inflammatory neurodegenerative disorders such as MS.

Additional files

Additional file 1: Table S1. Scoring of inflammatory infiltrates. Each level of the spinal cord was examined for the number and nature of infiltrates; sections were the same as those used to assess ARNT2 expression. The total infiltrate score was determined by adding the lesion score for all lesions in that section to obtain a total infiltrate score for each level. **Table S2.** List of antibodies used for western blotting (WB), immunocyto- (IC) and immunohistochemistry (IH) and primers for qPCR.

Additional file 2: Quantification of *Npas4* and *Bdnf* RNA in mouse spinal cords over the course of EAE. Tissues from 5 to 8 mice with similar disease scores were harvested at days 7, 10, 14, 18, 25, 32, and 45 as in Fig. 1a representing preclinical, onset, peak, recovery and times with some degree of worsening over time and analyzed by qPCR to obtain message levels normalized to β-actin.

Additional file 3: Table S3. Primary enriched neuronal cortical cultures have few glial cells. Breakdown of culture purity as well as cell distribution based on normalized ARNT2 intensity in primary cortical neuron-enriched cultures. Staining of enriched cortical cultures for neuronal (MAP2) and astrocytic (GFAP) markers. 3 independent experiments are shown to establish the threshold limits for ARNT2 staining intensity and distribution of staining intensities in $MAP2^+$ cells in primary cortical neuron-enriched cultures.

Additional file 4: qPCR to examine *Arnt2, Npas4, and Bdnf* expression following exposure of cortical neuronal cultures to H_2O_2. Values are normalized to β-actin. Bars represent average of 2 biological replicate/experiments. ARNT2 RNA levels remain largely unchanged.

Abbreviations

ARNT2: Aryl hydrocarbon receptor nuclear translocator 2; BDNF: Brain-derived neurotrophic factor; bHLH/PAS: Basic-helix-loop-helix period-ARNT-single minded protein; Bic: Bicuculline; DAPI: 4′,6-Diamidino-2-phenylindole; EAE: Experimental autoimmune encephalomyelitis; GFAP: Glial fibrillary acidic protein; H_2O_2: Hydrogen peroxide; MAP2: Microtubule-associated protein 2; MOG: Myelin oligodendroglial protein; NPAS4: Neuronal pas domain protein 4

Acknowledgements

Thank you to Jake Johnston, Emily Kamma, and Mahima Kapoor who assisted with aspects of data analyses. We thank Andrew Leung, Izabelle Gadawska, and Cheryl Whiting for technical contributions related to cell culturing and qPCR analyses, Sarah Neil for assisting with isolation and processing of EAE samples, and Adam Yu and Pascal St. Pierre for their assistance in establishing immunocytochemistry protocols and analyses.

Funding

This study was supported by Biomedical operating grant no. 1580 from the MS Society of Canada and by the Neuroprotection Fund and the MS Renewal Program Fund established by the Maureen and Milan Ilich Foundation through the VGH & UBC Hospital Foundation. JQ was supported by an MS Society of Canada Donald Paty Career Development Award. TR was supported by a Canada Graduate Scholarship-Master's and a MS Society of Canada MSc Studentship.

Authors' contributions

TR and PB contributed equally to this work. TR performed cell culture, immunocytochemistry, and western blotting experiments to analyze ARNT2 expression in vitro and conducted data collection and analyses as well as prepared a first draft of the manuscript. M-EB performed western blotting of EAE tissues. PB performed qPCR of the EAE tissues, all EAE tissue staining, image acquisition and analyses as well as additional in vitro culture to examine ARNT2 over time and in correlation with caspase by qPCR and immunocytochemistry over time, respectively. JQ performed EAE induction, animal scoring, and assisted with tissue harvesting and processing. JQ formulated the research plan and series of experiments to address the aims of the paper, oversaw the experimental approach and design, reviewed data and analyses for interpretation of the data, and oversaw the manuscript preparation including revising the manuscript critically for technical and scientific accuracy. All authors have reviewed the manuscript in entirety and are in agreement with the content of this work. All authors read and approved the final manuscript.

Consent for publication

Not applicable.

Competing interests

The authors declare that they have no competing interests.

References

1. Bersten DC, Bruning JB, Peet DJ, Whitelaw ML. Human variants in the neuronal basic helix-loop-helix/Per-Arnt-Sim (bHLH/PAS) transcription factor complex NPAS4/ARNT2 disrupt function. PLoS One. 2014;9:e85768.
2. Hao N, Bhakti VL, Peet DJ, Whitelaw ML. Reciprocal regulation of the basic helix-loop-helix/Per-Arnt-Sim partner proteins, Arnt and Arnt2, during neuronal differentiation. Nucleic Acids Res. 2013;41:5626–38.
3. Quintana FJ. Regulation of central nervous system autoimmunity by the aryl hydrocarbon receptor. Semin Immunopathol. 2013;35:627–35.
4. Quintana FJ, Sherr DH. Aryl hydrocarbon receptor control of adaptive immunity. Pharmacol Rev. 2013;65:1148–61.
5. Rothhammer V, Mascanfroni ID, Bunse L, Takenaka MC, Kenison JE, Mayo L, Chao CC, Patel B, Yan R, Blain M, et al. Type I interferons and microbial metabolites of tryptophan modulate astrocyte activity and central nervous system inflammation via the aryl hydrocarbon receptor. Nat Med. 2016;22:586 97.
6. Gandhi R, Kumar D, Burns EJ, Nadeau M, Dake B, Laroni A, Kozoriz D, Weiner HL, Quintana FJ. Activation of the aryl hydrocarbon receptor induces human type 1 regulatory T cell-like and Foxp3(+) regulatory T cells. Nat Immunol. 2010;11:846–53.
7. Hirose K, Morita M, Ema M, Mimura J, Hamada H, Fujii H, Saijo Y, Gotoh O, Sogawa K, Fujii-Kuriyama Y. cDNA cloning and tissue-specific expression of a novel basic helix-loop-helix/PAS factor (Arnt2) with close sequence similarity to the aryl hydrocarbon receptor nuclear translocator (Arnt). Mol Cell Biol. 1996;16:1706–13.
8. Holmes JL, Pollenz RS. Determination of aryl hydrocarbon receptor nuclear translocator protein concentration and subcellular localization in hepatic and nonhepatic cell culture lines: development of quantitative western blotting protocols for calculation of aryl hydrocarbon receptor and aryl hydrocarbon receptor nuclear translocator protein in total cell lysates. Mol Pharmacol. 1997;52:202–11.
9. Aitola MH, Pelto-Huikko MT. Expression of Arnt and Arnt2 mRNA in developing murine tissues. J Histochem Cytochem. 2003;51:41–54.
10. Drutel G, Heron A, Kathmann M, Gros C, Mace S, Plotkine M, Schwartz JC, Arrang JM. ARNT2, a transcription factor for brain neuron survival? Eur J Neurosci. 1999;11:1545–53.
11. Laiosa MD, Lai ZW, Thurmond TS, Fiore NC, DeRossi C, Holdener BC, Gasiewicz TA, Silverstone AE. 2,3,7,8-Tetrachlorodibenzo-p-dioxin causes alterations in lymphocyte development and thymic atrophy in hemopoietic chimeras generated from mice deficient in ARNT2. Toxicol Sci. 2002;69:117–24.
12. Hosoya T, Oda Y, Takahashi S, Morita M, Kawauchi S, Ema M, Yamamoto M, Fujii-Kuriyama Y. Defective development of secretory neurones in the hypothalamus of Arnt2-knockout mice. Genes Cells. 2001;6:361–74.
13. Keith B, Adelman DM, Simon MC. Targeted mutation of the murine arylhydrocarbon receptor nuclear translocator 2 (Arnt2) gene reveals partial redundancy with Arnt. Proc Natl Acad Sci U S A. 2001;98:6692–7.
14. Wines ME, Tiffany AM, Holdener BC. Physical localization of the mouse aryl hydrocarbon receptor nuclear translocator-2 (Arnt2) gene within the c112K deletion. Genomics. 1998;51:223–32.
15. Webb EA, AlMutair A, Kelberman D, Bacchelli C, Chanudet E, Lescai F, Andoniadou CL, Banyan A, Alsawaid A, Alrifai MT, et al. ARNT2 mutation causes hypopituitarism, post-natal microcephaly, visual and renal anomalies. Brain. 2013;136:3096–105.
16. Zhang Z, Fei P, Mu J, Li W, Song J. Hippocampal expression of aryl hydrocarbon receptor nuclear translocator 2 and neuronal PAS domain protein 4 in a rat model of depression. Neurol Sci. 2014;35:277–82.
17. Lin Y, Bloodgood BL, Hauser JL, Lapan AD, Koon AC, Kim TK, Hu LS, Malik AN, Greenberg ME. Activity-dependent regulation of inhibitory synapse development by Npas4. Nature. 2008;455:1198–204.
18. Pruunsild P, Sepp M, Orav E, Koppel I, Timmusk T. Identification of cis-elements and transcription factors regulating neuronal activity-dependent transcription of human BDNF gene. J Neurosci. 2011;31:3295–308.
19. Guidotti G, Calabrese F, Auletta F, Olivier J, Racagni G, Homberg J, Riva MA. Developmental influence of the serotonin transporter on the expression of npas4 and GABAergic markers: modulation by antidepressant treatment. Neuropsychopharmacology. 2012;37:746–58.
20. Mattson MP, Maudsley S, Martin B. BDNF and 5-HT: a dynamic duo in age-related neuronal plasticity and neurodegenerative disorders. Trends Neurosci. 2004;27:589–94.
21. Shamloo M, Soriano L, von Schack D, Rickhag M, Chin DJ, Gonzalez-Zulueta M, Gido G, Urfer R, Wieloch T, Nikolich K. Npas4, a novel helix-loop-helix PAS domain protein, is regulated in response to cerebral ischemia. Eur J Neurosci. 2006;24:2705–20.
22. Zhang SJ, Zou M, Lu L, Lau D, Ditzel DA, Delucinge-Vivier C, Aso Y, Descombes P, Bading H. Nuclear calcium signaling controls expression of a large gene pool: identification of a gene program for acquired neuroprotection induced by synaptic activity. PLoS Genet. 2009;5: e1000604.
23. Hester I, McKee S, Pelletier P, Thompson C, Storbeck C, Mears A, Schulz JB, Hakim AA, Sabourin LA. Transient expression of Nxf, a bHLH-PAS transactivator induced by neuronal preconditioning, confers neuroprotection in cultured cells. Brain Res. 2007;1135:1–11.
24. Frohman EM, Racke MK, Raine CS. Multiple sclerosis--the plaque and its pathogenesis. N Engl J Med. 2006;354:942–55.

25. Bjartmar C, Trapp BD. Axonal degeneration and progressive neurologic disability in multiple sclerosis. Neurotox Res. 2003;5:157–64.
26. Trapp BD, Peterson J, Ransohoff RM, Rudick R, Mork S, Bo L. Axonal transection in the lesions of multiple sclerosis. N Engl J Med. 1998;338:278–85.
27. Ferguson B, Matyszak MK, Esiri MM, Perry VH. Axonal damage in acute multiple sclerosis lesions. Brain. 1997;120(Pt 3):393–9.
28. Rashid W, Davies GR, Chard DT, Griffin CM, Altmann DR, Gordon R, Thompson AJ, Miller DH. Increasing cord atrophy in early relapsing-remitting multiple sclerosis: a 3 year study. J Neurol Neurosurg Psychiatry. 2006;77:51–5.
29. Chard DT, Griffin CM, Parker GJ, Kapoor R, Thompson AJ, Miller DH. Brain atrophy in clinically early relapsing-remitting multiple sclerosis. Brain. 2002; 125:327–37.
30. Barnett MH, Henderson AP, Prineas JW. The macrophage in MS: just a scavenger after all? Pathology and pathogenesis of the acute MS lesion. Mult Scler. 2006;12:121–32.
31. Sospedra M, Martin R. Immunology of multiple sclerosis. Annu Rev Immunol. 2005;23:683–747.
32. Kuhlmann T, Lingfeld G, Bitsch A, Schuchardt J, Bruck W. Acute axonal damage in multiple sclerosis is most extensive in early disease stages and decreases over time. Brain. 2002;125:2202–12.
33. Kutzelnigg A, Lucchinetti CF, Stadelmann C, Bruck W, Rauschka H, Bergmann M, Schmidbauer M, Parisi JE, Lassmann H. Cortical demyelination and diffuse white matter injury in multiple sclerosis. Brain. 2005;128:2705–12.
34. Ingle GT, Stevenson VL, Miller DH, Thompson AJ. Primary progressive multiple sclerosis: a 5-year clinical and MR study. Brain. 2003;126:2528–36.
35. van Horssen J, Witte ME, Schreibelt G, de Vries HE. Radical changes in multiple sclerosis pathogenesis. Biochim Biophys Acta. 2011;1812:141–50.
36. Hobom M, Storch MK, Weissert R, Maier K, Radhakrishnan A, Kramer B, Bahr M, Diem R. Mechanisms and time course of neuronal degeneration in experimental autoimmune encephalomyelitis. Brain Pathol. 2004;14:148–57.
37. Qi X, Lewin AS, Sun L, Hauswirth WW, Guy J. Mitochondrial protein nitration primes neurodegeneration in experimental autoimmune encephalomyelitis. J Biol Chem. 2006;281:31950–62.
38. Andrews HE, Nichols PP, Bates D, Turnbull DM. Mitochondrial dysfunction plays a key role in progressive axonal loss in multiple sclerosis. Med Hypotheses. 2005;64:669–77.
39. Su KG, Banker G, Bourdette D, Forte M. Axonal degeneration in multiple sclerosis: the mitochondrial hypothesis. Curr Neurol Neurosci Rep. 2009;9:411–7.
40. Mahad DJ, Ziabreva I, Campbell G, Lax N, White K, Hanson PS, Lassmann H, Turnbull DM. Mitochondrial changes within axons in multiple sclerosis. Brain. 2009;132:1161–74.
41. Neil S, Huh J, Baronas V, Li X, McFarland HF, Cherukuri M, Mitchell JB, Quandt JA. Oral administration of the nitroxide radical TEMPOL exhibits immunomodulatory and therapeutic properties in multiple sclerosis models. Brain Behav Immun. 2017;62:332–43.
42. Cassiani-Ingoni R, Muraro PA, Magnus T, Reichert-Scrivner S, Schmidt J, Huh J, Quandt JA, Bratincsak A, Shahar T, Eusebi F, et al. Disease progression after bone marrow transplantation in a model of multiple sclerosis is associated with chronic microglial and glial progenitor response. J Neuropathol Exp Neurol. 2007;66:637–49.
43. Aiga M, Levinson JN, Bamji SX. N-cadherin and neuroligins cooperate to regulate synapse formation in hippocampal cultures. J Biol Chem. 2011; 286:851–8.
44. Oyama Y, Chikahisa L, Ueha T, Kanemaru K, Noda K. Ginkgo biloba extract protects brain neurons against oxidative stress induced by hydrogen peroxide. Brain Res. 1996;712:349–52.
45. Koh J-Y, Wie MB, Gwag BJ, Sensi SL, Canzoniero LMT, Demaro J, Csernansky C, Choi DW. Staurosporine-induced neuronal apoptosis. Exp Neurol. 1995; 135:153–9.
46. Sternberger LA, Sternberger NH. Monoclonal antibodies distinguish phosphorylated and nonphosphorylated forms of neurofilaments in situ. Proc Natl Acad Sci U S A. 1983;80:6126–30.
47. Kaech S, Banker G. Culturing hippocampal neurons. Nat Protoc. 2006;1: 2406–15.
48. Krohn AJ, Preis E, Prehn JH. Staurosporine-induced apoptosis of cultured rat hippocampal neurons involves caspase-1-like proteases as upstream initiators and increased production of superoxide as a main downstream effector. J Neurosci. 1998;18:8186–97.
49. Nye SH, Squinto SP, Glass DJ, Stitt TN, Hantzopoulos P, Macchi MJ, Lindsay NS, Ip NY, Yancopoulos GD. K-252a and staurosporine selectively block autophosphorylation of neurotrophin receptors and neurotrophin-mediated responses. Mol Biol Cell. 1992;3:677–86.
50. Tiwari-Woodruff S, Morales LB, Lee R, Voskuhl RR. Differential neuroprotective and antiinflammatory effects of estrogen receptor (ER)alpha and ERbeta ligand treatment. Proc Natl Acad Sci U S A. 2007;104:14813–8.
51. Ciccarelli O, Barkhof F, Bodini B, Stefano ND, Golay X, Nicolay K, Pelletier D, Pouwels PJW, Smith SA, Wheeler-Kingshott CAM, et al. Pathogenesis of multiple sclerosis: insights from molecular and metabolic imaging. Lancet Neurol. 2014;13:807–22.
52. Imayoshi I, Kageyama R. Oscillatory control of bHLH factors in neural progenitors. Trends Neurosci. 2014;37:531–8.
53. Hao N, Whitelaw ML, Shearwin KE, Dodd IB, Chapman-Smith A. Identification of residues in the N-terminal PAS domains important for dimerization of Arnt and AhR. Nucleic Acids Res. 2011;39:3695–709.
54. Choy FC, Klaric TS, Koblar SA, Lewis MD. The role of the neuroprotective factor Npas4 in cerebral ischemia. Int J Mol Sci. 2015;16:29011–28.
55. Ernfors P, Lee KF, Jaenisch R. Mice lacking brain-derived neurotrophic factor develop with sensory deficits. Nature. 1994;368:147–50.
56. Jones KR, Farinas I, Backus C, Reichardt LF. Targeted disruption of the BDNF gene perturbs brain and sensory neuron development but not motor neuron development. Cell. 1994;76:989–99.
57. Binder DK, Scharfman HE. Brain-derived neurotrophic factor. Growth Factors. 2004;22:123–31.
58. Hall J, Thomas KL, Everitt BJ. Rapid and selective induction of BDNF expression in the hippocampus during contextual learning. Nat Neurosci. 2000;3:533–5.
59. Patterson SL, Abel T, Deuel TA, Martin KC, Rose JC, Kandel ER. Recombinant BDNF rescues deficits in basal synaptic transmission and hippocampal LTP in BDNF knockout mice. Neuron. 1996;16:1137–45.

10

Increased interleukin-27 cytokine expression in the central nervous system of multiple sclerosis patients

Patrice H. Lalive[1,2], Mario Kreutzfeldt[3], Odile Devergne[4], Imke Metz[5], Wolfgang Bruck[5], Doron Merkler[3] and Caroline Pot[2,6*]

Abstract

Background: Multiple sclerosis (MS) is an autoimmune disorder characterized by chronic inflammation, demyelination, and neuronal damage. During autoimmunity, cytokines are important mediators of the inflammation. In this line, interleukin-27 (IL-27) modulates inflammation and can be produced directly at inflammatory sites such as in the joints during rheumatoid arthritis or in the central nervous system (CNS) during MS. While in animal models of MS, treatment with IL-27 decreases the disease severity, its role in humans is not clearly established and it is not known if IL-27 could be detected in the cerebrospinal fluid (CSF) of MS patients.

Methods: In this study, we measured IL-27 levels using a quantitative enzyme-linked immunosorbent assay in CSF of patients with relapsing remitting multiple sclerosis (RRMS), isolated optic neuritis (ON) and non-inflammatory neurological disease (NIND) as well as in the sera of healthy donors (HD) and RRMS patients undergoing different disease modifying treatments. We further confirmed by immunohistology of patient biopsies the identity of IL-27 producing cells in the brain of active MS lesions.

Results: We observed that IL-27 levels are increased in the CSF but not in the sera of RRMS compared to HD. We confirmed that IL-27 is expressed in active MS plaques by astrocytes of MS patients.

Conclusions: Our results point toward a local secretion of IL-27 in the CNS that is increased during autoimmune processes. We propose that local production of IL-27 could sign the induction of a regulatory response that promotes inflammation's resolution. The effect of new immunomodulatory therapies on cerebral IL-27 production could be used to understand the biology of IL-27 in MS disease.

Keywords: Cytokines, Interleukin-27, Multiple sclerosis, Cerebrospinal fluid, Immunohistochemistry

Background

Multiple sclerosis (MS) is an autoimmune disorder characterized by demyelination, chronic inflammation, and neuronal damage. Among mediators recognized to contribute to inflammatory processes in the CNS, accumulating evidence indicates that members of interleukin-12 (IL-12) family of cytokines, which includes IL-12, IL-23, IL-35, and IL-27, are important mediators of inflammation. While IL-12 and IL-23 have clearly been demonstrated to be pro-inflammatory, IL-27 has been ascribed with additional anti-inflammatory properties. In this line, continuous infusion of IL-27 has been shown to dampen disease severity during the experimental autoimmune encephalomyelitis (EAE), an animal model for MS [1–3]. In addition, mice that lack the receptor for IL-27 or IL-27-downstream signaling transcription factors are characterized by more severe EAE disease compared to control mice [4, 5]. Translational human studies performed in vitro indicate that IL-27 secretion from dendritic cells (DCs) obtained from healthy donors can increase upon

* Correspondence: Caroline.Pot-Kreis@chuv.ch
[2]Department of Pathology and Immunology, Geneva University Hospital and University of Geneva, 1211 Geneva 4, Switzerland
[6]Laboratories of Neuroimmunology, Division of Neurology and Neuroscience Research Center, Department of Clinical Neurosciences, Lausanne University Hospital, 1011 Lausanne, Switzerland

exposure to the drug-modifying treatment IFN-β. Further, in vitro analysis proposed IL-27 as a marker to identify responders to IFN-β treatment [6] as IL-27 secretion was increased from ex vivo isolated plasmacytoid dendritic cells (*pDCs*) from MS patients treated with IFN-β for 1 month [7]. In this line, elevation of IL-27 has been observed in patients responding to glatiramer acetate therapy [8]. Those studies all point toward an anti-inflammatory function of IL-27 during CNS autoimmunity.

In addition to IL-27 secretion in the immune peripheral compartment, IL-27 can be produced directly at the sites of inflammation by local resident cells and antigen presenting cells (APC). In rheumatoid arthritis, increased IL-27 levels in the joint synovial fluid but not in the blood have been reported [9]. Furthermore, IL-27 can be secreted by resident cells of the CNS such as astrocytes or microglia cultured in vitro [10, 11]. IL-27 was shown to be expressed in astrocytes and microglia in MS brains [12]. However, it is not known if IL-27 could be detected directly in the CSF of RRMS patients. We here show that IL-27 production from the CNS can be directly assessed in CSF and in addition that it is increased in RRMS compared to other non-inflammatory neurological diseases or healthy controls. We further confirm that IL-27 is expressed in astrocytes from brain biopsies of MS patients presenting with active lesions.

Methods

CSF and sera

Cerebrospinal fluids (CSF), collected in excess during spinal taps performed for diagnosis purposes, were stored anonymously in a centralized biobank for retrospective research purposes. This research was conducted according to the regulations of the Act on Medical Research Involving Human Subjects of the Geneva University Hospital (HUGO.RE.DG.0010). This study was approved by The Geneva University Hospital Medical Ethical board (Authorization # 07-261R (NAC 07-102R).

The three CSF groups tested were composed of relapsing remitting multiple sclerosis (RRMS), isolated optic neuritis (ON), and non-inflammatory neurological diseases (NIND). NIND consisted of patients who underwent spinal tap for investigation of peripheral seventh nerve palsy or of headaches, which revealed to be non-inflammatory. For RRMS patients, the revised 2005 McDonald Criteria [13] were used to diagnose MS. Demographic and clinical characteristics, including gender, age, neurological symptoms and signs, and CSF white blood cell (WBC) count were retrieved from our CSF biobank database as previously described [14].

Sera were collected from healthy controls (HC) and RRMS patients under different disease-modifying treatments.

Analysis of IL-27 in the sera and CSF

IL-27 was measured using an enzyme immune-assay (Human IL-27 ELISA, Kit: Duo Set (R&D) Ref:DY2526).

EBI3 immunohistochemistry

Post-mortem samples and biopsies from the human MS brain were assessed. Formalin-fixed paraffin-embedded tissue was cut in 2-μm-thick sections. Sections were dewaxed, rehydrated, and subjected to antigen retrieval by heat pre-treatment using citrate buffer pH 6. Ebi3 antibody (clone 2G4H6, mouse monoclonal antibody IgG2a) was diluted 1:500 if visualized using EnVision$^+$ kit (DAKO) or 1:200 together with AffiniPure Goat Anti-Mouse IgG (H+L) AlexaFluor488 labeled antibody (Jackson Immunoresearch) for immunofluorescence. GFAP (DAKO, Z0334, rabbit) antibodies were directly labeled with AlexaFluor555 or AlexaFluor647 following the protocol of the antibody labeling kit (Invitrogen) and applied 1:100. Nuclei were counterstained by H&E for brightfield or by DAPI for fluorescence. Slides were acquired using the Panoramic 250 Flash II (3D-Histech) slide scanner.

Statistical analysis

Differences in variables were analyzed using ANOVA and Student's *t* tests (for normally distributed data) or Kruskal–Wallis and Mann–Whitney *U* tests (for non-normally distributed data) as appropriate.

Results

Increased production of IL-27 in CSF during RRMS is correlated with disease activity

Astrocytes have recently been proposed as a source of IL-27 secretion in active MS lesions [12], which would suggest that IL-27 is directly produced at the site of inflammation in the central nervous system. We therefore examined IL-27 secretion in CSF. Using the ELISA that specifically detects the cytokine IL-27, CSF concentrations of IL-27 were measured in untreated patients with RRMS ($n = 56$), with ON ($n = 29$), or with NIND ($n = 42$) (Fig. 1). The demographic feature characteristics of patients are shown in Table 1. NIND consisted of patients who underwent spinal tap for investigation of peripheral seventh nerve palsy ($n = 13$) or of headaches ($n = 29$), which revealed to be non-infectious and non-inflammatory.

Our results indicate a higher production of IL-27 in the CSF of RRMS patients compared to isolated ON and NIND ($p < 0.005$) (Fig. 1a). The spinal tap was performed at the time of diagnosis; therefore, none of the patients were under a disease-modifying treatment and only two patients had received corticoid treatment. The levels of IL-27 for those two patients were in the range of the other values.

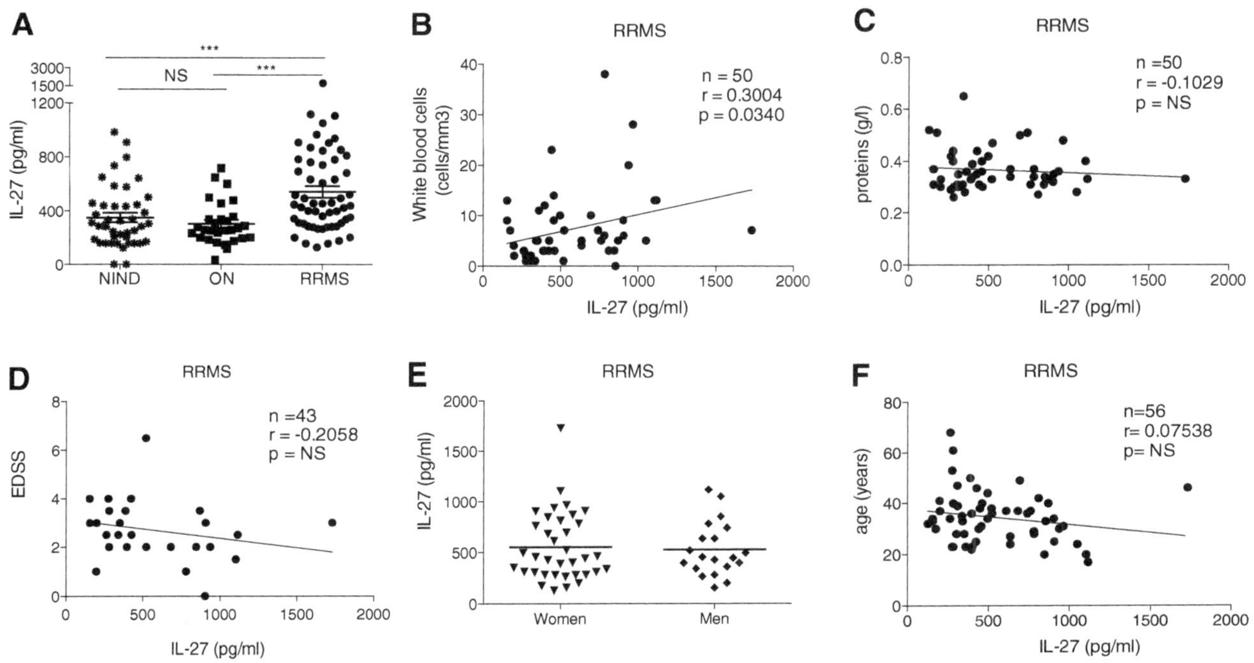

Fig. 1 Distribution of CSF IL-27 levels in patient subgroups. **a** The CSF IL-27 levels of all individual patients were measured using quantitative ELISA. Data are expressed in pg/mL. Only significant *p* values are shown in the graph ($p < 0.001$; Kruskal–Wallis test). *ON* optic neuritis, *RRMS* relapsing remitting multiple sclerosis, *NIND* non-inflammatory neurological diseases. Correlation between IL-27 and **b** white blood cells counts, **c** total proteins levels in the CSF, **d** EDSS score, **e** gender, and **f** age. Pearson product-moment correlation coefficients (*r*) and *p* values are shown

Significant correlation between IL-27 levels and WBC counts (Fig. 1b) but not with protein levels (Fig. 1c) were observed in the CSF of RRMS patients. Those results indicate a link between CNS inflammation and a local IL-27 secretion and argue against increased CSF IL-27 levels through blood-brain-barrier (BBB) leakage. The CSF levels of IL-27 were correlated to neither disease severity as indicated by the EDSS score (Fig. 1d) nor gender (Fig. 1e) nor age (Fig. 1f).

Table 1 Demographic and clinical characteristics of patients (CSF samples $n = 127$)

	NIND ($n = 42$)	ON ($n = 29$)	RRMS ($n = 56$)
Age (years), mean (±SD)	38.38 (±13.42)	33.03 (±11.72)	34.7 (±9.994)
Gender			
Women	20 (48%)	23 (80%)	35 (62.5%)
Men	22 (52%)	6 (20%)	21 (37.5%)
EDSS, mean	–	–	2.895 (±1.485)
Treatments			
DMT	–	0	0
Corticoids	–	0	2 (3.5%)

NIND non inflammatory neurological disease, *ON* optic neuritis, *RRMS* relapsing remitting multiple sclerosis, *EDSS* expanded disability status scale, *DMT* disease-modifying treatments

IL-27 CSF levels are correlated to oligoclonal bands positivity

The correlation between inflammatory parameters and IL-27 levels prompted us to further look at the correlation between oligoclonal IgG bands (OB) profile in the CSF and IL-27 levels. OB accompany CNS inflammation and are found in 95% of patients with MS. Interestingly, IL-27 CSF levels were lower in the few RRMS patients that did not present OB positivity (Fig. 2a). Those results lead us to explore the correlation between OB and IL-27 levels in ON patients. Although IL-27 levels were not elevated in ON patients compared to HC, ON patients with a positive OB pattern (that are at higher risk to develop MS) showed significant higher levels of IL-27 compared with ON patients with a negative OB pattern (Fig. 2b). Similar to RRMS patients, we noted in the CSF of ON patients a significant correlation between IL-27 levels and WBC (Fig. 2c), but not with protein levels (data not shown).

No significant change in IL-27 expression in the sera of RRMS-treated patients

In order to assess if the protein levels of IL-27 were increased in the immune peripheral compartment, IL-27 levels were measured by ELISA in the sera of HC donors ($n = 23$) and RRMS patients without treatment ($n = 30$)

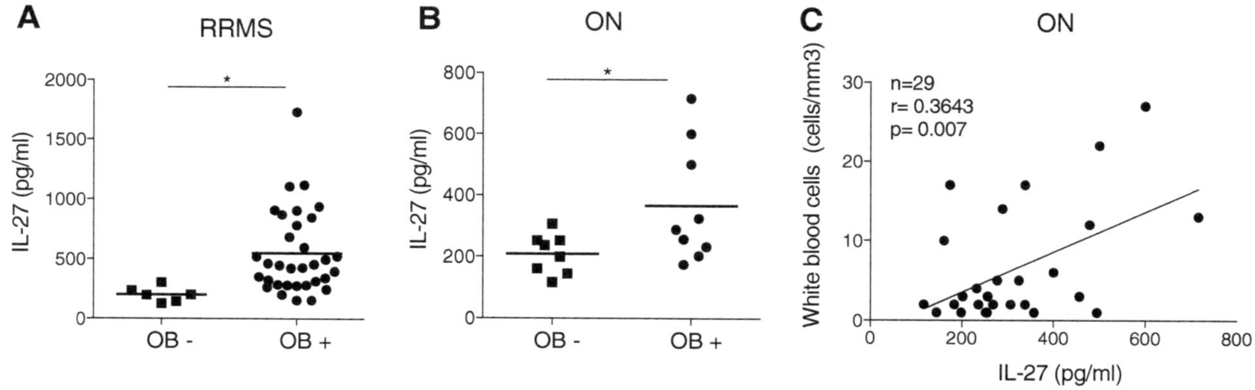

Fig. 2 Distribution of CSF IL-27 levels is correlated with positivity in oligoclonal IgG bands (OB). CSF IL-27 levels and OB pattern in **a** RRMS and **b** ON individual patients. **c** Correlation between IL-27 and white blood cells counts in ON patients

or treated with Interferon beta (IFN-β1a, n = 28), glatiramer acetate (GA, n = 24), or natalizumab (NTZ, n = 12). The demographic features and clinical characteristics of patients are shown in Table 2. By contrast to the CSF, IL-27 sera levels of RRMS patients were equivalent to those observed in HC and were not significantly influenced by disease-modifying treatments (Fig. 3).

IL-27 is expressed in the MS brain by astrocytes

We next investigated if IL-27 could be detected in human MS lesions similarly as has been previously described in autopsy MS lesions [12]. First, we assessed IL-27 expression by bright field immunohistochemistry using an antibody directed against EBI3 (a subunit of IL-27) on an autopsy MS lesion showing a hypocellular center and a more hypercellular rim (referred to as chronic-active lesion stage according to [15]). EBI3 immunoreactivity was mostly observed at the rim of the demyelinated lesion (Fig. 4a). At higher magnification, the morphology of EBI3 positive cells resembled astrocytes (Fig. 4b) which was further confirmed by fluorescence co-staining for EBI3 together with astrocyte specific marker GFAP (data not shown).

The notion that EBI3 immunoreactivity was prominent in more active lesion areas together with the observation that IL-27 expression was noted at high levels in the CSF at early stages of the disease prompted us to investigate EBI3 expression in histopathological early active lesion stages in MS biopsies [16, 17]. We focused here on pattern II early active MS lesion in biopsies, as described previously [18], derived from patients with relatively short disease duration with a mean duration of 5 years (±2.5 years) (Table 3). In these biopsies, we could detect EBI3 signal (although at variable intensity) that mostly co-localized with GFAP-expressing astrocytes in five out of six analyzed lesions (Table 3), one example being shown in Fig. 4c. Altogether these analyses suggest that astrocytes may represent the main cellular source of IL-27 in MS lesions which is in line with previous observations [12].

Discussion

This study shows that patients suffering from RRMS exhibit increased IL-27 expression solely in the CNS compartment as its levels were increased in RRMS patients compared to controls in CSF but not in sera. Interestingly, IL-27 was positively correlated with inflammatory markers in particular white blood cell count and OB positivity. The observation that IL-27 positively correlated with OB in ON patients points toward a role for IL-27 in early inflammation. Biochemical changes of the CSF compartment can be considered as a marker of the CNS inflammation due to its anatomical contact with the brain interstitial fluid. This corroborates with immunohistochemistry staining on cerebral MS biopsies of early active lesions, where astrocytes are found at the highest level. This is in agreement with CSF analysis and highlights a local secretion of IL-27 within the CNS during early neuroinflammation.

Table 2 Demographic characteristics of patients for serum analysis

	CTRL (n = 20)	Untreated (n = 22)	IFN-1a (n = 21)	GA (n = 24)	NTZ (n = 12)
Age, mean ± SEM	39.25 ± 0.5	35.05 ± 0.33	44.05 ± 0.43	37.05 ± 0.49	38.92 ± 0.75
Sex (men/women)	6/14	8/14	3/18	6/18	4/8

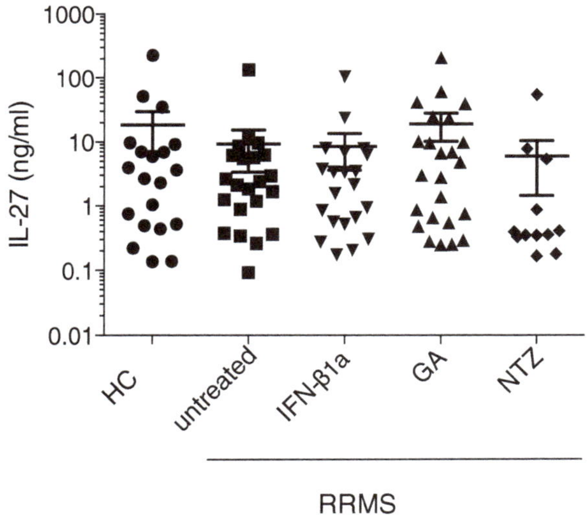

Fig. 3 IL-27 levels are similar in sera of healthy controls and RRMS patients. Sera were obtained from aged-matched healthy controls (HC) and patients with RRMS without treatment (untreated) or treated with interferon beta1a (INF-β1a), glatiramer acetate (GA), or natalizumab (NTZ)

IL-27 has been assigned with both pro- and anti-inflammatory functions [19]. The increased levels of IL-27 in the CSF that we observe in RRMS patient could either indicate that IL-27 is implicated in the causality of the disease with a pro-inflammatory role, or in opposition be regarded as a secondary host response that would be held to fight an ongoing disease. We are in favor of a regulatory role of IL-27, in line with murine models. Our observations that higher IL-27 levels in the CSF are not positively but on the contrary possibly negatively correlated with higher EDSS scores support this hypothesis. IL-27 levels could be regarded as part of a regulatory response held to counterpart the initial inflammation, but that might however be insufficiently maintained with disease evolution. An imbalance between inflammatory and regulatory signals could thus be linked with disease progression. This hypothesis is supported by the ability of IFN-β [6] and glatiramer acetate [8], two MS drug-modifying treatments, to stimulate IL-27 production which could itself be held as a marker to identify responders to those treatments [6]. Moreover, the elevated CSF IL-27 levels can be compared to the increased CSF IL-10 levels, a recognized anti-inflammatory cytokine, during RRMS [20]. IL-10 levels are not only increased in the CSF of MS patients compared to healthy subjects but also higher at an active stage compared to a relieving stage

Table 3 Description of cerebral biopsies

Samples	Gender	Age [years]	DD [years]	Lesion type	Pattern
MS-1	W	52.69	12.74	EA	II
MS-2	W	NA	NA	EA	II
MS-3	W	73.17	0.43	EA	II
MS-4	M	30.89	0.06	EA	II
MS-5	W	35.66	2.89	EA	II
MS-6	W	54.69	8.99	EA	II

W women, *M* men, *NA* not available, *EA* early active lesion

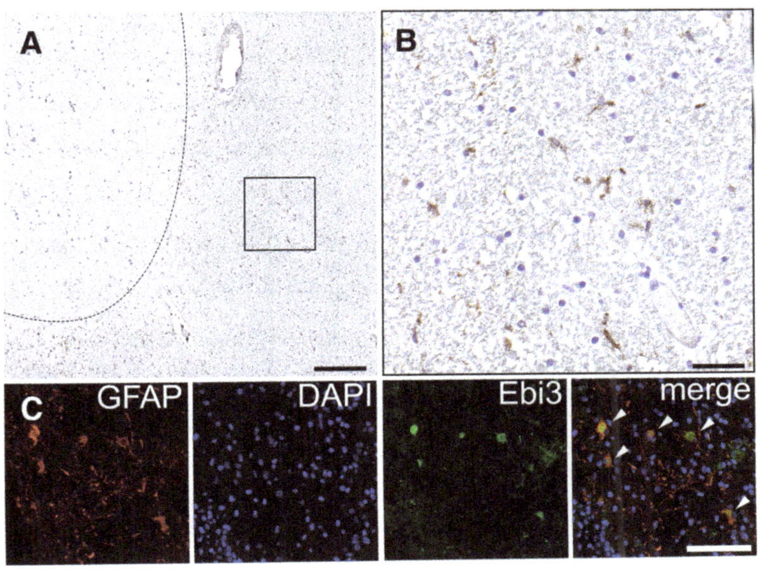

Fig. 4 IL-27 expression in MS plaques. **a** A chronic active lesion of a MS patient autopsy was stained for IL-27 using anti-EBI3 antibody visualized with DAB. The *dashed line* indicates the lesion border. **b** Enlarged detail crop from square region in **a**. **c** Representative fluorescence immunohistochemistry image of a biopsy showing an early active MS lesions co-immunostained for EBI3 (*green*) and astrocytes (GFAP, *red*). Nuclei were counterstained using DAPI (*blue*). *Arrowheads* in the merged image indicate EBI3, GFAP double positive cells. Scale bars: **a** = 200 μm; **b** = 40 μm; **c** = 100 μm

in MS patients [21], comforting the idea that the development of a regulatory response is present at early stages during neuroinflammation.

IL-27 is composed of two subunits, EBI3 and p28. A specific ELISA kit detection for IL-27 has been used that specifically detects the heterodimeric cytokine IL-27, but an antibody specific only for EBI3 was used for histology. While p28 is specific for IL-27, the EBI3 combined p35 composes IL-35 cytokine. We however believe that EBI3 staining is representative of IL-27 cytokine as it is typically produced by antigen-presenting cells (APCs) [22] while IL-35 is produced by lymphocytes, in particular Foxp3^{+} regulatory T-cells [23, 24] and regulatory B-cells [25]. In the CNS, we observed EBI3 expression in astrocytes but not in lymphocytes in MS plaques thus supporting our interpretation that IL-27 but not IL-35 is produced by astrocytes in the context of MS disease. In one of the six biopsies, we did not detect EBI3. This could indicate that EBI3 might not be uniformly expressed within the plaques. Alternatively, the detected epitope of EBI3 might be vulnerable to tissue fixation-related effects resulting in antigen masking that prevents antibody binding on paraffin-embedded tissue as used for this study; over-fixation might indeed lower epitope recognition by 2G4H6 mAb. Further studies are thus needed to corroborate our histological findings.

IL-27 has anti-inflammatory properties during autoimmune diseases. We propose that local production of IL-27 by astrocytes highlights the induction of a regulatory response that promotes inflammation's resolution that is the hallmark of early MS lesions. Lymphocytes, in particular infiltrating CD4^{+} T cells express highest levels of IL-27 receptor in the CNS, in a EAE mouse model [10] and in post-mortem tissue analysis [12] suggesting that IL-27 produced locally at the site of inflammation may regulate T cell responses during neuroinflammation.

Conclusions

Our study provides additional evidence that IL-27 may contribute to autoimmune processes in MS patients.

Abbreviations

CNS: Central nervous system; CSF: Cerebrospinal fluid; EAE: Experimental autoimmune encephalomyelitis; MS: Multiple sclerosis; OB: Oligoclonal IgG bands; ON: Isolated optic neuritis; RRMS: Relapsing remitting multiple sclerosis

Acknowledgements

The authors would like to acknowledge Catherine Juillard-Mochon for technical assistance.

Funding

P.H.L. received support from the Swiss National Foundation (#310030-153164), D.M. receives support by the Swiss National Science Foundation (310030_173010), and C.P. holds stipendiary professorships of the Swiss National Science Foundation (No. PP00P3_157426). P.H.L., D.M. and C.P. received supports from the Swiss Multiple Sclerosis Society.

Authors' contributions

PHL and CP designed and analyzed the experiments and wrote the manuscript. MK and DM performed histological analysis. OD provided EBI3 antibody and scientific assistance. IM and WB provided histological samples. All authors read and approved the final manuscript for publication.

Competing interests

The authors declare that they have no competing interests.

Author details

[1]Unit of Neuroimmunology and Neuromuscular Diseases, Division of Neurology, Department of Clinical Neurosciences, Geneva University Hospital, 1211 Geneva 4, Switzerland. [2]Department of Pathology and Immunology, Geneva University Hospital and University of Geneva, 1211 Geneva 4, Switzerland. [3]Department of Pathology and Immunology, Clinical Pathology Division, Geneva University Hospital and University of Geneva, 1211 Geneva 4, Switzerland. [4]Institut Necker Enfants Malades, INSERM U1151 CNRS UMR 8253, Université Paris Descartes, Sorbonne Paris Cité, 75 015 Paris, France. [5]Institute of Neuropathology, University Medical Center Göttingen, 37075 Göttingen, Germany. [6]Laboratories of Neuroimmunology, Division of Neurology and Neuroscience Research Center, Department of Clinical Neurosciences, Lausanne University Hospital, 1011 Lausanne, Switzerland.

References

1. Pot C, Apetoh L, Awasthi A, Kuchroo VK. Induction of regulatory Tr1 cells and inhibition of T(H)17 cells by IL-27. Semin Immunol. 2011;23(6):438–45.
2. Awasthi A, Carrier Y, Peron JP, Bettelli E, Kamanaka M, Flavell RA, et al. A dominant function for interleukin 27 in generating interleukin 10-producing anti-inflammatory T cells. Nat Immunol. 2007;8(12):1380–9.
3. Fitzgerald DC, Zhang GX, El-Behi M, Fonseca-Kelly Z, Li H, Yu S, et al. Suppression of autoimmune inflammation of the central nervous system by interleukin 10 secreted by interleukin 27-stimulated T cells. Nat Immunol. 2007;8(12):1372–9.
4. Fitzgerald DC, Ciric B, Touil T, Harle H, Grammatikopolou J, Das Sarma J, et al. Suppressive effect of IL-27 on encephalitogenic Th17 cells and the effector phase of experimental autoimmune encephalomyelitis. J Immunol. 2007;179(5):3268–75.
5. Peters A, Fowler KD, Chalmin F, Merkler D, Kuchroo VK, Pot C. IL-27 induces Th17 differentiation in the absence of STAT1 signaling. J Immunol. 2015; 195(9):4144–53.
6. Sweeney CM, Lonergan R, Basdeo SA, Kinsella K, Dungan LS, Higgins SC, et al. IL-27 mediates the response to IFN-beta therapy in multiple sclerosis patients by inhibiting Th17 cells. Brain Behav Immun. 2011;25(6):1170–81.
7. Severa M, Rizzo F, Giacomini E, Annibali V, Gafa V, Romano S, et al. IFN-beta therapy regulates TLR7-mediated response in plasmacytoid dendritic cells of multiple sclerosis patients influencing an anti-inflammatory status. J Interf Cytokine Res. 2015;35(9):668–81.
8. Mindur JE, Valenzuela RM, Yadav SK, Boppana S, Dhib-Jalbut S, Ito K. IL-27: a potential biomarker for responders to glatiramer acetate therapy. J Neuroimmunol. 2017;304:21–8.
9. Tanida S, Yoshitomi H, Ishikawa M, Kasahara T, Murata K, Shibuya H, et al. IL-27-producing CD14(+) cells infiltrate inflamed joints of rheumatoid arthritis and regulate inflammation and chemotactic migration. Cytokine. 2011;55(2):237–44.
10. Li J, Gran B, Zhang GX, Rostami A, Kamoun M. IL-27 subunits and its receptor (WSX-1) mRNAs are markedly up-regulated in inflammatory cells in the CNS during experimental autoimmune encephalomyelitis. J Neurol Sci. 2005;232(1–2):3–9.
11. Sonobe Y, Yawata I, Kawanokuchi J, Takeuchi H, Mizuno T, Suzumura A. Production of IL-27 and other IL-12 family cytokines by microglia and their subpopulations. Brain Res. 2005;1040(1–2):202–7.
12. Senecal V, Deblois G, Beauseigle D, Schneider R, Brandenburg J, Newcombe J, et al. Production of IL-27 in multiple sclerosis lesions by astrocytes and myeloid cells: modulation of local immune responses. Glia. 2016;64(4):553–69.
13. Polman CH, Reingold SC, Edan G, Filippi M, Hartung HP, Kappos L, et al. Diagnostic criteria for multiple sclerosis: 2005 revisions to the "McDonald Criteria". Ann Neurol. 2005;58(6):840–6.

14. Wullschleger A, Kapina V, Molnarfi N, Courvoisier DS, Seebach JD, Santiago-Raber ML, et al. Cerebrospinal fluid interleukin-6 in central nervous system inflammatory diseases. PLoS One. 2013;8(8):e72399.
15. Bo L, Mork S, Kong PA, Nyland H, Pardo CA, Trapp BD. Detection of MHC class II-antigens on macrophages and microglia, but not on astrocytes and endothelia in active multiple sclerosis lesions. J Neuroimmunol. 1994;51(2):135–46.
16. Bruck W, Porada P, Poser S, Rieckmann P, Hanefeld F, Kretzschmar HA, et al. Monocyte/macrophage differentiation in early multiple sclerosis lesions. Ann Neurol. 1995;38(5):788–96.
17. Bruck W, Schmied M, Suchanek G, Bruck Y, Breitschopf H, Poser S, et al. Oligodendrocytes in the early course of multiple sclerosis. Ann Neurol. 1994; 35(1):65–73.
18. Lucchinetti C, Bruck W, Parisi J, Scheithauer B, Rodriguez M, Lassmann H. Heterogeneity of multiple sclerosis lesions: implications for the pathogenesis of demyelination. Ann Neurol. 2000;47(6):707–17.
19. Yoshida H, Hunter CA. The immunobiology of interleukin-27. Annu Rev Immunol. 2015;33:417–43.
20. Sosvorova L, Kanceva R, Vcelak J, Kancheva L, Mohapl M, Starka L, et al. The comparison of selected cerebrospinal fluid and serum cytokine levels in patients with multiple sclerosis and normal pressure hydrocephalus. Neuro Endocrinol Lett. 2015;36(6):564–71.
21. Ji AL, Liu ZH, Chen WW, Huang WJ. The clinical significance of level changes of hs-CRP, IL-10 and TNF for patients with MS during active and relieving period. Eur Rev Med Pharmacol Sci. 2016;20(20):4274–6.
22. Pflanz S, Timans JC, Cheung J, Rosales R, Kanzler H, Gilbert J, et al. IL-27, a heterodimeric cytokine composed of EBI3 and p28 protein, induces proliferation of naive CD4(+) T cells. Immunity. 2002;16(6):779–90.
23. Collison LW, Pillai MR, Chaturvedi V, Vignali DAA. Regulatory T cell suppression is potentiated by target T cells in a cell contact, IL-35-and IL-10-dependent manner. J Immunol. 2009;182(10):6121–8.
24. Ye S, Wu J, Zhou L, Lv Z, Xie H, Zheng S. Interleukin-35: the future of hyperimmune-related diseases? J Interf Cytokine Res. 2013;33(6):285–91.
25. Shen P, Roch T, Lampropoulou V, O'Connor RA, Stervbo U, Hilgenberg E, et al. IL-35-producing B cells are critical regulators of immunity during autoimmune and infectious diseases. Nature. 2014;507(7492):366–70.

11

Rab32 connects ER stress to mitochondrial defects in multiple sclerosis

Yohannes Haile[1,6†], Xiaodan Deng[2†], Carolina Ortiz-Sandoval[1], Nasser Tahbaz[1], Aleksandra Janowicz[1], Jian-Qiang Lu[3], Bradley J. Kerr[4], Nicholas J. Gutowski[5], Janet E. Holley[5], Paul Eggleton[5], Fabrizio Giuliani[2*] and Thomas Simmen[1*]

Abstract

Background: Endoplasmic reticulum (ER) stress is a hallmark of neurodegenerative diseases such as multiple sclerosis (MS). However, this physiological mechanism has multiple manifestations that range from impaired clearance of unfolded proteins to altered mitochondrial dynamics and apoptosis. While connections between the triggering of the unfolded protein response (UPR) and downstream mitochondrial dysfunction are poorly understood, the membranous contacts between the ER and mitochondria, called the mitochondria-associated membrane (MAM), could provide a functional link between these two mechanisms. Therefore, we investigated whether the guanosine triphosphatase (GTPase) Rab32, a known regulator of the MAM, mitochondrial dynamics, and apoptosis, could be associated with ER stress as well as mitochondrial dysfunction.

Methods: We assessed Rab32 expression in MS patient and experimental autoimmune encephalomyelitis (EAE) tissue, via observation of mitochondria in primary neurons and via monitoring of survival of neuronal cells upon increased Rab32 expression.

Results: We found that the induction of Rab32 and other MAM proteins correlates with ER stress proteins in MS brain, as well as in EAE, and occurs in multiple central nervous system (CNS) cell types. We identify Rab32, known to increase in response to acute brain inflammation, as a novel unfolded protein response (UPR) target. High Rab32 expression shortens neurite length, alters mitochondria morphology, and accelerates apoptosis/necroptosis of human primary neurons and cell lines.

Conclusions: ER stress is strongly associated with Rab32 upregulation in the progression of MS, leading to mitochondrial dysfunction and neuronal death.

Keywords: Multiple sclerosis, Endoplasmic reticulum, Mitochondria, Unfolded protein response (UPR)

Background

At an advanced stage of MS, immunomodulating therapies are no longer effective, highlighting the need to understand the molecular basis of this disease. Like other neurodegenerative diseases that are associated with mitochondrial impairment [1], MS mitochondria can be dysfunctional, especially during disease progression [1] and its neurodegenerative phase [2, 3]. For instance, mitochondria no longer respire normally in progressive MS patients [4]. Dysfunctional mitochondria produce reactive oxygen species (ROS). As a consequence, mitochondrial ROS promote inflammation and shift mitochondrial dynamics towards fission [5]. This latter process requires dynamin-related protein 1 (Drp1), a ubiquitous guanosine triphosphatase (GTPase) [6]. While Drp1 is essential for post-mitotic neurons [7], its excessive activity can result in apoptosis [8]. Indeed, mitochondria increase in number in MS neurons undergoing demyelination [9], thus accelerating axonal degeneration [10]. Upstream causes of these mitochondrial defects are largely unknown. One potential mechanism involves the uncontrolled release of Ca^{2+} ions from the main cellular Ca^{2+} store, the endoplasmic reticulum

* Correspondence: giuliani@ualberta.ca; Thomas.Simmen@ualberta.ca
[†]Equal contributors
[2]Department of Medicine, Division of Neurology, University of Alberta, Edmonton, Canada
[1]Department of Cell Biology, University of Alberta, Edmonton, Canada

(ER), within the diseased neurons. This intracellular signaling mechanism ultimately promotes cell death via a mitochondrial mechanism [11, 12]. Lethal ER-mitochondria Ca^{2+} transfer is observed for instance following axotomy [13] or spinal cord injury [14].

In addition to disrupted mitochondrial dynamics, the induction of ER stress is another hallmark of MS [15, 16]. This process not only promotes ER-mitochondria crosstalk in general by increasing the apposition of the ER and mitochondria at the so-called mitochondria-associated membrane (MAM) [17–19], but could also promote neuronal death, thus contributing to the MS pathology [20].

A prominent MAM regulatory protein is Rab32. This GTPase localizes to the ER and mitochondria [21, 22], where it regulates ER-mitochondria interactions and mitochondrial dynamics [23]. Rab32 is induced upon brain inflammation in a mouse model [24]. Consistent with an important role in neuroinflammation, our data indicate that ER stress induces Rab32 and occurs in the MS brain. These findings increase our understanding of Rab32 role in impairment of neuronal mitochondrial dynamics and cell survival.

Methods

Antibodies

Antibodies used in this study were purchased as follows: anti-actin, anti-phospho-Drp1 Ser637 (Cell Signaling, Danvers, MA), anti-amyloid precursor protein, anti-glucose-regulated protein of 94 kDA (GRP94), anti-α tubulin, anti-receptor-interacting protein kinase (RIPK) (EMD-Millipore, Billerica, MA), anti-immunoglobulin-binding protein/glucose-regulated protein of 78 kDA (BiP/GRP78) (BD Biosciences, Franklin Lakes, NJ), anti-BiP/GRP78, anti-Drp1 (abcam, Cambridge, UK), anti-CD68 (Dako/Agilent, Markham, ON), anti-CCAAT/enhancer-binding protein (C/EBP) homologous protein (CHOP), anti-GRP75 (Pierce/Thermo, Waltham, MA), anti-CHOP (Enzo, Farmingdale, NY), anti-phosphofurin acidic cluster sorting protein 2 (PACS-2) (Protein Tech, Chicago, IL), anti-Rab32 (Sigma/Aldrich, St. Louis, MO), and anti-FLAG (Rockland, Limerick, PA). The antibody against calnexin has been described previously [25].

Isolation and maintenance of primary neuronal cultures

Cultures of human fetal neurons (HFN) were generated from 15–19-week fetal brains (obtained with consent from the University of Alberta Ethics Committee) as described [26].

Human frozen brain tissues and EAE mice tissue

For immunohistochemistry, snap-frozen blocks of post-mortem normal control (NC) or MS cerebral sub-ventricular deep white matter samples were obtained from the NeuroResource Tissue Bank, UCL Institute of Neurology, London, and UK MS Biobank, with next-of-kin informed consent for tissue donation and ethical approval from Central London REC1 (I.D.08/H0718/62) and approval for the study from the Local Research Ethics Committee (I.D.04/Q2102/111), UK MS brain bank charity number 1139257. A total of 12 MS patients (9 females, 3 males) who had been affected from secondary progressive (10), primary progressive (1) or relapsing progressive MS were used for this part of the study. Control tissue from individuals who had not been affected by disease (7) and 2 individuals who had been affected by Parkinson's disease was also examined. Control patients died of non-inflammatory diseases (cardiac failure, lung cancer, bladder cancer, prostate cancer, tongue cancer, myelodysplastic syndrome; for two control cases, the cause of death was not known). Further information is contained in Additional file 1.

For Western blot and immunofluorescence analysis, tissues of two frozen MS brains (patient 1: secondary progressive MS, aged 54, male; patient 2: relapsing-remitting MS, aged 45, male) were obtained from the MS Tissue Bank at the University of Alberta. Post-mortem brain tissues were collected and processed as described [27]. Frozen brain and spinal cord tissues of triplicate experimental autoimmune encephalomyelitis (EAE) mice, an animal model of MS, were generated with proper approvals as described [28]. Control samples showed no signs of nervous disease. Disease peak samples were from clinical grade 1, whereas post-peak samples were from clinical grade 4 (hind limb paralysis at time of dissection).

Lysate preparation and analysis from tissues and cell lines

Tissue lysates were prepared from the human frozen brain as well as from the spinal cords of EAE mice in 1× sodium dodecyl sulphate (SDS) extraction buffer (0.125 M Tris-HCK pH 6.8, 2% SDS, 10% glycerol, 5% β-ME), followed by sonication on a 550 Sonic Dismembrator (Fisher Scientific, Ottawa, ON). Supernatants were collected, and protein concentrations were measured by NanoDrop Spectrophotometer ND1000 (Thermo/Life Technologies) at an absorbance of 280 nm. Cellular lysates from SH-SY5Y cells were prepared as described [25].

RT-PCR

SH-SY5Y cells were cultured in mild hypoxia (4% O_2, grown in the presence of 4% O_2, 5% CO_2 balanced N_2, as is typical for brain tissue) in the presence of thapsigargin. After 24 h in culture, total RNA was extracted. The primers used for RT-PCR were as follows: Rab32 forward AGCAGGACTCTGGTGCGCCTG (position 211-231); Rab32 reverse CGGGCAGCTTCCTCTATG TTTATGTTATC (position 557-529). The result was normalized against the ribosomal 18S.

Immunohistochemistry

Sample sections were stained with hematoxylin and eosin (H&E) and luxol fast blue (LFB) as described [27]. Lesions were classified into acute (referring to tissue phenotype, see below), sub-acute, and chronic on the basis of the number and distribution of oil red-O-positive macrophages, the extent of demyelination, cellularity in the borders and parenchyma of lesions, and perivascular cuffing as described in our previous work [29]. Briefly, acute lesions were identified via demyelination, invading macrophages, hypercellularity at the lesion border, and cuffing around the blood vessels. Sub-acute lesions showed a demyelinated plaque with fewer macrophages, mostly at the lesion border, and less perivascular cuffing. A chronic lesion consisted of a hypocellular demyelinated plaque completely lacking of oil red-O-stained macrophages. Examination of MS brain tissue for Rab32 expression in specific cell types was performed employing enzyme immunohistochemistry using a Vectastain ABC system® (Vector Laboratories, Peterborough, UK), as described [30].

Transfection of constructs and shRNA, immunofluorescence, and quantification of apoptosis

mCherry-labeled Rab32 shRNA psi-mH1 plasmids (HSH001118) as well as scrambled control (CSHCTR001) were purchased from Genecopoeia (Rockland MD). FLAG-tagged Rab32 constructs were expressed from pcDNA3 as published [22] (wt, wild type; Q85L, dominant-active; T39N, dominant-negative) or transferred into the bi-cistronic pIRES2-EGFP plasmid (Clontech-Takara, Mountain View, CA) that allows for the expression of any protein, in parallel with nuclear EGFP. To do so, the described constructs contained in pcDNA3 were PCR-amplified using the SP6 and TS484 (ATATGCTAGC ACCATGGACTACAAGGACGACGATGACAAG) oligos following cuts with the 5' Nhe1 and 3' Xho1 sites. Primary neurons or SH-SY5Y neuronal cell lines were transfected by nucleofection (Lonza, Mississauga, ON). Immunofluorescence was performed as described [25]. To assay neurotoxicity, nuclear EGFP was used to identify transfected HFNs and SH-SY5Y. Apoptosis was then detected by Cy5-annexin V binding (BD Biosciences). Assays were repeated in the presence of bafilomycin (100 nM, Sigma-Aldrich), necrostatin-1 (Nec-1, 50 μM, Cayman Chemical), carbobenzoxy-valyl-alanyl-aspartyl-[O-methyl]- fluoromethylketone (zVAD-fmk) (10 μM, Enzo Life Sciences, Farmingdale, NY), or with a combination of nec-1 and zVAD-fmk.

Immunogold labeling

Cells were rinsed in PBS and fixed in 3% paraformaldehyde and 0.05% glutaraldehyde (GA) containing 2% sucrose. Next, free aldehyde groups were quenched with ammonium chloride (50 mM), and samples were permeabilized with saponin (0.1%). The samples were blocked (PBS + 1% BSA + 0.05% FSG + Saponin 0.05%) for an hour and then were incubated with mouse anti-FLAG in the blocking buffer overnight in a wet chamber. Following washes (0.2%BSA + 0.05%FSG + 0.05% saponin), the samples were incubated with the secondary antibody (Fluoronanogold Anti-mouse Fab'Alexa Fluor 488, cat. 7202; Nanoprobes, NY) for 3 h at RT and washed with PBS three times. The samples then were fixed (2% GA in PBS + 2% sucrose) for an hour, followed by three rinses in water. Following a 1-min incubation with Gold-Enhance EM Plus (Cat. 2114; Nanoprobes, NY), the samples were rinsed in water, scraped in 100 mM sodium cacodylate and pelleted. The pellet was incubated for 1 h with osmium tetroxide (1%), followed by overnight staining with uranyl acetate. After dehydration in increasing concentrations of ethanol and then propylene oxide treatments, the pellets were transferred to resin (Embed 812 kit, cat. 14120; Electron Microscopy Sciences, Hatfield, PA) and incubated at 60 °C for 48 h. Blocks were sectioned (70 nm) using Ultracut E (Reichert Jung) and imaged with a Philips 310 electron microscope, equipped with a digital camera (Mega View III Soft Imaging System, Emsis Gmbh, Muenster, Germany).

Results

Rab32 parallels ER stress within MS patient and EAE brains

Rab32 is enriched on the ER and mitochondria [31], where it determines various aspects of ER-mitochondria crosstalk [21, 23]. The recent discovery that Rab32 expression increases during brain inflammation in mice [24] and the connection between ER-mitochondria crosstalk and inflammation [32, 33] led us to hypothesize that Rab32 might play a role in the MS pathology. Thus, we examined autopsy tissue sections from the MS patient brains (Fig. 1a–c) for Rab32 expression. These results demonstrated that Rab32 was increased in lesions of MS brain tissues (Fig. 1d). Importantly, Rab32 was higher in active lesions where infiltrating macrophages and resident microglia were present. Consistent with the reported low expression of Rab32 in brain tissue [34, 35], very low levels of Rab32 were noticed in the normal-appearing white matter (NAWM, Fig. 1d). We next tested whether this increase in Rab32 paralleled an increase of proteins functionally connected to Rab32, including ER chaperones and proteins regulating ER-mitochondria interactions.

Consistent with the previous identification of ER stress as a hallmark of the MS CNS [16, 36], we detected increased expression of calnexin, BiP/GRP78, GRP94, and the CCAAT/enhancer-binding protein (C/EBP) homologous protein (CHOP) in active, but not chronic lesions

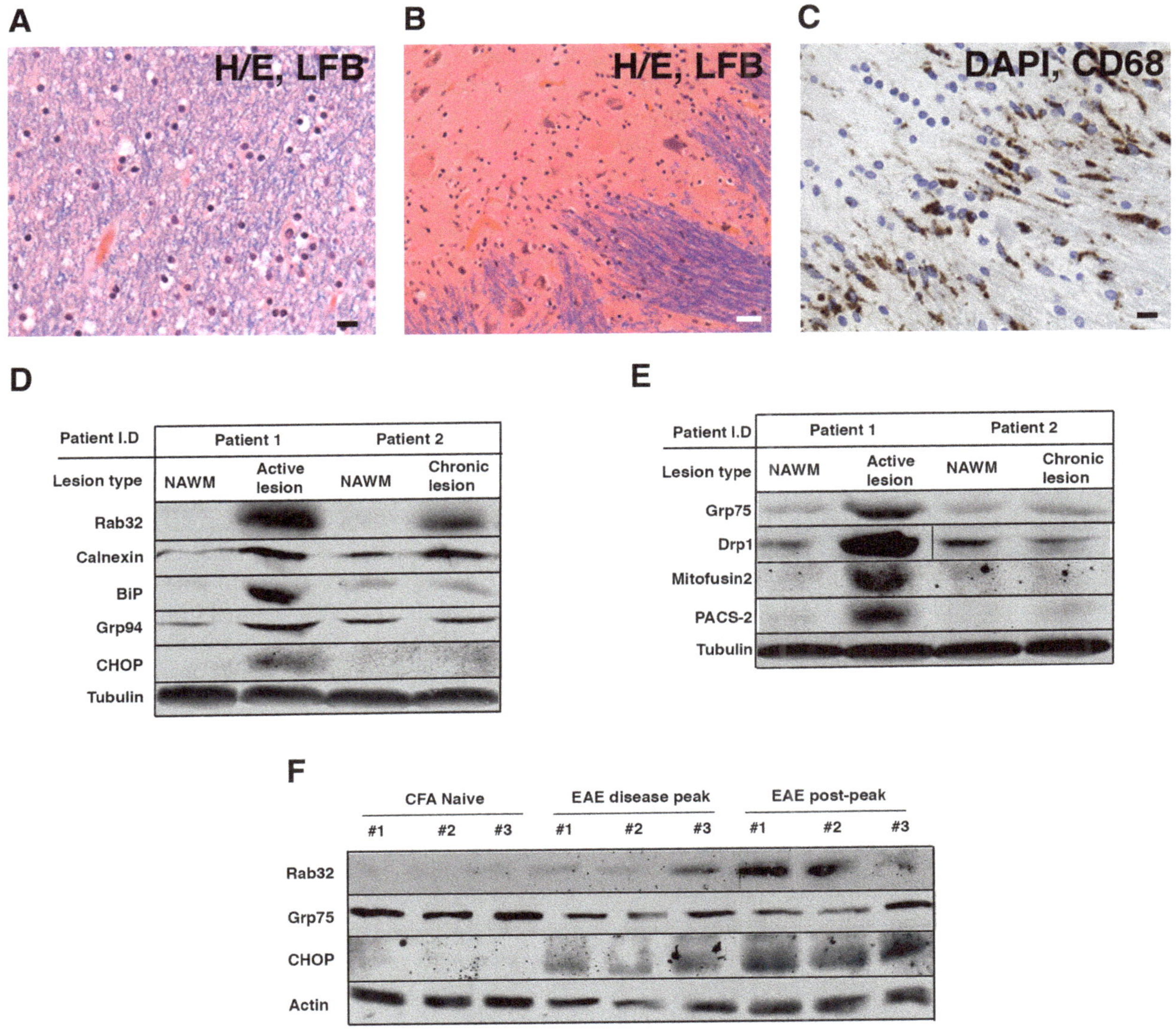

Fig. 1 Proteomic characterization of MS brain tissues. **a** Normal-appearing white matter (NAWM) in the right frontal lobe exhibiting intact LFB staining for myelin. **b** Identification of lesion and NAWM areas in autopsy tissue sections of an MS patient brain derived from a 44-year-old male patient. Hematoxylin and eosin staining in a chronic lesion in the pons shows a hypocellular center (*upper left*) containing neuronal cells with diminished LFB staining for myelin and hypercellular edge. **c** Abundant CD68-immunoreactive macrophages/microglia are detected in the hypercellular edge of the active lesion. **d** Western blotting analysis showing the amounts of Rab32, together with ER stress-related markers (calnexin, BiP/GRP78, GRP94, and CHOP (patient 1: secondary-progressive MS, patient 2: relapsing-remitting MS)). **e** Western blotting analysis showing the amounts of MAM-related proteins GRP75, Drp1, mitofusin2, and PACS-2. **f** Expression of Rab32 associated with selected marker proteins in EAE (GRP75 and CHOP) in tissues obtained from the spinal cords of EAE mice. Triplicate samples from CFA naive, EAE disease peak (clinical grade 1), and EAE post-peak (clinical grade 4) are shown

(Fig. 1d). Next, we tested whether other MAM regulatory proteins were upregulated as well. We probed for the tether proteins GRP75 and Mfn2 the MAM-associated mitochondria fission GTPase Drp1 and the MAM enrichment factor phosphofurin acidic cluster sorting protein 2 (PACS-2). Western blotting showed that all of the above proteins showed increased expression in active, but not chronic MS brain lesions (Fig. 1e). We extended our investigation into the animal model of MS, experimental autoimmune encephalomyelitis (EAE). Western blotting showed that high levels of brain-localized Rab32 occurred in the peak and post-peak period of EAE (Fig. 1f), reflecting the induction of Rab32 in both active and chronic lesions of MS brain.

Cell-type specific localization of Rab32 expression

We next examined which cell types harbor increased amounts of Rab32 in MS brain tissue and also expanded the number of patients in our study. To do so, we first stained for axonal and non-phosphorylated neurofilament that identifies cells as neurons, as well as for Rab32 and CHOP. Control brain tissue did not show significant Rab32 staining (Additional file 2). In contrast, our results shown in Fig. 2a–c demonstrate that high Rab32 expression was especially encountered at the border of active lesions of MS brains. Chronic lesions showed less expression of Rab32. In the merged images, the signals of Rab32 and neurofilament were only partially overlapping but were most pronounced in swollen axons at the active lesion border (arrows in Fig. 2a–c). Infiltrating immune cells (visible from their DAPI staining) surrounded these cells. We detected high amounts of CHOP in virtually the same set of cells that also over-expressed Rab32. Next, we evaluated to what extent microglial cells in MS brain expressed Rab32, using independent tissue samples, part of a 12-patient cohort (Figs. 2g–l and 3, Additional file 1). This showed that distinct staining for Rab32 was found within microglial cells in active lesions characterized by heavy myelin debris (stained black with DAB nickel chloride, Fig. 2g–i). Next, we discovered via double immunohistochemistry that in MS NAWM, Rab32 (brown) was localized to cells with the morphology of microglia and blood vessels, but not axons (blue/gray) (Fig. 3a, b). In contrast, in acute MS lesions (referring to tissue, Fig. 3c), we detected Rab32-positive microglia in the acute lesion border and adjacent NAWM (Fig. 3d–i). Interestingly, within the lesion area (Fig. 3h, f), we detected not only a mix of both Rab32 (brown)-positive cells and Rab32-negative macrophages (blue/gray) but also some Rab32-positive macrophages (black). Here, we also detected extensive overlap between staining for Rab32 (brown) and axons (blue/gray) (Fig. 3f–i). Together, using multiple patient tissue samples, our findings indicate that Rab32 increases dramatically in neurons and macrophages/microglia localized within active MS lesions and that high amounts of Rab32 coincide with the expression of CHOP. In contrast, chronic MS lesions show Rab32 predominantly in neurons.

Rab32 expression is under the control of the unfolded protein response (UPR)

Next, we aimed to understand what cell biological mechanism could give rise to high levels of this small GTPase. To investigate this question, we used in vitro approaches. First, we performed RT-PCR on the mRNA from SH-SY5Y cells incubated with and without 0.5 μM thapsigargin. This showed that the Rab32 mRNA increased by 2.6-fold upon ER stress (Fig. 4a). To corroborate this result at a protein level, we treated SH-SY5Y cells with tunicamycin in a 0–4-h time course under normoxic conditions or in presence of 4% oxygen. Western blotting revealed that 4% O_2, as is typical for brain tissue, increased expression of Rab32, but tunicamycin accentuated this increase Rab32 at 2 and 4 h (Fig. 4b). In parallel, we also assessed the expression of selected ER stress-related proteins, calnexin and CHOP. Both the amounts of calnexin and CHOP were only responsive to tunicamycin treatment. Therefore, Rab32 expression appears to be tied to the induction of ER stress and to a lesser degree hypoxia, as described previously for other proteins [37].

Rab32 interferes with neuronal mitochondrial dynamics and growth

To understand the functional readout of increased neuronal Rab32 transcription, we investigated whether Rab32 alters neuronal mitochondrial dynamics, as shown by others and us [21, 23]. Thus, we decided to express Rab32 constructs and interfering ribonucleic acid (RNAi) from bi-cistronic plasmids co-expressing nuclear EGFP. As a cellular model, we used primary human fetal neurons (HFNs) as well as SH-SY5Y neuroblastoma cells. Using the primary cells, we investigated neurite outgrowth of transfected neurons or control cells, as well as their mitochondria distribution following mitotracker-labeling. In contrast to control conditions (Fig. 5a), neurons transfected with dominant-active Rab32Q85L showed bulkier, less interconnected mitochondria units (Fig. 5b, see enlarged areas in Fig. 5a, b). Quantification revealed that transfection of neurons with Rab32WT and Rab32Q85L, but not dominant-negative Rab32T39N, indeed increased the numbers of mitochondria per length of neurite by 13 and 26%, respectively (Fig. 5c). However, this alteration of mitochondrial dynamics coincided with 12 and 22% shorter neurites in neurons expressing wild-type Rab32 and Rab32Q85L, respectively (Fig. 5d). Interestingly, knockdown of Rab32 did not have any effects for mitochondrial dynamics or neurite outgrowth, when normalized to scrambled control transfected cells (Fig. 5c, d). To investigate which effects on mitochondrial morphology resulted in the altered mitochondria density and neurite length, we transiently transfected SH-SY5Y cells with dominant-active FLAG-tagged Rab32Q85L, which showed the most significant changes. We then analyzed these cells via immunogold labeling of their FLAG signal to distinguish between transfected, over-expressing cells (top) and untransfected, control cells (bottom, Fig. 5e). This showed that Rab32Q85L promoted the formation of larger mitochondria with fewer cristae, concomitant with a 38% reduction in their cristae density per area (table, Fig. 5e). Our results imply that Rab32 alters mitochondrial dynamics in neurons and affects neurite outgrowth.

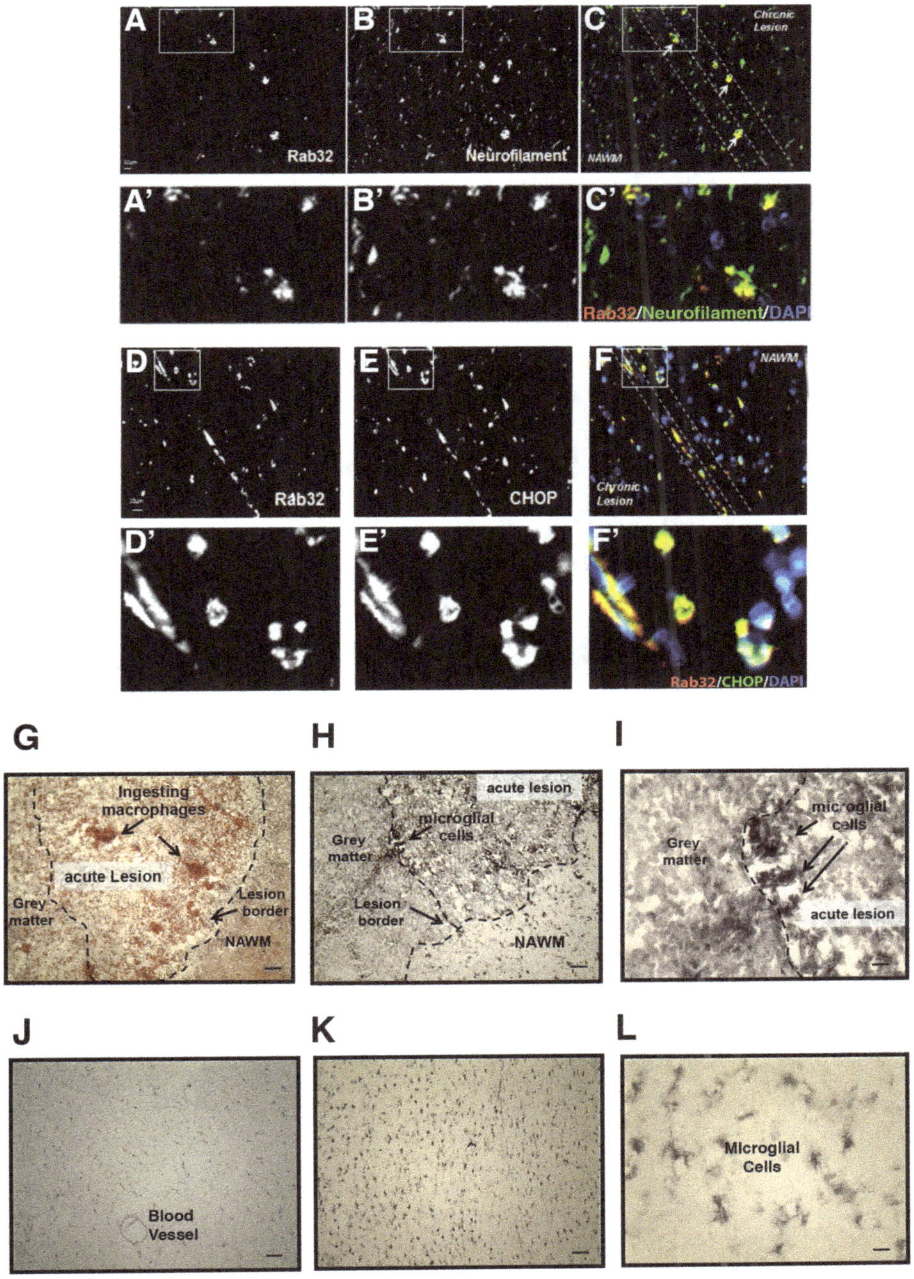

Fig. 2 Rab32 localization in active MS lesions. **a**–**f** Immunofluorescence stainings of patient brain tissue from secondary progressive MS showing Rab32 (**a**, **d**), neurofilament (**b**), merged Rab32/neurofilament, including DAPI (**c**), CHOP (**e**) and merged Rab32/CHOP, including DAPI (**f**). Enlarged areas in **a**–**f** are shown below (**A'**–**F'**). Active chronic lesion, lesion border, and NAWM were identified using H&E and LFB stain of adjacent sections as described in Fig. 1**a**–**c**. **g**–**l** Representative images from a 12-patient, 9-control study examining expression of RAB32 in 10 μm sections, containing an acute lesion of an MS patient (referring to tissue phenotype (**g**–**i**)) and white matter from control subjects (**j**–**l**). **g** Low power image (×100 mag) of clumps of macrophages ingesting myelin stained with oil red-O within the active border of an acute lesion (fresh frozen tissue) surrounded by gray matter and normal-appearing white matter (NAWM) demarked by *dotted line*. **h** RAB32 immunostained with DAB nickel chloride localized within the cell bodies of microglial cells at low magnification (×100 mag) and **i** at higher magnification (×400). **j** Weak RAB32 expression in the blood vessel and NAWM of a control subject. **k** Intermediate RAB32 staining in glial cells present in the NAWM of a separate control subject brain section (×100 mag) and **l** at ×400 magnification. Note the intensity of staining of RAB32 in microglial/macrophage cells in acute lesions of MS patient compared to control subjects. *Scale bars* in **a**, **b**, **d**, and **e** = 50 μm and 12.5 μm in **c** and **f**

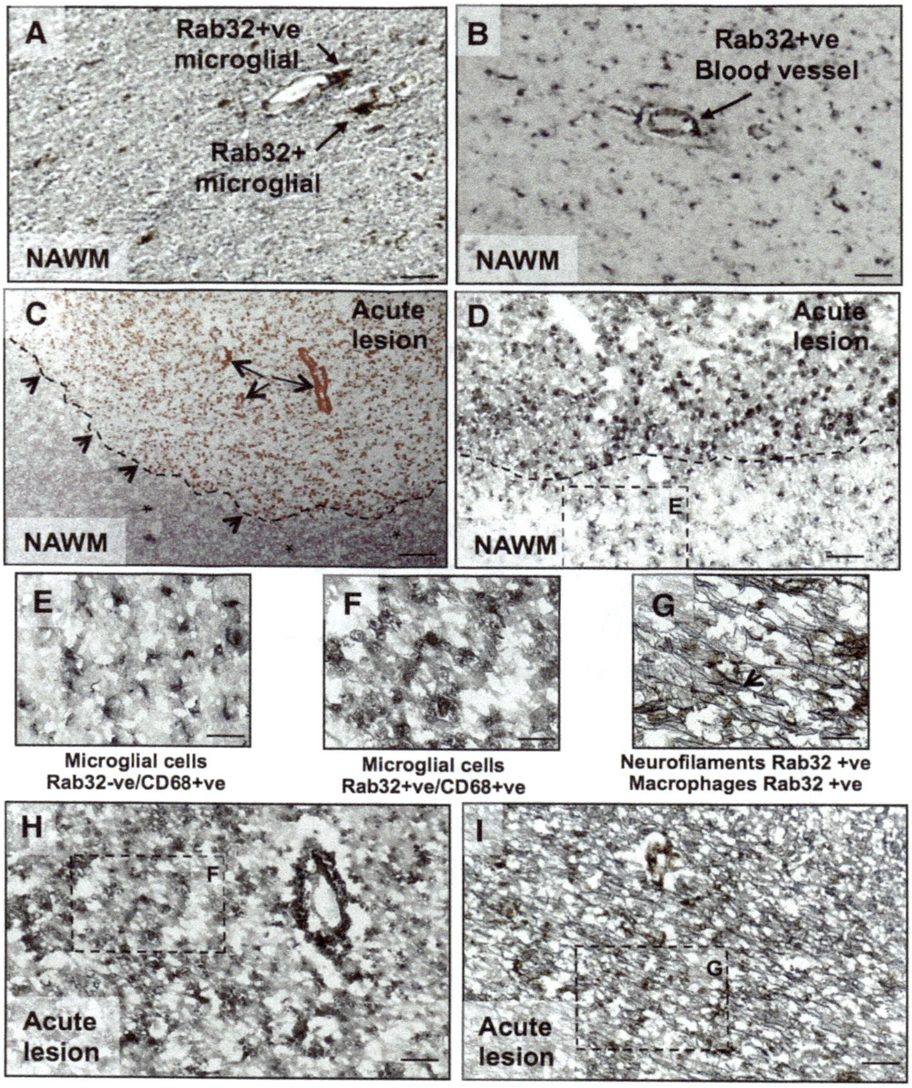

Fig. 3 Double immunohistochemistry confirms Rab32 staining in microglia/macrophages and axons in MS. Rab32 positive staining (*brown*) was investigated in microglia/macrophages (CD68, *blue/gray*) and axons (neurofilament, *blue/gray*) with co-localization producing a black stain. **a** Staining of MS NAWM; Rab32 (*brown*) staining of CD68-positive (+ve) microglia cells. **b** Rab32 expression was also observed in microvascular cells (*arrow*). **c** Oil red-O staining of an acute MS lesion. The *dashed line* and *small arrows* depict the lesion border, and red staining shows myelin ingestion by macrophages. The *large arrows* show the blood vessels. The *asterisk* depicts surrounding NAWM. **d** Rab32-positive (+ve) microglia in the acute lesion border and Rab32-negative (−ve) microglial cells in adjacent NAWM. The *dashed lines* represent the area shown at higher power. (see high-magnification *insets E, F*, and *G*). **e** Rab32-negative (−ve) CD68+ve microglial cells in NAWM. **h**, **i** Staining of acute lesion tissue labeled for Rab32 (*brown*), macrophages (*blue/gray*, **h**), and axons (*blue/gray*, **i**). **f** High magnification of CD68-positive (+ve) microglial cells staining for Rab32 in acute lesions. **g** High power magnification of axons (*blue/gray*, co-localized with Rab32 as *black*), in close proximity to Rab32-positive (+ve) macrophages (*brown*). *Scale bars* in **a** and **b** = 25 μm; **c**, **d**, **h**, and **i** = 50 μm; and 12.5 μm in **e**, **f**, and **g**

Long-term effect of Rab32 and its mutants on neuronal survival

Next, we focused on the role of Rab32 to control apoptosis onset [21] and investigated whether altered expression or activity of Rab32 would influence the survival of neurons. We assayed cell viability at 24, 48, and 72 h post-transfection and set the viability of control EGFP-expressing cells as 100%. At 24 h, we were unable to detect differences in the survival of cells with altered Rab32 expression levels or activity compared to control cells. However, the amounts of cells over-expressing any version of Rab32 started to decrease at 48 h after transfection (Fig. 6a). This trend accelerated at 72 h. In contrast, neurons expressing Rab32 RNAi as well

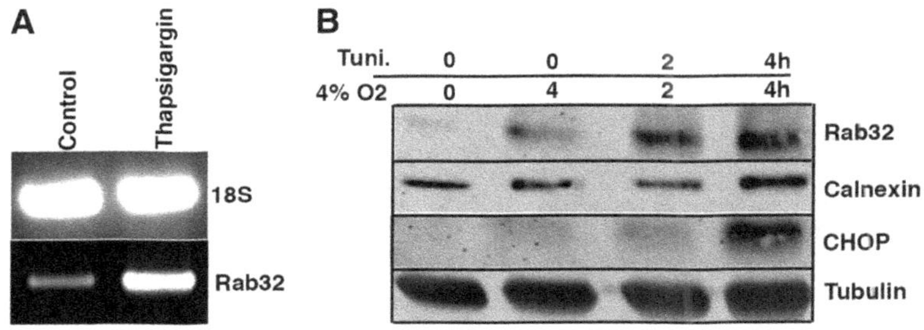

Fig. 4 Rab32 expression under conditions of ER stress. **a** RT-PCR showing the expression of Rab32 transcripts in thapsigargin-treated SH-SY5Y cells. **b** Western blot showing the expression of Rab32, calnexin, and CHOP in tunicamycin-treated SH-SY5Y cell lines cultured in 4% O_2 that corresponds to brain normoxia

as EGFP-only-expressing control cells did not show significant reductions in their viability (Fig. 6b). We repeated this survival assay using human SH-SY5Y neuroblastoma cells and found these cells to be even more dependent on Rab32 (Fig. 5c), regardless of whether it was active or inactive.

Caspase inhibition and necrostatin can block Rab32-directed neuronal death

We next aimed to investigate the mechanism(s) triggered by Rab32 that led to neuronal damage and death. To do so, we transfected SH-SY5Y cells and determined whether they subsequently underwent apoptosis. Twenty-four hours after transfection, we were unable to detect annexin V on the surface of control cells (Fig. 7a, first column), but cells transfected with Rab32WT, Rab32Q85L, and Rab32T39N (identified via bi-cistronically expressed EGFP) readily showed annexin V binding (Fig. 7a, as labeled; scale bar 20 μm). In addition to apoptosis, we also investigated whether the increased expression of Rab32 might induce necroptosis. First, we investigated whether Rab32 expression and activity levels could influence the amounts of receptor-interacting protein kinase (RIPK). Thus, we lysed the SH-SY5Y cells transfected with Rab32WT, Rab32Q85L, Rab32T39N, and shRab32 as well as EGFP-expressing controls. Western blot analysis showed that increased Rab32 expression led to increased amounts of RIPK1 (Fig. 7b). No difference could be detected upon Rab32 knockdown.

To determine the relative contribution of apoptosis and necroptosis to neuronal cell death upon Rab32 over-expression, we re-examined the survival of SH-SY5Y cells transfected with EGFP, shRab32, Rab32WT, and Rab32Q85L. We then repeated our survival assay in the presence of necrostatin-1 and zVAD-fmk and, as an additional control, bafilomycin that inhibits autophagy. Quantification of the surviving cells showed that the role or Rab32 in autophagy was not responsible for our observations. In contrast, necrostatin-1 and zVAD-fmk significantly inhibited the Rab32-induced neuronal damage and death, further increased upon combination of both inhibitors (Fig. 7c). Our results therefore indicate that Rab32 induces neuronal damage and death from a combination of apoptosis and necroptosis.

Discussion

In our study, we report that Rab32 serves as a novel marker of neurodegeneration in MS lesions, consistent with its previously detected induction in response to pro-inflammatory lipopolysaccharide (LPS) [24]. Interestingly, we found that Rab32 correlated with the inflammatory status of the tissues. In contrast to healthy tissue, which showed low levels of Rab32 as reported previously [34, 35], Rab32 was highly expressed in active lesions of both human MS patients and EAE mice; while not as high, expression of Rab32 was still elevated in chronic lesions. In terms of cell types, we have detected high amounts of Rab32 in neurons and microglial/macrophage cells.

Our investigation into a transcriptional regulation of Rab32 expression showed that this gene responds to ER stress. Since ER stress is well known to trigger inflammation and mitochondrial dysfunction, our observation that ER stress leads to Rab32 induction and subsequently alters mitochondrial dynamic as well as neuronal apoptosis induction identifies Rab32 as a protein of critical interest to MS research. Results presented in this study demonstrate that an increase of Rab32 in the inflamed brain directly promotes neuronal cell death from a combination of apoptosis and necroptosis. Interestingly, the putative role of Rab32 as an autophagy promoter [38] is not tied to this pro-death function of Rab32. While wild-type and active Rab32Q85L showed effects on mitochondrial morphology and neurite outgrowth, inactive Rab32T39N also compromised the survival of primary neurons as well as SH-SY5Y cells (Figs. 5 and 6), suggesting the mere upregulation of Rab32 is detrimental to neuronal function, potentially

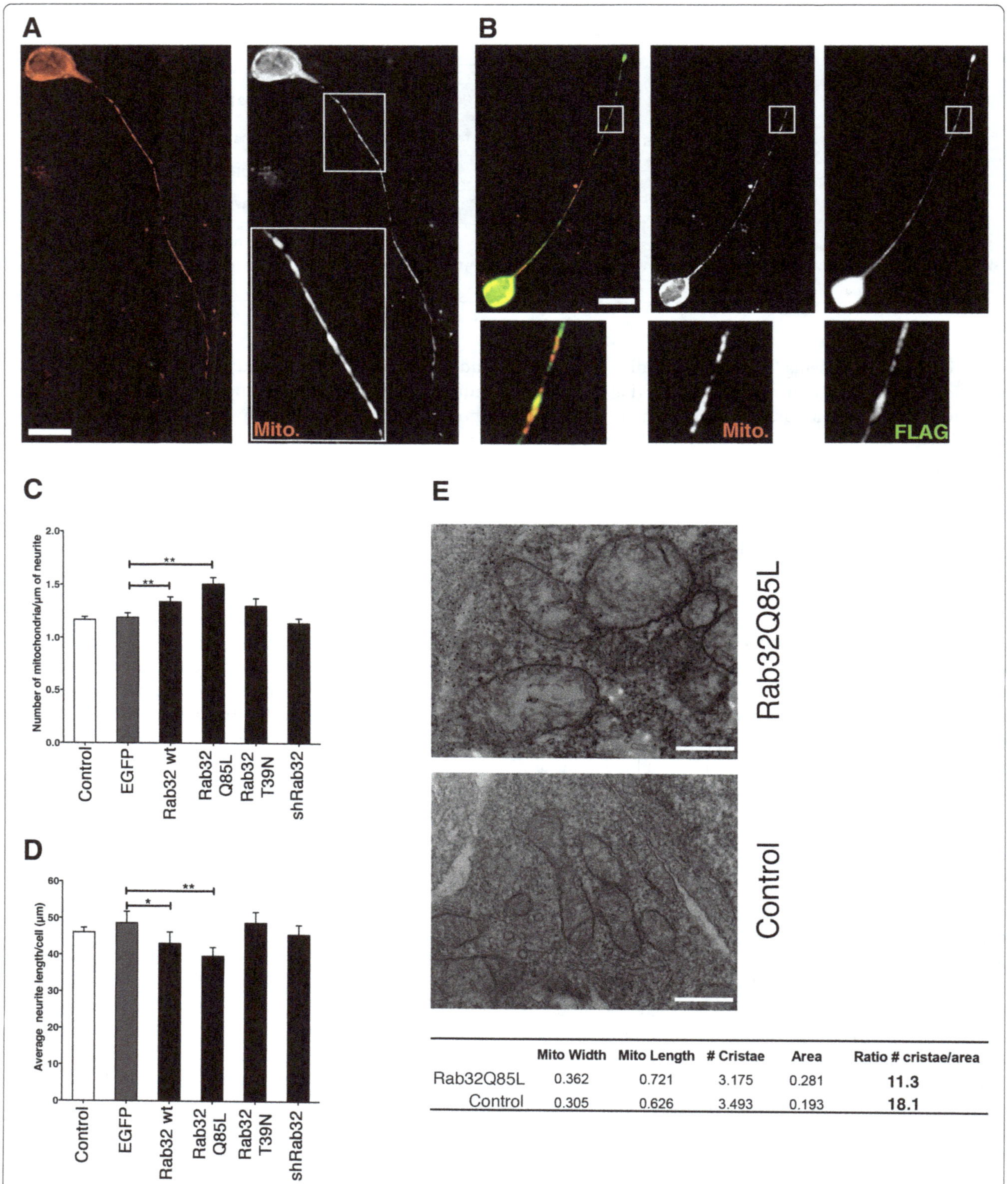

	Mito Width	Mito Length	# Cristae	Area	Ratio # cristae/area
Rab32Q85L	0.362	0.721	3.175	0.281	**11.3**
Control	0.305	0.626	3.493	0.193	**18.1**

Fig. 5 (See legend on next page.)

(See figure on previous page.)
Fig. 5 Assessment of Rab32-induced mitochondrial dynamics and neurite length in HFNs. **a**, **b** Primary human neurons were transfected with pDsRed2-Mito alone (Control: **a**) or co-transfected with pDsRed2-Mito and Rab32Q85L (**b**). Twenty-four hours post transfection, cells were processed for immunofluorescence microscopy. Mitochondria and FLAG distribution are shown as indicated. *Scale bar* 5 μm. **c** Quantification of the number of mitochondria within neurites, expressed as number of mitochondria per micrometer. **d** Quantification of the average neurite length/cell. For panels **c** and **d**, $n = 30$, $*p < 0.05$, and $**p < 0.01$, EGFP was used as an alternative control. **e** Immunoelectron microscopic determination of mitochondria phenotype. SH-SY5Y cells were transfected with FLAG-tagged Rab32Q85L, followed by immunogold detection of the FLAG signal. Mitochondria from expressing and control (non-expressing) cells were measured, and their number of cristae was determined (table below, units: μm). *Scale bar* 0.5 μm

due to shared functions of active and inactive Rab32. Moreover, our results reinforce the role of ER stress as an upstream trigger of inflammation, which is one of the main pathology drivers in the MS context. Interestingly, the inhibition of the UPR can improve myelination of some disease models [39] and also plays a critical role in the most promising approaches to treat neurodegeneration [40].

Rab32 is induced in parallel with known mediators or regulators of the MAM, namely, Grp75, PACS-2, Mitofusin 2, and Drp1 (Fig. 1). In contrast to Rab32, however, these MAM modulatory proteins were only

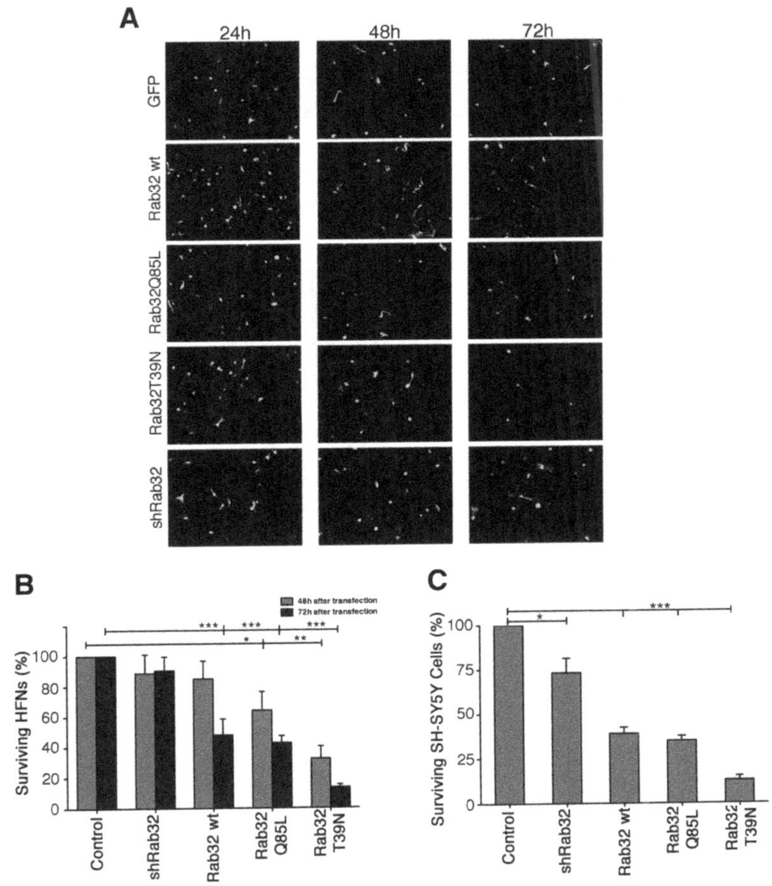

Fig. 6 Rab32-mediated neuronal killing assay. **a** HFNs were transfected with pIRES2-EGFP, or pIRES2-EGFP expressing Flag-tagged Rab32WT, Rab32Q85L, and Rab32T39N as well as the mCherry reporter-tagged shRab32. After 24, 48, and 72 h, neurons were fixed and analyzed under a fluorescent microscopy. Note: the *red color* of mCherry was converted to *green* for the sake of consistency with the rest of the micrographs. *Scale bar* 30 μm. **b** Rab32-mediated neuronal killing was evaluated at 48 and 72 h post-transfection. **c** SH-SY5Y cells were transfected with pIRES2-EGFP, or pIRES2-EGFP expressing Flag-tagged Rab32WT, Rab32Q85L, and Rab32T39N as well as the mCherry reporter-tagged shRab32. After 24 h in culture, the cells were fixed, and the percentage of surviving neurons in comparison to the control (EGFP) was analyzed. $n = 3$; $*p < 0.05$; $**p < 0.01$; $***p < 0.001$

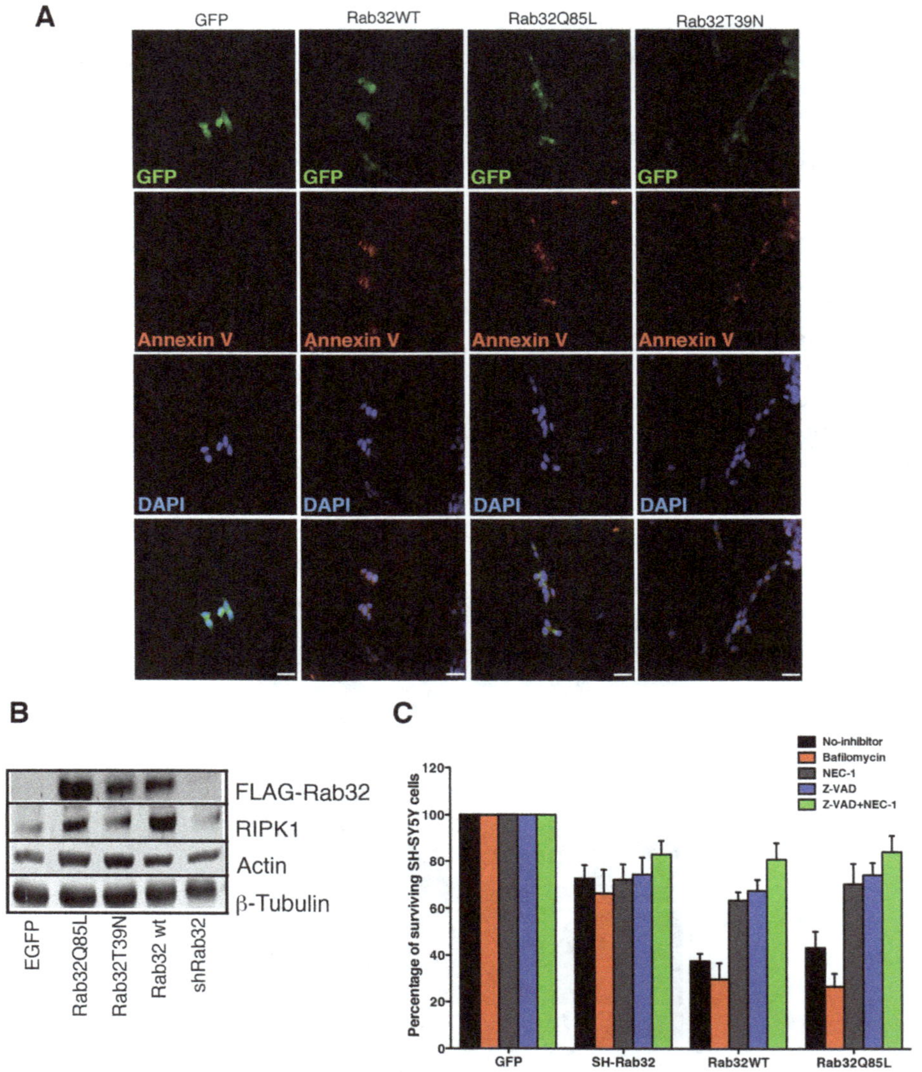

Fig. 7 Mechanisms of Rab32-mediated neuronal killing. **a** SH-SY5Y cells were transfected with pIRES2-EGFP, or pIRES2-EGFP expressing Flag-tagged Rab32WT, Rab32Q85L, and Rab32T39N. After 24 h in culture, cells were processed for Cy5-annexin V and stained with DAPI. *Scale bars* 20 μm. **b** Western blot analysis showing the expression of Rab32, RIPK1, actin, and tubulin in SH-SY5Y cells transfected with pIRES2-EGFP, or pIRES2-EGFP expressing Flag-tagged Rab32WT, Rab32Q85L, and Rab32T39N. **c** Quantification of surviving SH-SY5Y cells transfected with pIRES2-EGFP, or pIRES2-EGFP expressing Flag-tagged Rab32WT, Rab32Q85L, and Rab32T39N either under control conditions (*black*) or treated with autophagy (bafilomycin, *red*), necroptosis (necrostatin-1, *gray*), apoptosis inhibitors (zVAD-fmk, *blue*), as well as a combination of necrostatin-1 and zVAD-fmk (*green*). After 24 h in culture, the cells were fixed, and surviving neuronal cells were quantified. In each plasmid group, each treatment was compared to the untreated control (No-inhibitor). $n = 3$

induced in active, but not in chronic lesions. Nevertheless, this suggests that MAM functions, including the exchange of Ca^{2+} between the two organelles and mitochondrial dynamics, actively control neuronal decay within active MS lesions but reach a new equilibrium in chronic lesions.

Conclusions

Taken together, our results identify Rab32 as a new marker for active and chronic inflammatory lesions of the CNS in MS whose ER stress-triggered transcription leads to altered mitochondrial dynamics and neuronal cell death. Future research will have to investigate whether the inhibition of Rab32 production in the inflamed CNS could inhibit neurodegeneration in vivo.

Abbreviations

ALS: Amyotrophic lateral sclerosis; BiP/GRP78: Immunoglobulin-binding protein/glucose-regulated protein of 78 kDA; CHOP: CCAAT/enhancer-binding protein (C/EBP) homologous protein; CNS: Central nervous system; DAPI: 4′,6-Diamidino-2-phenylindole; Drp1: Dynamin-related protein 1; EAE: Experimental autoimmune encephalomyelitis; EGFP: Enhanced green fluorescent protein;

ER: Endoplasmic reticulum; GRP94: Glucose-regulated protein of 94 kDA; GTPase: Guanosine triphosphatase; H&E: Hematoxylin and eosin; HFN: Human fetal neurons; LPS: Lipopolysaccharide; MAM: Mitochondria-associated membrane; MS: Multiple sclerosis; NAWM: Normal-appearing white matter; NC: Normal control; PACS-2: Phosphofurin acidic cluster sorting protein 2; RIPK: Receptor-interacting protein kinase; RNAi: Interfering ribonucleic acid; ROS: Reactive oxygen species; RT-PCR: Reverse transcription polymerase chain reaction; SDS: Sodium dodecyl sulphate; UK: United Kingdom; UPR: Unfolded protein response; zVAD-fmk: carbobenzoxy-valyl-alanyl-aspartyl-[O-methyl]-fluoromethylketone

Acknowledgements
We thank Trefa M. Abdullah for the expert technical assistance and Sol Herrera for the useful discussions. We are indebted to Chris Power for providing some patient samples.

Funding
The study was supported by CIHR (MOP 133541 to TS and FG) and MS Society of Canada (FG) and a Royal Devon and Exeter Foundation Trust Hospital research grant (PE, JEH & NJG).

Authors' contributions
The experiments were performed by YH, XD, COS, NT, AJ, NJG, and JEH. The tissue samples from patients and animals were collected under the supervision of JQL, BJK, PE, and FG. FG and TS designed the study. TS wrote the manuscript, with editing assistance provided by PE and FG. All authors read and approved the final manuscript.

Competing interests
The authors declare that they have no competing interests.

Consent for publication
All authors have read the manuscript and consent of its publication.

Author details
[1]Department of Cell Biology, University of Alberta, Edmonton, Canada. [2]Department of Medicine, Division of Neurology, University of Alberta, Edmonton, Canada. [3]Department of Laboratory Medicine and Pathology, University of Alberta, Edmonton, Canada. [4]Department of Anesthesiology and Pain Medicine, University of Alberta, Edmonton, Canada. [5]University of Exeter Medical School & Neurology Department, Royal Devon & Exeter Hospital, Exeter, UK. [6]Present address: Alberta Diabetes Institute, University of Alberta, Edmonton, Canada.

References
1. Piaceri I, Rinnoci V, Bagnoli S, Failli Y, Sorbi S. Mitochondria and Alzheimer's disease. J Neurol Sci. 2012;322(1-2):31–4.
2. Nikić I, Merkler D, Sorbara C, Brinkoetter M, Kreutzfeldt M, Bareyre FM, Brück W, Bishop D, Misgeld T, Kerschensteiner M. A reversible form of axon damage in experimental autoimmune encephalomyelitis and multiple sclerosis. Nat Med. 2011;17(4):495–9.
3. Witte ME, Mahad DJ, Lassmann H, van Horssen J. Mitochondrial dysfunction contributes to neurodegeneration in multiple sclerosis. Trends Mol Med. 2014;20(3):179–87.
4. Campbell GR, Worrall JT, Mahad DJ. The central role of mitochondria in axonal degeneration in multiple sclerosis. Mult Scler. 2014;20(14):1806–13.
5. Wang X, Jiang W, Yan Y, Gong T, Han J, Tian Z, Zhou R. RNA viruses promote activation of the NLRP3 inflammasome through a RIP1-RIP3-DRP1 signaling pathway. Nat Immunol. 2014;15(12):1126–33.
6. Reddy PH, Reddy TP, Manczak M, Calkins MJ, Shirendeb U, Mao P. Dynamin-related protein 1 and mitochondrial fragmentation in neurodegenerative diseases. Brain Res Rev. 2011;67(1-2):103–18.
7. Kageyama Y, Zhang Z, Roda R, Fukaya M, Wakabayashi J, Wakabayashi N, Kensler TW, Reddy PH, Iijima M, Sesaki H. Mitochondrial division ensures the survival of postmitotic neurons by suppressing oxidative damage. J Cell Biol. 2012;197(4):535–51.
8. Frank S, Gaume B, Bergmann-Leitner ES, Leitner WW, Robert EG, Catez F, Smith CL, Youle RJ. The role of dynamin-related protein 1, a mediator of mitochondrial fission, in apoptosis. Dev Cell. 2001;1(4):515–25.
9. Chen H, Chan DC. Mitochondrial dynamics—fusion, fission, movement, and mitophagy—in neurodegenerative diseases. Hum Mol Genet. 2009;18(R2):R169–176.
10. Witte ME, Geurts JJG, de Vries HE, van der Valk P, van Horssen J. Mitochondrial dysfunction: a potential link between neuroinflammation and neurodegeneration? Mitochondrion. 2010;10(5):411–8.
11. Decuypere JP, Monaco G, Bultynck G, Missiaen L, De Smedt H, Parys JB. The IP(3) receptor-mitochondria connection in apoptosis and autophagy. Biochim Biophys Acta. 2011;1813(5):1003–13.
12. Patterson RL, Boehning D, Snyder SH. Inositol 1,4,5-trisphosphate receptors as signal integrators. Annu Rev Biochem. 2004;73:437–65.
13. Villegas R, Martinez NW, Lillo J, Pihan P, Hernandez D, Twiss JL, Court FA. Calcium release from intra-axonal endoplasmic reticulum leads to axon degeneration through mitochondrial dysfunction. J Neurosci. 2014;34(21):7179–89.
14. Stirling DP, Cummins K, Wayne Chen SR, Stys P. Axoplasmic reticulum Ca(2+) release causes secondary degeneration of spinal axons. Ann Neurol. 2014;75(2):220–9.
15. Roussel BD, Kruppa AJ, Miranda E, Crowther DC, Lomas DA, Marciniak SJ. Endoplasmic reticulum dysfunction in neurological disease. Lancet Neurol. 2013;12(1):105–18.
16. Cunnea P, Mhaille AN, McQuaid S, Farrell M, McMahon J, FitzGerald U. Expression profiles of endoplasmic reticulum stress-related molecules in demyelinating lesions and multiple sclerosis. Mult Scler. 2011;17(7):808–18.
17. Bravo R, Vicencio JM, Parra V, Troncoso R, Munoz JP, Bui M, Quiroga C, Rodriguez AE, Verdejo HE, Ferreira J, et al. Increased ER-mitochondrial coupling promotes mitochondrial respiration and bioenergetics during early phases of ER stress. J Cell Sci. 2011;124(Pt 13):2143–52.
18. Csordas G, Renken C, Varnai P, Walter L, Weaver D, Buttle KF, Balla T, Mannella CA, Hajnóczky G. Structural and functional features and significance of the physical linkage between ER and mitochondria. J Cell Biol. 2006;174:915–21.
19. Csordas G, Varnai P, Golenar T, Roy S, Purkins G, Schneider TG, Balla T, Hajnoczky G. Imaging interorganelle contacts and local calcium dynamics at the ER-mitochondrial interface. Mol Cell. 2010;39(1):121–32.
20. Simmen T, Lynes EM, Gesson K, Thomas G. Oxidative protein folding in the endoplasmic reticulum: tight links to the mitochondria-associated membrane (MAM). Biochim Biophys Acta. 2010;1798(8):1465–73.
21. Bui M, Gilady SY, Fitzsimmons RE, Benson MD, Lynes EM, Gesson K, Alto NM, Strack S, Scott JD, Simmen T. Rab32 modulates apoptosis onset and mitochondria-associated membrane (MAM) properties. J Biol Chem. 2010;285(41):31590–602.
22. Alto NM, Soderling J, Scott JD. Rab32 is an A-kinase anchoring protein and participates in mitochondrial dynamics. J Cell Biol. 2002;158(4):659–68.
23. Ortiz-Sandoval CG, Hughes SC, Dacks JB, Simmen T. Interaction with the effector dynamin-related protein 1 (Drp1) is an ancient function of Rab32 subfamily proteins. Cell Logist. 2014;4(4):e986399.
24. Liang Y, Lin S, Zou L, Zhou H, Zhang J, Su B, Wan Y. Expression profiling of Rab GTPases reveals the involvement of Rab20 and Rab32 in acute brain inflammation in mice. Neurosci Lett. 2012;572(2):110–4.
25. Lynes EM, Bui M, Yap MC, Benson MD, Schneider B, Ellgaard L, Berthiaume LG, Simmen T. Palmitoylated TMX and calnexin target to the mitochondria-associated membrane. EMBO J. 2012;31(2):457–70.
26. Haile Y, Simmen KC, Pasichnyk D, Touret N, Simmen T, Lu JQ, Bleackley RC, Giuliani F. Granule-derived granzyme B mediates the vulnerability of human neurons to T cell-induced neurotoxicity. J Immunol. 2011;187(9):4861–72.
27. Lu JQ, Wilson B, Yong VW, Pugh J, Menta V. Immune cell infiltrates in atypical teratoid/rhabdoid tumors. Can J Neurol Sci. 2012;39(5):605–12.
28. Lieu A, Tenorio G, Kerr BJ. Protein kinase C gamma (PKCgamma) as a novel marker to assess the functional status of the corticospinal tract in experimental autoimmune encephalomyelitis (EAE). J Neuroimmunol. 2013;256(1-2):43–8.
29. Holley JE, Bremer E, Kendall AC, de Bruyn M, Helfrich W, Tarr JM, Newcombe J, Gutowski NJ, Eggleton P. CD20+inflammatory T-cells are present in blood and brain of multiple sclerosis patients and can be selectively targeted for apoptotic elimination. Mult Scler Relat Disord. 2014;3(5):650–8.

30. Holley JE, Newcombe J, Whatmore JL, Gutowski NJ. Increased blood vessel density and endothelial cell proliferation in multiple sclerosis cerebral white matter. Neurosci Lett. 2010;470(1):65–70.
31. Ortiz Sandoval C, Simmen T. Rab proteins of the endoplasmic reticulum: functions and interactors. Biochem Soc Trans. 2012;40(6):1426–32.
32. Murakami T, Ockinger J, Yu J, Byles V, McColl A, Hofer AM, Horng T. Critical role for calcium mobilization in activation of the NLRP3 inflammasome. Proc Natl Acad Sci U S A. 2012;109(28):11282–7.
33. Zhou R, Yazdi AS, Menu P, Tschopp J. A role for mitochondria in NLRP3 inflammasome activation. Nature. 2011;469(7329):221–5.
34. Bao X, Faris AE, Jang EK, Haslam RJ. Molecular cloning, bacterial expression and properties of Rab31 and Rab32 New blood platelet Rab proteins. Eur J Biochem. 2002;271:259–71.
35. Cohen-Solal KA, Sood R, Marin Y, Crespo-Carbone SM, Sinsimer D, Martino JJ, Robbins C, Makalowska I, Trent J, Chen S. Identification and characterization of mouse Rab32 by mRNA and protein expression analysis. Biochim Biophys Acta. 2003;1651(1-2):68–75.
36. Deslauriers AM, Afkhami-Goli A, Paul AM, Bhat RK, Acharjee S, Ellestad KK, Noorbakhsh F, Michalak M, Power C. Neuroinflammation and endoplasmic reticulum stress are coregulated by crocin to prevent demyelination and neurodegeneration. J Immunol. 2011;187(9):4788–99.
37. McMahon JM, McQuaid S, Reynolds R, FitzGerald UF. Increased expression of ER stress- and hypoxia-associated molecules in grey matter lesions in multiple sclerosis. Mult Scler. 2012;18(10):1437–47.
38. Hirota Y, Tanaka Y. A small GTPase, human Rab32, is required for the formation of autophagic vacuoles under basal conditions. Cell Mol Life Sci. 2009;66(17):2913–32.
39. D'Antonio M, Musner N, Scapin C, Ungaro D, Del Carro U, Ron D, Feltri ML, Wrabetz L. Resetting translational homeostasis restores myelination in Charcot-Marie-Tooth disease type 1B mice. J Exp Med. 2013;210(4):821–38.
40. Halliday M, Mallucci GR. Review: modulating the unfolded protein response to prevent neurodegeneration and enhance memory. Neuropathol Appl Neurobiol. 2015;41(4):414–27.

12

A comparison of brain magnetic resonance imaging lesions in multiple sclerosis by race with reference to disability progression

Yuri Nakamura[1], Laura Gaetano[2,3], Takuya Matsushita[1], Altermatt Anna[2,4], Till Sprenger[5], Ernst-Wilhelm Radue[6], Jens Wuerfel[2,4], Lorena Bauer[2,7], Michael Amann[2,3,8], Koji Shinoda[1], Noriko Isobe[9], Ryo Yamasaki[1], Takahiko Saida[10,11], Ludwig Kappos[3] and Jun-ichi Kira[1*]

Abstract

Background: We compared the magnetic resonance imaging (MRI) features between Japanese and Caucasian patients with multiple sclerosis (MS), and identified the relationships between MRI features and disability.

Methods: From the baseline data of phase II fingolimod trials, 95 Japanese and 246 Caucasian relapsing-remitting MS patients were enrolled. The number, volume, and distribution of brain MRI lesions were evaluated using T2-weighted (T2W) images. Cross-sectional total normalized brain volume (NBV), normalized cortical gray matter volume, normalized deep gray matter volume (NDGMV), normalized white matter volume (NWMV), and normalized thalamic volume were measured.

Results: Japanese patients had significantly lower Expanded Disability Status Scale (EDSS) scores than Caucasian patients (mean 2.0 vs. 2.3, $p = 0.008$), despite a similar disease duration. Japanese patients showed a trend towards fewer T2W-lesions (median 50 vs. 65, $p = 0.08$) and significantly lower frequencies of cerebellar and parietal lobe lesions ($p = 0.02$ for both) than Caucasian patients. There were no differences in T2W-lesion volume between races, whereas Japanese patients had a significantly larger T2W-lesion volume per lesion compared with Caucasian patients (median 140 mm^3 vs. 85 mm^3, $p < 0.0001$). T2W-lesion volumes were positively correlated with EDSS scores in Japanese patients ($p < 0.0001$). In both races, NBV, normalized cortical gray matter volume, NDGMV, and thalamic volume were negatively correlated with disease duration and EDSS scores ($p < 0.01$ for all). NWMV was negatively correlated with disease duration and EDSS scores only in Caucasian patients ($p = 0.03$ and $p = 0.004$, respectively). NBV, NDGMV, NWMV, and thalamic volume were consistently smaller in Japanese compared with Caucasian patients throughout the entire examined disease duration ($p = 0.046$, $p = 0.01$, $p = 0.005$, and $p = 0.04$, respectively). Japanese patients had a significantly faster reduction in NDGMV ($p = 0.001$), particularly for thalamic volume ($p = 0.001$), with disease duration compared with Caucasian patients.

Conclusions: Gray matter atrophy is a common denominator for disability in Japanese and Caucasian patients. Additional contributory factors for disability include T2W-lesion volume in Japanese patients and white matter atrophy in Caucasian patients. Less frequent parietal and cerebellar involvement with fewer T2W-lesions may underlie milder disability in Japanese patients.

Keywords: Brain lesions, Brain volume, Disability, Magnetic resonance imaging, Multiple sclerosis, Progression, Race

* Correspondence: kira@neuro.med.kyushu-u.ac.jp
[1]Department of Neurology, Neurological Institute, Graduate School of Medical Sciences, Kyushu University, 3-1-1 Maidashi, Higashi-ku, Fukuoka 812-8582, Japan

Background

Multiple sclerosis (MS) is an autoimmune demyelinating disorder of the central nervous system, caused by a complex interaction between environmental and genetic factors. As such, the clinical and magnetic resonance imaging (MRI) features of MS are likely influenced by differences in genetic backgrounds between racial groups. Indeed, individuals with African ancestry, who develop MS less frequently than those with European ancestry [1], show more rapid disease progression after MS onset [2, 3].

The prevalence of MS is also low in individuals with Asian ancestry, including Japanese people. To our knowledge, only one study has conducted a direct comparison of disease severity between British and Japanese MS patients. This institutional study, which took place after the discovery of a specific biomarker for neuromyelitis optica (neuromyelitis optica IgG) revealed that Japanese MS patients exhibited milder disability compared with Caucasian patients [4]. The fourth nationwide survey of MS in Japan also showed that only 49.5% of patients with the conventional form of MS had brain lesions fulfilling the Barkhof criteria [5] after an average disease duration of 10.4 years [6]. This proportion was much lower than that for Caucasian patients, with 74% of patients with early relapsing-remitting MS (RRMS) [7], and approximately 50% of patients with clinically isolated syndrome [8], having brain lesions fulfilling the Barkhof criteria after a disease duration of 2 years.

Two studies have suggested that Japanese patients with MS may have lower cerebellar involvement and fewer intra-cortical lesions, as revealed by MRI, than Caucasian patients [9, 10]. In addition, although the Swanton modified criteria can predict the conversion from a clinically isolated syndrome to clinically definite MS according to baseline MRI findings with high sensitivity and accuracy in Western countries [11, 12], the sensitivity of these criteria was reported to be far lower in Asian individuals [13]. These observations suggest that the milder MS severity found in Japanese compared with Caucasian individuals may relate to a lower frequency of brain lesions.

To our knowledge, no studies have performed a direct MRI comparison between Asian and Caucasian MS patients using the same imaging protocol. Thus, in the present study, we directly compared brain MRI findings in Japanese and Caucasian MS patients, using pooled baseline data from the phase II fingolimod trials in Japan and Western countries, obtained using a standardized MRI protocol, with the aim to clarify the mechanisms of the milder disease course in Japanese MS patients.

Methods

Patients

We examined brain MRI from a population of patients with RRMS selected from pooled baseline data from phase II fingolimod trials for treatment of MS. The trials were conducted at 32 centers in 10 European countries and Canada, and at 43 centers in Japan. All participants from Europe and Canada were Caucasian, and all participants from Japan were Japanese. The eligibility criteria for the core studies were previously described in detail [14, 15]. In brief, participants were between 18 and 60 years of age, with a clinical diagnosis of relapsing MS. Patients had at least one of the following: one or more relapses in the previous year before enrollment, two or more relapses in the previous 2 years, and at least one contrast-enhanced T1-weighted (T1W) brain lesion on baseline MRI. Patients also had at least one T2-weighted (T2W) brain lesion, were neurologically stable without relapse, and had a Kurtzke's Expanded Disability Status Scale (EDSS) score [16] ranging from 0 to 6. Exclusion criteria were use of corticosteroids (within the previous 30 days), immunomodulatory therapy (within the prior 3 months), or immunosuppressive treatment (e.g., azathioprine or methotrexate within the past 6 months).

We collected baseline demographic and clinical data including sex, age, disease duration from the initial symptom, EDSS score, Multiple Sclerosis Severity Score (MSSS), and previous MS treatment exposure such as disease-modifying drugs (DMDs) or immunosuppressive therapy. Of the participants who met the baseline eligibility criteria for the phase II fingolimod clinical trial, 167 Japanese and 250 Caucasian patients had RRMS. In the Japanese RRMS group, 70 patients did not consent to take part in the present study and were not included. Clinical parameters from two of the Japanese patients were unavailable, and these patients were excluded from this study. In the Caucasian RRMS group, four patients were excluded as their baseline scans or clinical parameters were unavailable. Demographics and MRI parameters were available for a total of 95 Japanese and 246 Caucasian patients. All participants provided written informed consent, and the research protocol for the study was approved by the Kyushu University Ethics Committee.

Image acquisition

MRI images were obtained using 1.5 T scanners with interleaved axial 3.0-mm-thick slices, field of view = 25 cm, and matrix = 128 × 128. The imaging protocol included axial proton density (repetition time [TR] 2800–3800 ms; echo time [TE] 14–40) and T2W fast/turbo spin echo (TR 2800–3800 ms; TE 80–1200 ms). Additionally, T1W conventional spin echo (TR 500–650 ms; TE 10–20 ms) and post-contrast T1W spin-echo images (TR 500–650 ms; TE 10–20 ms) were obtained.

MRI analysis

Trained and experienced technicians at the Medical Image Analysis Center (MIAC, Basel, Switzerland), who were blinded to clinical information, conducted T2W-lesion segmentation on T2W images using semi-automatic thresholding contour software with an interactive digital analysis program (AMIRA V.3.1.1; Mercury Computer Systems Inc., Hillsboro, OR, USA). To compare the number, volume, and distribution of T2W-lesions between the Japanese and Caucasian cohorts, we selected only patients with MRI scans that completely covered the regions from the medulla to the top of the parietal lobe. Scans from 93 Japanese and 72 Caucasian patients were available for evaluation of total T2W-lesion number and volume. We also used this dataset to calculate the average T2W-lesion volume in individuals (dividing the total T2W-lesion volume by the number of T2W-lesions) in the Japanese and Caucasian cohorts. The distribution and location of T2W-lesions were determined as follows. Segmented hyper-intense T2W-lesions in native space were linearly registered to the T1 images, which were then registered to the Montreal Neurological Institute (MNI) standard space template using a linear and nonlinear transformation method. The resulting transformation matrix was applied to the T2W-lesion mask previously registered to T1 images. We conducted a quality assessment of the procedure, and patients without successful registration to the standard were excluded from the analysis. Once the T2W-lesions were translated to MNI space, we automatically assessed the presence or absence of lesions in each brain lobe according to the Talairach atlas (i.e., frontal lobe, occipital lobe, parietal lobe, temporal lobe, limbic area, sub-lobar area, cerebellum, and brainstem), as well as the number and volume of lesions in the whole brain.

We used the entire cohort to measure total normalized brain volume (NBV), normalized cortical (NCGMV) and deep gray matter volume (NDGMV), and normalized white matter volume (NWMV) using the Structural Image Evaluation Using Normalization of Atrophy X (SIENAX) program [17]. This software uses a fully automated algorithm to estimate cross-sectional brain volume using a single time-point scan [18], performs segmentation of the brain from non-brain tissue in the head, and estimates the outer skull surface. The brain and skull images are then registered to a standard space brain and skull image derived from the MNI152 standard image. This step enables estimation of the volumetric scaling factor used for normalization of head size. To increase the reproducibility among patients, NBV, NWMV, NCGMV, and NDGMV were assessed in the 70-mm central area of the brain (z-block; MNI152 z-coordinates − 10-mm bottom to + 60-mm top). Finally, we separately assessed the normalized thalamic volume from the NDGMV using the FMRIB's Integrated Registration and Segmentation Tool algorithm [19]. We performed a quality assessment to ensure the correct segmentation of each compartment.

T2W-lesions of 68 Japanese and 57 Caucasian patients were successfully registered to the MNI space and included in the final analysis. When comparing clinical features between the Japanese and Caucasian subgroups for evaluation of T2W-lesion distribution, we found similar trends in the demographic features to those in the total study population (data not shown). Based on white matter, cortical, and deep gray matter segmentation, scans from 83 Japanese and 233 Caucasian patients were available for NBV comparison, from 45 Japanese and 148 Caucasian patients for evaluation of NWMV, from 52 Japanese and 165 Caucasian patients for evaluation of NCGMV, and from 73 Japanese and 207 Caucasian patients for evaluation of NDGMV and normalized thalamic volume. When comparing clinical features in the Japanese and Caucasian subgroups of brain volume measurement, we found similar trends to the demographic features (data not shown).

Statistical analyses

All analyses were performed using statistical software (JMP 13.0.0; SAS Institute Inc., Cary, NC, USA) or R. The Fisher's exact probability test was used to compare categorical variables, while the Mann–Whitney U test was used to compare continuous variables, including age, age at onset, disease duration from the first symptom, EDSS score, MSSS, and MRI parameters, between Japanese and Caucasian patients. Race-based differences in MRI parameters, number and volumes of T2W-lesions, individual T2W-lesion size, NBV, NWMV, NCGMV, NDGMV, and normalized thalamic volume were assessed by multivariate linear regression analyses adjusting for age, sex, disease duration from the initial symptom, and MS treatment exposure. To meet the normality assumption for the regression model, the cube root transformation was applied to the number or volume of the total T2W-lesions, or individual T2W-lesion size prior to data analysis. Correlations of EDSS scores with brain volumes were examined using Spearman's correlation. Linear regression analysis was used to examine the association of disease duration with brain volume. We also performed a test of homogeneity of slope to examine differences in the rate of brain volume reduction with disease duration, and a test of homogeneity of intercept to examine differences in brain volume at the early course of the disease, between the two racial groups. Statistical significance was set at $p < 0.05$. A statistical trend was assumed if $p < 0.1$.

Results

Clinical characteristics

The demographics and clinical characteristics of the Japanese and Caucasian groups are shown in Table 1 (see "Entire study population"). The proportion of

Table 1 Comparison of baseline characteristics between Japanese and Caucasian patients with MS

	Entire study population			Population for T2W-lesion evaluation		
	Japanese patients ($n = 95$)	Caucasian patients ($n = 246$)	p	Japanese patients ($n = 93$)	Caucasian patients ($n = 72$)	p
Female (%)	65 (68.4)	179 (72.8)	0.43	65 (69.9)	48 (66.7)	0.74
Age at time of the MRI, years[a]	34.2 ± 8.3	36.9 ± 9.5	0.03	34.0 ± 8.3	35.9 ± 9.8	0.24
Age at first symptom, years[a]	26.9 ± 8.9	29.0 ± 8.5	0.03	26.6 ± 8.7	28.3 ± 8.6	0.15
Duration of disease from first symptom, years[a]	7.4 ± 6.4	7.9 ± 7.2	0.60	7.4 ± 6.4	7.7 ± 8.1	0.75
EDSS scores[a]	2.0 ± 1.7	2.3 ± 1.2	0.008	1.9 ± 1.7	2.2 ± 1.3	0.10
MSSS[a]	3.24 ± 2.61	3.84 ± 2.09	0.01	3.19 ± 2.60	3.78 ± 1.92	0.04
Previous exposure of DMDs or immunosuppressive therapy, *n* (%)	54 (56.8)	70 (28.5)	< 0.0001	53 (57.0)	22 (30.6)	0.0009
Patients with contrast-enhanced lesions, *n* (%)	53 (55.8)	126 (51.2)	0.47	52 (55.9)	40 (55.6)	1.00

[a]Values are expressed as mean ± standard deviation
DMDs Disease modifying drugs, *EDSS* Kurtzke's Expanded Disability Status Scale, *MS* multiple sclerosis, *MSSS* Multiple Sclerosis Severity Score, *T2W* T2-weighted

women and duration of disease from the first symptom were similar between the Japanese and Caucasian groups. In the total study population, Japanese patients were younger at the time of MRI scans (mean 34.2 vs. 36.9 years, respectively; $p = 0.03$) and at the onset of the first symptom (mean 26.9 vs. 29.0 years, respectively; $p = 0.03$), and had lower EDSS scores (mean 2.0 vs. 2.3, respectively; $p = 0.008$) and MSSS (mean 3.24 vs. 3.84, respectively; $p = 0.01$), compared with Caucasian patients. The proportion of patients with previous MS treatment exposure, including DMDs or immunosuppressive therapy, was significantly higher in Japanese patients compared with Caucasian patients (56.8% vs. 28.5%, respectively; $p < 0.0001$). The demographics of the subset used for the T2W-lesion evaluation are summarized in Table 1 (see "Population for T2W-lesion evaluation"). Japanese patients in this subset also had significantly lower MSSS (mean 3.19 vs. 3.78, respectively; $p = 0.04$) and a higher frequency of previous MS treatment exposure (57.0% vs. 30.6%, respectively; $p = 0.0009$) compared with Caucasian patients.

Comparison of MRI findings between Japanese and Caucasian patients with MS

After adjusting for age, sex, duration of disease from the first symptom, and previous MS treatment exposure, Japanese patients showed a trend towards fewer T2W-lesions than Caucasian patients (median 50 vs. 65, respectively; $p = 0.08$; Table 2). However, there were no significant differences in the volume of T2W-lesions between the two groups (median 7.8 cm^3 vs. 5.3 cm^3, respectively; $p = 0.12$). Japanese patients had a significantly larger mean volume per lesion compared with Caucasian patients (median 140 mm^3 vs. 85 mm^3, respectively; $p < 0.0001$). The proportion of patients with cerebellar lesions was significantly lower in Japanese patients compared with Caucasian patients (45.6% vs. 66.7%, respectively; $p = 0.02$; Fig. 1), which was also observed for patients with lesions in the parietal lobe (89.7% vs. 100%, respectively; $p = 0.02$). There were no differences in any other brain regions between the two groups.

After adjusting for confounding factors, Japanese patients had significantly smaller NBV, NWMV, and NDGMV compared with Caucasian patients (NBV median 954.1 cm^3 vs. 977.9 cm^3, respectively; $p < 0.0001$; NWMV median 466.1 cm^3 vs. 487.7 cm^3, respectively, $p < 0.0001$; NDGMV median 36.7 cm^3 vs. 41.4 cm^3, respectively; $p < 0.0001$; Table 2). Among NDGMV, normalized thalamic volume of Japanese patients was also significantly smaller than that of Caucasian patients (median 17.3 cm^3 vs. 18.9 cm^3, respectively; $p < 0.0001$). Japanese patients also showed a trend towards a smaller NCGMV compared with Caucasian patients (median 438.3 cm^3 vs. 452.0 cm^3, respectively; $p = 0.08$).

Correlation of brain MRI metrics with EDSS scores in Japanese and Caucasian MS patients

EDSS scores were correlated with T2W-lesion volumes in Japanese patients ($r_s = 0.46$, $p < 0.0001$; Fig. 2a), but not Caucasian patients ($r_s = 0.12$, $p = 0.33$; Fig. 2g). NBV, NCGMV, and NDGMV were significantly correlated with EDSS scores in both Japanese patients (NBV $r_s = -0.33$, $p = 0.002$; NCGMV $r_s = -0.44$, $p = 0.001$; NDGMV $r_s = -0.48$, $p < 0.0001$; Fig. 2b–d) and Caucasian patients (NBV $r_s = -0.48$, $p < 0.0001$; NCGMV $r_s = -0.38$, $p < 0.0001$; NDGMV $r_s = -0.38$, $p < 0.0001$; Fig. 2h–j). In both populations, EDSS scores were also negatively correlated with normalized thalamic volume (Japanese $r_s = -0.47$, $p < 0.0001$; Caucasian $r_s = -0.34$, $p < 0.0001$; Fig. 2e and k). There was a weak correlation of

Table 2 Comparison of baseline brain MRI features between Japanese and Caucasian patients with MS

	Mean	Median (IQR)	Mean	Median (IQR)	*p*
	Japanese patients (*n* = 93)		Caucasian patients (*n* = 72)		
Number of T2W-lesions	62	50 (27–96)	73	65 (24–108)	0.08
T2W-lesion volumes (cm^3)	11.5	7.8 (2.3–16.9)	8.0	5.3 (2.4–12.2)	0.12
Each T2W-lesion volume (mm^3)	174	140 (78–224)	118	85 (63–138)	< 0.0001
	Japanese patients (*n* = 83)		Caucasian patients (*n* = 233)		
NBV (cm^3)	942.6	954.1 (903.9–980.2)	972.9	977.9 (940.4–1002.6)	< 0.0001
	Japanese patients (*n* = 45)		Caucasian patients (n = 148)		
NWMV (cm^3)	467.4	466.1 (446.5–486.1)	486.9	487.7 (473.2–501.4)	< 0.0001
	Japanese patients (*n* = 52)		Caucasian patients (*n* = 165)		
NCGMV (cm^3)	441.3	438.3 (418.6–473.1)	449.8	452.0 (429.9–471.7)	0.08
	Japanese patients (*n* = 73)		Caucasian patients (*n* = 207)		
NDGMV (cm^3)	37.0	36.7 (33.3–40.6)	40.8	41.4 (38.0–43.8)	< 0.0001
Normalized thalamic volume (cm^3)	17.2	17.3 (15.7–19.0)	18.8	18.9 (17.6–20.2)	< 0.0001

Statistical comparisons were performed using linear regression with adjustments for age, sex, duration of disease from the first symptom, and exposure to previous MS treatment. We calculated the average T2W-lesion volume by dividing overall T2W-lesion volume by the number of T2W-lesions in individual patients
IQR interquartile range, *MRI* Magnetic resonance imaging, *MS* multiple sclerosis, *NBV* normalized brain volume, *NCGMV* normalized cortical gray matter volume, *NDGMV* normalized deep gray matter volume, *NWMV* normalized white matter volume

NWMV with EDSS scores in Caucasian patients (r_s = – 0.24, $p = 0.004$; Fig. 2l), but not in Japanese patients ($r_s = 0.08$, $p = 0.62$; Fig. 2f).

Association of brain volume with disease duration in MS patients

To assess the trajectory of brain volume reduction with respect to disease duration from the first symptom, we analyzed the association of disease duration with brain volume. NBV (Japanese $R^2 = 0.20$, $p < 0.0001$; Caucasian $R^2 = 0.15$, $p < 0.0001$), NCGMV (Japanese $R^2 = 0.14$, $p = 0.005$; Caucasian $R^2 = 0.10$, $p < 0.0001$), and NDGMV (Japanese $R^2 = 0.34$, $p < 0.0001$; Caucasian $R^2 = 0.14$, $p < 0.0001$) were negatively associated with disease duration in both cohorts (Fig. 3a–c). Normalized thalamic volume was also negatively associated with disease duration in both cohorts (Japanese $R^2 = 0.33$, $p < 0.0001$; Caucasian $R^2 = 0.13$, $p < 0.0001$; Fig. 3d). By contrast, NWMV was weakly and negatively correlated with disease duration in Caucasian patients ($R^2 = 0.03$, $p = 0.03$; Fig. 3e), but not Japanese patients ($R^2 = 0.05$, $p = 0.16$).

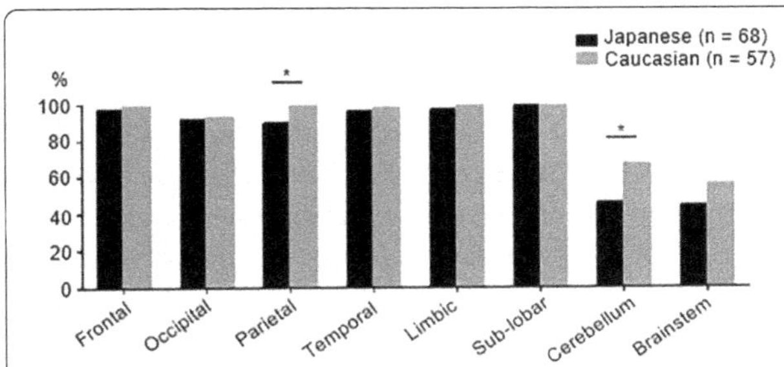

Fig. 1 Distribution of lesions between Japanese and Caucasian patients with multiple sclerosis (MS). The proportion of patients with lesions in each brain region is shown. The proportion of patients with lesions in the cerebellum and parietal lobe was significantly lower in the Japanese group (black bar) compared with the Caucasian group (gray bar). "Sub-lobar" includes the basal ganglia and surrounding white matter. *$p < 0.05$

Finally, we used a test for homogeneity of slope to compare trends in the association of brain volume with disease duration among the Japanese and Caucasian patients. Japanese patients had a significantly faster reduction in NDGMV including normalized thalamic volume and normalized thalamic volume alone with disease duration when compared with Caucasian patients ($p = 0.001$ for both). Japanese patients also had a marginally faster reduction in NBV with disease duration compared with Caucasian patients ($p = 0.06$). These findings suggest the potential for faster deep gray matter atrophy in Japanese MS patients. NBV, NDGMV, NWMV, and normalized thalamic volume were consistently smaller in Japanese patients compared with Caucasian patients throughout the entire examined disease duration ($p = 0.046$, $p = 0.01$, $p = 0.005$, and $p = 0.04$, respectively), suggesting an inherently smaller volume of deep gray matter, white matter, and the whole brain in Japanese MS patients. NCGMV was similar between the two racial groups in the early course of the disease, and did not differ significantly in terms of the reduction slope ($p = 0.87$ and $p = 0.22$, respectively).

To exclude the impact of outliers who had a disease duration of ≥ 10 years, we also evaluated the association

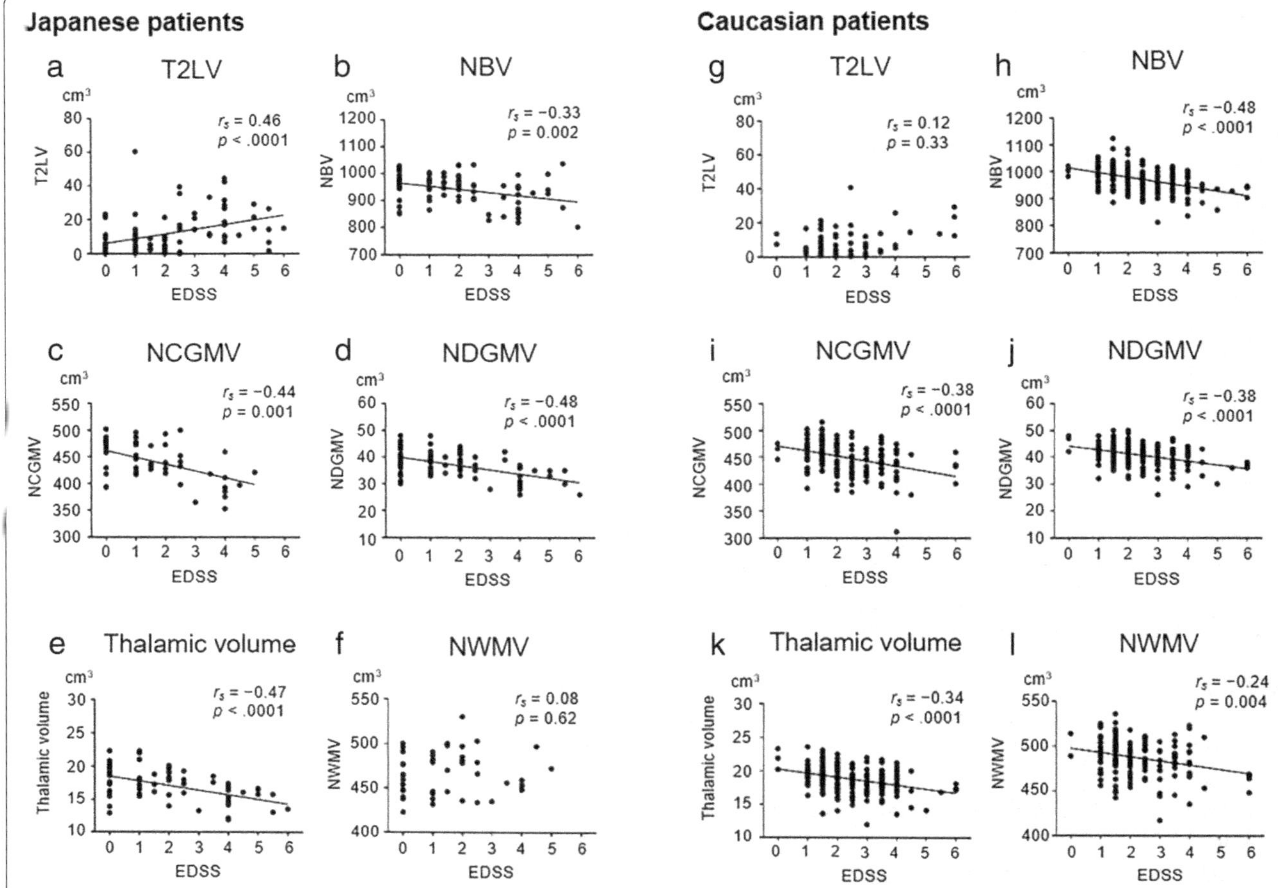

Fig. 2 Correlations of Expanded Disability Status Scale (EDSS) scores with brain lesions or volume in patients with MS. Correlations of EDSS scores with T2W-lesion volumes (T2LV), normalized brain volume (NBV), normalized white matter volume (NWMV), normalized cortical gray matter volume (NCGMV), normalized thalamic volume, or normalized deep gray matter volume (NDGMV) in Japanese (**a–f**) and Caucasian patients (**g–l**). The lines represent the linear regression of the data. r_s = Spearman's rank correlation coefficient

of disease duration with brain volumes in MS patients with a disease duration of < 10 years. Even after excluding patients with a disease duration of ≥ 10 years, NBV (Japanese $R^2 = 0.26$, $p < 0.0001$; Caucasian $R^2 = 0.13$, $p < 0.0001$), NCGMV (Japanese $R^2 = 0.13$, $p = 0.02$; Caucasian $R^2 = 0.11$, $p = 0.0003$), NDGMV (Japanese $R^2 = 0.36$, $p < 0.0001$; Caucasian $R^2 = 0.04$, $p = 0.02$), and normalized thalamic volume (Japanese $R^2 = 0.41$, $p < 0.0001$; Caucasian $R^2 = 0.05$, $p = 0.01$) were negatively associated with disease duration in both cohorts (Fig. 4a–d). By contrast, NWMV was not associated with disease duration in either cohort (Fig. 4e). A test of homogeneity of slopes showed significant differences in NBV ($p = 0.02$), NDGMV ($p = 0.0002$), and normalized thalamic volume ($p < 0.0001$) between the two groups. Thus, the exclusion of outliners with a disease duration of ≥ 10 years showed a stronger trend towards Japanese patients having a faster reduction in NBV, NDGMV, and normalized thalamic volume with disease duration than Caucasian patients.

Discussion

This study represents the first direct comparison of brain MRI findings between Japanese and Caucasian MS patients with similar disease duration using a standardized imaging protocol. The similarities in brain MRI findings between Japanese and Caucasian patients were as follows: (1) both Japanese and Caucasian patients had similar total T2W-lesion volumes, and (2) NBV, NCGMV, NDGMV, and normalized thalamic volume were negatively correlated with disease duration and EDSS scores in both racial groups. The differences in brain MRI findings were as follows: (1) Japanese patients had a larger individual lesion size compared with Caucasian patients, although Japanese patients tended to have fewer T2W-lesions. (2) Cerebellar and parietal lobe lesions were less common in Japanese patients compared with Caucasian patients. (3) There was a positive correlation of T2W-lesion volumes with EDSS scores in Japanese patients, but not in Caucasian patients. (4) NBV, NWMV, NDGMV, and normalized thalamic

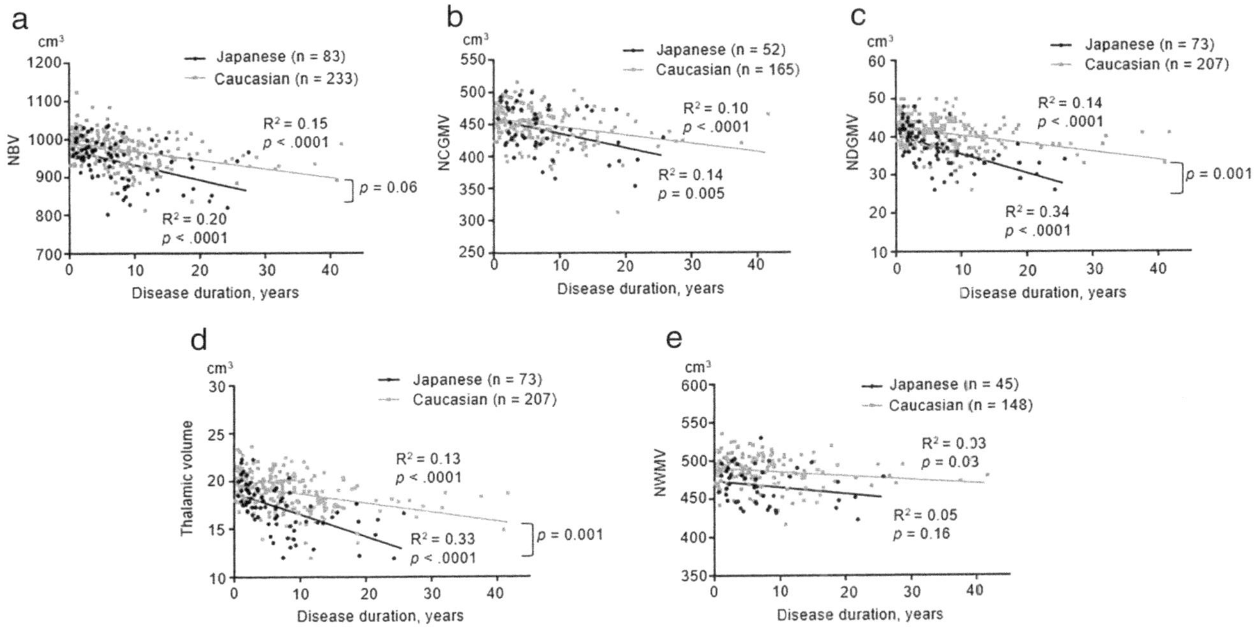

Fig. 3 Relationship between disease duration and brain volumes in MS. Scatter plots show the relationship between disease duration and brain volumes (NBV, NCGMV, NDGMV, normalized thalamic volume, or NWMV; **a–e**) in Japanese (black dots) and Caucasian patients (gray dots). The solid lines represent the linear regression of the data. A test of homogeneity of slopes shows significant differences in NDGMV and normalized thalamic volume between the groups ($p = 0.001$ for both), and a statistically different trend in NBV between the groups ($p = 0.06$). A test of homogeneity of intercept demonstrated that NBV, NWMV, NDGMV, and normalized thalamic volume were consistently smaller in Japanese versus Caucasian patients throughout the entire disease duration examined ($p = 0.046$, $p = 0.005$, $p = 0.01$, and $p = 0.04$, respectively), while NCGMV was similar between the two racial groups in the early course of the disease. R^2 = coefficient of determination

volume were significantly and consistently smaller in the Japanese cohort compared with Caucasian patients, while there were no differences in NCGMV. (5) The reduction in NDGMV, including normalized thalamic volume and normalized thalamic volume alone with disease duration, was faster in Japanese versus Caucasian patients. (6) NWMV was significantly and negatively correlated with EDSS and disease duration in Caucasian patients, but not in Japanese patients.

The Japanese and Caucasian MS patients in our study cohort consisted mainly of patients in the relatively early stage of RRMS, as those with progressive MS and severe disability were excluded. Although the disease duration was similar, both EDSS scores and MSSS were significantly lower in Japanese versus Caucasian patients, consistent with a previous report [4]. The average age at onset and MRI examination was slightly lower in Japanese versus Caucasian patients, although the effects of onset age on disability progression speed remain controversial [20, 21]. Indeed, it is unlikely that such a subtle difference in age had a significant impact on differences in disability between the two racial groups. Prior use of DMDs and immunosuppressants was significantly higher in Japanese versus Caucasian patients in our study (56.8% vs. 28.5%, respectively) and in the aforementioned study (83.2% vs. 17.0%, respectively) [4]. Given that DMDs and immunosuppressants have suppressive effects on relapse and new lesion formation, especially in early RRMS patients, more frequent use of these drugs may explain the lower level of disability observed in Japanese patients. Given this consideration, we carefully interpreted our MRI findings in relation to disability.

In MS, T2W-lesions are attributable to a variety of pathological reactions, including inflammatory demyelination, gliosis, edema, and axonal swelling and loss [22, 23], whereas brain volume loss reflects neuro-axonal degeneration [24]. Both processes contribute to disability progression. Inflammation was proposed to occur in the early course of MS, while neuro-axonal degeneration plays a critical role, and is more closely related to disability, in the later progressive stage [25, 26]. Nevertheless, a recent study provided evidence of early and persisting neuro-axonal degeneration throughout MS [27]. In the present study, although T2W-lesion volumes were similar between the Japanese and Caucasian patients, there was a trend towards a reduction in total T2W-lesion numbers in Japanese patients, and significantly lower frequencies of cerebellar and parietal lobe lesions. Fewer lesions in these structures may partly account for the lower degree of disability observed in

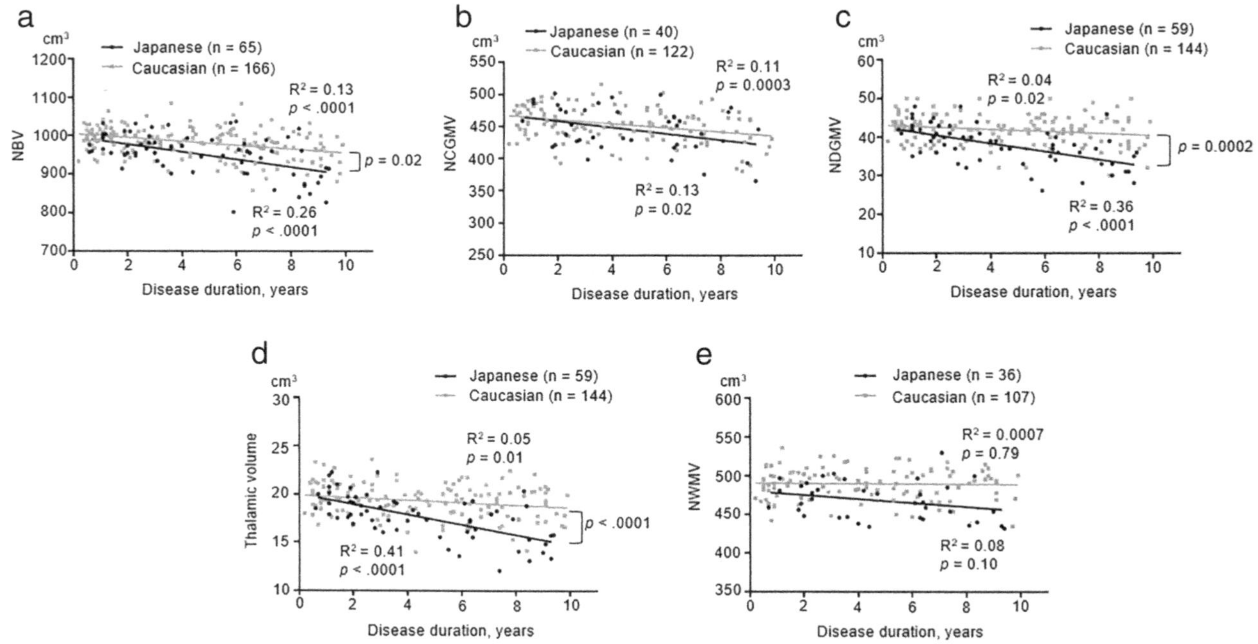

Fig. 4 Relationship between disease duration and brain volumes in MS with a disease duration of < 10 years. Scatter plots show the relationship between disease duration and brain volumes (NBV, NCGMV, NDGMV, normalized thalamic volume, or NWMV; **a–e**) in Japanese (black dots) and Caucasian patients (gray dots). The solid lines represent the linear regression of the data. A test of homogeneity of slopes showed significant differences in NBV ($p = 0.02$), NDGMV ($p = 0.0002$), and normalized thalamic volume ($p < 0.0001$) between the two groups. R^2 = coefficient of determination

Japanese patients. In particular, early cerebellar involvement is a predictor for disability progression in MS, given the abundant connections between the cerebellum and many cerebral cortical areas [28]. Additionally, the parietal lobe was reported to be associated with both physical disability and cognitive decline in MS [29, 30].

Genetic background may also influence the number of brain lesions in MS patients. We previously reported that MS patients with HLA-DRB1*04:05, one of the strongest and most common susceptibility alleles for MS in Japanese individuals, but which is rare in general European populations, showed decreased Barkhof criteria fulfillment and fewer intracortical lesions compared with those without DRB1*04:05 [10, 31, 32]. Thus, the relatively high proportion of DRB1*04:05 carriers in Japanese MS patients (approximately 30–40% in our previous report [31]) may explain the lower number of brain MRI lesions and lower degree of disability in this population. However, as described, the wide use of DMDs during the early course of disease in Japanese MS patients may also influence disability and lesion formation.

Surprisingly, Japanese patients had larger individual lesion sizes compared with Caucasian patients. In Asian MS patients, tumefactive MS may be more frequent, with an occurrence of 6.3% versus 0.1–1.4% in Western MS patients [33–35]. The development of tumefactive demyelinating lesions is attributed to the failure of focal immune-regulation against inflammatory insults that underlie MS lesion formation [36]. Although the molecular mechanisms that produce larger demyelinating lesions are unclear, demyelinating lesions may tend to expand in Japanese patients once developed. Indeed, the significant positive correlation of T2W-lesion volumes with EDSS scores in Japanese patients suggests that acute inflammation leading to T2W-lesion formation may contribute to disability in this population, and that early introduction of DMDs may be of particular benefit. Interestingly, T2W-lesion volumes, but not NWMV, correlated with EDSS scores in Japanese patients. Conversely, NWMV, but not T2W-lesion volumes, correlated with disability in Caucasian patients. This discrepancy may be based on the idea that white matter atrophy reflects a degenerative process, but is partly independent of the genesis of T2W-lesions produced by acute inflammation [24, 37]. Acute inflammation leading to T2W-lesion formation is important in Japanese patients, while white matter degeneration may contribute to disability in Caucasian patients.

In patients from Western countries, brain atrophy is significantly correlated with overall disability as evaluated by EDSS and the Multiple Sclerosis Functional Composite scores [38, 39]. In particular, gray matter atrophy was the most significant MRI variable influencing disability in Western MS patients [40]. In agreement with these observations, our study demonstrated that NBV was significantly correlated with EDSS scores, and that the correlations of NCGMV with EDSS scores, and of NDGMV with EDSS scores, were more significant than that of NWMV with EDSS scores. Additionally, normalized thalamic volume was significantly correlated with EDSS scores in both cohorts. Azevedo et al. reported that thalamic atrophy is an excellent marker for neurodegeneration in MS [27]. Therefore, gray matter atrophy including thalamic atrophy appears to be critical for determining disability between racial groups, and NCGMV, NDGMV, and normalized thalamic volume may be excellent biomarkers for disease severity across race.

Unexpectedly, we found that Japanese patients had a lower NBV, NWMV, NDGMV, and normalized thalamic volume than Caucasian patients throughout the entire disease duration, despite milder disability. To our knowledge, there are no studies that directly compare brain volume, including deep gray matter volume, between Caucasians and Japanese. However, Japanese MS patients may have an inherently smaller brain size, including the deep gray matter and white matter, after applying the normalization procedures. As white matter volume accounts for the largest proportion of whole brain volume, the initial or inherent difference in NWMV may largely explain the difference in NBV between the two groups. By contrast, the faster reduction in NDGMV and the normalized thalamic volume observed in Japanese versus Caucasian patients suggests that deep gray matter, especially the thalamus, may be lost earlier in the disease process in Japanese patients. In a comparative study of African American and Caucasian patients with MS, thalamic volume was significantly smaller in Caucasian patients, although they had lower EDSS scores than African American patients [41]. Thus, while the speed of deep gray matter loss, especially thalamic volume loss, may vary between the racial groups, its influence on physical disability may be limited, at least in the early course of the disease. However, the influence of deep gray matter degradation on cognitive function should be carefully evaluated in long-term follow-up studies.

Our study has several limitations. First, as we compared T2W-lesions between racial subgroups extracted from the entire study population, the sample sizes became relatively small. However, as the clinical characteristics between the subgroups were essentially the same as those in the entire study population, we consider the selection bias to be minimal. Although 72 of the 167 Japanese participants in the phase II fingolimod clinical trial were excluded because of lack of informed consent and data unavailability, the clinical characteristics of 95 patients enrolled in the present study were similar to that reported for the whole cohort [15]. Thus, we consider that this selection bias did not severely distort our data. Second, we could not compare the imaging measures with age-matched healthy controls in each population, as the phase II fingolimod clinical trials did not include healthy controls. Given that brain atrophy is related to normal aging processes [42] and the influence of genetic background on brain structure [43], a comparison with healthy controls is necessary to adjust for racial background in future studies. Third, we applied the MNI152 standard template, based on data from 152 individuals from Western countries, to normalize the measures for head size in both racial groups. Although this template is the most widely used in research studies and clinical trials, bias and error may occur when applying it to Japanese populations. Finally, spinal cord data were not available in this study, as the phase II fingolimod clinical trials were not designed to include spinal cord MRI. As physical disability in MS also relates to spinal cord atrophy [44], we are now prospectively measuring spinal cord cross-sectional areas and whole brain parenchymal volume in our cohort. This study will provide more information on the relationship of disability progression with neuroimaging findings.

Conclusions

In conclusion, the cerebellum and parietal lobe are less frequently involved in Japanese MS patients compared with Caucasian patients, which may relate to milder levels of disability. Larger individual lesion sizes and a positive correlation of T2W-lesion volumes with EDSS scores in Japanese MS patients may relate to the greater role of inflammation in determining disability in Japanese than in Caucasian patients. However, brain volumes, especially gray matter volumes, are negatively associated with disease duration and disability in both Japanese and Caucasian patients, suggesting that gray matter atrophy is a common denominator for disability, and that it may be useful for evaluating disease progression. Finally, the possibility that Japanese MS patients have faster deep gray matter volume loss over time compared with Caucasian MS patients warrants future longitudinal studies.

Abbreviations

DMDs: Disease-modifying drugs; EDSS: Expanded Disability Status Scale; MNI: Montreal Neurological Institute; MRI: Magnetic resonance imaging; MS: Multiple sclerosis; MSSS: Multiple Sclerosis Severity Score; NBV: Normalized brain volume; NCGMV: Normalized cortical gray matter volume; NDGMV: Normalized deep gray matter volume; NMO: Neuromyelitis optica; NWMV: Normalized white matter volume; RRMS: Relapsing-remitting MS, T1W: T1-weighted; T2W: T2-weighted

Acknowledgements

We thank the patients who joined this study, the experts at MIAC for technical assistance, Dr. Junji Kishimoto (Centre for Clinical and Translational Research,

Kyushu University Hospital, Kyushu University) for assistance with statistical analyses, and Sydney Koke (MFA) from Edanz Group (www.edanzediting.com/ac) for editing a draft of this manuscript.

Funding

This study was supported in part by a Health and Labour Sciences Research Grant on Intractable Diseases (H29-Nanchitou (Nan)-Ippan-043) from the Ministry of Health, Labour, and Welfare, Japan, by the "Practical Research Project for Rare/Intractable Diseases" from the Japan Agency for Medical Research and Development, AMED, Japan, by a research grant from the Japanese Multiple Sclerosis Society, by a research grant from the Japan Intractable Disease Research Foundation, by 'Glial Assembly' Grants-in-Aid for Scientific Research on Innovative Areas (MEXT KAKENHI Grant Number 25117012) from the Ministry of Education, Culture, Sports, Science and Technology of Japan, by a Grant-in-Aid for Scientific Research (A) (JSPS KAKENHI Grant Number 16H02657), by a Grant-in-Aid for Scientific Research (C) (JSPS KAKENHI Grant Numbers 16 K09694), by a Grant-in-Aid for Scientific Research (C) (JSPS KAKENHI Grant Number 15 K09341), and by a Grant-in-Aid for Young Scientists (B) (JSPS KAKENHI Grant Number 17 K16125) from the Japan Society for the Promotion of Science, Japan. None of the funding bodies played any role in the study design, data collection and analysis, data interpretation, or writing of the manuscript.

Authors' contributions

YN contributed to study concept and design, drafting the manuscript and figures, analysis and interpretation of data. LG contributed to study concept and design and analysis and interpretation of data. AA, LB, MA, KS, NI, and RY contributed to analysis and interpretation of data. JW, TSp, EWR, TSa, and LK contributed to study concept and design and interpretation of data. TM contributed to analysis and interpretation of data and drafting the manuscript. JK contributed to study concept and design, drafting the manuscript, analysis and interpretation of data, and study supervision. All authors read and approved the final manuscript.

Consent for publication

Not applicable.

Competing interests

YN, AA, LB, and MA declare that they have no competing interests. LG reports personal fees from Novartis AG. TM received a grant and payment from Bayer Schering Pharma and Takeda Pharmaceutical Company for manuscript preparation and for development of educational presentations, and also received speaker honoraria payments from Mitsubishi Tanabe Pharma, Bayer Schering Pharma, and Biogen Idec Japan. Till S received previous and/or current payments for consulting, speaking activities (Actelion, Biogen Idec, Electrocore, Sanofi Genzyme, Mitsubishi Pharma, Teva, Novartis), and grants (EFIC-Grünenthal, Novartis Pharmaceuticals Switzerland, Swiss MS Society, Swiss National Research Foundation). EWR received speaker honoraria and travel compensation from Bayer Schering, Biogen, Fondazione Italiana Sclerosi Multipla, Genzyme, Novartis, Merck Serono, MorphoSys, and Synthon; consulted for Bayer Schering, Biogen Idec, Fondazione Italiana Sclerosi Multipla, Genzyme, Novartis, Merck Serono, Synthon, and MorphoSys; and received institutional research support from Novartis, Biogen Idec, Actelion, Basilea, SAKK, and Synarc. JW is CEO of MIAC AG. He served on scientific advisory board for Actelion, Genzyme, Novartis, Teva, and Roche; he received travel support and/or speaker honoraria from Bayer, Biogen, and Novartis; he received research support from the EU (Horizon2020), the German Ministry of Education and Research and the German Ministry of Economy. KS has received grants from the Japan Intractable Disease Research Foundation, Japanese Multiple Sclerosis Society, and the Japan Society for the Promotion of Science; and received personal fees from Takeda Pharmaceutical Company and Biogen Japan. NI has received grants and personal fees from Tanabe Mitsubishi Pharma, Bayer Yakuhin, Ltd., and Japan Blood Products Organization. RY has received grants from the Japan Society for the Promotion of Science, Bayer Schering Pharma, Biogen Idec Japan, Novartis Pharma, and Mitsubishi Tanabe Pharma; and received research support from the Ministry of Education, Culture, Sports, Science and Technology of Japan and the Ministry of Health, Labour, and Welfare, Japan. Takahiko S has received funding from, held board membership of, spoken at scientific meetings for, prepared manuscripts for, and had consulting agreements with Astellas Pharma, Bayer Schering, Biogen Japan, Daiichi Sankyo, Eisai, Kaketsuken, Merck Serono, Mitsubishi Tanabe Pharma, Nihon Pharmaceutical, Novartis Pharma, Ono Pharmaceutical, Sanofi, TDS Japan, and Teijin. LK's Institution (University Hospital Basel) received exclusive research support at the Department of Neurology, including steering committee, advisory board, and consultancy fees from Actelion, Alkermes, Almirall, Bayer, Biogen, df-mp, Excemed, GeNeuro SA, Genzyme, Merck, Mitsubishi Pharma, Novartis, Receptos, Roche, Sanofi-Aventis, Santhera, Teva, and Vianex, and royalties from Neurostatus products. For educational activities of the Department, the institution received honoraria from Allergan, Almirall, Bayer, Biogen, Excemed, Genzyme, Merck, Novartis, Pfizer, Sanofi-Aventis, Teva, and UCB. LK has served as principal investigator for the following drug studies: BOLD EXT, EXPAND (BAF312, Novartis), DECIDE, DECIDE EXT (Daclizumab HYP, Biogen), ENDORSE (BG00012, Biogen), FINGORETT, FTYUMBRELLA, INFORMS, INFORMS EXT LONGTERM (Fingolimod, Novartis), MOMENTUM (Amiselimod, Mitsubishi) OCRELIZUMAB PHASE II EXT, OPERA, ORATORIO (Ocrelizumab, Roche), REFLEXION (IFN β-1a, Merck), STRATA EXT (Natalizumab, Biogen Idec), and TERIFLUNOMIDE EXT (Teriflunomide, Sanofi-Aventis). Research at the MS center in Basel was supported by grants from Bayer, Biogen, Novartis, the Swiss MS Society, the Swiss National Research Foundation, the European Union, and Roche Research Foundations. The institution has also received grants for patient services from Bayer, Merck, and Teva. JK has received grants from the Ministry of Health, Labour, and Welfare, Japan, the Ministry of Education, Culture, Sports, Science and Technology of Japan, the Japan Society for the Promotion of Science, the Japan Agency for Medical Research and Development, AMED, Japan; and received grants and personal fees from Biogen Idec Japan, Bayer Healthcare, Novartis Pharma, and Mitsubishi Tanabe Pharma, Eisai, Sanofi, Nobelpharma, Otsuka Pharmaceutical, Chugai Pharmaceutical Company, and Teijin Pharma. This independent academic research was supported by Novartis Pharma A.G., Novartis Pharma K.K., and Mitsubishi Tanabe Pharma Corporation, who provided baseline demographic data for the patients analyzed. Novartis and Mitsubishi Tanabe Pharma Corporation played no role in the design, methods, data management, or analysis of the study, or in the decision to publish.

Author details

[1]Department of Neurology, Neurological Institute, Graduate School of Medical Sciences, Kyushu University, 3-1-1 Maidashi, Higashi-ku, Fukuoka 812-8582, Japan. [2]Medical Image Analysis Center (MIAC AG), Marktgasse 8, 4051 Basel, Switzerland. [3]Neurology and Department of Biomedicine, University Hospital Basel, Spitalstrasse 21, 4031 Basel, Switzerland. [4]Department of Biomedical Engineering, University of Basel, Marktgasse 8, 4051 Basel, Switzerland. [5]DKD Helios Klinik Wiesbaden, Aukammallee 33, 65191 Wiesbaden, Germany. [6]Biomedical Research and Education GmbH, Mittlere Strasse 91, 4031 Basel, Switzerland. [7]Klinikum rechts der Isar, Department of Neurology, Technical University of Munich, Ismaninger Str. 22, 81675 Munich, Germany. [8]Division of Diagnostic and Interventional Neuroradiology, Department of Radiology, University Hospital Basel, Spitalstrasse 21, 4031 Basel, Switzerland. [9]Department of Neurological Therapeutics, Neurological Institute, Graduate School of Medical Sciences, Kyushu University, 3-1-1 Maidashi, Higashi-ku, Fukuoka 812-8582, Japan. [10]Institute of Neurotherapeutics, 16-1 Nishinokyoukasugachou, Nakagyo-ku, Kyoto 604-8453, Japan. [11]Department of Neurology, Kyoto Min-Iren-Central Hospital, 16-1 Nishinokyoukasugachou, Nakagyo-ku, Kyoto 604-8453, Japan.

References

1. Alter M. Multiple sclerosis in the Negro. Arch Neurol. 1962;7:83–91.
2. Cree BAC, Khan O, Bourdette D, Goodin DS, Cohen JA, Marrie RA, et al. Clinical characteristics of African Americans vs Caucasian Americans with multiple sclerosis. Neurology. 2004;63:2039–45.
3. Kister I, Chamot E, Bacon JH, Niewczyk PM, De Guzman RA, Apatoff B, et al. Rapid disease course in African Americans with multiple sclerosis. Neurology. 2010;75:217–23.

4. Piccolo L, Kumar G, Nakashima I, Misu T, Kong Y, Wakerley B, et al. Multiple sclerosis in Japan appears to be a milder disease compared to the UK. J Neurol. 2015;262:831–6.
5. Barkhof F, Filippi M, Miller DH, Scheltens P, Campi A, Polman CH, et al. Comparison of MRI criteria at first presentation to predict conversion to clinically definite multiple sclerosis. Brain. 1997;120:2059–69.
6. Ishizu T, Kira J, Osoegawa M, Fukazawa T, Kikuchi S, Fujihara K, et al. Heterogeneity and continuum of multiple sclerosis phenotypes in Japanese according to the results of the fourth nationwide survey. J Neurol Sci. 2009; 280:22–8.
7. Gieß RM, Pfuhl C, Behrens JR, Rasche L, Freitag E, Khalighy N, et al. Epstein-Barr virus antibodies in serum and DNA load in saliva are not associated with radiological or clinical disease activity in patients with early multiple sclerosis. PLoS One. 2017;12:e0175279.
8. Barkhof F, Rocca M, Francis G, Van Waesberghe J-HTM, Uitdehaag BMJ, Hommes OR, et al. Validation of diagnostic magnetic resonance imaging criteria for multiple sclerosis and response to interferon beta1a. Ann Neurol. 2003;53:718–24.
9. Nakashima I, Fujihara K, Okita N, Takase S, Itoyama Y. Clinical and MRI study of brain stem and cerebellar involvement in Japanese patients with multiple sclerosis. J Neurol Neurosurg Psychiatry. 1999;67:153–7.
10. Shinoda K, Matsushita T, Nakamura Y, Masaki K, Yamasaki R, Yamaguchi H, et al. HLA-DRB1*04:05 allele is associated with intracortical lesions on three-dimensional double inversion recovery images in Japanese patients with multiple sclerosis. Mult Scler. 2018;24:710–20.
11. Polman CH, Reingold SC, Banwell B, Clanet M, Cohen JA, Filippi M, et al. Diagnostic criteria for multiple sclerosis: 2010 revisions to the McDonald criteria. Ann Neurol. 2011;69:292–302. https://doi.org/10.1002/ana.22366.
12. Swanton JK, Fernando K, Dalton CM, Miszkiel KA, Thompson AJ, Plant GT, et al. Modification of MRI criteria for multiple sclerosis in patients with clinically isolated syndromes. J Neurol Neurosurg Psychiatry. 2006;77: 830–3.
13. Lo CC, Kao HH, Chen SS, Hsueh CC, Lin WW, Hsu WW, et al. Prediction of conversion from clinically isolated syndrome to clinically definite multiple sclerosis according to baseline MRI findings: comparison of revised McDonald criteria and Swanton modified criteria. J Neurol Neurosurg Psychiatry. 2009;80:1107–9.
14. Kappos L, Antel J, Comi G, Montalban X, O'Connor P, Polman CH, et al. Oral fingolimod (FTY720) for relapsing multiple sclerosis. N Engl J Med. 2006; 355:1124–40.
15. Saida T, Kikuchi S, Itoyama Y, Hao Q, Kurosawa T, Nagato K, et al. A randomized, controlled trial of fingolimod (FTY720) in Japanese patients with multiple sclerosis. Mult Scler. 2012;18:1269–77.
16. Kurtzke JF. Rating neurologic impairment in multiple sclerosis: an expanded disability status scale (EDSS). Neurology. 1983;33:1444–52.
17. Smith SM. Fast robust automated brain extraction. Hum Brain Mapp. 2002; 17:143–55.
18. Smith SM, Zhang Y, Jenkinson M, Chen J, Matthews PM, Federico A, et al. Accurate, robust, and automated longitudinal and cross-sectional brain change analysis. NeuroImage. 2002;17:479–89.
19. Patenaude B, Smith SM, Kennedy DN, Jenkinson M. A Bayesian model of shape and appearance for subcortical brain segmentation. NeuroImage. 2011;56:907–22.
20. Confavreux C, Vukusic S. Age at disability milestones in multiple sclerosis. Brain. 2006;129:595–605.
21. Scalfari A, Neuhaus A, Daumer M, Ebers GC, Muraro PA. Age and disability accumulation in multiple sclerosis. Neurology. 2011;77:1246–52.
22. Moore GRW, Leung E, MacKay AL, Vavasour IM, Whittall KP, Cover KS, et al. A pathology-MRI study of the short-T2 component in formalin-fixed multiple sclerosis brain. Neurology. 2000;55:1506–10.
23. Fisher E, Chang A, Fox RJ, Tkach JA, Svarovsky T, Nakamura K, et al. Imaging correlates of axonal swelling in chronic multiple sclerosis brains. Ann Neurol. 2007;62:219–28.
24. Bermel RA, Bakshi R. The measurement and clinical relevance of brain atrophy in multiple sclerosis. Lancet Neurol. 2006;5:158–70.
25. Li DK, Held U, Petkau J, Daumer M, Barkhof F, Fazekas F, et al. MRI T2 lesion burden in multiple sclerosis: a plateauing relationship with clinical disability. Neurology. 2006;66:1384–9.
26. Fisniku LK, Brex PAP, Altmann DRDR, Miszkiel KA, Benton CEC, Lanyon R, et al. Disability and T2 MRI lesions: a 20-year follow-up of patients with relapse onset of multiple sclerosis. Brain. 2008;131:808–17.
27. Azevedo CJ, Cen SY, Khadka S, Liu S, Kornak J, Shi Y, et al. Thalamic atrophy in multiple sclerosis: a magnetic resonance imaging marker of neurodegeneration throughout disease. Ann Neurol. 2018;83:223–34.
28. Bergamaschi R. Prognosis of multiple sclerosis: clinical factors predicting the late evolution for an early treatment decision. Expert Rev Neurother. 2006;6:357–64.
29. Hackmack K, Weygandt M, Wuerfel J, Pfueller CF, Bellmann-Strobl J, Paul F, et al. Can we overcome the "clinico-radiological paradox" in multiple sclerosis? J Neurol. 2012;259:2151–60.
30. van Munster CE, Jonkman LE, Weinstein HC, Uitdehaag BM, Geurts JJ. Gray matter damage in multiple sclerosis: impact on clinical symptoms. Neuroscience. 2015;303:446–61.
31. Nakamura Y, Matsushita T, Sato S, Niino M, Fukazawa T, Yoshimura S, et al. Latitude and HLA-DRB1*04:05 independently influence disease severity in Japanese multiple sclerosis: a cross-sectional study. J Neuroinflammation. 2016;13:239.
32. Yoshimura S, Isobe N, Yonekawa T, Matsushita T, Masaki K, Sato S, et al. Genetic and infectious profiles of Japanese multiple sclerosis patients. PLoS One. 2012;7:e48592.
33. Kuan Y-C, Wang K-C, Yuan W-H, Tsai C-P. Tumefactive multiple sclerosis in Taiwan. PLoS One. 2013;8:e69919.
34. Poser S, Lüer W, Bruhn H, Frahm J, Brück Y, Felgenhauer K. Acute demyelinating disease. Classification and non-invasive diagnosis Acta Neurol. Scandinavica 1992;86:579–585.
35. Sánchez P, Meca-Lallana V, Barbosa A, Manzanares R, Palmí I, Vivancos J. Tumefactive demyelinating lesions of 15 patients: clinico-radiological features, management and review of the literature. J Neurol Sci. 2017;381:32–8.
36. Hardy TA, Tobin WO, Lucchinetti CF. Exploring the overlap between multiple sclerosis, tumefactive demyelination and Baló's concentric sclerosis. Mult Scler J. 2016;22:986–92.
37. Grassiot B, Desgranges B, Eustache F Defer G. Quantification and clinical relevance of brain atrophy in multiple sclerosis: a review. J Neurol. 2009;256:1397–412.
38. Fisher E, Rudick RA, Simon JH, Cutter G Baier M, Lee J-C, et al. Eight-year follow-up study of brain atrophy in patients with MS. Neurology. 2002; 59:1412–20.
39. Maghzi AH, Revirajan N, Julian LJ, Spain R, Mowry EM, Liu S, et al. Magnetic resonance imaging correlates of clinical outcomes in early multiple sclerosis. Mult Scler Relat Disord. 2014;3:720–7.
40. Tedeschi G, Lavorgna L, Russo P, Prinster A, Dinacci D, Savettieri G, et al. Brain atrophy and lesion load in a large population of patients with multiple sclerosis. Neurology. 2005;65:280–5.
41. Al-Kawaz M, Monohan E, Morris E, Perumal JS, Nealon N, Vartanian T, et al. Differential impact of multiple sclerosis on cortical and deep gray matter structures in African Americans and Caucasian Americans. J Neuroimaging. 2017;27:333–8.
42. Giorgio A, Santelli L, Tomassini V, Bosnell R, Smith S, De Stefano N, et al. Age-related changes in grey and white matter structure throughout adulthood. NeuroImage. 2010;51:943–51.
43. Eyler LT, Prom-Wormley E, Panizzon MS, Kaup AR, Fennema-Notestine C, Neale MC, et al. Genetic and environmental contributions to regional cortical surface area in humans: a magnetic resonance imaging twin study. Cereb Cortex. 2011;21:2313–21.
44. Lukas C, Knol DL, Sombekke MH, Bellenberg B, Hahn HK, Popescu V, et al. Cervical spinal cord volume loss is related to clinical disability progression in multiple sclerosis. J Neurol Neurosurg Psychiatry. 2015;86:410–8.

13

Differential effects of FTY720 on the B cell compartment in a mouse model of multiple sclerosis

Kathrin Bail[1†], Quirin Notz[1†], Damiano M. Rovituso[1], Andrea Schampel[1], Marie Wunsch[1], Tobias Koeniger[1], Verena Schropp[6], Richa Bharti[2], Claus-Juergen Scholz[2,3], Konrad U. Foerstner[2], Christoph Kleinschnitz[4,5] and Stefanie Kuerten[1,6*]

Abstract

Background: MP4-induced experimental autoimmune encephalomyelitis (EAE) is a mouse model of multiple sclerosis (MS), which enables targeted research on B cells, currently much discussed protagonists in MS pathogenesis. Here, we used this model to study the impact of the $S1P_1$ receptor modulator FTY720 (fingolimod) on the autoreactive B cell and antibody response both in the periphery and the central nervous system (CNS).

Methods: MP4-immunized mice were treated orally with FTY720 for 30 days at the peak of disease or 50 days after EAE onset. The subsequent disease course was monitored and the MP4-specific B cell/antibody response was measured by ELISPOT and ELISA. RNA sequencing was performed to determine any effects on B cell-relevant gene expression. $S1P_1$ receptor expression by peripheral T and B cells, B cell subset distribution in the spleen and B cell infiltration into the CNS were studied by flow cytometry. The formation of B cell aggregates and of tertiary lymphoid organs (TLOs) was evaluated by histology and immunohistochemistry. Potential direct effects of FTY720 on B cell aggregation were studied in vitro.

Results: FTY720 significantly attenuated clinical EAE when treatment was initiated at the peak of EAE. While there was a significant reduction in the number of T cells in the blood after FTY720 treatment, B cells were only slightly diminished. Yet, there was evidence for the modulation of B cell receptor-mediated signaling upon FTY720 treatment. In addition, we detected a significant increase in the percentage of $B220^+$ B cells in the spleen both in acute and chronic EAE. Whereas acute treatment completely abrogated B cell aggregate formation in the CNS, the numbers of infiltrating B cells and plasma cells were comparable between vehicle- and FTY720-treated mice. In addition, there was no effect on already developed aggregates in chronic EAE. In vitro B cell aggregation assays suggested the absence of a direct effect of FTY720 on B cell aggregation. However, FTY720 impacted the evolution of B cell aggregates into TLOs.

Conclusions: The data suggest differential effects of FTY720 on the B cell compartment in MP4-induced EAE.

Keywords: B cells, EAE, Fingolimod, FTY720, Multiple sclerosis, TLO

* Correspondence: stefanie.kuerten@fau.de
†Equal contributors
[1]Department of Anatomy and Cell Biology, University of Würzburg, Würzburg, Germany
[6]Institute of Anatomy and Cell Biology, Friedrich-Alexander University Erlangen-Nürnberg, Erlangen, Germany

Background

Multiple sclerosis (MS) is a neuroinflammatory and demyelinating disease of the central nervous system (CNS) that leads to irreversible neurological deficits and premature retirement predominantly in young adults [1]. Still today, the etiology of the disease has remained unclear, but an interaction between genetic, environmental, and infectious agents is assumed to play a role in disease initiation and maintenance [1]. For decades, autoreactive T cells were primarily thought to mediate MS [2]. However, an additional crucial role of B cells in the pathogenesis of MS is underlined by clinical as well as immunological observations. B cell depletion with anti-CD20 antibodies ameliorated both clinical symptoms and magnetic resonance imaging (MRI) activity in MS patients [3–5]. Therapeutic plasma exchange was more likely to be beneficial in patients with MS lesions that showed complement and immunoglobulin depositions [6]. CNS-reactive B cells were detected in the peripheral blood of MS patients [7] and clonally expanded B cells were found in the CNS and cerebrospinal fluid (CSF) [8]. Along these lines, oligoclonal bands (OCBs) indicate intrathecal antibody synthesis [2] and antibody depositions with concurrent complement activation represent the most frequently observed pattern of demyelination in MS brain lesions [9]. We have introduced a B cell-/antibody-dependent model of experimental autoimmune encephalomyelitis (EAE), which is based upon active immunization of C57BL/6 (B6) mice with MP4, a fusion protein of myelin basic protein (MBP) and proteolipid protein (PLP) [10]. One of the hallmark features of the model is the development of B cell aggregates mainly in the cerebellum, which evolve into tertiary lymphoid organs (TLOs) in the chronic stage of the disease and resemble secondary lymphoid organs (SLOs) both in morphology and function [11]. Similar findings were recently reported in a spontaneous model of EAE showing that B cells actively participate in the CNS immune response in meningeal ectopic lymphoid tissue [12]. B cell aggregates have also been described in the meninges of post mortem brain sections of patients with secondary progressive MS (SP-MS) [13] and were associated with an early disease onset, a severe disease course and cortical histopathology [14, 15]. Unfortunately, treatment options for SP-MS are very limited and therefore approved drugs for relapsing-remitting MS (RR-MS) are currently re-evaluated in ongoing studies [16]. FTY720, also known as fingolimod, was the first oral drug for the treatment of RR-MS. FTY720 significantly reduces relapse rates and gadolinium-enhancing MRI lesions [17]. Pharmacologically, FTY720 is a $S1P_1$ receptor modulator and traps lymphocytes in SLOs, resulting in a reduction of inflammatory cells both in the circulation and CNS [18]. In addition, other $S1P_1$ subtype receptor-mediated effects on oligodendrocytes, astrocytes, neurons, microglia, or on the blood-brain-barrier (BBB) via interaction with endothelial cells were discussed [19]. These potential effects of FTY720 included reduced leakiness of the BBB, stimulation of astrocyte migration or the promotion of oligodendrocyte precursor cell survival [19]. Furthermore, sphingolipids seem to play an important role in neurogenesis and remyelination, and therefore, FTY720 may also influence these pathways [19]. However, so far, there is no evidence for an impact of FTY720 on B and T lymphocyte effector function [20]. The aim of this study was to evaluate the effect of FTY720 on autoreactive B cells in the MP4-EAE model in terms of autoantibody production, B cell subset distribution and the formation of B cell aggregates in the CNS. Our results demonstrate that only an early application of FTY720 was capable of ameliorating clinical disease and preventing the formation of B cell aggregates in vivo. Drug administration during the chronic stage of the disease remained ineffective on these parameters, but displayed an inhibitory effect on B cell aggregate transformation into TLOs.

Methods

Mice

Female 6-week-old B6 mice were purchased from Envigo (The Netherlands) and maintained at the animal facility of the Zentrum für Zahn-, Mund- und Kiefergesundheit at the University of Würzburg under specific pathogen-free conditions. Mice were fed a standard rodent diet (Altromin Spezialfutter GmbH & Co. KG, Lage, Germany) and had free access to pathogen-free water. From the time when mice displayed paralytic signs, food and water were offered at ground level. All animal experiments complied with the German Law on the Protection of Animals and the "Principles of laboratory animal care" (NIH publication no. 86–23, revised 1985). The treatments were performed according to a protocol that was approved by the Regierung von Unterfranken, Germany (approval number 91/14).

Induction and clinical assessment of EAE

The MBP-PLP fusion protein MP4 was obtained from Alexion Pharmaceuticals (Cheshire, CT, USA). By mixing mannide monooleate (Sigma-Aldrich, St. Louis, MO, USA) and paraffin oil (EMScience, Gibbstown, NJ, USA) at a ratio of 1:9, incomplete Freund's adjuvant (IFA) was prepared. The addition of *Mycobacterium tuberculosis* H37 Ra (Difco Laboratories, Franklin Lakes, NJ, USA) at 5 mg/ml into IFA resulted in complete Freund's adjuvant (CFA). Mice were immunized subcutaneously in both sides of the flank with 200 µg MP4 in 200 µl CFA. Mice received intraperitoneal injections of 200 ng pertussis toxin (List Biological Laboratories, Hornby, ONT,

Canada) on the day of immunization and 48 h later. The clinical assessment was based on the standard EAE scoring system: (0) no disease, (1) floppy tail, (2) hind limb weakness, (3) full hind limb paralysis, (4) quadriplegia, and (5) death. Mice that were in between the clear--cut gradations of clinical signs were scored in increments of 0.5.

Drug administration and grouping

MP4-immunized mice received a daily oral dose of 1 mg/kg body weight (BW) FTY720 (Sigma-Aldrich) diluted in 25% ethanol in *Aqua dest.* Control mice were MP4-immunized and treated with 20 μl of the vehicle solution only. Treatment was administered at the same time each day by pipetting the total volume of 20 μl into the mouth of each mouse as shown in Additional file 1. Treatment was started either at the peak of acute EAE or 50 days after EAE onset and was maintained for ~30 days except otherwise stated. For grouping of the mice, the scores at the beginning of the treatment were matched so that there was no significant difference between FTY720- and vehicle-treated mice (Additional file 2). Since the vehicle solution contained ethanol, we performed histological analysis on the liver to exclude any side effects due to the treatment (Additional file 1). We did not observe any signs of liver inflammation or fibrosis in MP4-immunized animals treated with FTY720 or vehicle solution, respectively.

Tissue sampling

Blood from the tail vein was collected for flow cytometry. Mice were then sacrificed with CO_2, blood from the inferior vena cava was used for ELISA, and draining inguinal lymph nodes from one side were dissected for ELISPOT analysis. The spleen was used for extended flow cytomery analysis. The animals were perfused with 4% paraformaldehyde (PFA, AppliChem, St. Louis, MO, USA). Afterwards, cerebella and inguinal lymph nodes from the other side were removed and embedded in paraffin.

B cell enzyme-linked immunospot assay (ELISPOT)

MultiScreen®HTS 96-well ELISPOT plates (Merck Millipore, Darmstadt, Germany) were coated overnight with either 10 μg/ml MP4 (Alexion Pharmaceuticals, Inc.) or 15 μg/ml anti-mouse IgG (MabTech, Nacka Strand, Sweden), while coating with sterile PBS (Sigma-Aldrich) served as a negative control. Plates were blocked with 10% fetal bovine serum (FBS; Gibco, Thermo Fisher Scientific, Waltham, MA, USA) in sterile PBS at room temperature for 2 h. Inguinal lymph nodes were disintegrated mechanically and filtered through a 70 μm cell strainer (Corning Inc., Corning, NY, USA). Cells were washed twice with complete RPMI-1640 medium (Gibco), subsequently resuspended in HL-1 medium (Lonza, Basel, Switzerland) containing 1% L-glutamine (Sigma-Aldrich) and 1% penicillin/streptomycin (Sigma-Aldrich) and plated at 1×10^6 cells/well followed by incubation at 37 °C and 7% CO_2 for 24 h. Biotinylated goat anti-mouse IgG (Dako, Glostrop, Denmark) served as secondary antibody at 1:2000 dilution in 0.5% FBS/PBS + 0.025% Tween at 4 °C overnight. Plates were washed and incubated with streptavidin-alkaline phosphatase (Vector) at 1:800 dilution in 0.5% FBS/PBS for 2 h. Vector Blue substrate (Vector) was used for development. The spots were counted on an ImmunoSpot Series 6 UV Analyzer (CTL-Europe, Bonn, Germany).

ELISA

ELISA plates (Nunclon Delta Surface; Nalge Nunc International, Rochester, NY, USA) were coated with MP4 at 3 μg/ml in PBS at 4 °C overnight. Plates were washed with PBS + 0.05% Tween and blocked with 1% milk powder (MP) in 0.05% PBS + 0.05% Tween at room temperature for 2 h. Serum samples were plated at 1:1000 dilution in 1% MP and incubated at 4 °C overnight. Negative controls contained 1% MP only. After renewed washing, biotinylated anti-mouse IgG (diluted 1:800 in 0.1% MP; eBioscience, San Diego, CA, USA) was added to the plates for overnight incubation at 4 °C. After incubation with avidin-horseradish peroxidase (diluted 1:1000 in 0.1% MP; BD Biosciences, San Jose, CA, USA) at room temperature for 2 h, plates were developed with tetramethylbenzidine (eBioscience). The reaction was stopped with 0.16 M sulfuric acid and read at 450 nm using a Perkin Elmer (Waltham, MA, USA) Victor 3 1420 Multilabel Counter with Wallac 1420 software version 3.00 revision 5.

RNA-seq expression profiling

The complementary DNA (cDNA) libraries for all samples of isolated B cells were prepared using standard Illumina protocol, following the manufacturer's instructions. B cells were purified from the spleens of MP4-immunized mice using a commercially available Mouse B Cell Isolation Kit (Miltenyi Biotec, Bergisch Gladbach, Germany). Subsequently, all libraries were sequenced with a high output 1×75 cycles kit using the Illumina Nextseq 500 sequencing platform that generated 75 bp long single-end reads. A total of ~400 million raw reads were produced that were processed and analyzed. The generated raw reads were processed using FastQC 0.11.3 for assessing read quality, amount of duplicates, and presence of adapter sequences. After this, the Illumina TruSeq adaptors were cleaved using cutadapt (version 1.12), and resulting reads were further trimmed keeping a quality drop value below a mean of Q20. Further, the processed sequences were mapped to the murine genome (mm12, GRCm38) using the short read aligner STAR-2.5.2b with genome and annotation files retrieved from GENCODE. For all the studied samples, the proportion of reads mapped to the mouse reference genome ranged between 86 and 89% in total. The sequences aligning to specific genes were quantified using bedtools subcommand intersect (version 2.15.0). Next, the differentially expressed genes were identified using DESeq2 (version 1.16.1). Only the genes having a Benjamini-Hochberg corrected p value below 0.05 were classified as significantly differentially expressed (DEGs). The data were visualized as MA plot using DESeq2's function plotMA. To ascertain the biological relevance of the global transcriptomic differences between the sampling groups, KEGG-based enrichment analysis of DEGs was done using clusterProfiler. The RNA-seq data presented in this work has been deposited at the NCBI Gene Expression Omnibus and can be accessed through GEO series accession number GSE101753 (https://www.ncbi.nlm.nih.gov/geo/query/acc.cgi?acc=GSE101753).

Flow cytometry of CD4$^+$ T cells and CD19$^+$ B cells in the blood

Blood of FTY720- and vehicle-treated mice was drawn from the tail vein and 40 μl of heparin were added. After erythrocyte lysis using an ammonium chloride-based red blood cell lysis buffer, cells were washed and incubated with BD Horizon™ Fixable Viability Stain 450 (FVS450; BD Biosciences, San Jose, CA, USA) at 4 °C for 30 min. Afterwards, cells were stained with anti-CD4 and anti-CD19 antibodies at 4 °C for 30 min (Additional file 3). Analysis was done on a FACS Canto™ II (BD Biosciences) at a flow rate of 2000 events per second, and each tube was run until 50,000 or 100,000 live events were recorded. Data were evaluated using FlowJo version 10.0.6 (Tree Star, Inc., Ashland, OR, USA). We excluded dead cells before a single gate on the FSC-H (forward scatter height)/FSC-A (forward scatter area) profile was set. Afterwards monocytes were excluded. B cells were characterized as CD19$^+$CD4$^-$ and T cells as CD19$^-$CD4$^+$ applying a CD4/CD19 bivariate gate. Gates were first set identically for all samples and adjusted individually according to unstained samples.

Flow cytometry of S1P$_1^+$ T and B cells in lymph nodes and blood

Naïve female B6 mice were treated with 1 mg/kg BW FTY720 or vehicle solution for 10 consecutive days. Blood was obtained by cardiac puncture, and 5 μl of 0.5 M EDTA (AppliChem) was added. Erythrocyte lysis was performed using an ammonium chloride-based red blood cell lysis buffer. Lymph nodes were disintegrated mechanically and filtered through a 70 μm Falcon cell strainer (Corning Inc.). All samples were incubated with BD Horizon™ FVS450 (BD Biosciences) at 4 °C for 30 min. Afterwards, cells were stained with anti-CD4, anti-CD19, and anti-S1P$_1$ antibodies at 4 °C for 30 min (Additional file 3). Analysis was done on a FACS Canto™ II (BD Biosciences) at a flow rate of 2000 events per second. Each sample was run until at least 10,000 (blood) or 100,000 (lymph nodes) live events were recorded. Data were evaluated using FlowJo version 10.0.6 (Tree Star, Inc.). We excluded dead cells before a single gate on the FSC-H (forward scatter height)/FSC-A (forward scatter area) profile was set followed by a single cell gate on the SSC-H (sideward scatter height)/SSC-A (sideward scatter area) profile. B cells were characterized as CD19$^+$CD4$^-$ and T cells as CD19$^-$CD4$^+$ applying a CD4/CD19 bivariate gate. Afterwards, S1P$_1^+$ T and B cells were identified. Gates were first set identically for all samples and adjusted individually according to unstained samples and fluorescence minus one controls (for S1P$_1$).

Flow cytometry of B cell subsets in the spleen

Spleens of FTY720- and vehicle-treated mice were disintegrated mechanically and filtered through a 70 μm Falcon cell strainer (Corning Inc.). After erythrocyte lysis using an ammonium chloride-based red blood cell lysis buffer, cells were washed and incubated with BD Horizon™ Fixable Viability Stain 780 (FVS780; BD Biosciences) at 4 °C for 30 min. Subsequently, samples were stained with the following anti-mouse antibodies at 4 °C for 30 min (Additional file 3): anti-CD5, anti-CD23, anti-CD43, anti-CD73, anti-CD80, anti-CD138, and anti-B220/CD45R. Analysis was performed on a FACS Canto™ II (BD Biosciences) at a flow rate of 2000 events per second, and each tube was run until 50,000 or 100,000 live events were recorded. Recorded data were evaluated using FlowJo version 10.0.6 (Tree Star, Inc.). We excluded dead cells before a single gate on the FSC-H (forward scatter height)/FSC-A (forward scatter area) profile was set. B220$^+$ B cell subgroups were characterized as naïve B cells (CD43$^-$CD73$^-$CD80$^-$CD138$^-$), regulatory B cells (CD5$^+$CD23$^{+/-}$CD43$^-$), B1a cells (CD5$^+$CD23$^-$CD43$^+$), B1b cells (CD5$^-$CD23$^-$CD43$^+$), and B memory cells (CD5$^-$CD23$^-$CD73$^+$CD80$^+$CD138$^{+/-}$). To identify plasma cells (CD73$^-$CD80$^-$CD138$^+$B220$^-$), we set a B220/CD138 bivariate gate. Gates were first set identically for all samples and adjusted individually according to unstained samples and fluorescent minus one controls (for CD73, CD80, CD138).

Flow cytometry of B cell subsets in the CNS

Periventricular cerebral tissue, cerebellum, and spinal cord of FTY720- and vehicle-treated mice were dissected and homogenized in 1 x HBSS$^{+/+}$ (Gibco). After preparation of the stock isotonic Percoll, composed of

Percoll™ Plus (GE Healthcare) and $10 \times HBSS^{-/-}$ (Gibco), the cell suspension was mixed with the stock to get a 30% solution. Additionally, a 70% solution was prepared by diluting the stock isotonic Percoll with $1 \times HBSS^{-/-}$ (Gibco). To achieve a density gradient, the 30% solution was slowly pipetted onto the 70% solution and centrifuged at × 500*g* and 18 °C for 30 min without break. Cells were then isolated from the interlayer and washed in $1 \times HBSS^{+/+}$ (Gibco). Afterwards, cells were resuspended in PBS and incubated with BD Horizon™ FVS780 (BD Biosciences) at 4 °C for 30 min. Subsequently, samples were stained with the following anti-mouse antibodies at 4 °C for 30 min (Additional file 3): anti-CD5, anti-CD23, anti-CD43, anti-CD73, anti-CD80, anti-CD138, and anti-B220/CD45R. Analysis was performed on a FACS Canto™ II (BD Biosciences) at a flow rate of 2000 events per second and each tube was run until 50,000 live events were recorded. Recorded data were evaluated using FlowJo version 10.0.6 (Tree Star, Inc.). We excluded dead cells before a single gate on the FSC-H (forward scatter height)/FSC-A (forward scatter area) profile was set. To identify plasma cells ($CD138^{+}$ $B220^{-}$) and $B220^{+}$ B cells, we set a B220/CD138 bivariate gate. Gates were first set identically for all samples and adjusted individually according to unstained samples.

Histological analysis (immunohistochemistry)

Lymph nodes were used as a control tissue and processed into 39 serial sections at 5 µm. The cerebella were cut into 84 serial sections at 5 µm and every eighth section was immunohistochemically stained with anti-B220/anti-CD3 antibodies in order to screen for the presence of inflammatory infiltrates. In case the sections were positive for B cell aggregates, the consecutive sections served for further characterization of lymphoid neogenesis using anti-CXCL13, -FDC-SP, -Ig, and -PNAd antibodies (Additional file 4). Hematoxylin/eosin stained sections were analyzed with ImageJ version 1.50b (National Institutes of Health, USA) to assess the size of the parenchymal area. The diaminobenzidine (DAB) staining protocol consisted of the following steps: paraffin-embedded sections were rehydrated and endogenous peroxidase was blocked. After citrate buffer-mediated epitope retrieval and protein blocking, the primary antibodies (Additional file 5) were incubated at 4 °C overnight. Biotinylated anti-rabbit, anti-rat, or anti-goat IgG (diluted 1:250 in PBS, Vector Laboratories, Burlingame, CA, USA) were used as secondary antibodies and incubated at room temperature for 1 h. For CD3/FDC-SP detection, the sections were additionally incubated with rabbit-peroxidase-anti-peroxidase complex (rb-PAP, Jackson ImmunoResearch Laboratories, West Grove, PA, USA, diluted 1:250 in PBS) for 30 min in the dark. The sections were developed with a horseradish peroxidase-based VECTASTAIN ABC Kit (Vector) and monitored under microscopic control in a solution containing nickel sulfate, glucose, ammonium chloride, DAB (Sigma-Aldrich), and glucose oxidase (Sigma-Aldrich). In case of CD3/B220 double staining, alkaline phosphatase-conjugated streptavidin (Vector) and Vector Blue Subtrate Kit (Vector) were additionally used. The sections were examined with a DM 2000 LED microscope (Leica, Wetzlar, Deutschland). B cell aggregates were classified by the aforementioned markers indicating lymphoid neogenesis. Positive staining of one marker categorized the aggregate as low-grade, of two or three markers as mid-grade, and the detection of all four markers as high-grade aggregate. Aggregates lacking all markers were identified as aggregates without lymphoid characteristics.

Murine in vitro B cell aggregation assays

Spleens from 6 to 10-week-old naïve non-immunized female B6 mice ($n = 6$) were disintegrated mechanically and filtered through a 70 µm Falcon cell strainer (Corning Inc.) to obtain six individual samples. Cells were washed three times and resuspended in RPMI-1640 medium (Gibco). B cells were obtained through negative selection by using the Mouse B Lymphocyte Enrichment Set-DM (BD Biosciences) according to the vendor's protocol and four wells with 5×10^5 cells/well per mouse were plated onto a 96-well microplate (Greiner Bio-One, Frickenhausen, Germany). RPMI-1640 (Gibco) containing 1% L-glutamine (Sigma-Aldrich) and 1% penicillin/streptomycin (Sigma-Aldrich) was used as cell culture medium. FTY720 was added at a concentration of 8 µM. Vehicle solution at a corresponding volume was used as a control. After 90 min of pre-incubation at 37 °C and 7% CO_2 on a shaker, cell activation was achieved by adding 0.25 µg/ml lipopolysaccharide (LPS, Sigma-Aldrich) and 5 U/ml recombinant murine interleukin-4 (IL-4, PeproTech, Rocky Hill, NJ, USA) followed by an incubation for 72 h. Well images were acquired with a Leica DM IL LED microscope (Leica) at ×200 magnification before FTY720 or vehicle solution was added, after 90 min of incubation and at the end of the 72 h incubation period. Images were evaluated using ImageJ Version 1.50b and its plugins ITCN (Centre for Bio-image Informatics, Santa Barbara, CA, USA) and Cell Counter (University of Sheffield, Sheffield, UK).

Statistical analysis

GraphPadPrism 6.0 (GraphPad Software, Inc., La Jolla, CA, USA) was used for statistical analysis. Differences between groups were assessed using Mann-Whitney test. Three levels of statistical significance were differentiated: $^{*}p \leq 0.05$, $^{**}p \leq 0.01$ and $^{***}p \leq 0.001$. Mean values and the standard error of the mean (SEM) are shown in the graphs.

Results

FTY720 treatment attenuates acute but not chronic EAE

B6 mice were immunized with MP4 and received daily oral treatment with either 1 mg/kg BW FTY720 or vehicle, respectively, either at the peak of the disease or 50 days after disease onset. EAE onset in all treated cohorts was 19.05 ± 3.20 days post immunization, and treatment started at a mean EAE score of 2.19 ± 0.19 in the FTY720 group compared to a mean EAE score of 2.29 ± 0.19 in the vehicle group ($p = 0.90$). Detailed information on the disease course are provided in Additional file 2. FTY720 treatment at the peak of disease significantly attenuated clinical EAE as early as day 7 of application (Fig. 1a, c). This significant amelioration of the disease course was continuously seen from day 17 on until the end of the experiment, which was 27.65 days (±1.09 days) after treatment onset. In contrast, FTY720 treatment 50 days after onset of disease did not result in any significant differences in EAE scores when compared to the control group (Fig. 1b, d). To determine whether treatment with FTY720 triggered the drug-related reduction in peripheral lymphocyte counts, we performed flow cytometry of $CD4^+$ T cells and $CD19^+$ T cells on tail vein blood that was collected at end of the treatment period. The proportion of $CD4^+$ T cells was significantly reduced in the peripheral blood of FTY720-treated mice ($n_{FTY720} = 6$, $n_{vehicle} = 8$ with $p < 0.001$), while the percentage of $CD19^+$ B cells was not significantly altered ($p = 0.18$, Fig. 1e, f). One explanation for the diminished effect of FTY720 on B cells could be lower $S1P_1$ receptor expression compared to T cells. However, our results rather indicate that there were

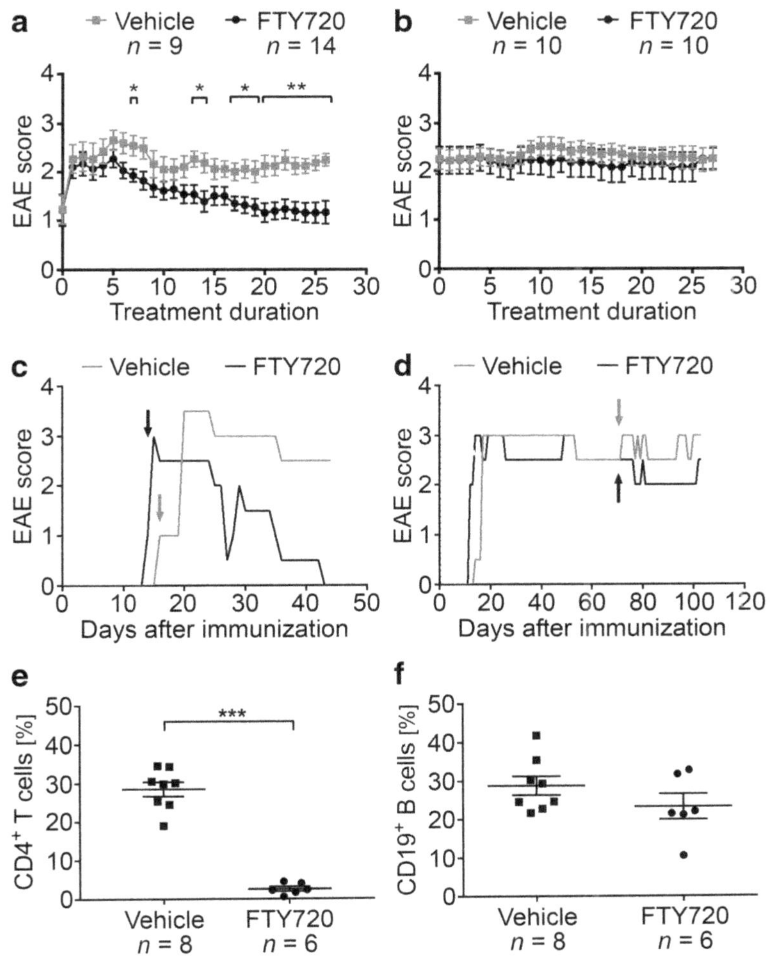

Fig. 1 Disease course in mice treated with FTY720 either in the acute or chronic stage of EAE. MP4-immunized mice were treated with 1 mg/kg BW FTY720 or vehicle **a** at the peak of the disease or **b** 50 days after EAE onset. **c, d** Representative disease course of individual animals treated during **c** acute or **d** chronic EAE. *Arrows* indicate treatment onset. **e, f** Flow cytometry of $CD4^+$ T cells and $CD19^+$ B cells in the blood after treatment with FTY720 compared to vehicle. Mice were treated 50 days after disease onset. $^*p < 0.05$, $^{**}p < 0.01$, $^{***}p < 0.001$, Mann-Whitney test. *Bars* in **a** and **b** show mean values ± SEM

no differences in the extent of $S1P_1$ receptor expression on T and B cells in blood and lymph nodes of FTY720- and vehicle-treated mice (Additional file 6).

FTY720 treatment neither affects the MP4-specific B cell and antibody response nor B cell function in general

Next, we set out to study whether there was a potential impact of FTY720 on B cell function. To this end, we collected serum and draining inguinal lymph nodes either at the end of the acute or the chronic treatment period and performed measurements of MP4-specific antibody production by ELISPOT and ELISA. Fig. 2 shows that there was no difference in the number of total or MP4-specific IgG producing B cells in FTY720- and vehicle-treated mice (Fig. 2a, b). Comparable results were obtained for the detection of MP4-specific antibodies (Fig. 2c, d).

In a next step, we investigated the effect of FTY720 on B cell gene expression profiles by performing RNA sequencing (Fig. 3). To this end, we purified B cells from the spleens of MP4-immunized mice that were treated at the peak of EAE with either FTY720 ($n = 5$) or vehicle ($n = 4$). Analysis was performed for genes that are relevant for B cell receptor (BCR)-mediated signaling. When focusing on genes that showed a $\log_2$ fold-change and had a p value below 0.05 some differences between FTY720- and vehicle-treated mice were evident. On the one hand, there was a significant downregulation of Lyn and Syk, which are involved in the transmission of signals from the BCR [21]. In addition, Ifitm1 expression was decreased after FTY720 treatment. Ifitm1 has been described to reduce the threshold of BCR engagement needed for cell stimulation in conjunction with interactions involving CD81 and the BCR [22]. On the other hand, we observed an upregulation of factors involved in apoptotic cell death including Card11 [23], Fos [24] and Rasgrp3 [25] suggesting pro-apoptotic effects of FTY720.

Effects of FTY720 on B cell emigration from SLOs

To study the effect of FTY720 on B cells in greater detail, we performed flow cytometry on spleen cells of MP4-immunized mice that were treated either with FTY720 ($n = 6$) or vehicle ($n = 4$) for 22.90 ± 1.83 days at the peak of disease (Fig. 4) or for 30.71 ± 0.16 days during chronic EAE (50 days after EAE onset) ($n_{FTY720} = 10$; $n_{vehicle} = 7$) (Fig. 5). Mice that received treatment at the peak of disease showed significantly altered percentages of total $B220^+$ B cells and of naïve B cells. Vehicle-treated animals harbored 7.09% $B220^+$ B cells compared to 36.42% in FTY720-treated animals ($p = 0.02$). While a mean percentage of 49.70% naïve B cells was observed in vehicle-treated animals, FTY720-treated mice showed

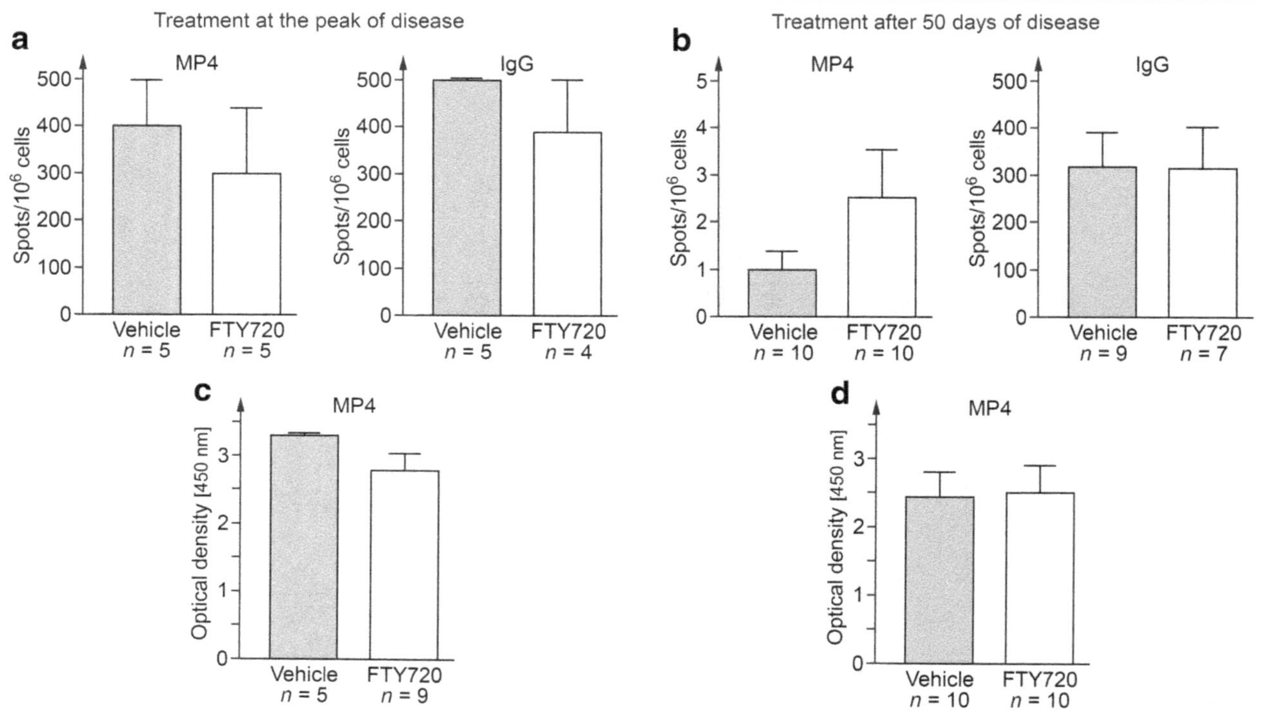

Fig. 2 Measurements of MP4-specific B cells and antibody production. B cell ELISPOT was performed on draining inguinal lymph nodes of MP4-immunized mice to detect total or MP4-specific IgG during **a** acute or **b** chronic EAE. MP4-specific serum antibodies were measured by ELISA during **c** acute or **d** chronic treatment. Mice were treated either with 1 mg/kg BW FTY720 or vehicle. *Bars* show means ± SEM

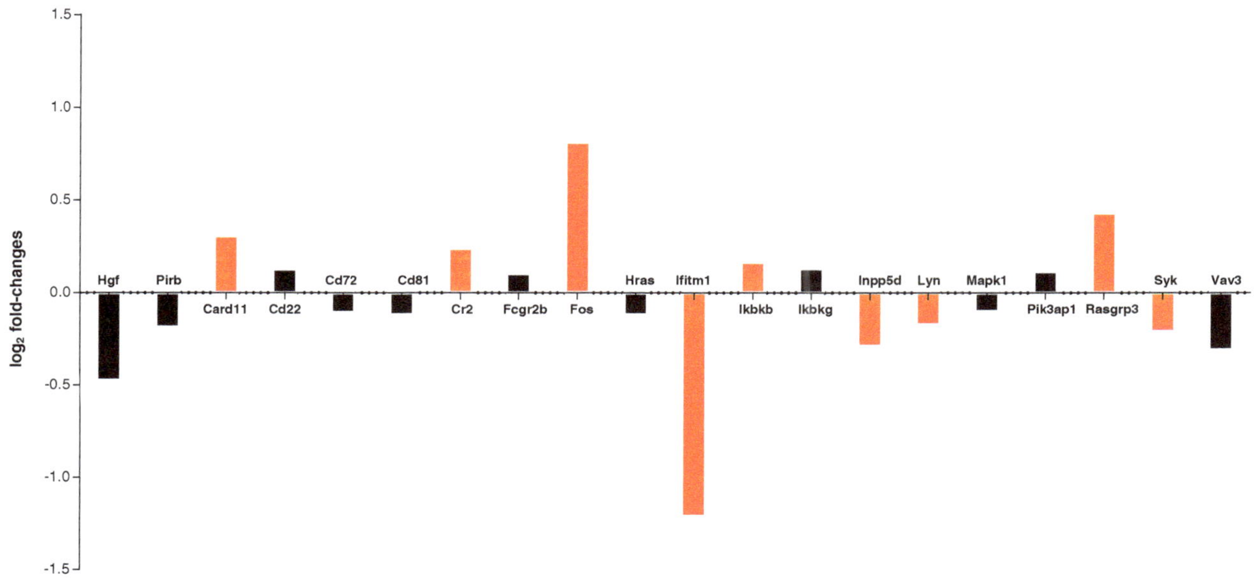

Fig. 3 RNA sequencing analysis of isolated B cells from the spleens of MP4-immunized B6 mice that were treated with FTY720 ($n = 5$) or vehicle ($n = 4$), respectively, at the peak of EAE. Differential expression analysis results for B cell-related genes are shown. Log_2 fold-changes of the comparison between vehicle- vs. drug-treated samples ($n = 3$ replicates each) calculated by DESeq2 for genes associated with BCR signaling in KEGG are plotted. Results with an adjusted p value below 0.05 are colored in *orange* while the remaining ones are colored in *blue*

a significant decrease to 38.60% ($p = 0.02$). Furthermore, we detected a significant increase in the percentage of $CD23^-$ regulatory B cells after treatment with FTY720 (compare 1.07 to 2.31%; $p = 0.02$) (Fig. 4). In mice that were treated after 50 days of EAE, a significant increase was observed only for the overall population of $B220^+$ cells. While vehicle-treated mice possessed 23.63% $B220^+$ cells, this percentage increased to 34.13% in the FTY720 group ($p = 0.03$) (Fig. 5). To investigate the effects of FTY720 on B cell infiltration into the CNS of MP4-immunized mice, flow cytometry was performed on the brain, cerebellum, and spinal cord of mice that were treated at the peak of EAE with either vehicle ($n = 4$) or FTY720 ($n = 6$). Due to the low number of cells, detailed subset analysis could not be performed, but there were no differences in the percentages of plasma cells and of $B220^+$ B cells comparing the two groups (Additional file 7).

Treatment with FTY720 affects the development but not maintenance of B cell aggregates in the CNS

In addition to investigating the effects of FTY720 treatment on the peripheral B cell response, we also explored the impact of FTY720 on B cell aggregation in the CNS. To this end, the cerebella of MP4-immunized mice were assessed after ~30 days of treatment, which started either at the peak of acute EAE or 50 days after disease onset. Overall, three different kinds of inflammatory infiltrates were investigated (Fig. 6a–d): non-B cell infiltrates, diffuse B cell infiltrates, or B cell aggregates. Non-B cell infiltrates were characterized by perivascular $CD3^+$ T cells in a loose arrangement, while similar structures with presence of additional $B220^+$ B cells were defined as diffuse B cell infiltrates. B cell aggregates showed a tight and compartmentalized perivascular cluster of cells that contained at least one third B cells. Mice treated with FTY720 during acute EAE showed a significant reduction in the overall number of inflammatory infiltrates per parenchymal area (Fig. 6e; $p = 0.001$). This significant decrease also pertained to the different categories of inflammation (non-B cell infiltrates: $p = 0.006$; diffuse B cell infiltrates: $p = 0.001$; B cell aggregates: $p < 0.001$). Interestingly, in five of the nine mice treated during acute EAE we did not find any infiltrates, and in none of the remaining four mice B cell aggregates were detected. In contrast, mice which were treated after 50 days of EAE did not show a significant difference in the total number of infiltrates per parenchymal area ($p = 0.075$), diffuse B cell infiltrates ($p = 0.123$) or B cell aggregates ($p = 0.978$), when compared to the vehicle-treated group. However, there was a significant reduction in the number of non-B cell infiltrates per area in FTY720-treated mice ($p = 0.007$). B cell aggregates were further subdivided into B cell aggregates with or without evidence for lymphoid neogenesis based on the expression of CXCL13 and the presence of follicular dendritic cells (FDC), plasma cells (Ig^+), and/or $PNAd^+$ high endothelial venules (HEV). Since no B cell aggregates were detected in mice treated with FTY720 during acute EAE, the analysis of lymphoid

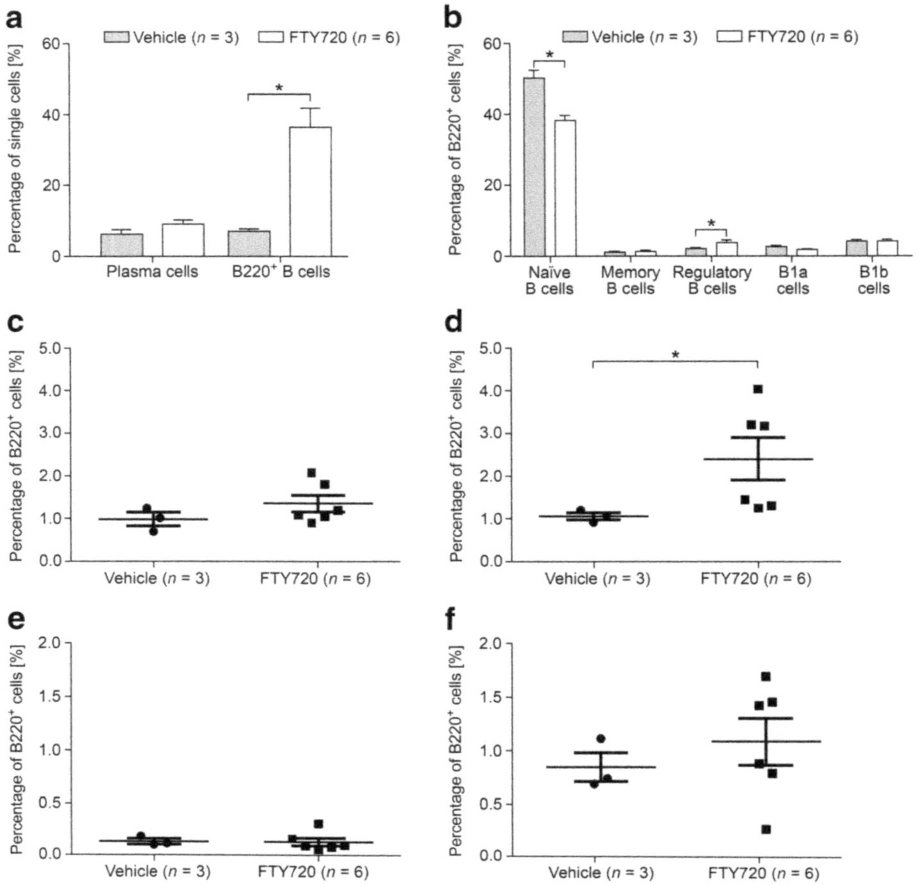

Fig. 4 B cell subsets were measured by flow cytometry in the spleens of MP4-immunized mice that were treated at the peak of disease with 1 mg/kg BW FTY720 or vehicle, respectively. **a** Percentages of plasma cells and of $B220^+$ B cells. **b** Percentages of the different $B220^+$ B cell subsets. More detailed analysis of the percentages of **c** $CD23^+$ regulatory B cells, **d** $CD23^-$ regulatory B cells, **e** $CD138^+$ memory B cells, and **f** $CD138^-$ memory B cells. *Bars* show means ± SEM. *$p < 0.05$, Mann-Whitney test

neogenesis was limited to the vehicle group. All four characteristics found in lymphoid tissue-like structures were observed except for $PNAd^+$ HEVs. As a consequence, mid-grade aggregates were the most common infiltrates at this stage of EAE. Overall, >70% of B cell aggregates showed features of lymphoid neogenesis. In mice treated after 50 days of disease with vehicle solution, all B cell aggregates displayed markers of lymphoid follicle-like structures and one high-grade B cell aggregate was observed. Interestingly, after treatment with FTY720 in chronic EAE, the absence of high-grade aggregates, a higher number of low-grade aggregates and the presence of an aggregate without any lymphoid features indicated an attenuating effect of FTY720 on lymphoid neogenesis. Statistical significance was reached for the reduction in mid-grade aggregates in FTY720- compared to vehicle-treated animals ($p = 0.04$). The differences in TLO marker distribution are summarized in Additional file 8.

No direct effect of FTY720 on B cell aggregation in vitro

Using an in vitro assay, we further investigated a potential direct effect of FTY720 on B cell aggregation. B cells were purified from $n = 6$ naïve non-immunized B6 mice, pre-incubated with 8 μM FTY720 or vehicle for 90 min, and aggregation was subsequently induced using a combination of LPS and IL-4. The percentage of single cells was determined after 72 h of incubation. As shown in Fig. 7, there was no difference comparing FTY720- and vehicle-treated B cells after in vitro aggregation.

Discussion

The aim of our study was to investigate the therapeutic effect of FTY720 on B cells in the B cell-/antibody-dependent MP4-EAE model. We employed two different treatment strategies: mice were either treated at the peak of EAE or during chronic disease. Our readout parameters of interest comprised global effects of FTY720 on B cells in addition to effects on MP4-specific antibody

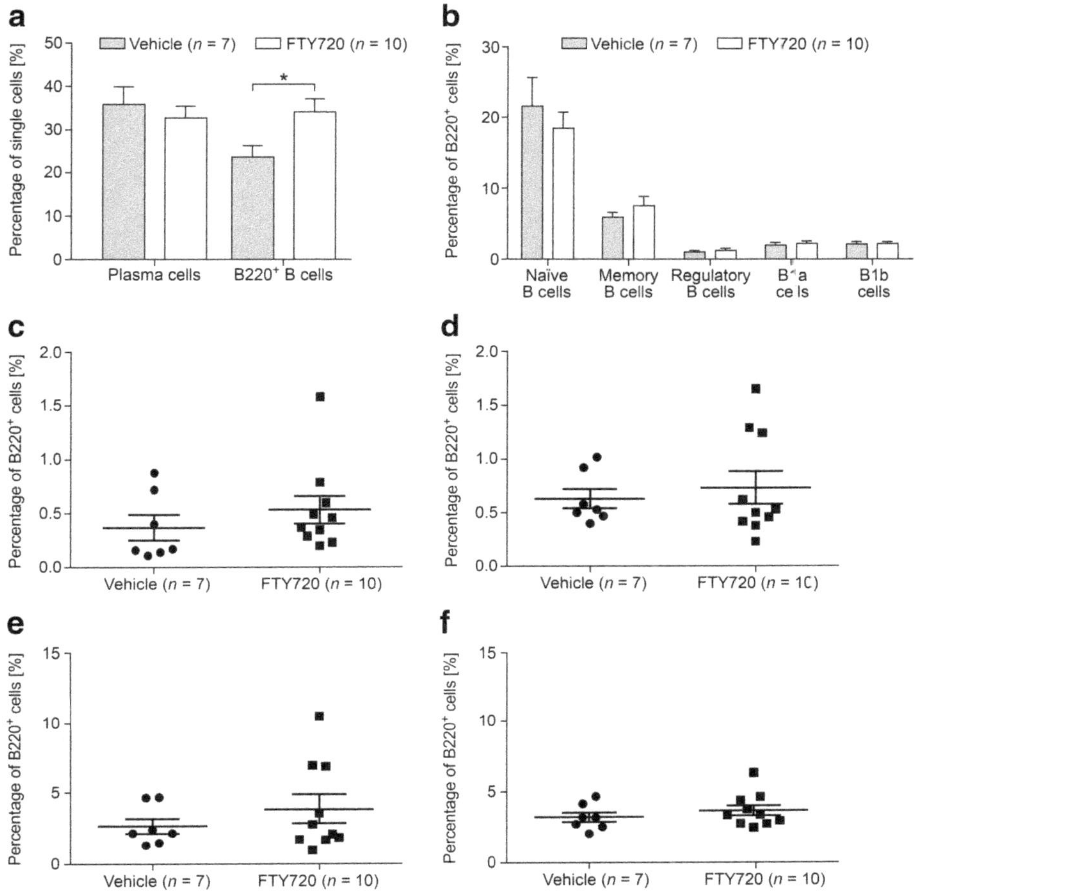

Fig. 5 B cell subsets were measured by flow cytometry in the spleens of MP4-immunized mice that were treated 50 days after EAE onset with 1 mg/kg BW FTY720 or vehicle, respectively. **a** Percentages of plasma cells and $B220^+$ B cells. **b** Percentages of the different $B220^+$ B cell subsets. More detailed analysis of the percentages of **c** $CD23^+$ regulatory B cells, **d** $CD23^-$ regulatory B cells, **e** $CD138^+$ memory B cells, and **f** $CD138^-$ memory B cells. *Bars* show means ± SEM. *$p < 0.05$, Mann-Whitney test

production, B cell subset distribution in SLOs, and B cell aggregation in the CNS.

FTY720 is an orally administered S1P receptor modulator (functional antagonist) and currently approved for the treatment of RR-MS. Its main mode of action is thought to be mediated by internalization and degradation of the $S1P_1$ receptor on lymphocytes, consequently trapping them in SLOs [26, 27]. As a consequence, less autoreactive lymphocytes are able to migrate into the CNS and to participate in inflammatory and neurodegenerative processes [28, 29]. While effects of FTY720 on T cells have been described in detail [30–32], only limited data are available on the effects on B cells. In-depth studies on B cell-specific effects of FTY720, however, are of outmost importance considering the crucial role of B cells in the pathogenesis of MS and the recent most promising advances in the development of B cell-depleting therapies [3–5, 33]. In particular, the notion that the development of B cell aggregates and the consecutive evolvement into TLOs is a hallmark feature of SP-MS and at least partly linked to clinical disease progression [14] demands further studies on the effect of FTY720 on these structures.

In a first set of experiments, we explored the effects of FTY720 on peripheral B cell function. Measuring both MP4-reactive and total IgG production, we did not detect any differences between FTY720- or vehicle-treated mice. These data are in line with early experiments examining the immunosuppressive effect of FTY720 in the context of organ transplantation [20, 34]. Pinschewer et al. investigated the humoral response of B6 mice in a viral infection model, showing that FTY720 did not affect B cell antibody secretion [34]. Furthermore, they measured the vesicular stomatitis virus antibody titer after immunization and transient FTY720 treatment and did not find a difference compared to the untreated control animals. This led to the conclusion that B memory cells were not impaired by the drug [34]. Activation, proliferation, and effector

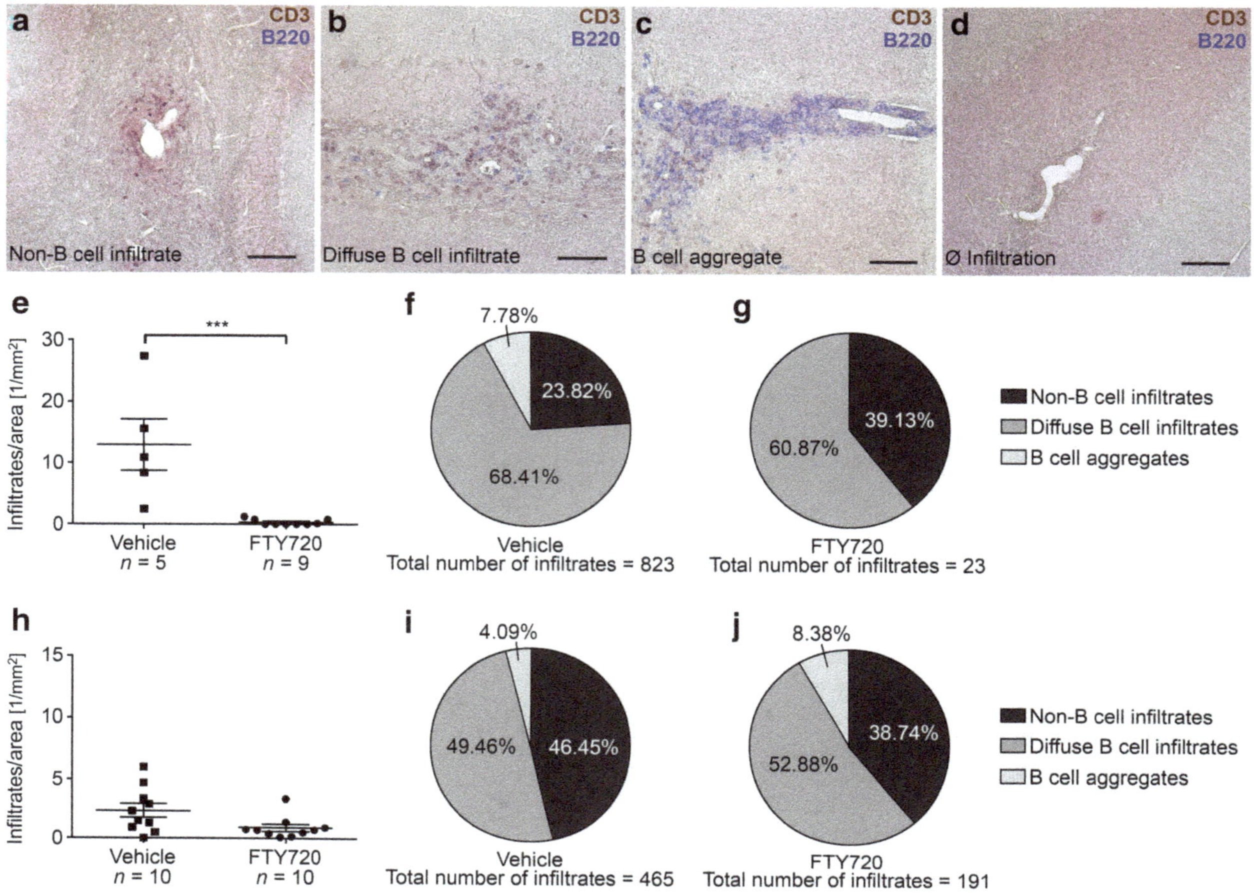

Fig. 6 Histological analysis of B cell aggregates in the cerebella of MP4-immunized mice. **a–d** CD3/B220 double staining of representative cerebellar sections of a mouse treated with vehicle solution at the peak of disease. The panels demonstrate the different infiltrate categories. *Bars* represent 100 µm. **e–g** Quantification of the number of infiltrates per parenchymal area and distribution of infiltrate categories in mice treated either with 1 mg/kg BW FTY720 or vehicle at the peak of disease. **h–j** Quantification of the number of infiltrates per parenchymal area and distribution of infiltrate categories in mice treated 50 days after disease onset. Graphs show means ± SEM. *$p < 0.05$, **$p < 0.01$, Mann-Whitney test

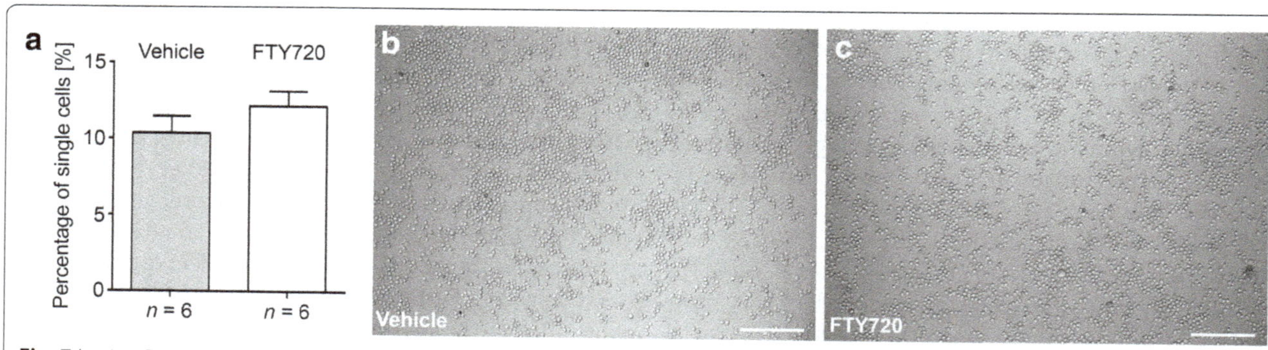

Fig. 7 In vitro B cell aggregation assay. B cells were purified from naïve B6 mice and pre-incubated with 8 µM FTY720 or corresponding vehicle solution for 90 min. B cells were then stimulated with 0.25 µg/ml LPS and 5 U/ml IL-4 for 72 h to induce aggregation. **a** Percentage of single cells at the end of the culture period. Graphs show means ± SEM. **b**, **c** Representative images of B cell aggregation under each of the two culture conditions. *Scale bars* represent 100 µm

functions of human B cells were also not influenced by FTY720 treatment [20]. However, it should be noted that Grützke et al. proposed a direct effect of FTY720 on B cell migration, as they found an increased migratory activity in in vitro BBB experiments comparing B cells from FTY720-treated MS patients with those of untreated controls [35].

In our study, RNA sequencing revealed differential effects of FTY720 on isolated B cells from MP4-immunized mice. These included the downregulation of Lyn, Syk, and Ifitm1 indicating the modulation of BCR-mediated signaling [21] as well as a potential pro-apoptotic mode of action of the drug [23–25]. Pro-apoptotic effects of FTY720 on B cells have been described before–however, it was also noted that this effect was much less pronounced in B cells compared to T cells, most likely due to the fact that B cells have more abundant anti-apoptotic protein Bcl-2 [36].

When performing B cell subset analysis by flow cytometry, we found that the percentage of $CD4^+$ T cells was significantly diminished in the peripheral blood, while $CD19^+$ B cell numbers were not. On the one hand, these data are in line with the aforementioned relative resistance of B cells to apoptosis induction by FTY720 [36] and also with a study published by Matloubian et al., who proposed that $CD19^+$ B cells are less dependent on $S1P_1$-mediated egress than $CD4^+$ T cells [27]. On the other hand, our data partly contradict the significant decrease of $CD19^+$ B cells in human PBMCs of MS patients receiving FTY720 [37–39] –partly because we still detected a significantly increased number of total $B220^+$ B cells in the spleen, which suggests a B cell-specific effect of FTY720 although this effect might not have been visible to its full extent in the peripheral blood. Interestingly, in previous reports, FTY720 treatment had only little impact on the number of B cells in the CSF, the extent of intrathecal IgG synthesis, and the presence of OCBs [38]. Also, in our study, there was no difference in the number of B cells and plasma cells in the CNS comparing vehicle- and FTY720-treated mice. When analyzing different B cell subsets, FTY720-treated MS patients showed an increase in $CD19^+IgD^+CD27^-$ naïve B cells in the peripheral blood [35]. In line with these data, we noticed that $B220^+CD43^-CD73^-CD80^-CD138^-$ naïve B cells were significantly decreased in the spleen after FTY720 treatment in MP4-induced EAE. Furthermore, Grützke et al. detected a strongly increased ratio of regulatory B cells in the peripheral blood of MS patients [35]. In our model, the percentages of splenic $CD23^-$ regulatory B cells were increased in mice treated with FTY720 at the peak of disease, but not in chronic EAE. Since these cells might represent marginal zone-bound regulatory B cells that are permanently located in the white pulp of the spleen, this increase could be explained by activation caused by the inflammatory milieu [40]. Other B cell subsets remained unaffected in FTY720-treated animals. Since there is no sufficient data on S1P receptor expression on murine lymphocyte subsets, we have no final explanation for potential discrepancies between our data and the results obtained in the human studies. However, it should be noted that we used a more detailed panel of extracellular markers for flow cytometry experiments than in the human studies. To our knowledge, we are the first to offer extensive data on the influence of FTY720 on splenic B cell subsets in a B cell-dependent EAE model. To investigate $S1P_1$ receptor expression on T and B cells after treatment with FTY720, we conducted flow cytometry analyses of lymph nodes and blood and detected no significant differences. Yet, $S1P_1^+CD4^+$ T cells and in particular $S1P_1^+CD19^+$ B cells were elevated in the blood compared to the lymph nodes, which is in line with the results of Matloubian et al. [27]. In addition, Sinha et al. [41] suggested that S1P-mediated chemotaxis is of minor importance for B cell egress from SLOs. Their proposed model of B cell lymph node transit describes a rather complex interaction of $S1P_1$ and $S1P_3$ and the overall activation status of the cell, which might also explain the lack of effect of FTY720 treatment on peripheral B cell numbers.

The most remarkable effect of FTY720 in our study was achieved when treatment was initiated during acute EAE. Treatment during acute EAE both significantly ameliorated clinical EAE and prevented the formation of B cell aggregates in the CNS. To determine whether the effect on B cell aggregates was due to a direct effect on B cells or rather a "bystander" phenomenon, we performed in vitro assays on purified mouse B cells demonstrating a lack of inhibitory effect of FTY720 on B cell aggregation. Since not only B cell aggregates but also global cerebellar inflammation was significantly reduced after FTY720 treatment, we suggest that the inhibition of T cell infiltration was a key reason for the absence of B cell aggregate formation in the CNS in the acute treatment cohort. Peters and colleagues have previously shown that T_H17 cells are required for B cell aggregate formation [42], and we have demonstrated the presence of T_H17 cells in the vicinity of TLOs in the MP4 model [11]. Along these lines, FTY720 was shown to significantly suppress the ability of T cells to be polarized to T_H17 in vitro [43]. Interestingly, there was no effect of FTY720 on the maintenance of already developed B cell aggregates in chronic EAE.

However, we noted a significant reduction in the evolution of B cell aggregates into TLOs, suggesting that the drug may either directly affect lymphoid neogenesis through yet unknown pathways or that T_H17 cells may also be required for TLO evolution.

It is currently debated whether CNS B cell aggregates need constant lymphocyte supply from the periphery. Studies investigating the effects of the anti-VLA4 antibody natalizumab have reported that OCBs indicating local antibody production vanished in a proportion of natalizumab-treated patients [44]. If one assumes that OCBs are at least in part associated with TLOs as local source for plasmablasts, it is conceivable that blockage of the BBB by natalizumab [45, 46] triggered TLO disruption. Our data, however, rather suggest that TLOs are inert and stable structures that are not directly dependent on supply from the outside once established. Along these lines, there are currently no substantial data on any of the approved MS therapies and on autologous hematopoetic stem cell transplantation that they have an effect on OCBs in the CSF. If TLOs are indeed stable, it will be highly relevant to determine whether TLOs are actually required or important for disease perpetuation.

Conclusions

Taken together, this study used MP4-induced EAE as a B cell- and antibody-dependent model of MS to explore potential B cell-specific effects of FTY720. The data suggest that these effects pertained to the modulation of BCR signaling, a decreased egress of $B220^+$ B cells from SLOs and to a decrease in the evolution of CNS B cell aggregates into TLOs. Since the next generation drug siponimod is currently being tested in SP-MS with promising results, future studies will have to elucidate whether this drug has even more pronounced effects on B cells and B cell aggregates and whether such effects are beneficial for both the treatment of RR- and SP-MS.

Additional files

Additional file 1: Oral treatment of mice with vehicle or 1 mg/kg BW FTY720 (a). (b) Macroscopic image of the liver after 30 days of treatment with vehicle solution. (c) HE staining of the liver and (d) higher magnification of the image. (e) Macroscopic image of the liver after 30 days of treatment with FTY720. (f) HE staining of the liver and (g) higher magnification of the image. Scale bars represent 200 μm in (c) and (f) and 100 μm in (d) and (g). Results are representative of $n = 10$ mice treated with vehicle solution and $n = 12$ mice treated with FTY720.

Additional file 2: Clinical parameters of EAE in mice treated either with FTY720 or vehicle.

Additional file 3: Antibodies used for flow cytometry.

Additional file 4: B cell aggregates in the cerebellar parenchyma show different characteristics of lymphoid neogenesis. (a) HE staining, (b) CD3/B220 double staining, (c-f) CXCL13, FDC-SP, Ig, and PNAd DAB staining. Scale bars represent 100 μm.

Additional file 5: Antibodies used for immunohistochemistry.

Additional file 6: Flow cytometry of $S1P_1^+$ T and B cells. Cells were measured in the blood (a) and lymph nodes (b) of naïve B6 mice that were treated either with 1 mg/kg BW FTY720 or vehicle for 10 consecutive days. Bars show means ± SEM.

Additional file 7: Flow cytometry analysis of plasma cells and of $B220^+$ B cells in the CNS. Cells were measured in periventricular brain, cerebellar, and spinal cord tissue of MP4-immunized mice that were treated at the peak of disease with either 1 mg/kg BW FTY720 or vehicle. Bars show means ± SEM.

Additional file 8: TLO marker distribution in mice treated with vehicle at the peak of disease (a, b). Treatment with vehicle (c, d) or FTY720 (e, f) was initiated 50 days after EAE onset.

Abbreviations

B6: C57BL/6; BBB: Blood-brain-barrier; BCR: B cell receptor; BW: Body weight; CNS: Central nervous system; CSF: Cerebrospinal fluid; CXCL13: Chemokine ligand 13; DAB: Diaminobenzidine; DEG: Differentially expressed gene; EAE: Experimental autoimmune encephalomyelitis; FDC: Follicular dendritic cell; HE: Hematoxylin and eosin; HEV: High endothelial venule; Ig: Immunglobulin; LPS: Lipopolysaccharide; IL-4: Interleukin-4; MBP: Myelin basic protein; MOG: Myelin oligodendrocyte glycoprotein; MP: Milk powder; MP4: MBP-PLP fusion protein; MS: Multiple sclerosis; OCB: Oligoclonal bands; PBS: Phosphate-buffered saline; PFA: Paraformaldehyde; PLP: Proteolipid protein; PNAd: Peripheral node addressin; RR-MS: Relapsing-remitting MS; SLO: Secondary lymphoid organ; SP-MS: Secondary progressive MS; TLO: Tertiary lymphoid organ

Acknowledgements

We would like to thank Alla Ganscher and Brigitte Treffny for excellent technical support, Michael Christof for graphical procession of the figures and Süleyman Ergün for valuable discussion.

Funding

This study was funded by a research grant from Novartis.

Authors' contributions

KB and QN conducted the ELISA and ELISPOT experiments, immunohistochemistry, and statistical analyses. They also drafted the manuscript. KB and SK conducted the in vitro B cell aggregation assays. DMR, KB, TK, and VS conducted the flow cytometry experiments. MW immunized and scored the mice. AS and TK contributed to the experimental design of the study as well as scored and treated the mice. RB, CJS, and KUF conducted the RNA sequencing experiments and analysis. SK was responsible for the design of the study, the interpretation of the results, and wrote the manuscript. All authors read and approved the final manuscript.

Consent for publication

Not applicable.

Competing interests

The authors declare that they have no competing interests.

Author details

[1]Department of Anatomy and Cell Biology, University of Würzburg, Würzburg, Germany. [2]Core Unit Systems Medicine, University Hospitals of

Würzburg, Würzburg, Germany. [3]LIMES Institute, University of Bonn, Bonn, Germany. [4]Department of Neurology, University Hospital Würzburg, Würzburg, Germany. [5]Department of Neurology, University Hospital Essen, Essen, Germany. [6]Institute of Anatomy and Cell Biology, Friedrich-Alexander University Erlangen-Nürnberg, Erlangen, Germany.

References

1. Sospedra M, Martin R. Immunology of multiple sclerosis. Annu Rev Immunol. 2005;23:683–747.
2. Franciotta D, Salvetti M, Lolli F, Serafini B, Aloisi F. B cells and multiple sclerosis. Lancet Neurol. 2008;7:852–8.
3. Hauser SL, Waubant E, Arnold DL, Vollmer T, Antel J, Fox RJ, Bar-Or A, Panzara M, Sarkar N, Agarwal S, Langer-Gould A, Smith CH. B-cell depletion with rituximab in relapsing-remitting multiple sclerosis. N Engl J Med. 2008; 358:676–88.
4. Hauser SL, Bar-Or A, Comi G, Giovannoni G, Hartung HP, Hemmer B, Lublin F, Montalban X, Rammohan KW, Selmaj K, Traboulsee A, Wolinsky JS, Arnold DL, Klingelschmitt G, Masterman D, Fontoura P, Belachew S, Chin P, Mairon N, Garren H, Kappos L. Ocrelizumab versus interferon beta-1a in relapsing multiple sclerosis. N Engl J Med. 2017;376:221–34.
5. Montalban X, Hauser SL, Kappos L, Arnold DL, Bar-Or A, Comi G, de Seze J, Giovannoni G, Hartung HP, Hemmer B, Lublin F, Rammohan KW, Selmaj K, Traboulsee A, Sauter A, Masterman D, Fontoura P, Belachew S, Garren H, Mairon N, Chin P, Wolinsky JS. Ocrelizumab versus placebo in primary progressive multiple sclerosis. N Engl J Med. 2017;376:209–20.
6. Keegan M, Konig F, McClelland R, Bruck W, Morales Y, Bitsch A, Panitch H, Lassmann H, Weinshenker B, Rodriguez M, Parisi J, Lucchinetti CF. Relation between humoral pathological changes in multiple sclerosis and response to therapeutic plasma exchange. Lancet. 2005;366:579–82.
7. Kuerten S, Pommerschein G, Barth SK, Hohmann C, Milles B, Sammer FW, Duffy CE, Wunsch M, Rovituso DM, Schroeter M, Addicks K, Kaiser CC, Lehmann PV. Identification of a B cell-dependent subpopulation of multiple sclerosis by measurements of brain-reactive B cells in the blood. Clin Immunol. 2014;152:20–4.
8. Stangel M, Fredrikson S, Meinl E, Petzold A, Stuve O, Tumani H. The utility of cerebrospinal fluid analysis in patients with multiple sclerosis. Nat Rev Neurol. 2013;9:267–76.
9. Lucchinetti C, Bruck W, Parisi J, Scheithauer B, Rodriguez M, Lassmann H. Heterogeneity of multiple sclerosis lesions: implications for the pathogenesis of demyelination. Ann Neurol. 2000;47:707–17.
10. Kuerten S, Lichtenegger FS, Faas S, Angelov DN, Tary-Lehmann M, Lehmann PV. MBP-PLP fusion protein-induced EAE in C57BL/6 mice. J Neuroimmunol. 2006;177:99–111.
11. Kuerten S, Schickel A, Kerkloh C, Recks MS, Addicks K, Ruddle NH, Lehmann PV. Tertiary lymphoid organ development coincides with determinant spreading of the myelin-specific T cell response. Acta Neuropathol. 2012; 124:861–73.
12. Lehmann-Horn K, Wang SZ, Sagan SA, Zamvil SS, von Budingen HC. B cell repertoire expansion occurs in meningeal ectopic lymphoid tissue. JCI Insight. 2016;1, e87234.
13. Serafini B, Rosicarelli B, Magliozzi R, Stigliano E, Aloisi F. Detection of ectopic B-cell follicles with germinal centers in the meninges of patients with secondary progressive multiple sclerosis. Brain Pathol. 2004;14:164–74.
14. Magliozzi R, Howell O, Vora A, Serafini B, Nicholas R, Puopolo M, Reynolds R, Aloisi F. Meningeal B-cell follicles in secondary progressive multiple sclerosis associate with early onset of disease and severe cortical pathology. Brain. 2007;130:1089–104.
15. Howell OW, Reeves CA, Nicholas R, Carassiti D, Radotra B, Gentleman SM, Serafini B, Aloisi F, Roncaroli F, Magliozzi R, Reynolds R. Meningeal inflammation is widespread and linked to cortical pathology in multiple sclerosis. Brain. 2011;134:2755–71.
16. Kappos L, Bar-Or A, Cree B, Fox R, Giovannoni G, Gold R, Vermersch P, Arnould S, Sidorenko T, Wolf C, Wallstroem E, Dahlke F. Efficacy and safety of siponimod in secondary progressive multiple sclerosis--results of the placebo controlled, double-blind, Phase III EXPAND study. 32nd Congress of the European Committee for Treatment and Research in Multiple Sclerosis. September 14 -17, 2016. London, UK
17. Kappos L, Antel J, Comi G, Montalban X, O'Connor P, Polman CH, Haas T, Korn AA, Karlsson G, Radue EW. Oral fingolimod (FTY720) for relapsing multiple sclerosis. N Engl J Med. 2006;355:1124–40.
18. Cohen JA, Chun J. Mechanisms of fingolimod's efficacy and adverse effects in multiple sclerosis. Ann Neurol. 2011;69:759–77.
19. Groves A, Kihara Y, Chun J. Fingolimod: direct CNS effects of sphingosine 1-phosphate (S1P) receptor modulation and implications in multiple sclerosis therapy. J Neurol Sci. 2013;328:9–18.
20. Brinkmann V, Chen S, Feng L, Pinschewer D, Nikolova Z, Hof R. FTY720 alters lymphocyte homing and protects allografts without inducing general immunosuppression. Transplant Proc. 2001;33:530–1.
21. Takata M, Sabe H, Hata A, Inazu T, Homma Y, Nukada T, Yamamura H, Kurosaki T. Tyrosine kinases Lyn and Syk regulate B cell receptor-coupled Ca^{2+} mobilization through distinct pathways. EMBO J. 1994;13:1341–9.
22. Levy S, Todd SC, Maecker HT. CD81 (TAPA-1): a molecule involved in signal transduction and cell adhesion in the immune system. Ann Rev Immunol. 1998;16:89–109.
23. Bertin J, Wang L, Guo Y, Jacobson MD, Poyet JL, Srinivasula SM, Merriam S, DiStefano PS, Alnemri ES. CARD11 and CARD14 Are novel caspase recruitment domain (CARD)/membrane-associated guanylate kinase (MAGUK) family members that interact with BCL10 and activate NF-κB. J Biol Chem. 2001;276:11877–82.
24. Preston GA, Lyon TT, Yin Y, Lang JE, Solomon G, Annab L, Srinivasan DG, Alcorta DA, Barrett JC. Induction of apoptosis by c-Fos protein. Mol Cell Biol. 1996;16:211–18.
25. Limnander A, Depeille P, Freedman TS, Liou J, Leitges M, Kurosaki T, Roose JP, Weiss A. STIM1, PKC-δ and RasGFP set a threshold for proapoptotic Erk signaling during B cell development. Nat Immunol. 2011;12:425–33.
26. Brinkmann V, Cyster JG, Hla T. FTY720: sphingosine 1-phosphate receptor-1 in the control of lymphocyte egress and endothelial barrier function. Am J Transplant. 2004;4:1019–25.
27. Matloubian M, Lo CG, Cinamon G, Lesneski MJ, Xu Y, Brinkmann V, Allende ML, Proia RL, Cyster JG. Lymphocyte egress from thymus and peripheral lymphoid organs is dependent on S1P receptor 1. Nature. 2004;427:355–60.
28. Fujino M, Funeshima N, Kitazawa Y, Kimura H, Amemiya H, Suzuki S, Li XK. Amelioration of experimental autoimmune encephalomyelitis in Lewis rats by FTY720 treatment. J Pharmacol Exp Ther. 2003;305:70–7.
29. Massberg S, von Andrian UH. Fingolimod and sphingosine-1-phosphate--modifiers of lymphocyte migration. N Engl J Med. 2006;355:1088–91.
30. Metzler B, Gfeller P, Wieczorek G, Li J, Nuesslein-Hildesheim B, Katopodis A, Mueller M, Brinkmann V. Modulation of T cell homeostasis and alloreactivity under continuous FTY720 exposure. Int Immunol. 2008;20:633–44.
31. Mehling M, Brinkmann V, Antel J, Bar-Or A, Goebels N, Vedrine C, Kristofic C, Kuhle J, Lindberg RL, Kappos L. FTY720 therapy exerts differential effects on T cell subsets in multiple sclerosis. Neurology. 2008;71:1261–7.
32. Brinkmann V. FTY720 (fingolimod) in multiple sclerosis: therapeutic effects in the immune and the central nervous system. Br J Pharmacol. 2009;158:1173–82.
33. Hauser SL, Bar-Or A, Comi G, Giovannoni G, Hartung HP, Hemmer B, Lublin F, Montalban X, Rammohan KW, Selmaj K, Traboulsee A, Wolinsky JS, Arnold DL, Klingelschmitt G, Masterman D, Fontoura P, Belachew S, Chin P, Mairon N, Garren H, Kappos L, OPERA I and OPERA II Clinical Investigators. Ocrelizumab versus interferon-beta1a in relapsing multiple sclerosis. N Engl J Med. 2017;376:221–34.
34 Pinschewer DD, Ochsenbein AF, Odermatt B, Brinkmann V, Hengartner H, Zinkernagel RM. FTY720 immunosuppression impairs effector T cell peripheral homing without affecting induction, expansion, and memory. J Immunol. 2000;164:5761–70.
35 Grutzke B, Hucke S, Gross CC, Herold MV, Posevitz-Fejfar A, Wildemann BT, Kieseier BC, Dehmel T, Wiendl H, Klotz L. Fingolimod treatment promotes regulatory phenotype and function of B cells. Ann Clin Transl Neurol. 2015; 2:119–30.
36 Nagahara Y, Ikekita M, Shinomiya T. T cell selective apoptosis by a novel immunosuppressant, FTY720, is closely regulated with Bcl-2. Br J Pharamcol. 2002;137:953–62.
37 Claes N, Dhaeze T, Fraussen J, Broux B, Van Wijmeersch B, Stinissen P, Hupperts R, Hellings N, Somers V. Compositional changes of B and T cell subtypes during fingolimod treatment in multiple sclerosis patients: a 12-month follow-up study. PLoS One. 2014;9, e111115.
38 Kowarik MC, Pellkofer HL, Cepok S, Korn T, Kumpfel T, Buck D, Hohlfeld R, Berthele A, Hemmer B. Differential effects of fingolimod (FTY720) on immune cells in the CSF and blood of patients with MS. Neurology. 2011;76:1214–21.
39 Nakamura M, Matsuoka T, Chihara N, Miyake S, Sato W, Araki M, Okamoto T,

Lin Y, Ogawa M, Murata M, Aranami T, Yamamura T. Differential effects of fingolimod on B-cell populations in multiple sclerosis. Mult Scler. 2014;20: 1371–80.
40 Gray M, Miles K, Salter D, Gray D, Savill J. Apoptotic cells protect mice from autoimmune inflammation by the induction of regulatory B cells. Proc Natl Acad Sci U S A. 2007;104:14080–5.
41 Sinha RK, Park C, Hwang IY, Davis MD, Kehrl JH. B lymphocytes exit lymph nodes through cortical lymphatic sinusoids by a mechanism independent of sphingosine-1-phosphate-mediated chemotaxis. Immunity. 2009;30:434–46.
42 Peters A, Pitcher LA, Sullivan JM, Mitsdoerffer M, Acton SE, Franz B, Wucherpfennig K, Turley S, Carroll MC, Sobel RA, Bettelli E, Kuchroo VK. Th17 cells induce ectopic lymphoid follicles in central nervous system tissue inflammation. Immunity. 2011;35:986–96.
43 Garris CS, Wu L, Acharya S, Arac A, Blaho VA, Huang Y, Moon BS, Axtell RC, Ho PP, Steinberg GK, Lewis DB, Sobel RA, Han DK, Steinman L, Snyder MP, Hla T, Han MH. Defective sphingosine 1-phosphate receptor 1 (S1P1) phosphorylation exacerbates T_H17-mediated autoimmune neuroinflammation. Nat Immunol. 2013;14:1166–72.
44 von Glehn F, Farias AS, de Oliveira AC, Damasceno A, Longhini AL, Oliveira EC, Damasceno BP, Santos LM, Brandao CO. Disappearance of cerebrospinal fluid oligoclonal bands after natalizumab treatment of multiple sclerosis patients. Mult Scler. 2012;18:1038–41.
45 Yednock TA, Cannon C, Fritz LC, Sanchez-Madrid F, Steinman L, Karin N. Prevention of experimental autoimmune encephalomyelitis by antibodies against alpha 4 beta 1 integrin. Nature. 1992;356:63–6.
46 Hoepner R, Faissner S, Salmen A, Gold R, Chan A. Efficacy and side effects of natalizumab therapy in patients with multiple sclerosis. J Cent Nerv Syst Dis. 2014;6:41–9.

14

Relationship of acute axonal damage, Wallerian degeneration, and clinical disability in multiple sclerosis

Shailender Singh[1†], Tobias Dallenga[1,2†], Anne Winkler[1], Shanu Roemer[1,3], Brigitte Maruschak[1], Heike Siebert[1], Wolfgang Brück[1†] and Christine Stadelmann[1*†]

Abstract

Background: Axonal damage and loss substantially contribute to the incremental accumulation of clinical disability in progressive multiple sclerosis. Here, we assessed the amount of Wallerian degeneration in brain tissue of multiple sclerosis patients in relation to demyelinating lesion activity and asked whether a transient blockade of Wallerian degeneration decreases axonal loss and clinical disability in a mouse model of inflammatory demyelination.

Methods: Wallerian degeneration and acute axonal damage were determined immunohistochemically in the periplaque white matter of multiple sclerosis patients with early actively demyelinating lesions, chronic active lesions, and inactive lesions. Furthermore, we studied the effects of Wallerian degeneration blockage on clinical severity, inflammatory pathology, acute axonal damage, and long-term axonal loss in experimental autoimmune encephalomyelitis using Wallerian degeneration slow (Wld^S) mutant mice.

Results: The highest numbers of axons undergoing Wallerian degeneration were found in the perilesional white matter of multiple sclerosis patients early in the disease course and with actively demyelinating lesions. Furthermore, Wallerian degeneration was more abundant in patients harboring chronic active as compared to chronic inactive lesions. No co-localization of neuropeptide Y-Y1 receptor, a *bona fide* immunohistochemical marker of Wallerian degeneration, with amyloid precursor protein, frequently used as an indicator of acute axonal transport disturbance, was observed in human and mouse tissue, indicating distinct axon-degenerative processes. Experimentally, a delay of Wallerian degeneration, as observed in Wld^S mice, did not result in a reduction of clinical disability or acute axonal damage in experimental autoimmune encephalomyelitis, further supporting that acute axonal damage as reflected by axonal transport disturbances does not share common molecular mechanisms with Wallerian degeneration. Furthermore, delaying Wallerian degeneration did not result in a net rescue of axons in late lesion stages of experimental autoimmune encephalomyelitis.

Conclusions: Our data indicate that in multiple sclerosis, ongoing demyelination in focal lesions is associated with axonal degeneration in the perilesional white matter, supporting a role for focal pathology in diffuse white matter damage. Also, our results suggest that interfering with Wallerian degeneration in inflammatory demyelination does not suffice to prevent acute axonal damage and finally axonal loss.

Keywords: Multiple sclerosis, Experimental autoimmune encephalomyelitis, Wallerian degeneration, Axonal damage, Wld^S

* Correspondence: cstadelmann@med.uni-goettingen.de
[†]Equal contributors
[1]Institute of Neuropathology, University Medical Center, Göttingen, Germany

Background

Axonal damage and loss are the key structural features in multiple sclerosis patients and the most important correlates of persistent disability [1–3]. Also, the insidious clinical worsening in later stages of the disease, often independent of newly formed lesions and largely non-responsive to immunomodulatory treatments, but reflected in important brain and cervical spinal atrophy, is considered due to cumulative axonal loss [4–7]. Reports on axonal loss in the normal-appearing white matter (NAWM) and spinal cord range from ~20 to 55%, whereas in chronic multiple sclerosis lesions, axonal reduction of up to 70% has been reported [8]. Axonal degeneration can occur via several mechanisms, the most prominent being anterograde (or Wallerian) and retrograde ("dying back") degeneration [9]. Inflammation-associated axonal transport disturbances, so-called "focal axonal degeneration," may precede axonal transection and ensuing axonal self-destruction by Wallerian degeneration [10].

Axonal transport disturbances, as visualized by the accumulation of anterogradely transported proteins such as amyloid precursor protein (APP) and synaptophysin, are often used as indicators of "acute axonal damage," and the density of APP-positive axonal profiles is highest in the earliest stages of multiple sclerosis lesion formation [2, 11, 12]. Axons with transport disturbance are also present at relatively high density in the rims of chronic active, smoldering lesions and may be found in the NAWM [2, 13, 14]. Whether and to which extent axonal transport disturbances are reversible or lead to definite, irreversible axonal transection, is not yet clear. Correlations of APP-positive axonal profiles with the density of macrophages have been repeatedly shown for early lesions; however, in chronic disease, also a correlation with T cells was observed [2, 14–16].

In experimental models of inflammatory demyelination, the accumulation of organelles and proteins in axons corresponds to "focal axonal degeneration," i.e., localized axonal swelling. Importantly, a proportion of axons showing focal axonal degeneration finally undergo transection and degenerate [10]. In experimental autoimmune encephalomyelitis (EAE), the progression to axonal transection is largely prevented by treatment with ROS/NOS scavengers, and axonal morphology is restored in the majority of treated axons studied [17]. Demyelination is not a prerequisite for focal axonal degeneration, supporting the contribution of highly lipid-soluble reactive species to axonal damage [10, 17–19]. Of note, however, chronic axonal transport disturbances may lead to distal axonal "malnutrition" and dying back, highlighting the importance of early therapeutic intervention [17].

Axons proceeding from focally disturbed axonal transport to axonal transection undergo a series of orderly events, namely, an acute retraction process, both proximally and distally, termed acute axonal degeneration, followed by classical Wallerian degeneration of the distal axon part [20]. Both processes are, at least in part, mediated by similar molecular mechanisms and contribute to the important physical "gap" between the proximal and distal axon stump rendering regenerative attempts challenging. As of yet, it is not well understood when the majority of Wallerian degeneration, the final process of axonal self-destruction, takes place in multiple sclerosis. In particular, it has not been explored whether Wallerian degeneration is abundant in the chronic disease stage of the disease.

Thus, to better understand the dynamics of axonal loss in patients with multiple sclerosis, we set out to study the timing and extent of Wallerian degeneration in patients with short- and long-standing disease harboring early- and late-stage lesions. Furthermore, experimentally, we strived to determine whether delaying Wallerian degeneration helps to decrease inflammatory axonal damage in a model of multiple sclerosis. Our data indicate that axonal transection and ensuing axonal self-destruction is most pronounced in the periplaque white matter of patients with early demyelinating lesions. Of note, however, also the presence of chronic active lesions associates with a high density of neuropeptide Y-Y1 receptor (NPY-Y1R)-positive axonal profiles, underlining the notion that focal demyelinated lesions are the key contributors to axonal demise in the periplaque and normal-appearing white matter. Experimentally, we find that neither acute axonal damage nor persistent axonal loss is ameliorated in focal EAE lesions in Wallerian degeneration slow (*Wld^S*) compared to wild-type (WT) mice, indicating limited sharing of molecular mechanisms between acute axonal transport disturbance and Wallerian degeneration [21]. Our study underlines the role of focal white matter lesions for axonal loss in the NAWM of patients with multiple sclerosis and supports the concept of early pharmacological interventions to prevent highly vulnerable, transport-deficient axons showing signs of focal axonal degeneration from transection.

Methods

Brain tissue from patients with multiple sclerosis

We investigated paraffin-embedded archival brain tissue from 17 autopsied multiple sclerosis patients and 14 biopsied patients diagnosed with inflammatory demyelination consistent with multiple sclerosis. A total of 34 [16] tissue specimens, which included non-demyelinated white matter regions, were used for the study. All biopsy samples analyzed contained non-demyelinated periplaque white matter (PPWM) areas contiguous with early/late active ($n = 6$) or inactive ($n = 9$) lesions. For direct comparison, non-demyelinated white matter tissue adjacent to 5 active lesions, 7 chronic active, and 7 chronic inactive lesions was analyzed in multiple sclerosis autopsy tissue. All lesions fulfilled the criteria for the diagnosis of multiple sclerosis [22]. Lesional activity was determined using previously described criteria [23]. The biopsies were performed in different neurosurgical centers to exclude neoplastic or infectious diseases. Specimens were sent to the Department of Neuropathology in Göttingen, Germany, for a second opinion. The patients' clinical characteristics are summarized in Table 1.

Brain tissue from stroke patients

Axonal transport disturbances and Wallerian degeneration are typical and abundant after brain ischemia. To study the spatial relation of the two phenomena in a prototypic human disease, we analyzed archival paraffin-embedded brain biopsy tissue from four patients (three females, one male; median age = 54 years; range 49–63 years) with ischemic stroke lesions. Lesions were characterized by tissue necrosis as evidenced by massive axonal loss and dense macrophage infiltration. Axonal swellings in a typical ischemic pattern were abundant at the lesion borders.

Mice

Female 8–10-week-old *Wld*^{S} (C57BL/6 OlaHsd) and C57BL/6 mice were obtained from the Harlan Laboratories, UK. The *Wld*^{S} mouse strain is characterized by an 85-kb tandem triplication on chromosome four that occurred as a spontaneous mutation in the B6 strain in the 1940s, leading to the expression of an Ube4b/Nmnat chimeric protein. Mutant mice do not show a spontaneous phenotype. All mice had free access to water and chow and were included in the experiments after at least 5 days of acclimatization.

Table 1 Characteristics of multiple sclerosis patients included in the study

Sex; female $n = 16$, male $n = 15$
Age; 47 years (median), 19–76 (range)
Clinical diagnosis[a]
Clinically isolated syndrome suggestive of multiple sclerosis; $n = 9$ (9 biopsies)
Primary progressive multiple sclerosis; $n = 6$ (6 autopsies)
Relapsing-remitting multiple sclerosis; $n = 4$ (4 biopsies)
Secondary progressive multiple sclerosis; $n = 9$ (1 biopsy, 8 autopsies)
Disease duration of biopsied patients[b]; 42 days (median), 9–540 days (range)
Disease duration of autopsied patients[b]; 19 years (median), 6–34 years (range)

[a]Clinical course was not available for three autopsy patients
[b]Time from the first symptoms to biopsy/autopsy

EAE induction and clinical evaluation

EAE was induced by subcutaneous injection of 200 μg myelin oligodendrocyte glycoprotein (MOG)-peptide$_{35-55}$ emulsified in complete Freund's adjuvant (CFA) containing 1 mg/ml inactivated *Mycobacterium tuberculosis*. Control mice were injected with CFA alone. Three hundred nanogram pertussis toxin was injected i.p. at day 0 and day 2 after immunization. Clinical deficits were assessed daily by a blinded observer using the following scoring system: 0=no symptoms, 0.5=partial tail paresis, 1.0=complete tail paralysis, 1.5=slight hind limb paresis, 2.0=distinct hind limb paresis, 2.5=severe hind limb paresis, 3.0=complete hind limb paralysis, 3.5=slight forelimb paresis, 4.0=tetraparesis, 4.5=moribund, and 5.0=death. Mice were euthanized when reaching a score of 3.5.

Histopathology

At the end of the EAE experiments, animals were deeply anesthetized and perfused with phosphate buffered saline (PBS) (pH 7.4) followed by 4% paraformaldehyde (PFA) in PBS. The spinal cords (SC) were dissected, and at least eight transverse sections were embedded in paraffin. One to three micrometer-thick sections were stained with hematoxylin-eosin (HE), Luxol Fast Blue/periodic acid Schiff's reagent (LFB/PAS), and Bielschowsky silver impregnation to determine inflammation, demyelination, and axonal loss. Immunohistochemistry (IHC) was performed using the primary antibodies listed in Table 2. For antigen retrieval, tissue slices were microwaved in 10 mM citrate buffer (pH 6.0) 3 × 5 min. Bound antibodies were visualized using an appropriate biotinylated secondary antibody and an avidin-peroxidase-DAB technique. Negative control sections were incubated without primary antibodies or with irrelevant primary antibodies of the respective isotypes. Slices were counterstained with hemalaun and cover-slipped. Double fluorescence labeling with two mouse monoclonal primary antibodies was carried out as described previously [24].

Mouse sciatic nerve transection

Four female C57BL/6 mice were used to study sciatic nerve axotomy. They were deeply anesthetized by intraperitoneal injection of ketamine hydrochloride ("Ketanest Inresa," 50 mg/ml, Inresa, Freiburg, Germany) mixed with xylazine hydrochloride ("Rompun" 2%, Bayer, Leverkusen, Germany) in a ratio of 2:1 (0.4 mg Ketanest and 2 mg Rompun for each mouse). Skin and muscles above the right femur were opened by fine scissors, and the sciatic nerve was completely transected. Subsequently, muscle and skin were closed by suture (Ethicon). The mice were kept for 6 days under a 12-h dark-light cycle and given food and water ad libitum. The animals were perfused transcardially with PBS and 4% PFA, and the sciatic nerves

Table 2 Antibodies used for immunohistochemistry

Target	Antibody type (clone)	Dilution	Pre-treatment	Source
Amyloid precursor protein (APP)	Mouse mAb (22C11)	1:2000	Citrate MW	Chemicon International, USA
Neuropeptide Y receptor Y1 (NPY-Y1R)	Rabbit polyAb #96106	1:1000	Tris-EDTA MW	CURE/UCLA, USA
Myelin basic protein (MBP)	Rabbit polyAb	1:1000	None	DakoCytomation, Denmark
MBP peptic fragment 70–89	Mouse mAb (SMI94)	1:5000	Steam	Covance Inc., USA
Myelin proteolipid protein (PLP)	Mouse mAb (Plpc 1)	1:500	Citrate MW	Biozol, Germany
Myelin oligodendrocyte glycoprotein (MOG)	Rat polyAb	1:1000	Citrate MW	[75]
Myelin-associated glycoprotein (MAG)	Rabbit polyAb	1:10	Citrate MW	[76]
2′,3′-Cyclic-nucleotide 3′-phosphodiesterase (CNPase)	Mouse mAb (SMI91)	1:200	Citrate MW	Covance Inc., USA
Monocytes, activated microglia	Mouse mAb (KiM1P)	1:5000	Citrate MW	[77]
Early-activated macrophages (S100A9)	Rabbit polyAb	1:500	Citrate MW	[78]
Phosphorylated NFs	Mouse mAb (SMI31)	1:10000	Citrate MW	Covance Inc., USA
Non-phosphorylated NFs	Mouse mAb (SMI32)	1:1000	Citrate MW	Covance Inc., USA
Hypo-phosphorylated NFs	Mouse mAb (SMI35)	1:10000	Citrate MW	Covance Inc., USA
NF-low-molecular-weight (NF68)	Mouse mAb (NR4)	1:100	Citrate MW	Sigma Chemical Company, USA
NF-high-molecular-weight (NF200)	Mouse mAb (N52)	1:400	Citrate MW	Sigma Chemical Company, USA
Growth-associated protein 43 (GAP43)	Mouse mAb (9-1E12)	1:4000	Citrate MW	Chemicon International, USA
Synaptophysin (protein p38)	Mouse mAb (SY38)	1:10	Citrate MW	DakoCytomation, Denmark

NF neurofilament, *mAb* monoclonal antibody, *polyAb* polyclonal antibody, *MW* microwave pre-treatment

dissected. The contralateral nerves and a sciatic nerve from an animal without axotomy served as controls. Sciatic nerves were post-fixed in 4% PFA overnight and embedded in paraffin. Microtome sections of 1–3 μm thickness were de-paraffinized, pre-treated by cooking in citrate buffer (pH 6) for 10 min, and subjected to IHC.

Data acquisition and analysis

Tissue sections were analyzed using an Olympus BX51 fluorescence microscope equipped with a DP71 CCD camera (Olympus Optical Co, Ltd., Hamburg, Germany), a Zeiss Cell Observer microscope with an AxioCam ICc 3 CCD camera (Carl Zeiss MicroImaging, Ltd., Göttingen, Germany), or by confocal laser scanning microscopy with a Fluoview 1000 Olympus microscope. Transverse spinal cord (SC) sections at the cervical, thoracic, lumbar, and sacral levels were used for quantitative analysis. The extent of acute axonal damage of axons undergoing Wallerian degeneration and the density of healthy phosphorylated axons was calculated by counting APP^{+}, NPY-Y1R^{+}, or SMI31^{+} profiles in spinal cross sections within at least five white matter lesions per mouse at ×400 magnification using an ocular counting grid. Counts are given as immunopositive axonal profiles per square millimeter. Relative axonal densities within lesions were determined in sections stained with Bielschowsky's silver impregnation by using an axonal counting grid with 25 cross-points [25]. The number of axons intersecting with the crossing points was determined as a fraction of the total number of cross-points at a magnification of ×1000, under oil immersion. The value obtained in control animals was set to 100%. The degree of axon reduction in the lesion is given as the percentage of axon density compared with the control animals. To determine the extent of demyelination, digital images of LFB/PAS-stained SC cross sections were recorded through an Olympus light microscope with a CCD DP71 camera at ×100 magnification. Using the computer program Cell^F (Soft Imaging Systems®), demyelinated white matter areas were measured, and the percentage with respect to total white matter was calculated. The inflammatory index was defined as the mean number of perivascular infiltrates within the SC parenchyma of 8–10 spinal cross sections per animal. All the images were prepared in Adobe Photoshop CS4 Version 11.0.2.

Statistical analysis

Statistical analyses were carried out using Microsoft Office Excel 2007 and GraphPad Prism (GraphPad Software, La Jolla, USA). After normality testing, an unpaired *t* test was applied to determine potential differences in the mean clinical severity scores of WT and Wld^S mice at day 20 and day 40 after disease onset. Histological data were analyzed by the non-parametric Mann-Whitney *U* test; animals in two groups (i.e., Wld^S and WT) were compared on the basis of closely matched clinical scores. The influence of genotype and disease stage on inflammation and demyelination was determined using a two-way-ANOVA. Statistical significance was defined as $p < 0.05$. All quantitative morphological data are expressed as mean ± standard error of the mean (SEM) in the EAE studies.

Results

Prevalence of Wallerian degeneration in patients with early- and late-stage multiple sclerosis

Wallerian degeneration is thought to reflect a clinically relevant component of disability and disease progression in multiple sclerosis. However, the contribution of Wallerian degeneration to multiple sclerosis pathology is not yet known. Here, we studied the occurrence and extent of Wallerian degeneration in biopsy multiple sclerosis tissue from patients with short duration as well as in autopsied patients with chronic multiple sclerosis. Using NPY-Y1R immunohistochemistry, Wallerian degeneration was quantified in areas of PPWM brain tissue from 31 multiple sclerosis patients. We observed widespread occurrence of NPY-Y1R^{+} degenerating axonal fibers in non-demyelinated PPWM areas in multiple sclerosis patients (Fig. 1). Patients were divided into early and chronic disease groups according to disease duration, i.e., time from the first symptoms to biopsy/autopsy. The number of NPY-Y1R^{+} axons in multiple sclerosis PPWM was significantly higher in the early as compared to the chronic disease stage (early; 113.6 ± 7, chronic; 4.6 ± 0.8 profiles/mm^2; $^{***}p < 0.001$). In early multiple sclerosis, the number of axons undergoing Wallerian degeneration was significantly higher in PPWM connected to active lesions as compared to early inactive lesions (PPWM-active; 129.1 ± 5, early inactive; 85.9 ± 5 profiles/mm^2; $^{**}p < 0.01$). Indeed, even in chronic disease stages, the number of axons undergoing Wallerian degeneration was significantly lower in PPWM areas of chronic inactive lesions (1.4 ± 0.6 profiles/mm^2) compared

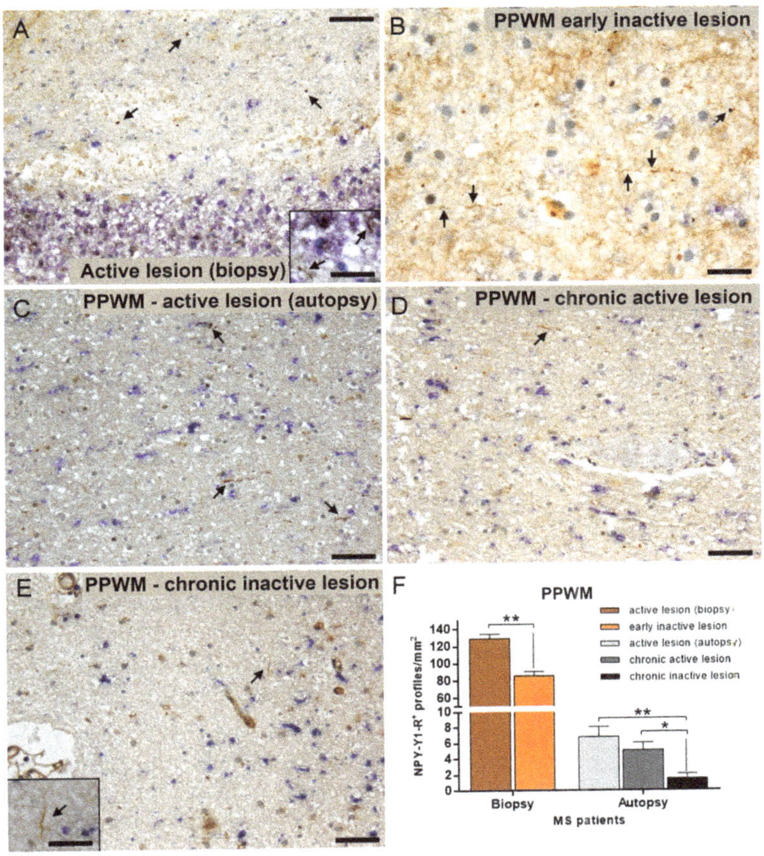

Fig. 1 Wallerian degeneration is most frequent in the PPWM of lesions with ongoing demyelinating activity. NPY-Y1R IHC was performed on multiple sclerosis biopsy and autopsy tissue samples containing active, early inactive, chronic active, and chronic inactive lesions (**a**–**e**). Double IHC of NPY-Y1R (*red*, **a**) with the pan-macrophage marker KiM1P (*blue*, **a**) showed very little evidence for Wallerian degeneration (*arrows*) in the actively demyelinating lesion edge of a multiple sclerosis biopsy (**a**, *inset*). The density of NPY-Y1R^{+} axonal profiles indicating Wallerian degeneration was significantly higher in PPWM areas of active and chronic active lesions compared to early inactive and chronic inactive lesions in both early and chronic multiple sclerosis patients (**f**). Significantly higher numbers of NPY-Y1R^{+} axonal profiles (*arrows*) were detected in the PPWM of early multiple sclerosis patients (biopsies; **a**–**b**, **f**) compared to chronic multiple sclerosis patients (autopsies; **c**–**f**). *Error bars*=SEM, $^{*}p < 0.05$, $^{**}p < 0.01$, $^{***}p < 0.001$. *Scale bars*; **a** 100 μm; **b** 25 μm, **c**–**e** 50 μm; (*inset* **a**, **e**) 10 μm

to PPWM of active (6.8 ± 1.3 profiles/mm^2; $^{**}p < 0.01$), and chronic active lesions (5.1 ± 0.9 profiles/mm^2; $^{*}p = 0.03$). Our findings in brains of patients with multiple sclerosis indicate a high incidence of Wallerian degeneration in early stages of multiple sclerosis, which may be related to axonal transections in focal demyelinated lesions.

No difference in MOG_{35-55} EAE course and severity between *Wld*^{S} and WT mice

To assess the impact of the *Wld*^{S} fusion gene on inflammatory disease severity, MOG_{35-55} EAE was induced in *Wld*^{S} mutant and WT C57BL/6 mice. No statistically significant difference in disease severity, i.e., mean disease score ± SD (standard deviation) was observed between *Wld*^{S} and WT mice on specifically testing the acute (day 20, $p = 0.94$) and chronic (day 40, $p = 0.85$) disease phase (Fig. 2) [26]. Also, the mean maximal cumulative score 40 days after disease onset was comparable in WT (2.5 ± 0.32) and *Wld*^{S} (2.31 ± 0.28) mice. A qualitative histopathological analysis revealed an increase in lesion sizes from day 20 to day 40 after disease onset in both experimental groups. Experiments were repeated at least three times, and consistent results were obtained.

Analysis of inflammation and demyelination in MOG_{35-55}-induced EAE in *Wld*^{S} and WT mice

Differences in lesion acuteness and extent of inflammation and demyelination might obscure differences in the extent of axonal vulnerability between the two mouse strains. We thus examined the number of perivascular and subpial inflammatory infiltrates per SC cross section (inflammatory index) and the percentage of demyelinated white matter in *Wld*^{S} vs. WT mice with acute EAE (Fig. 3a–f). The mean inflammatory index was 4.8 ± 0.8 in *Wld*^{S} and 4.9 ± 0.7 in WT mice (Fig. 3c); the mean demyelinated white matter area was $5.4 \pm 1.3\%$ in *Wld*^{S} and $5.7 \pm 0.7\%$ in WT mice (Fig. 3f). Inflammatory index and demyelination after immunization with MOG_{35-55} in *Wld*^{S} and WT mice were thus virtually the same, making a direct comparison of axonal pathology between the two mouse strains possible [27]. To ensure that lesions with similar inflammatory demyelinating activity were examined for axonal damage and loss, IHC for the early macrophage activation antigen S100A9 was performed, and all animals were found to have active lesions with recent monocyte invasion [28]. Also, morphometry on H&E and LFB/PAS stained sections of *Wld*^{S} and WT mice with chronic EAE revealed no significant differences with regard to inflammation (mean inflammatory index *Wld*^{S}; 1.3 ± 0.5 and WT; 1.4 ± 0.3 inflammatory infiltrates per spinal cord cross section) or demyelination (mean demyelinated white matter *Wld*^{S}; $3.3 \pm 1.2\%$ and WT; $2.7 \pm 0.9\%$) between the strains (Fig. 3g-l). However, a significant decrease in the extent of inflammation and a trend towards reduced demyelination from day 20 to day 40 after disease onset was observed for both experimental groups (two-way ANOVA; inflammatory index, F (1, 25), $p = 0.0002$); demyelination, F (1, 25), $p = 0.0519$).

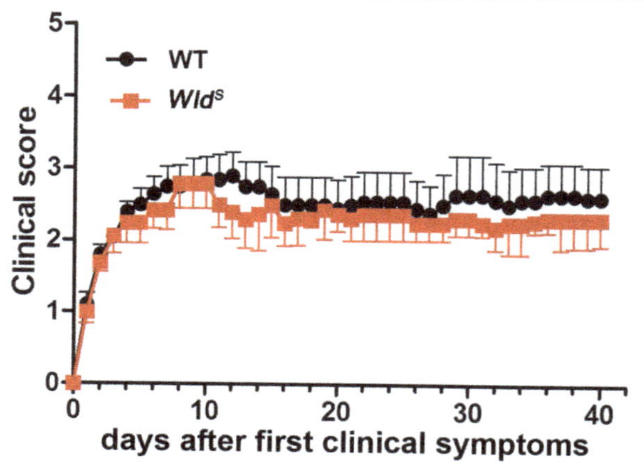

Fig. 2 The *Wld*^{S} mutation does not influence the clinical severity of EAE. EAE severity in *Wld*^{S} ($n = 18$) and WT ($n = 19$) mice was similar in both the acute and chronic disease stage. Mean disease score ± SD during 40 days after disease onset are shown. The graph contains scores from three independent experiments. The days after development of the first clinical symptoms are plotted on the *x*-axis

Similar amount of acute axonal damage in *Wld*^{S} and WT EAE mice

The clinical deficit in an acute inflammatory demyelinating disease may not reflect the extent of structural axonal damage due to the effects of cytokines and edema on ion homeostasis and axonal conduction. In fact, elevated cytokine levels in the CNS could affect neuroaxonal function and may at least be partly responsible for the clinical manifestations during acute exacerbation of multiple sclerosis and EAE [29, 30]. Therefore, to identify the extent of acute axonal damage in *Wld*^{S} mutant and WT mice, we applied antibodies to APP (Fig. 4a–d) to visualize axons with impaired axonal transport. In the acute as well as chronic disease stage, the densities of APP$^+$ axonal profiles in inflammatory demyelinated lesions did not differ between *Wld*^{S} and WT mice [*Wld*^{S}; 370 ± 58, WT; 424 ± 37 APP$^+$ profiles/mm^2 (acute, $p = 0.46$); *Wld*^{S}; 350 ± 47, WT; 387 ± 64 APP$^+$ profiles/mm^2 (chronic, $p = 0.79$)], thus indicating that axons are damaged to a similar degree in both mouse strains, irrespective of the genotype and disease phase (Fig. 4e).

Less Wallerian degeneration in the acute stage of EAE in *Wld*^{S} mutant mice

As characterized previously [31, 32], the NPY-Y1R antiserum recognized elongated and ovoid axonal structures in *Wld*^{S} and WT EAE mice (Fig. 4f–g). In acute disease,

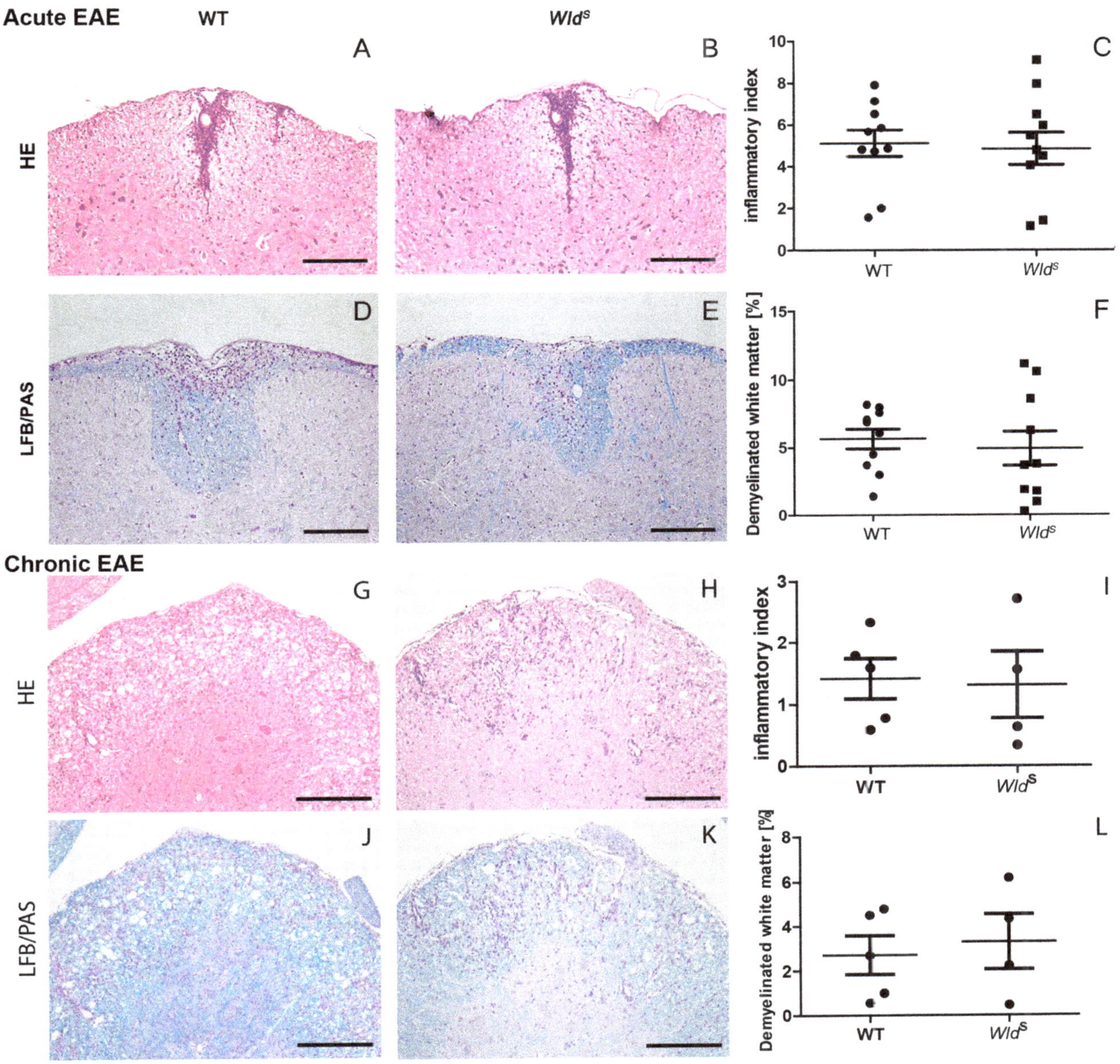

Fig. 3 Similar extent of inflammation and demyelination in *Wld^S* and WT mice in acute and chronic MOG_{35-55}-EAE. The mean number of inflammatory infiltrates per spinal cord (SC) cross section (H&E; **a**–**c**; **g**–**i**), and the percentage of demyelinated wh te matter (LFB/PAS; **d**–**f**; **j**–**l**) did not differ between *Wld^S* and WT mice in the acute as well as the chronic disease stage (d20 and d40). *Error bars*=SEM. *Scale bars*=(**a**, **b**, **d**, and **e**) 100 μm; (**g**, **h**, **j**, and **k**) 200 μm

a mean of 67 ± 13 NPY-Y1R$^+$ axonal profiles/mm^2 in *Wld^S* mutant mice and 1153 ± 241 NPY-Y1R$^+$ axonal profiles/mm^2 in WT mice were detected (Fig. 4f–g and j), indicating markedly reduced Wallerian degeneration in *Wld^S* mice in the acute phase of the disease (*$p = 0.02$). In contrast, no significant difference in Wallerian degeneration was observed in the chronic disease phase; 535 ± 154 NPY-Y1R$^+$ axonal profiles per square millimeter were detected in *Wld^S* mice and 633 ± 164 per mm^2 in *Wld^S* mice ($p = 0.69$) (Fig. 4h–j). Intriguingly, a significant increase in the densities of NPY-Y1R$^+$ axonal profiles was observed in chronic *Wld^S* EAE mice as compared to the acute stage (*$p = 0.03$). This implies that axon degenerative mechanisms in *Wld^S* mice are averted primarily during the acute stage of an autoimmune inflammatory demyelinating attack.

NPY-Y1R immunoreactivity specifically identifies Wallerian degeneration in EAE and stroke

To examine whether the Wallerian degeneration-induced expression of NPY-Y1R is associated with degenerating

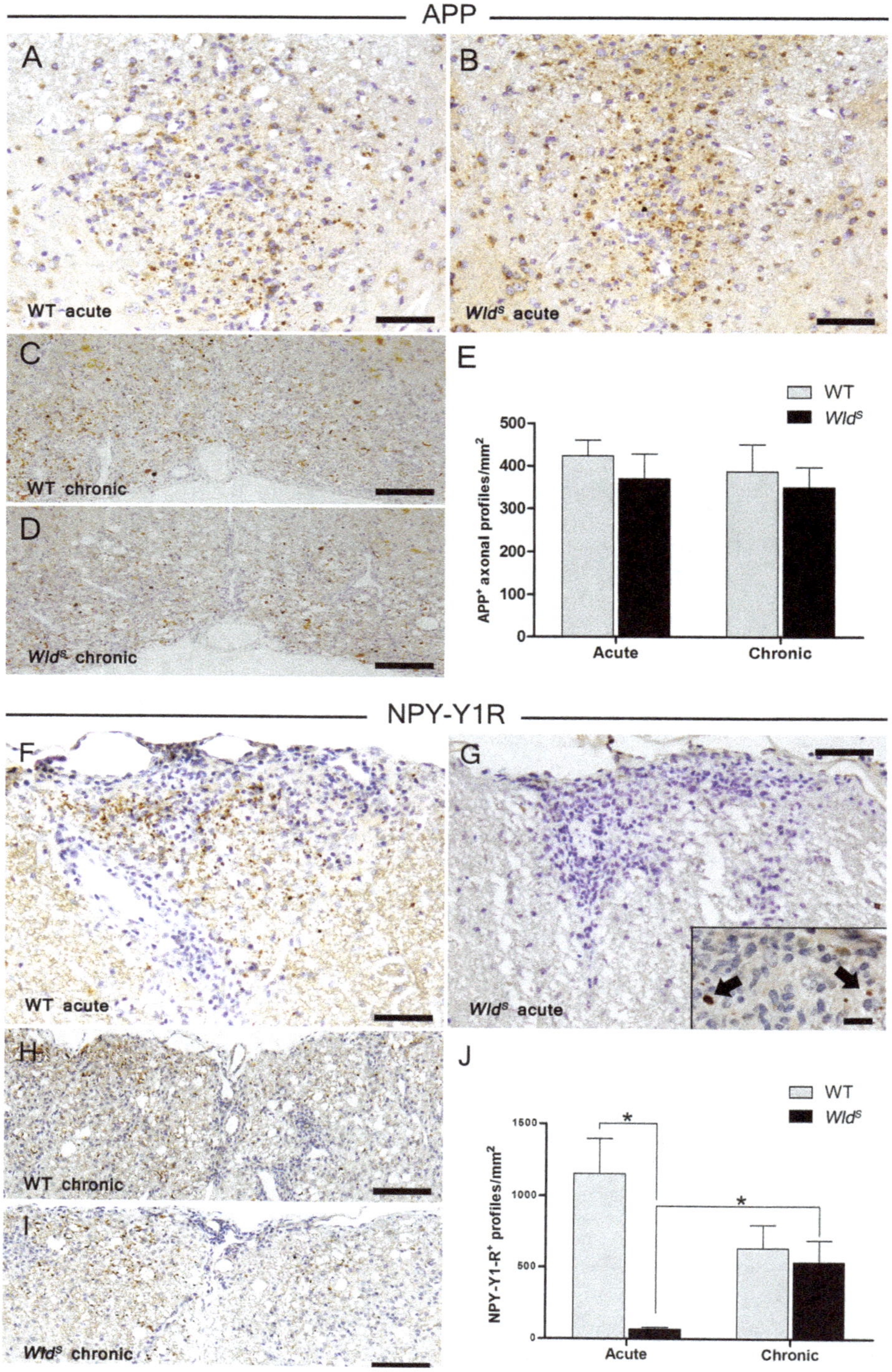

Fig. 4 Similar extent of acute axonal damage but markedly reduced Wallerian degeneration in *Wld*^{S} mice with acute EAE. Comparable densities of APP$^+$ axonal profiles were found in spinal EAE lesions of *Wld*^{S} and WT mice in both the acute and chronic disease stage (**a**–**e**). In contrast, significantly fewer NPY-Y1R$^+$ axonal profiles were observed in *Wld*^{S} as compared to WT mice in acute EAE (**f**–**g** and **j**). In the chronic stage, the densities of NPY-Y1R-immunoreactive axonal profiles were comparable between *Wld*^{S} and WT mice (**h**–**j**). *Error bars*=SEM, *$p < 0.05$, $n = 15$ animals per group. *Scale bars*=(**a**–**b**) 100 µm; (*inset* **b**) 50 µm; (**c**–**d**) 200 µm; (**f**–**g**) 150 µm; (**h**–**i**) 200 µm

axonal structures, immunofluorescence double labelings were performed in mouse EAE lesions (Fig. 5). We observed only rarely a co-localization of NPY-Y1R immunoreactivity with accumulated APP in axons (Fig. 5a–c). Also, NPY-Y1R expression did not co-localize with phosphorylated neurofilaments (NFs) of healthy axons detected by the SMI31 antibody (Fig. 5d–f), dephosphorylated NFs of damaged axons detected by the SMI32 antibody (Fig. 5g–i), and the low-molecular-weight NF-68 (Additional file 1). Hypophosphorylated NFs found in normal axons recognized by the SMI35 antibody were only occasionally co-localized with NPY-Y1R$^+$ axons (Additional file 1). However, substantial co-localization of NPY-Y1R was observed with the high-molecular-weight NF-200, detected by the N52 antibody (Fig. 5j–l, Table 2). Besides axonal degeneration, Wallerian degeneration is characterized by disintegration of myelin with the formation of the pathognomonic myelin ovoids [33]. Hence, to assess whether the antigen detected by the anti-NPY-Y1R antiserum is associated with myelin

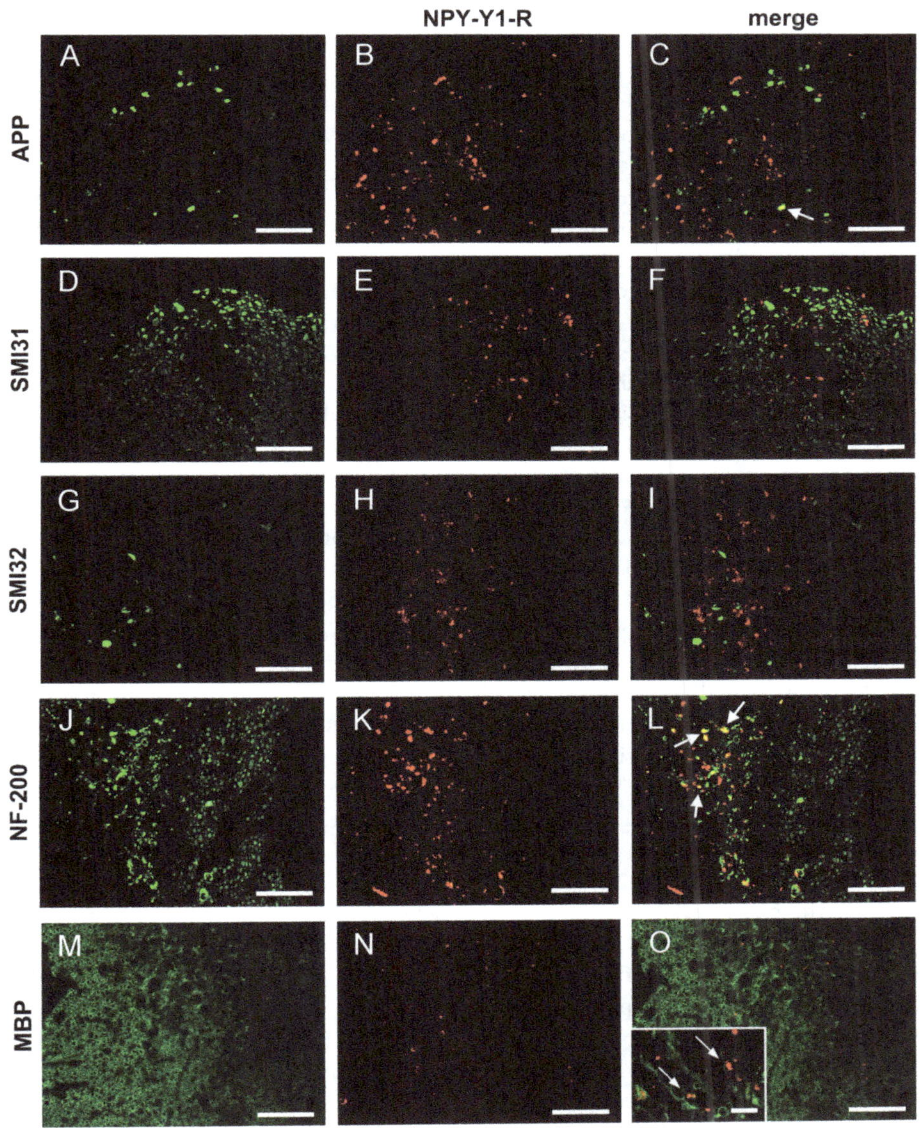

Fig. 5 NPY-Y1R does not co-localize with markers of axonal transport disturbance, neurofilament dephosphorylation or myelin proteins in EAE lesions. Immunofluorescence double labeling performed on EAE lesions in WT mice revealed only rare co-localization of NPY-Y1R (*red*) and early axonal transport deficits indicated by APP accumulation (*green*) (**a**–**c**, *arrow*). NPY-Y1R immunoreact vity also did not co-localize with phosphorylated neurofilaments (NF) of healthy axons (SMI31, *green*) (**d**–**f**) or de-, resp. non-phosphorylated NF predominantly found in damaged axons (SMI32, *green*) (**g**–**i**), but partly with the NF high molecular weight (NF-200, *green*) subunit (**j**–**l**, *arrows*). Double IHC of NPY-Y1R (**n**, *red*) with MBP (**m**, *green*) did not reveal any co-localization (**o**, *inset*). *Inset* in (**o**) shows NPY-Y1R$^+$ axons, in part enwrapped by myelin, at high magnification (*arrows*). *Scale bars*=(**a**–**o**) 200 μm; (*inset* **o**) 10 μm

ovoids, we performed fluorescent double IHC with antibodies against myelin basic protein (MBP), myelin proteolipid protein (PLP), MOG, myelin-associated glycoprotein (MAG), and 2′,3′-Cyclic-nucleotide 3′-phosphodiesterase (CNPase) in spinal EAE lesions from WT mice (Fig. 5m–o, Additional file 2). NPY-Y1R did not co-localize with any of the myelin proteins. In addition, to test whether this spatial co-localization pattern is also observed in areas of Wallerian degeneration after stroke, human ischemic brain lesions were double-labeled for NPY-Y1R and axonal markers (data not shown). In line with our findings in mouse EAE, co-localization of NPY-Y1R and NF-200 was observed, but not of NPY-Y1R and APP or SMI32.

NPY-Y1R$^+$ axonal structures are enwrapped by myelin in early experimental sciatic nerve transection

Wallerian degeneration after mouse sciatic nerve axotomy features a rapid degeneration of axons during the first 6 days after injury [34, 35]. Double immunofluorescence on mouse sciatic nerve 6 days after transection showed significantly more elongated and ovoid NPY-Y1R$^+$ axonal structures enwrapped by MBP$^+$ myelin sheaths than degenerated axons lacking any myelin (Additional file 3). This further supports that NPY-Y1R expression is present on axonal structures, but not myelin, in both the CNS and PNS, thus identifying comparatively early stages of Wallerian degeneration.

Axonal loss is similar in *Wld^S* and WT mice in the chronic disease phase

We hypothesized that the lower numbers of axons undergoing Wallerian degeneration in the early disease stage might lead to less net axonal loss in established EAE lesions of *Wld^S* mice. Healthy SMI31$^+$ axons as well as relative axonal densities (Bielschowsky silver impregnation) were determined in EAE lesions (Fig. 6). In the acute stage, the number of healthy SMI31$^+$ axons was significantly higher in *Wld^S* compared to WT lesions (*Wld^S*; 2658 ± 335, WT; 1156 ± 265 SMI31$^+$ profiles/mm^2; $^*p = 0.02$), whereas the counts were very similar in the chronic stage (*Wld^S*; 193 ± 21, WT; 173 ± 14 SMI31$^+$ profiles/mm^2; $p = 0.39$) (Fig. 6a and c). Furthermore, the densities of healthy axons in both genotypes were significantly higher in the acute compared to the chronic stage (*Wld^S*; $^*p = 0.03$; WT; $^*p = 0.01$). Importantly, axons after an inflammatory attack may become dephosphorylated but do not necessarily vanish. Therefore, we next quantified axons in defined lesion areas after Bielschowsky silver impregnation (Fig. 6b and d). Relative axonal densities were significantly higher in *Wld^S* mice than WT mice in the acute stage (*Wld^S*; 91.52 ± 2.3%, WT; 76.34 ± 2.3%; $^*p = 0.04$) but virtually identical in the chronic stage (*Wld^S*; 56.8 ± 8.4%, WT; 55.1 ± 11.6%; $p = 0.93$). Moreover, comparable with the SMI31$^+$ counts, relative axonal densities of silver impregnated axons in *Wld^S* mice were significantly lower in the chronic than in the acute stage ($^*p = 0.03$). This clearly indicates that the *Wld^S* mutation did not protect against long-term inflammatory axonal loss. Hence, consistent with other CNS lesion paradigms tested [36–38], our results suggest that also in inflammatory demyelination, Wallerian degeneration is merely slowed down or delayed in *Wld^S* mice.

Markers for axonal regeneration and synaptic plasticity are not co-expressed with NPY-Y1R in degenerating axons

De- and regenerative processes in axons may be closely related. We thus tested whether markers putatively associated with axonal regeneration are co-expressed with NPY-Y1R. Growth-associated protein 43 (GAP43) and synaptophysin (Syn) are synaptic proteins that are associated with axonal sprouting and synaptogenesis in various neurodegenerative diseases and may accumulate in regenerating neurons and axons. Therefore, expression of GAP43 and Syn in damaged axons could reflect a regenerative attempt [24]. However, immunofluorescence double labelings on WT EAE spinal lesions did not reveal any co-localizations of NPY-Y1R with GAP43 (Additional file 4 A-C) or Syn (Additional file 4 D-F).

Discussion

The extent of axonal loss is the most important predictor of permanent clinical deficits in multiple sclerosis [39–41]. Wallerian degeneration of axons transected in focal inflammatory demyelinated lesions contributes to the loss of neural structures. Here, we demonstrate a clear relationship between lesion demyelinating activity and Wallerian degeneration in non-demyelinated multiple sclerosis white matter. Furthermore, we find that the extent of Wallerian degeneration is most extensive in early disease stages supporting the interrelation between inflammation and neurodegeneration in multiple sclerosis [24, 42, 43]. In addition, in the present study, we hypothesized that *Wld^S* mutant mice would present with less axonal damage and reduced disability in MOG$_{35-55}$ EAE compared to WT mice. However, surprisingly, *Wld^S* and WT mice showed a similar disease course, and the degree of inflammation, demyelination, and acute axonal damage was comparable in the early as well as in the more advanced disease stage. Immunohistochemical staining with the anti-NPY-Y1R antibody demonstrated abundant Wallerian degeneration in WT mice in the early and chronic disease stage but identified only very few axons undergoing Wallerian degeneration in *Wld^S* mice in the acute disease stage. Furthermore, the net axonal loss was comparable in the chronic disease

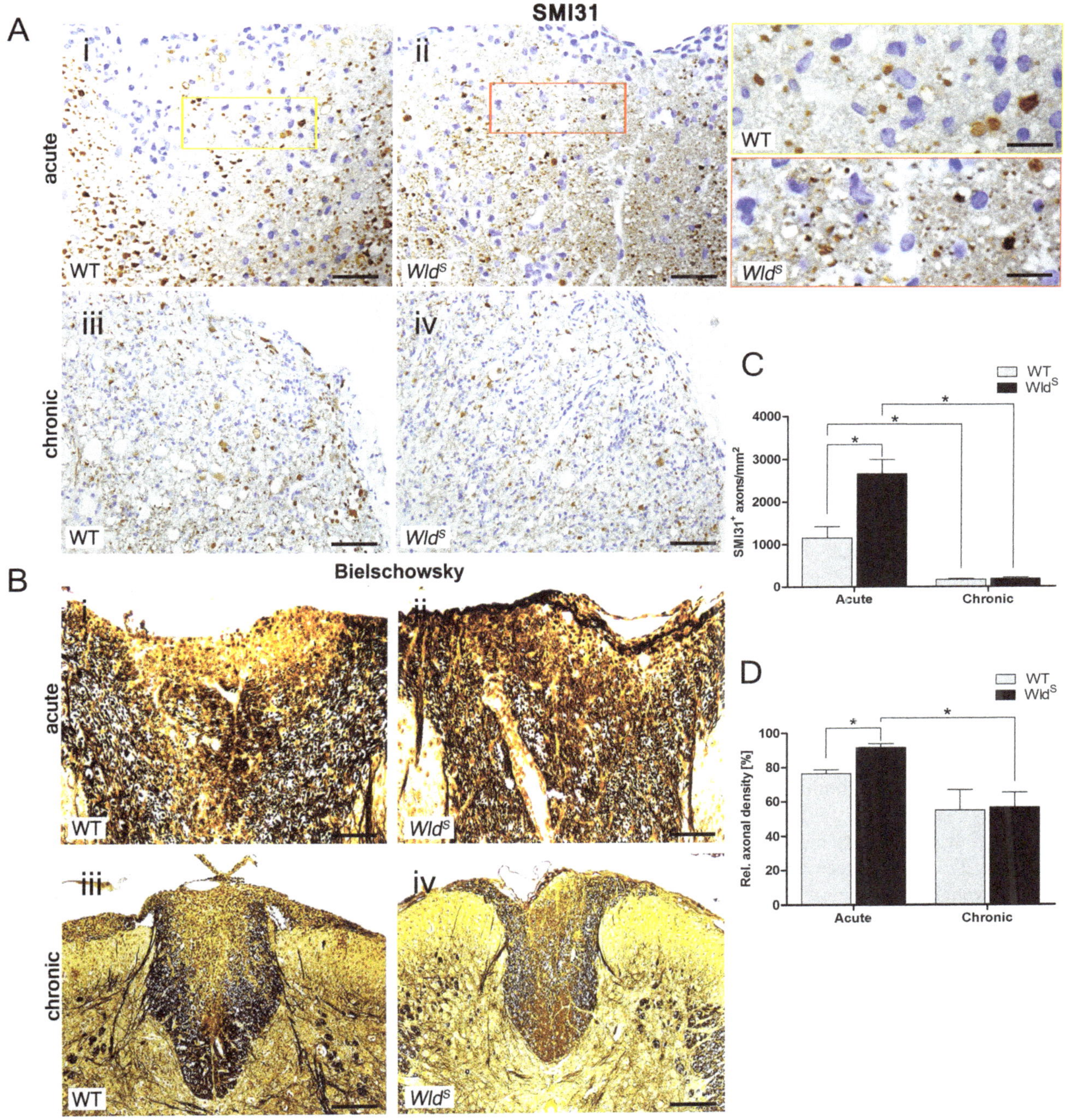

Fig. 6 Less axonal loss in the acute disease phase in *Wld^S* mutant mice. SC cross sections of *Wld^S* mutant and WT mice with EAE were stained with anti-SMI31 antibody (**a**) and Bielschowsky's silver impregnation (**b**) showing axonal loss in white matter lesions 20 days (acute) and 40 days (chronic) after disease onset. Quantification of SMI31$^+$ phosphorylated axons revealed that the densities of intact healthy axons were significantly higher in *Wld^S* mice as compared to WT mice in acute stage disease (**a** *i–ii*, **c**). However, similarly dense SMI31$^+$ profiles were observed in the chronic stage (**a** *iii–iv*; lateral funiculus, **c**). Densities of SMI31$^+$ profiles significantly decreased in both *Wld^S* and WT mice from the acute to the chronic disease stage (**a, c**). Similarly, Bielschowsky's silver impregnation displayed significantly higher relative axonal densities in *Wld^S* mice only in the acute stage (**b** *i–ii*, **d**); again, axonal loss in *Wld^S* mice was significantly more pronounced in the chronic than in the acute disease stage (**b**, **d**). *Yellow and red boxes* in (**a** *i–ii*) are higher magnifications of lesion areas with SMI31 immunostaining in acute disease. *Error bars*=SEM, $n = 15$ animals per group, $^*p < 0.05$. *Scale bars*=(**a** *i–ii*) 100 μm; (**a** *iii–iv*, **b** *i–ii*) 150 μm; (**b** *iii–iv*) 200 μm; (*insets* **a** *i–ii*) 25 μm

stage in both genotypes. Our data thus indicate that the *Wld*^{S} gene markedly delays Wallerian degeneration after inflammatory axonal damage but does not ameliorate disability resulting from EAE or cumulative axon loss.

Previous studies investigating axotomy-induced CNS Wallerian degeneration proposed three distinct phases: first, the sudden fragmentation (after 10–20 min) of both the distal and proximal axon close to the site of injury; second, the slow axonal retraction resulting in bulb formation at the axon ends with the distal stump remaining anatomically integrated and functional, and third, a proximal stable fragment while the distal fragment undergoes secondary degeneration, i.e., swelling, connection thinning, and rapid granularization [20, 44–47]. Convincing evidence for the distinct molecular basis of these processes was recently obtained in studies performed in *Wld*^{S} mutant mice. Kerschensteiner and colleagues could show that the *Wld*^{S} mutation prevented the onset of sudden fragmentation in transected CNS axons [20]. Also, expression of the *Wld*^{S} gene remarkably protracted the slow retraction phase in which the axon distal to the transection site remains morphologically intact and retains its physiologic function [34, 38, 48, 49].

Modulation of ion channels expressed in axons under inflammatory demyelinating conditions was shown to amend axonal degeneration [50–52]. Interestingly, it has been demonstrated that Wallerian degeneration of the distal stump is a Ca^{2+}-mediated process [53, 54]. The rise in intra-axonal ROS production in the distal stump after transection is diminished in the *Wld*^{S} mutation, which thus may entail preserved mitochondrial function and energy supply [55]. Hence, the fast fragmentation and slow retraction, but not the late rapid granularization, are ROS dependent. This is in agreement with the notion that the delay in axonal degeneration observed in *Wld*^{S} axons is only transient. Mitochondrial dysfunction, energy failure, and ensuing Ca^{2+} overload have been implicated as the final common pathways in inflammatory axonal damage, leading to the activation of intra-axonal proteases, cytoskeletal degradation, and axonal degeneration and loss [56, 57]. Therefore, the *Wld*^{S} mutation might be well suited to protect axons in an inflammatory demyelinating milieu, even beyond its well-described effect on the classical axonal self-destruction after transection. In our study, however, the densities of acutely damaged axons in inflammatory lesions were similar in *Wld*^{S} and WT mice, in both the acute and chronic disease stages, suggesting that the inflammatory insult surpassed the axonoprotective capacities of the *Wld*^{S} phenotype.

Our data show that the occurrence of Wallerian degeneration in multiple sclerosis is related to the density of axons with transport deficits observed in the tissue: Wallerian degeneration is most abundant in the periplaque white matter of patients early in the disease course harboring macrophage-rich focal lesions with ongoing myelin degradation. To the contrary, only few axons undergoing Wallerian degeneration were observed in late-stage patients with predominantly chronic inactive lesions. Noteworthy and as reported previously, chronic active lesions represent an area of ongoing demyelination and focal axonal degeneration [2, 14, 58]. In line, elevated levels of axons undergoing Wallerian degeneration were detected in the corresponding periplaque and normal-appearing white matter. Although our work cannot definitely exclude the presence of focal axonal degeneration in non-lesional areas, it clearly shows that the extent of Wallerian degeneration is related to focal demyelinating pathology. Furthermore, our work highlights the relevance of axonoprotective treatments, also in patients with more advanced disease, where smoldering lesions are most common.

Coleman and colleagues [59, 60] observed that the *Wld*^{S} mutation also inhibits degenerative axonal swellings in gracile axonal dystrophy (*gad*) mice, a mutant mouse strain characterized by a "dying-back" type axonal degeneration and the formation of axonal spheroids. In contrast, we studied axonal pathology under inflammatory demyelinating conditions. NOS and ROS released by activated macrophages have been implicated in acute axonal transport disturbance, even in myelinated axons, and may contribute to mitochondrial damage and Ca^{2+} overload, leading to a vicious cycle of energy failure and cytoskeletal degradation [10]. Our results suggest that the intra-axonal protective mechanisms operating in *Wld*^{S} mice, e.g., antioxidation and increased Ca^{2+} buffering capacity, are not sufficient to prevent or diminish axonal swellings during a myelin-specific T cell-mediated autoimmune attack. Prior studies showed that the *Wld*^{S} protection mechanism is intrinsic to the axon [47, 61, 62]. However, recently, an upregulation of CD200 was observed in *Wld*^{S} mice, which may play a critical role in reducing microglia-mediated neuroaxonal damage in the CNS [63–65]. Taken together, our results indicate that in inflammatory demyelination, axonal transport deficits and cumulative loss of axons are not restrained in *Wld*^{S} mice.

Irrespective of disease-related or mechanical transection of axons, the common downstream mechanisms of axonal degeneration include energy failure, increased Ca^{2+} influx and activation of calpains, resulting in the degradation of axon components [66–68]. As early as in the 1980s, it has been shown that NPY along with its Y1 receptor modulates increased Ca^{2+} concentrations in cultured dorsal root ganglion (DRG) neurons [69, 70]. NPY is widely distributed in the CNS and PNS, albeit NPY and its receptor Y1 are not expressed in the same population of neurons. However, both are upregulated in axonal processes of DRG neurons after nerve injury in rodents [71–74]. It seems therefore possible that NPY-Y1R plays a role in limiting the early destructive processes in damaged axons. In this study, we observed an important delay in NPY-Y1R expression in axons of *Wld^S^* mice with EAE, which is in line with the reduced Ca^{2+} influx in transected *Wld^S^* axons. Intriguingly, the increased Ca^{2+} buffering capacity of *Wld^S^* mitochondria shows a gradual decrease over time in the distal stump [53]. Hence, the intra-axonal protective mechanisms appear to decrease with time after transection in *Wld^S^* axons. Indeed, we observed substantially decreased immunoreactivity of NPY-Y1R in inflammatory SC lesions of *Wld^S^* mice in the acute stage as compared to the chronic stage. Our results thus support the use of anti-NPY-Y1R antibodies as a bona fide marker for Wallerian degeneration.

Conclusions

The present study provides evidence that axonal degeneration in multiple sclerosis is closely related to the occurrence of focal axonal transport disturbances, to focal demyelination and thus to phagocyte activation. Our experimental data indicate that the *Wld^S^* phenotype does not prevent axonal swellings in inflammatory demyelination and fails to provide sufficient long-term protection of CNS axons in a model of multiple sclerosis. Although we observed an important delay in Wallerian degeneration, this did not result in disease attenuation or a net rescue of axons in *Wld^S^* mice. Hence, in our model, a delay in Wallerian degeneration does not correlate with immediate clinical amelioration of inflammatory axon damage. Further molecular studies into the axonoprotective mechanisms elicited in the *Wld^S^* mutant are required to find a way to impede axonal degeneration and eventually restore axonal integrity and function.

Additional files

Additional file 1: NPY-Y1R+ axon undergoing Wallerian degeneration do not co-localize with hypophosphorylated and low-molecular-weight NF in EAE. Double-labeling fluorescent IHC reveals that NPY-Y1R$^+$ degenerating axons are only rarely labeled with antibodies recognizing hypophosphorylated NF (SMI35) (A-C). No colocalization is observed with the 68 kDa low-molecular-weight NF (D-F) in WT EAE lesional and perilesional tissue. *Scale bars*=(A-F) 100 μm.

Additional file 2: Axons undergoing Wallerian degeneration are at least in part myelinated in EAE lesions. No co-localization of NPY-Y1R immunoreactivity with myelin proteins, i.e., PLP (A-C), MOG (D-F), MAG (G-I), and CNPase (J-L) was observed by fluorescence double IHC in WT EAE mice, which further confirms that the antiserum against NPY-Y1R applied does not detect an antigen situated within the myelin sheath or myelin ovoids. Insets in (A-C) represent NPY-Y1R$^+$ degenerating fiber(s) in largely intact myelinated tracts, as determined by anti-PLP IHC. *Scale bars*=(A-L) 200 μm; (insets A-C) 10 μm.

Additional file 3: NPY-Y1R IHC labels myelin ovoids typical of Wallerian degeneration in mouse sciatic nerve transection. Elongated, beaded NPY-Y1R$^+$ (red, A) axonal structures surrounded by MBP$^+$ myelin sheaths (green, B) are seen in longitudinal sections of mouse sciatic nerve 6 days after and distal to the transection (C, arrows). Oil-immersion magnification (×1000) revealed that NPY-Y1R$^+$ axons were enwrapped with myelin (MBP) indicating myelin ovoid formation, typical of Wallerian degeneration (D-F). ($p < 0.05$; G). *Scale bars*=(A-C) 100 μm; (D-F) 20 μm.

Additional file 4: Neuroaxonal regenerative markers are not co-expressed in axons undergoing Wallerian degeneration. Axonal structures immunopositive for GAP43 (A-C) and Synaptophysin (Syn) (D-F) did not co-localize with NPY-Y1R$^+$ degenerating axons in WT EAE lesions by immunofluorescent double labeling. Syn expression was mostly limited to gray matter regions of the SC in WT EAE. *Scale bars*=(A-F) 100 μm.

Abbreviations

APP: Amyloid precursor protein; EAE: Experimental autoimmune encephalomyelitis; NAWM: Normal-appearing white matter; NPY-Y1R: Neuropeptide Y-Y1 receptor; PPWM: Periplaque white matter; *Wld^S^*: Wallerian degeneration slow

Acknowledgements

We thank Katja Schulz for expert technical assistance and Cynthia Bunker for language editing.

Funding

This work was supported by the Deutsche Forschungsgemeinschaft (DFG) Transregional Collaborative Research group (TRR-SFB) 43 "The brain as a target of inflammatory processes" (CS and WB) and the Gemeinnützige Hertie Foundation (to CS). SS was supported by a European Union (ENC-Network) grant.

Authors' contributions

SS and TD analyzed the data and wrote the manuscript. SS, TD, SR, AW, BM, and HS performed the experiments. SS, TD, AW, WB, and CS participated in the design, analyzed the data, and prepared the figures. WB and CS supervised the study and reviewed the manuscript. All authors contributed to discussion of the results and edited and approved the final version.

Competing interests

The authors declare that they have no competing interests.

Consent for publication

Not applicable.

Author details

[1]Institute of Neuropathology, University Medical Center, Göttingen, Germany. [2]Cellular Microbiology, Research Center Borstel, Borstel, Germany. [3]Department of Neurology, Rigshospitalet. Copenhagen, Denmark.

References

1. De Stefano N, Matthews PM, Antel JP, Preul M, Francis G, Arnold DL. Chemical pathology of acute demyelinating lesions and its correlation with disability. Ann Neurol. 1995;38:901–9.
2. Ferguson B, Matyszak MK, Esiri MM, Perry VH. Axonal damage in acute multiple sclerosis lesions. Brain. 1997;120(Pt 3):393–9.
3. Trapp BD, Peterson J, Ransohoff RM, Rudick R, Mork S, Bo L. Axonal transection in the lesions of multiple sclerosis. N Engl J Med.

1998;338:278–85.
4. Losseff NA, Webb SL, O'Riordan JI, Page R, Wang L, Barker GJ, Tofts PS, McDonald WI, Miller DH, Thompson AJ. Spinal cord atrophy and disability in multiple sclerosis. A new reproducible and sensitive MRI method with potential to monitor disease progression. Brain. 1996;119(Pt 3):701–8.
5. Tallantyre EC, Bo L, Al-Rawashdeh O, Owens T, Polman CH, Lowe JS, Evangelou N. Clinico-pathological evidence that axonal loss underlies disability in progressive multiple sclerosis. Mult Scler. 2010;16:406–11.
6. Mahad DH, Trapp BD, Lassmann H. Pathological mechanisms in progressive multiple sclerosis. Lancet Neurol. 2015;14:183–93.
7. Kearney H, Miller DH, Ciccarelli O. Spinal cord MRI in multiple sclerosis—diagnostic, prognostic and clinical value. Nat Rev Neurol. 2015;11:327–38.
8. Tallantyre EC, Bo L, Al-Rawashdeh O, Owens T, Polman CH, Lowe J, Evangelou N. Greater loss of axons in primary progressive multiple sclerosis plaques compared to secondary progressive disease. Brain. 2009;132:1190–9.
9. Simons M, Misgeld T, Kerschensteiner M. A unified cell biological perspective on axon-myelin injury. J Cell Biol. 2014;206:335–45.
10. Nikic I, Merkler D, Sorbara C, Brinkoetter M, Kreutzfeldt M, Bareyre FM, Bruck W, Bishop D, Misgeld T, Kerschensteiner M. A reversible form of axon damage in experimental autoimmune encephalomyelitis and multiple sclerosis. Nat Med. 2011;17:495–9.
11. Gentleman SM, Nash MJ, Sweeting CJ, Graham DI, Roberts GW. Beta-amyloid precursor protein (beta APP) as a marker for axonal injury after head injury. Neurosci Lett. 1993;160:139–44.
12. Kuhlmann T, Lingfeld G, Bitsch A, Schuchardt J, Bruck W. Acute axonal damage in multiple sclerosis is most extensive in early disease stages and decreases over time. Brain. 2002;125:2202–12.
13. Kutzelnigg A, Lucchinetti CF, Stadelmann C, Bruck W, Rauschka H, Bergmann M, Schmidbauer M, Parisi JE, Lassmann H. Cortical demyelination and diffuse white matter injury in multiple sclerosis. Brain. 2005;128:2705–12.
14. Frischer JM, Bramow S, Dal-Bianco A, Lucchinetti CF, Rauschka H, Schmidbauer M, Laursen H, Sorensen PS, Lassmann H. The relation between inflammation and neurodegeneration in multiple sclerosis brains. Brain. 2009;132:1175–89.
15. Bitsch A, Schuchardt J, Bunkowski S, Kuhlmann T, Bruck W. Acute axonal injury in multiple sclerosis. Correlation with demyelination and inflammation. Brain. 2000;123(Pt 6):1174–83.
16. Pfeifenbring S, Bunyan RF, Metz I, Rover C, Huppke P, Gartner J, Lucchinetti CF, Bruck W. Extensive acute axonal damage in pediatric multiple sclerosis lesions. Ann Neurol. 2015;77:655–67.
17. Sorbara CD, Wagner NE, Ladwig A, Nikic I, Merkler D, Kleele T, Marinkovic P, Naumann R, Godinho L, Bareyre FM, et al. Pervasive axonal transport deficits in multiple sclerosis models. Neuron. 2014;84:1183–90.
18. Smith KJ, Lassmann H. The role of nitric oxide in multiple sclerosis. Lancet Neurol. 2002;1:232–41.
19. Haider L, Fischer MT, Frischer JM, Bauer J, Hoftberger R, Botond G, Esterbauer H, Binder CJ, Witztum JL, Lassmann H. Oxidative damage in multiple sclerosis lesions. Brain. 2011;134:1914–24.
20. Kerschensteiner M, Schwab ME, Lichtman JW, Misgeld T. In vivo imaging of axonal degeneration and regeneration in the injured spinal cord. Nat Med. 2005;11:572–7.
21. Marinkovic P, Reuter MS, Brill MS, Godinho L, Kerschensteiner M, Misgeld T. Axonal transport deficits and degeneration can evolve independently in mouse models of amyotrophic lateral sclerosis. Proc Natl Acad Sci U S A. 2012;109:4296–301.
22. Kutzelnigg A, Lassmann H. Pathology of multiple sclerosis and related inflammatory demyelinating diseases. Handb Clin Neurol. 2014;122:15–58.
23. Bruck W, Porada P, Poser S, Rieckmann P, Hanefeld F, Kretzschmar HA, Lassmann H. Monocyte/macrophage differentiation in early multiple sclerosis lesions. Ann Neurol. 1995;38:788–96.
24. Schirmer L, Albert M, Buss A, Schulz-Schaeffer WJ, Antel JP, Bruck W, Stadelmann C. Substantial early, but nonprogressive neuronal loss in multiple sclerosis (MS) spinal cord. Ann Neurol. 2009;66:698–704.
25. Bruck W, Bitsch A, Kolenda H, Bruck Y, Stiefel M, Lassmann H. Inflammatory central nervous system demyelination: correlation of magnetic resonance imaging findings with lesion pathology. Ann Neurol. 1997;42:783–93.
26. Kaneko S, Wang J, Kaneko M, Yiu G, Hurrell JM, Chitnis T, Khoury SJ, He Z. Protecting axonal degeneration by increasing nicotinamide adenine dinucleotide levels in experimental autoimmune encephalomyelitis models. J Neurosci. 2006;26:9794–804.
27. Takada H, Yuasa S, Araki T. Demyelination can proceed independently of axonal degradation during Wallerian degeneration in wlds mice. Eur J Neurosci. 2011;34:531–7.
28. Nogai A, Siffrin V, Bonhagen K, Pfueller CF, Hohnstein T, Volkmer-Engert R, Bruck W, Stadelmann C, Kamradt T. Lipopolysaccharide injection induces relapses of experimental autoimmune encephalomyelitis in nontransgenic mice via bystander activation of autoreactive CD4+ cells. J Immunol. 2005;175:959–66.
29. Maimone D, Gregory S, Arnason BG, Reder AT. Cytokine levels in the cerebrospinal fluid and serum of patients with multiple sclerosis. J Neuroimmunol. 1991;32:67–74.
30. Czirr E, Wyss-Coray T. The immunology of neurodegeneration. J Clin Invest. 2012;122:1156–63.
31. Dziedzic T, Metz I, Dallenga T, Konig FB, Muller S, Stadelmann C, Bruck W. Wallerian degeneration: a major component of early axonal pathology in multiple sclerosis. Brain Pathol. 2010;20:976–85.
32. Singh S, Metz I, Amor S, van der Valk P, Stadelmann C, Bruck W. Microglial nodules in early multiple sclerosis white matter are associated with degenerating axons. Acta Neuropathol. 2013;125:595–608.
33. Vargas ME, Barres BA. Why is Wallerian degeneration in the CNS so slow? Annu Rev Neurosci. 2007;30:153–79.
34. Perry VH, Brown MC, Lunn ER. Very slow retrograde and wallerian degeneration in the CNS of C57BL/Ola mice. Eur J Neurosci. 1991;3:102–5.
35. Siebert H, Bruck W. The role of cytokines and adhesion molecules in axon degeneration after peripheral nerve axotomy: a study in different knockout mice. Brain Res. 2003;960:152–6.
36. Waxman SG, Black JA, Ransom BR, Stys PK. Protection of the axonal cytoskeleton in anoxic optic nerve by decreased extracellular calcium. Brain Res. 1993;614:137–45.
37. George EB, Glass JD, Griffin JW. Axotomy-induced axonal degeneration is mediated by calcium influx through ion-specific channels. J Neurosci. 1995;15:6445–52.
38. Mack TG, Reiner M, Beirowski B, Mi W, Emanuelli M, Wagner D, Thomson D, Gillingwater T, Court F, Conforti L, et al. Wallerian degeneration of injured axons and synapses is delayed by a Ube4b/Nmnat chimeric gene. Nat Neurosci. 2001;4:1199–206.
39. Bjartmar C, Kidd G, Mork S, Rudick R, Trapp BD. Neurological disability correlates with spinal cord axonal loss and reduced N-acetyl aspartate in chronic multiple sclerosis patients. Ann Neurol. 2000;48:893–901.
40. De Stefano N, Narayanan S, Francis SJ, Smith S, Mortilla M, Tartaglia MC, Bartolozzi ML, Guidi L, Federico A, Arnold DL. Diffuse axonal and tissue injury in patients with multiple sclerosis with low cerebral lesion load and no disability. Arch Neurol. 2002;59:1565–71.
41. Filippi M, Bozzali M, Rovaris M, Gonen O, Kesavadas C, Ghezzi A, Martinelli V, Grossman RI, Scotti G, Comi G, Falini A. Evidence for widespread axonal damage at the earliest clinical stage of multiple sclerosis. Brain. 2003;126:433–7.
42. Vogt J, Paul F, Aktas O, Muller-Wielsch K, Dorr J, Dorr S, Bharathi BS, Glumm R, Schmitz C, Steinbusch H, et al. Lower motor neuron loss in multiple sclerosis and experimental autoimmune encephalomyelitis. Ann Neurol. 2009;66:310–22.
43. Ellwardt E, Zipp F. Molecular mechanisms linking neuroinflammation and neurodegeneration in MS. Exp Neurol. 2014;262 Pt A:8–17.
44. Lubinska L. Patterns of Wallerian degeneration of myelinated fibres in short and long peripheral stumps and in isolated segments of rat phrenic nerve. Interpretation of the role of axoplasmic flow of the trophic factor. Brain Res. 1982;233:227–40.
45. Tsao JW, Brown MC, Carden MJ, McLean WG, Perry VH. Loss of the compound action potential: an electrophysiological, biochemical and morphological study of early events in axonal degeneration in the C57BL/Ola mouse. Eur J Neurosci. 1994;6:516–24.
46. Griffin JW, George EB, ST H, Glass JD. Axonal degeneration and disorders of the axonal cytoskeleton. In: Waxman SG, Kocsis JD, Stys PK, editors. The axon: structure, function and pathophysiology. NY: Oxford University Press; 1995. p. 3750–90.
47. Wang JT, Medress ZA, Barres BA. Axon degeneration: molecular mechanisms of a self-destruction pathway. J Cell Biol. 2012;196:7–18.
48. Tsao JW, George EB, Griffin JW. Temperature modulation reveals three distinct stages of Wallerian degeneration. J Neurosci. 1999;19:4718–26.
49. Gillingwater TH, Ribchester RR. Compartmental neurodegeneration and synaptic plasticity in the Wld(s) mutant mouse. J Physiol. 2001;534:627–39.

50. Craner MJ, Newcombe J, Black JA, Hartle C, Cuzner ML, Waxman SG. Molecular changes in neurons in multiple sclerosis: altered axonal expression of Nav1.2 and Nav1.6 sodium channels and Na+/Ca2+ exchanger. Proc Natl Acad Sci U S A. 2004;101:8168–73.
51. Friese MA, Craner MJ, Etzensperger R, Vergo S, Wemmie JA, Welsh MJ, Vincent A, Fugger L. Acid-sensing ion channel-1 contributes to axonal degeneration in autoimmune inflammation of the central nervous system. Nat Med. 2007;13:1483–9.
52. Schattling B, Steinbach K, Thies E, Kruse M, Menigoz A, Ufer F, Flockerzi V, Bruck W, Pongs O, Vennekens R, et al. TRPM4 cation channel mediates axonal and neuronal degeneration in experimental autoimmune encephalomyelitis and multiple sclerosis. Nat Med. 2012;18:1805–11.
53. Adalbert R, Morreale G, Paizs M, Conforti L, Walker SA, Roderick HL, Bootman MD, Siklos L, Coleman MP. Intra-axonal calcium changes after axotomy in wild-type and slow Wallerian degeneration axons. Neuroscience. 2012;225:44–54.
54. Avery MA, Rooney TM, Pandya JD, Wishart TM, Gillingwater TH, Geddes JW, Sullivan PG, Freeman MR. WldS prevents axon degeneration through increased mitochondrial flux and enhanced mitochondrial Ca2+ buffering. Curr Biol. 2012;22:596–600.
55. O'Donnell KC, Vargas ME, Sagasti A. WldS and PGC-1alpha regulate mitochondrial transport and oxidation state after axonal injury. J Neurosci. 2013;33:14778–90.
56. Breckwoldt MO, Pfister FM, Bradley PM, Marinkovic P, Williams PR, Brill MS, Plomer B, Schmalz A, St Clair DK, Naumann R, et al. Multiparametric optical analysis of mitochondrial redox signals during neuronal physiology and pathology in vivo. Nat Med. 2014;20:555–60.
57. Friese MA, Schattling B, Fugger L. Mechanisms of neurodegeneration and axonal dysfunction in multiple sclerosis. Nat Rev Neurol. 2014;10:225–38.
58. Prineas JW, Kwon EE, Cho ES, Sharer LR, Barnett MH, Oleszak EL, Hoffman B, Morgan BP. Immunopathology of secondary-progressive multiple sclerosis. Ann Neurol. 2001;50:646–57.
59. Mi W, Beirowski B, Gillingwater TH, Adalbert R, Wagner D, Grumme D, Osaka H, Conforti L, Arnhold S, Addicks K, et al. The slow Wallerian degeneration gene, WldS, inhibits axonal spheroid pathology in gracile axonal dystrophy mice. Brain. 2005;128:405–16.
60. Beirowski B, Nogradi A, Babetto E, Garcia-Alias G, Coleman MP. Mechanisms of axonal spheroid formation in central nervous system Wallerian degeneration. J Neuropathol Exp Neurol. 2010;69:455–72.
61. Glass JD, Brushart TM, George EB, Griffin JW. Prolonged survival of transected nerve fibres in C57BL/Ola mice is an intrinsic characteristic of the axon. J Neurocytol. 1993;22:311–21.
62. Raff MC, Whitmore AV, Finn JT. Axonal self-destruction and neurodegeneration. Science. 2002;296:868–71.
63. Wright GJ, Cherwinski H, Foster-Cuevas M, Brooke G, Puklavec MJ, Bigler M, Song Y, Jenmalm M, Gorman D, McClanahan T, et al. Characterization of the CD200 receptor family in mice and humans and their interactions with CD200. J Immunol. 2003;171:3034–46.
64. Hoek RM, Ruuls SR, Murphy CA, Wright GJ, Goddard R, Zurawski SM, Blom B, Homola ME, Streit WJ, Brown MH, et al. Down-regulation of the macrophage lineage through interaction with OX2 (CD200). Science. 2000;290:1768–71.
65. Chitnis T, Imitola J, Wang Y, Elyaman W, Chawla P, Sharuk M, Raddassi K, Bronson RT, Khoury SJ. Elevated neuronal expression of CD200 protects Wlds mice from inflammation-mediated neurodegeneration. Am J Pathol. 2007;170:1695–712.
66. Coleman M. Axon degeneration mechanisms: commonality amid diversity. Nat Rev Neurosci. 2005;6:889–98.
67. Barrientos SA, Martinez NW, Yoo S, Jara JS, Zamorano S, Hetz C, Twiss JL, Alvarez J, Court FA. Axonal degeneration is mediated by the mitochondrial permeability transition pore. J Neurosci. 2011;31:966–78.
68. Stirling DP, Cummins K, Wayne Chen SR, Stys P. Axoplasmic reticulum Ca(2+) release causes secondary degeneration of spinal axons. Ann Neurol. 2014;75:220–9.
69. Walker MW, Ewald DA, Perney TM, Miller RJ. Neuropeptide Y modulates neurotransmitter release and Ca2+ currents in rat sensory neurons. J Neurosci. 1988;8:2438–46.
70. Perney TM, Miller RJ. Two different G-proteins mediate neuropeptide Y and bradykinin-stimulated phospholipid breakdown in cultured rat sensory neurons. J Biol Chem. 1989;264:7317–27.
71. Dumont Y, Martel JC, Fournier A, St-Pierre S, Quirion R. Neuropeptide Y and neuropeptide Y receptor subtypes in brain and peripheral tissues. Prog Neurobiol. 1992;38:125–67.
72. Wahlestedt C, Reis DJ. Neuropeptide Y-related peptides and their receptors—are the receptors potential therapeutic drug targets? Annu Rev Pharmacol Toxicol. 1993;33:309–52.
73. Brumovsky PR, Shi TJ, Matsuda H, Kopp J, Villar MJ, Hokfelt T. NPY Y1 receptors are present in axonal processes of DRG neurons. Exp Neurol. 2002;174:1–10.
74. Obata K, Yamanaka H, Dai Y, Mizushima T, Fukuoka T, Tokunaga A, Noguchi K. Differential activation of MAPK in injured and uninjured DRG neurons following chronic constriction injury of the sciatic nerve in rats. Eur J Neurosci. 2004;20:2881–95.
75. Wrzos C, Winkler A, Metz I, Kayser DM, Thal DR, Wegner C, Bruck W, Nessler S, Bennett JL, Stadelmann C. Early loss of oligodendrocytes in human and experimental neuromyelitis optica lesions. Acta Neuropathol. 2014;127:523–38.
76. Matthieu JM, Waehneldt TV, Eschmann N. Myelin-associated glycoprotein and myelin basic protein are present in central and peripheral nerve myelin throughout phylogeny. Neurochem Int. 1986;8:521–6.
77. Radzun HJ, Hansmann ML, Heidebrecht HJ, Bodewadt-Radzun S, Wacker HH, Kreipe H, Lumbeck H, Hernandez C, Kuhn C, Parwaresch MR. Detection of a monocyte/macrophage differentiation antigen in routinely processed paraffin-embedded tissues by monoclonal antibody Ki-M1P. Lab Invest. 1991;65:306–15.
78. Nacken W, Sopalla C, Propper C, Sorg C, Kerkhoff C. Biochemical characterization of the murine S100A9 (MRP14) protein suggests that it is functionally equivalent to its human counterpart despite its low degree of sequence homology. Eur J Biochem. 2000;267:560–5.

15

[^{18}F]FSPG-PET reveals increased cystine/glutamate antiporter (xc-) activity in a mouse model of multiple sclerosis

Aileen Hoehne[1†], Michelle L. James[1,2†], Israt S. Alam[1], John A. Ronald[1], Bernadette Schneider[1], Aloma D'Souza[1], Timothy H. Witney[1], Lauren E. Andrews[1], Haley C. Cropper[1], Deepak Behera[1], Gayatri Gowrishankar[1], Zhaoqing Ding[2], Tony Wyss-Coray[2], Frederick T. Chin[1], Sandip Biswal[1] and Sanjiv S. Gambhir[1,3*]

Abstract

Background: The cystine/glutamate antiporter (xc-) has been implicated in several neurological disorders and, specifically, in multiple sclerosis (MS) as a mediator of glutamate excitotoxicity and proinflammatory immune responses. We aimed to evaluate an xc-specific positron emission tomography (PET) radiotracer, (4*S*)-4-(3-[^{18}F]fluoropropyl)-L-glutamate ([^{18}F]FSPG), for its ability to allow non-invasive monitoring of xc- activity in a mouse model of MS.

Methods: Experimental autoimmune encephalomyelitis (EAE) was induced in C57BL/6 mice by subcutaneous injection of myelin oligodendrocyte glycoprotein (MOG_{35-55}) peptide in complete Freund's adjuvant (CFA) followed by pertussis toxin. Control mice received CFA emulsion and pertussis toxin without MOG peptide, while a separate cohort of naïve mice received no treatment. PET studies were performed to investigate the kinetics and distribution of [^{18}F]FSPG in naïve, control, pre-symptomatic, and symptomatic EAE mice, compared to ^{18}F-fluorodeoxyglucose ([^{18}F]FDG). After final PET scans, each mouse was perfused and radioactivity in dissected tissues was measured using a gamma counter. Central nervous system (CNS) tissues were further analyzed using ex vivo autoradiography or western blot. [^{18}F]FSPG uptake in human monocytes, and T cells pre- and post-activation was investigated in vitro.

Results: [^{18}F]FSPG was found to be more sensitive than [^{18}F]FDG at detecting pathological changes in the spinal cord and brain of EAE mice. Even before clinical signs of disease, a small but significant increase in [^{18}F]FSPG signal was observed in the spinal cord of EAE mice compared to controls. This increase in PET signal became more pronounced in symptomatic EAE mice and was confirmed by ex vivo biodistribution and autoradiography. Likewise, in the brain of symptomatic EAE mice, [^{18}F]FSPG uptake was significantly higher than controls, with the largest changes observed in the cerebellum. Western blot analyses of CNS tissues revealed a significant correlation between light chain of xc- (xCT) protein levels, the subunit of xc- credited with its transporter activity, and [^{18}F]FSPG-PET signal. In vitro [^{18}F]FSPG uptake studies suggest that both activated monocytes and T cells contribute to the observed in vivo PET signal.

Conclusion: These data highlight the promise of [^{18}F]FSPG-PET as a technique to provide insights into neuroimmune interactions in MS and the in vivo role of xc- in the development and progression of this disease, thus warranting further investigation.

Keywords: FSPG, PET, Multiple sclerosis, EAE mice, Xc-

* Correspondence: sgambhir@stanford.edu
†Equal contributors
[1]Molecular Imaging Program at Stanford (MIPS), Department of Radiology, Stanford University, Stanford, CA 94305, USA
[3]Department of Bioengineering, Department of Materials Science & Engineering, Stanford University, Stanford, CA 94305, USA

Background

The key pathological hallmarks of multiple sclerosis (MS) include demyelination, oligodendrocyte cell death, microglial activation, peripheral immune cell infiltration, and axonal degeneration in the central nervous system (CNS) [1]. Over the past two decades, an increasing amount of data has emerged suggesting that oxidative stress also plays a key role in the pathogenesis of MS [2]. It is known that upregulation of cystine/glutamate antiporter (xc-) is an oxidative stress response by cells in an attempt to increase availability of the glutathione biosynthesis precursor cystine for improved reactive oxygen species (ROS) detoxification [3]. Under certain pathological conditions accompanied by dysregulation of glutamate homeostasis, increased cystine influx through xc- leads to elevated extracellular levels of the neurotransmitter glutamate [4]. Glutamate excitotoxicity is known to contribute to oligodendrocyte and tissue damage in MS by over-activating glutamate receptors [5]. In 2011, Pampliega and colleagues reported that the light chain of the heterodimeric xc- transmembrane protein (known as xCT) responsible for its transporter activity is upregulated in the spinal cord of mice and rats with experimental autoimmune encephalomyelitis (EAE), the most widely characterized rodent model of MS, as well as human MS postmortem tissue [6]. A recent study by Merckx and colleagues suggests that it is the peripheral immune cells expressing xc-, known to infiltrate the CNS in MS, rather than the resident immune cells that directly contribute to glutamate release and excitotoxicity [7].

Recently, Martin and colleagues described the use of a previously reported ^{18}F-labeled small molecule xc- substrate—known as (4S)-4-(3-[^{18}F]fluoropropyl)-L-glutamate ([^{18}F]FSPG)—for imaging xc- activity in EAE rats using PET [8]. While these studies highlighted the promise of [^{18}F]FSPG-PET imaging as a non-invasive biomarker of MS disease status and for therapy monitoring, the authors did not investigate the relationship between the observed increased PET signal in EAE rats and levels of target expression. Here, we propose to expand upon our previous work with [^{18}F]FSPG in MS rodent models [9] by conducting the first investigation of correlation between [^{18}F]FSPG-PET signal and levels of xCT in EAE, alongside human immune cell uptake studies, with the aim of improving understanding of the molecular and cellular significance of [^{18}F]FSPG signal in EAE and MS. Since the Lewis rat model of EAE does not undergo demyelination [10] (a hallmark feature of human MS), we conducted [^{18}F]FSPG-PET imaging in an EAE mouse model that does undergo demyelination, with the aim of obtaining clinically relevant and translatable information concerning this tracer's potential use in MS.

The primary goal of the present studies was therefore to evaluate [^{18}F]FSPG for its ability to detect alterations in xc- antiporter activity in EAE mice at different stages of disease via PET imaging and to correlate PET findings with xCT protein levels in affected CNS tissues.

Methods

Study design

Since there were no prior reports of [^{18}F]FSPG-PET imaging in EAE mice, we began by performing pilot dynamic PET/CT imaging studies in symptomatic EAE (score 1.0–3.5) versus naive mice to gain an understanding of the in vivo distribution and kinetics of [^{18}F]FSPG. Next, we compared the uptake pattern of [^{18}F]FSPG with that of the widely used clinical PET tracer, ^{18}F-fluorodeoxyglucose ([^{18}F]FDG), previously shown to have increased uptake in activated immune cells and/or CNS lesions in EAE rodent models and MS patients [11, 12]. The utility of [^{18}F]FDG-PET in MS is limited due to the high/fluctuating basal uptake of this radiotracer in CNS tissues of MS patients, which generates ambiguity in the detection of [^{18}F]FDG accumulation in lesions [13, 14]; hence, the need to assess whether [^{18}F]FSPG uptake could serve as a more sensitive marker of pathological changes in CNS tissues of EAE mice.

Following these initial comparison studies, we performed longitudinal experiments to characterize [^{18}F]FSPG uptake in CNS tissues at the pre-symptomatic versus symptomatic stages of EAE disease and to examine the relationship between imaging signal and xCT protein levels. Lastly, as a prelude to future clinical studies with [^{18}F]FSPG, we investigated the uptake of [^{18}F]FSPG in activated human monocytes and T cells—which have both been implicated in the pathogenesis of EAE/MS. We chose to use human cells for these studies to add a translational dimension to our work with the goal of obtaining insights into the extent that specific immune cell types contribute to [^{18}F]FSPG-PET signal in MS.

Radiochemistry

[^{18}F]FSPG was synthesized according to previous methods [15] in 45–70 min with a radiochemical yield of 36 ± 17% (decay-corrected to end of bombardment), specific activity 48.47 ± 16.65 GBq/μmol (end of synthesis) and radiochemical purity > 90% ($n = 13$). Clinical grade [^{18}F]FDG was supplied by the Radiochemistry Facility at Stanford University.

EAE immunization

Animal procedures were approved by Stanford University Institutional Animal Care and Use Committee. Female C57BL/6 mice (10–12 weeks old) were immunized subcutaneously with 100 μg of myelin oligodendrocyte glycoprotein fragment$_{35-55}$ (MOG_{35-55}) peptide (Stanford Protein and Nucleic Acid Biotechnology Facility) emulsified in complete Freund's adjuvant (CFA; 200 µg mycobacterium tuberculosis, BD Difco Adjuvants). Mice received an intravenous injection of 100 ng pertussis toxin (List Biological Laboratories Inc.) at the time of immunization and 48 h later. Control mice received a CFA/PBS emulsion without MOG peptide and the same amount of pertussis toxin. Mice were weighed, examined daily for clinical signs of EAE, and scored according to the following criteria: score of 0, no paralysis; 0.5, partial loss of tail tone; 1, complete loss of tail tone; 1.5, complete tail paralysis accompanied by weakness in one hind limb; 2, hind limb weakness or paresis; 2.5, paralysis of at least one hind limb or no weight bearing on hind limbs (dragging) but with some leg movement; 3, complete hind limb paralysis; 3.5, hind limb paralysis, unable to right itself when placed on its side; 4, hind limb paralysis and forelimb paresis; 4.5, moribund; and 5, dead. Mice were euthanized at the end of the day once they reached a score of 4.0 and immediately after reaching 4.5.

PET imaging studies

Naïve, control, and EAE mice were administered [^{18}F]FSPG (~ 9.25 MBq) or [^{18}F]FDG (~ 4.63 MBq) via tail vein injection. Mice receiving [^{18}F]FDG were fasted 5–6 h prior to radiotracer administration and were all given an equal volume of saline i.p. to prevent dehydration. PET imaging of anesthetized mice (1–2% isoflurane) was performed using a microPET/CT hybrid scanner (Inveon, Siemens). All PET images were reconstructed using 2 iterations of three-dimensional ordered subset expectation maximization algorithm (12 subsets) and 18 iterations of the accelerated version of 3D-MAP (i.e., FASTMAP), with a matrix size of 128 × 128 × 159. Attenuation correction was applied to datasets from CT image acquired just prior to each PET scan. No partial volume corrections were performed. Dynamic PET scans were acquired in list mode format over 90 min, starting just prior to radiotracer injection. The resulting data was sorted into 0.5-mm sinogram bins and 19 time frames for image reconstruction (4 × 15 s, 4 × 60 s, 11 × 300 s). For subsequent studies, static PET scans (10 min) were acquired at ~ 70 min after injection of the radiotracer.

Image files were co-registered and analyzed with VivoQuant (version 2.0, inviCRO) (Additional file 1: Figure S1a–c). For VivoQuant analyses, the spine from each mouse was isolated by use of the Otsu thresholding technique and the obtained region of interest (ROI) made immutable. An ROI of the spinal cord was then drawn using the segmented spine as a guide. Corresponding PET data were collected for the whole spinal cord ROI, which was drawn from the caudal end of the skull to the pelvis. For analysis of regional variations in PET signal, the spinal cord was divided, using L1–L5 as landmarks, into two cervical/thoracic and lumbar ROIs, for which separate data were collected. For analysis of the brain, a three-dimensional mouse brain atlas was fitted to the PET/CT images and radioactivity concentrations were obtained using ROIs for the major brain regions (Additional file 1: Figure S1d). From this data, the percentage of injected dose per gram (%ID/g) was calculated for the spinal cord and atlas-based brain regions.

Tissue collection for ex vivo biodistribution, autoradiography, and Western assays

While still under anesthesia, blood samples (200–400 µL) were collected via cardiac puncture immediately prior to perfusing mice with PBS. After mice had been euthanized, tissues of interest were quickly removed at 110 min post-injection of tracer.

For ex vivo biodistribution assays, tissues were placed in tubes for gamma counting and weighed. Tissue-associated radioactivity was assessed via an automated gamma counter (Cobra II Auto-Gamma counter; Packard Biosciences Co.) and decay-corrected to time of tracer injection using diluted aliquots of the initial administered dose as standards.

A subset of the spinal cords and brains were analyzed via ex vivo digital autoradiography ($n = 1$ for EAE, score 3.0–3.5 and $n = 1$ for naïve mice per tracer). Following perfusion, the brain was removed and embedded in optimal cutting temperature (O.C.T.) compound (Tissue-Tek, Sakura, USA). Subsequently, 20-µm-thick sagittal brain sections were cut using a cryostat microtome HM500 (Microm, Germany). The sections were mounted on microscope slides (Fisherbrand Superfrost™ Plus Microscope Slides), air-dried for 10 min, and then exposed to ^{18}F-sensitive storage phosphor screens (Perkin Elmer, USA) for 12 h at 4 °C. The image plates were analyzed using a Typhoon 9410 Variable Mode Imager (Amersham Biosciences, USA), and images were visualized and processed by ImageJ (image processing and analysis software in java, version 1.45s). Anatomy of brain sections was confirmed by staining the exact same sections with Nissl (cresyl violet acetate, Sigma Aldrich). Briefly, dehydrated mounted sections were cleared in xylene for 15 min, rehydrated, immersed in 0.5% cresyl violet acetate (Sigma Aldrich) solution for 10 min, rinsed, dehydrated, and coverslipped. Whole spinal cords were also analyzed via autoradiography using same storage phosphor screens and Typhoon imager.

For Western blotting, the spinal cords were cut into thoracic/cervical and lumbar segments and the right hemisphere of the brain was collected. Tissue samples were immediately frozen in liquid nitrogen and stored at − 80 °C.

Western blotting

Tissue samples were homogenized using a total protein extraction kit (BioChain) following the manufacturer's instructions. Protein concentration in lysates was determined by bicinchoninic acid (BCA) protein assay (Pierce). Rabbit anti-xCT antibody (1:2000 dilution, Novus NB300-318) was used according to a standard western blotting protocol. After enhanced chemiluminescence (ECL) exposure, blots were washed and re-probed with rabbit anti-actin antibody (Cell Signaling Technology 4967S; 1:5000) as a loading control. To verify efficient extraction of xCT from the membrane during tissue lysis, an anti-Na,K-ATPase antibody (Cell Signaling Technology 3010S; 1:5000) was used as an additional control for western blotting [16]. Blots were scanned and signal was quantified using ImageJ (National Institutes of Health).

Isolation and activation of primary human immune cells

Peripheral mononuclear blood cells (PMBCs) were isolated from the whole blood of healthy donors (Stanford Blood Center) via density gradient method (Ficoll Paque PLUS, GE Healthcare). T cells or monocytes were isolated from the PMBC fraction by negative selection (Naïve Pan T Cell Isolation Kit/Monocyte Isolation Kit II, Miltenyi Biotech). Purity of obtained fractions was assessed by staining with CD3-VioBLue and CD14-FITC antibodies (Miltenyi Biotech) for T cells and monocytes respectively. The number of stained cells was then counted as a percentage of total cell number using a fluorescence microscope (EVOS FL Cell Imaging System, Life Technologies).

T cells were maintained in TexMACS medium (Miltenyi Biotech) and an aliquot was activated for 48 h prior to the radiotracer uptake assay using a T Cell Activation/Expansion Kit human (Miltenyi Biotech) according to manufacturer's instructions. Monocytes were maintained in RPMI medium containing 10% heat-inactivated FBS and 1% penicillin-streptomycin (all from Life Technologies), and an aliquot was also activated for 48 h prior to the uptake assay with lipopolysaccharide (LPS; 100 ng/mL, *Escherichia coli* O11:B4, Sigma Aldrich). Activation was confirmed by assessing changes in morphology of activated versus resting cells.

Cell uptake studies using primary human immune cells

Cells were counted, washed with Hank's Balanced Salt solution (HBSS) and re-suspended at $5–10 \times 10^6$ cells/mL in HBSS. Five hundred microliters of aliquots of cell suspensions were allowed to recover for 15 min at 37 °C and 5% CO_2. Five hundred microliters of pre-warmed [^{18}F]FSPG solution (1.5 MBq/mL in HBSS) was then added to each tube. After incubation for 60 min at 37 °C and 5% CO_2, an aliquot of each cell suspension was layered over 200 μL of a 3:1 mixture of silicon oil and mineral oil in a dolphin tube on ice as previously described [17]. Tubes were spun for 3 min at 10,000*g*, and after freezing in liquid nitrogen, the tips containing the cell pellets were cut into gamma counter tubes. Cell-associated radioactivity was assessed using a gamma counter (Cobra II Auto-Gamma counter; Packard Biosciences Co.) and normalized to both the total activity added and cell number.

Statistical analysis

Statistical analyses were performed using GraphPad (version 6). Data are expressed as mean ± standard deviation, unless otherwise indicated. Two-tailed Mann-Whitney *U* tests were used for group comparisons and a p value < 0.05 was considered significant. Two-tailed Wilcoxon matched-pairs signed rank tests were used to analyze repeated measurements in the longitudinal PET study. A Bonferroni-adjusted p value of < 0.017 was considered significant when performing multiple comparisons. Correlation analyses were performed using linear regression with goodness of fit designated by R^2 value, 95% confidence levels.

Results

[^{18}F]FSPG distribution and kinetics in EAE mice using dynamic PET imaging

Time-activity curves obtained from dynamic PET data (Additional file 2: Figure S2) revealed significantly higher [^{18}F]FSPG accumulation in the spinal cords of EAE compared to those of naïve mice, from as early as 8 min after tracer administration until the end of scan ($p = 0.0043$, 75 min post-injection), and a strong trend toward higher uptake in the brain ($p = 0.0571$, 75 min post-injection). While [^{18}F]FSPG appeared to wash out of tissues from naïve mice over time, it continued to accumulate in the tissues of EAE mice, with a plateau observed in the spinal cords starting at approximately 60 min after injection. An imaging time point at 75 min post-injection was chosen for all subsequent studies to allow for optimal tracer accumulation in target tissues and clearance from non-target tissues.

[^{18}F]FSPG is more sensitive than [^{18}F]FDG at detecting molecular changes in the spinal cord and brain of EAE mice

Results from ex vivo biodistribution studies demonstrated a significant elevation in [^{18}F]FSPG uptake in most EAE tissues compared to that in naïve mice (Fig. 1). The greatest difference in [^{18}F]FSPG tissue uptake was seen in the spinal cord, with 1.07 ± 0.70 %ID/g in EAE ($n = 9$, score 2.6 ± 0.9) and 0.05 ± 0.01 %ID/g in naïve mice ($n = 7$), $p = 0.0007$. [^{18}F]FSPG uptake was significantly higher in the kidney and brain of EAE compared to naïve mice (kidney: 67.8 ± 40.2 %ID/g vs. 6.7 ± 3.9 %ID/g, $p = 0.0002$; brain: 0.36 ± 0.11 %ID/g vs. 0.18 ± 0.07 %ID/g, $p = 0.0059$). In contrast, there was no significant

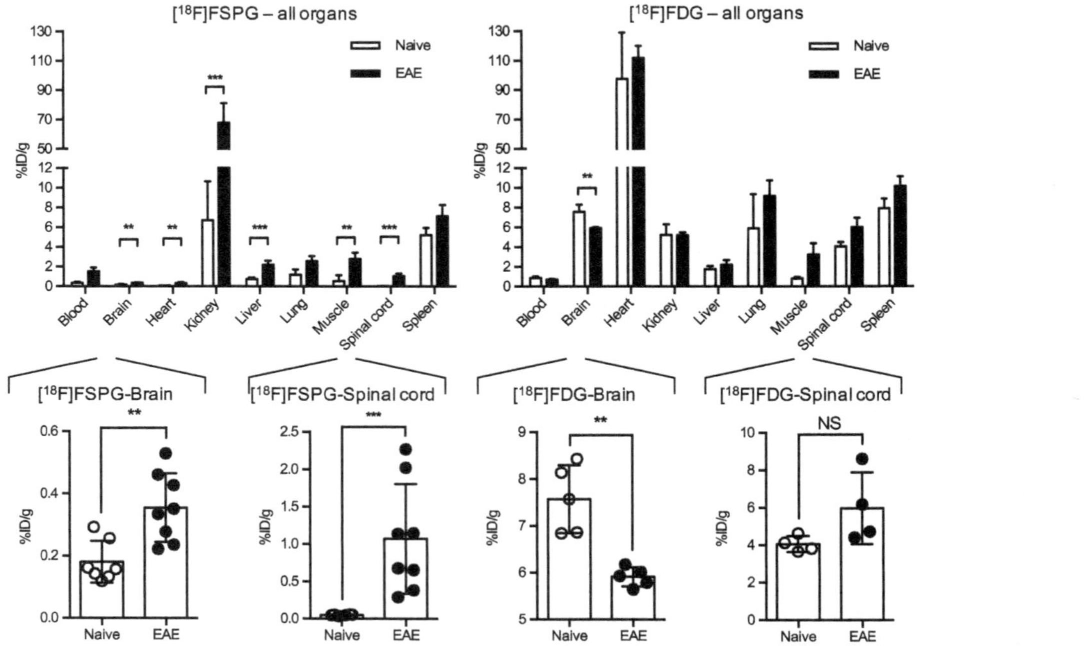

Fig. 1 Ex vivo biodistribution of [^{18}F]FSPG and [^{18}F]FDG in EAE and naive mice. Ex vivo data was obtained 110 min after radiotracer injection ($n = 5$–9, mean %ID/g ± SD) with magnified views of uptake in brain and spinal cord. EAE scores: 2.6 ± 0.9 and 3.2 ± 0.3 for [^{18}F]FSPG and [^{18}F]FDG groups respectively. ***p 0.0001–0.001, **p 0.001–0.01

difference in [^{18}F]FDG uptake in most EAE tissues compared to naïve mice (Fig. 1). The only significant difference in [^{18}F]FDG uptake was observed in the brain whereby there was a lower accumulation in EAE mice (5.9 ± 0.2 %ID/g) compared to the brains of naïve mice (7.6 ± 0.7 %ID/g, $p = 0.0079$).

Ex vivo autoradiography images corroborated PET and biodistribution findings, illustrating elevated [^{18}F]FSPG uptake in the spinal cords of EAE versus naïve mice (Additional file 3: Figure S3A), and a moderate increase in [^{18}F]FDG uptake in distinct foci of EAE mice (Additional file 3: Figure S3B). Qualitative autoradiography of selected brains revealed visually higher [^{18}F]FSPG uptake in the cerebellum, hippocampus (especially in the dentate gyrus), midbrain reticular nucleus, optic chiasm, posterior complex of the thalamus, and sensory-related substructures of the medulla of EAE compared to naïve mice. In contrast, there was lower global [^{18}F]FDG brain uptake in EAE versus naïve mice, most notably in the cortex and olfactory bulb.

In vivo [^{18}F]FSPG-PET imaging reveals increased xc- activity in CNS tissues of EAE mice

Next, we performed a longitudinal study to characterize [^{18}F]FSPG uptake at the pre-symptomatic versus symptomatic stage of disease. Since our pilot studies highlighted a tenfold increase in [^{18}F]FSPG uptake in EAE mouse kidneys, alongside the increased uptake in the spinal cord and brain, it appeared that [^{18}F]FSPG clearance might be affected in EAE mice. To address this, we generated an additional group of control mice with an identical immunization procedure to EAE mice but without administration of MOG peptide antigen. Additionally, we anesthetized mice just prior to PET imaging to allow additional time for clearance of the radiotracer.

For longitudinal studies, mice underwent an initial static PET/CT scan (~ 70 min post-injection of [^{18}F]FSPG) at the pre-symptomatic stage of disease on day 6 or 7 following immunization (Fig. 2a shows disease time course and PET imaging time points). Subsequent PET/CT imaging and biodistribution was performed between days 14 and 18 post-immunization for control and EAE mice after the latter reached a clinical score of 1.0–3.5.

Longitudinal studies revealed a significant increase in [^{18}F]FSPG-PET signal in the spinal cords of EAE mice exhibiting no clinical symptoms (score 0, 1 week post-immunization—Figs. 2 and 3; 1.2 ± 0.1-fold increase, $p = 0.0047$) that later went on to develop pronounced EAE within the next 4–8 days. After the onset of disease, an even greater increase in [^{18}F]FSPG uptake was observed in the whole spinal cord of EAE mice compared to that of controls (2.1 ± 0.2-fold higher, $p = 0.0002$). Higher absolute [^{18}F]FSPG uptake in the lumbar versus cervical/thoracic spinal cord region was observed (Figs. 2 and 3),

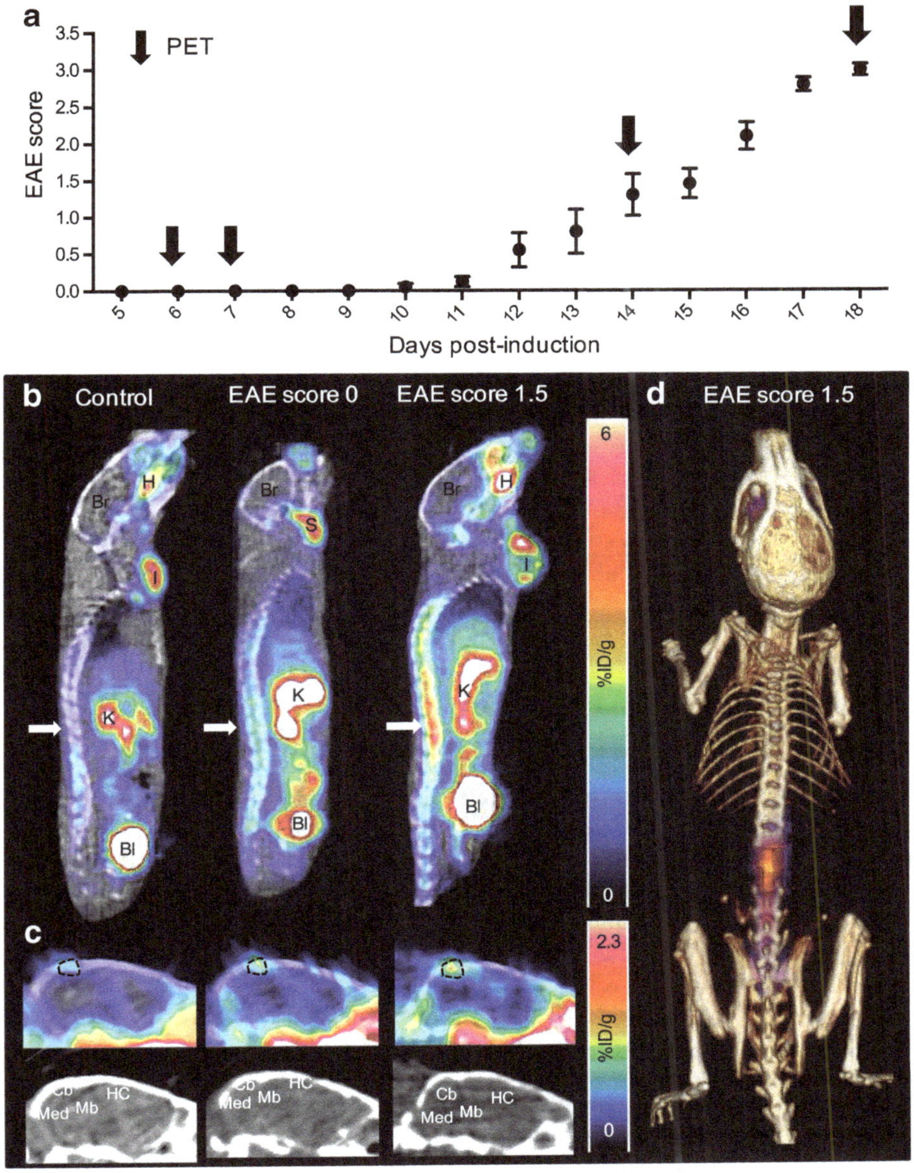

Fig. 2 Elevated [^{18}F]FSPG-PET signal in EAE mice at early stages of disease. **a** Disease scores of mice induced with EAE over 18 days. Arrows indicate PET/CT imaging time points and scores are represented as mean score ± SEM. **b** Representative sagittal PET/CT images of control, pre-symptomatic EAE (score 0), and EAE mice with early stage disease symptoms (score 1.5). Arrows indicate spinal cord uptake. Bl—bladder, Br—brain, H—Haderian glands, I—immunization site, K—kidneys, S—salivary glands. **c** Representative sagittal PET/CT images of identical brain sections of control, pre-symptomatic EAE (score 0), and symptomatic EAE (score 1.5) mice. Cb—cerebellum, HC—hippocampus, Mb—midbrain, Med—medulla. Dotted lines highlight region containing possible meningeal vessel(s). **d** Representative PET/CT volume rendering technique (VRT) image of EAE mouse (score 1.5). PET signal outside spinal column and skull was removed for better visualization of [^{18}F]FSPG uptake in areas of interest

while the fold-changes were in the same range (i.e., 1.2 ± 0.1 [$p = 0.0225$] and 1.3 ± 0.1 [$p = 0.0310$] in week 1 and 2.0 ± 0.2 [$p = 0.0005$] and 2.3 ± 0.3 [$p = 0.0002$] in week 2, for cervical/thoracic and lumbar spinal cord, respectively). Although a trend toward higher [^{18}F]FSPG uptake in the spinal cord of mice with lower clinical scores was observed, this was not statistically significant. The post-symptomatic signal in the whole spinal cord of EAE mice was 1.8 ± 0.2-fold higher than the pre-symptomatic signal ($p = 0.0002$), and the signal in control mice did not change over time ($p = 0.5625$).

PET image analysis of brain regions revealed significantly elevated uptake in the cerebellum, hippocampus, medulla, and midbrain of symptomatic EAE versus control mice—with the most marked fold-changes in the

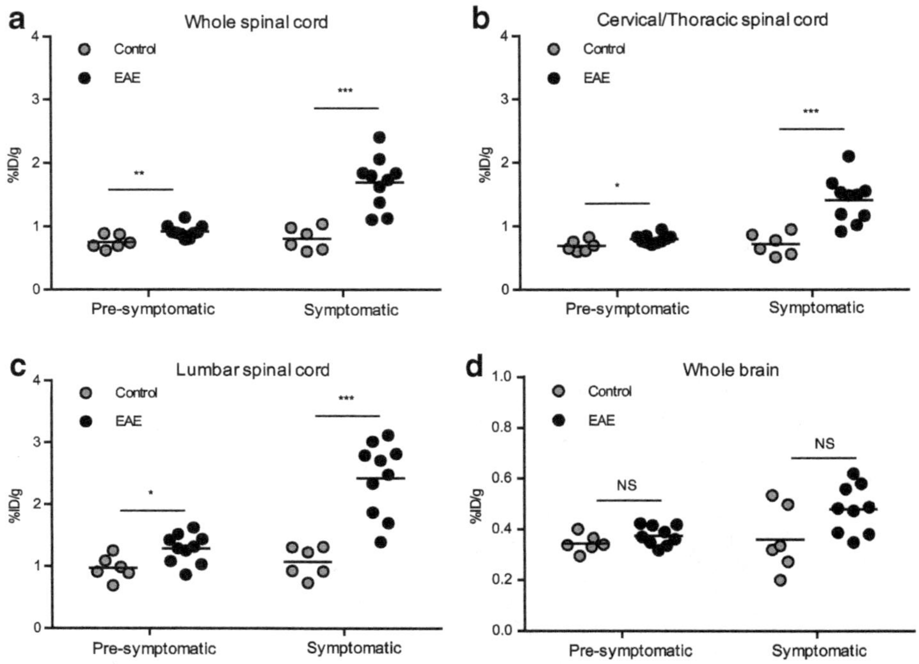

Fig. 3 Quantification of [^{18}F]FSPG-PET signal in CNS tissues of pre-symptomatic and symptomatic EAE versus control mice. Static PET imaging was performed 75 min post-injection of radiotracer (n = 6–10) and signal was quantified in the **a** whole spinal cord, **b** cervical/thoracic spinal cord, **c** lumbar spinal cord, and **d** whole brain. ***p 0.0001–0.001, **p 0.001–0.01, *p 0.01–0.05, NS—non-significant

cerebellum (Table 1). Interestingly, there was a region of radiotracer uptake present in the PET images of EAE mice, which appeared to be just outside the brain (dotted lines in Fig. 2c, see Additional file 4: Figure S4 for coronal brain slices) and became more intense when mice became symptomatic.

Elevated [^{18}F]FSPG-PET signal in EAE CNS tissues compared to control mice was further confirmed by ex vivo gamma counting of tissues from the same mice (Additional file 5: Fig. S5). Spinal cord [^{18}F]FSPG uptake was 0.69 ± 0.35 %ID/g (n = 9) in EAE compared to 0.04 ± 0.01 %ID/g in control mice (n = 8, p < 0.0001), with a similar fold-difference (16.2 ± 3.2) to what we previously observed in pilot studies using naïve mice. Brain uptake was also significantly higher in EAE mice compared to controls (0.15 ± 0.05 %ID/g vs. 0.07 ± 0.03 %ID/g, 2.2 ± 0.4-fold, p = 0.0012). Other significant differences in [^{18}F]FSPG uptake were observed in the blood (EAE: 0.37 ± 0.15 %ID/g vs. control: 0.20 ± 0.02 %ID/g, p = 0.0044) and kidneys (EAE: 6.7 ± 2.4 %ID/g vs. control: 3.8 ± 1.2 %ID/g, p = 0.0155).

[^{18}F]FSPG-PET signal correlates with elevated xCT protein levels in EAE CNS tissues

xCT protein levels were assessed by Western blot of the brain, cervical/thoracic, and lumbar cord tissues collected after [^{18}F]FSPG-PET/CT imaging (Fig. 4 and Additional file 6: Figure S6). Results from these studies revealed a strong correlation between [^{18}F]FSPG-PET signal and xCT protein levels in the cervical/thoracic spinal cord (R^2 = 0.80, p = 0.0002), and a moderate correlation in the lumbar spinal cord (R^2 = 0.46, p = 0.0143) and brain (right hemisphere, R^2 = 0.6664, p = 0.0012). xCT expression in the brain and cervical/thoracic and lumbar spinal cords from control versus naïve mice were not significantly different (p > 0.05, n = 3–4 per group; Additional file 7: Figure S7).

[^{18}F]FSPG uptake is increased in isolated primary human immune cells upon activation

Finally, we investigated the uptake of [^{18}F]FSPG in primary human T cells and monocytes; the immune cell types which are implicated in the pathogenesis of EAE. Data from these studies revealed a dramatic increase in [^{18}F]FSPG uptake in activated compared to resting T cells (75-fold, p < 0.0001) and in activated versus resting human monocytes (2.3-fold, p = 0.0079, Fig. 5). The absolute level of [^{18}F]FSPG uptake in activated monocytes (0.284 ± 0.006%uptake/10^5 cells), however, was fourfold higher than that in activated T cells (0.070 ± 0.004%uptake/10^5 cells).

Discussion

Cystine/glutamate antiporter, xc-, has been implicated in several neurological disorders and, specifically, in MS as a mediator of glutamate excitotoxicity and immune regulation [4]. Recent studies demonstrated that the

Table 1 Uptake values (%ID/g) for different brain regions in pre-symptomatic and symptomatic mice and fold differences with respect to the same quantitation in control mice

Brain regions	1 week post-immunization (pre-symptomatic mice)		2 weeks post-immunization (mice with clinical signs of EAE)	
	%ID/g in EAE mice	Fold-differences EAE vs. controls	%ID/g in EAE mice	Fold-differences EAE vs. controls
Whole brain	0.38 ± 0.04	1.1 ± 0.1^{NS}	0.48 ± 0.09	1.3 ± 0.2^{NS}
Cerebellum	0.36 ± 0.06	1.1 ± 0.1^{NS}	0.45 ± 0.10	1.6 ± 0.2**
Cortex	0.30 ± 0.04	1.1 ± 0.1^{NS}	0.34 ± 0.08	1.2 ± 0.2^{NS}
Hippocampus	0.32 ± 0.04	1.1 ± 0.1^{NS}	0.38 ± 0.09	1.4 ± 0.2*
Hypothalamus	0.76 ± 0.13	1.2 ± 0.1*	0.97 ± 0.19	1.2 ± 0.2^{NS}
Medulla	0.54 ± 0.08	1.1 ± 0.1^{NS}	0.67 ± 0.17	1.5 ± 0.2*
Midbrain	0.29 ± 0.04	1.1 ± 0.1^{NS}	0.35 ± 0.10	1.5 ± 0.2*
Olfactory bulb	0.64 ± 0.15	1.1 ± 0.1^{NS}	0.97 ± 0.30	1.3 ± 0.3^{NS}
Pallidum	0.45 ± 0.07	1.2 ± 0.1*	0.61 ± 0.13	1.2 ± 0.3^{NS}
Pons	0.44 ± 0.07	1.0 ± 0.1^{NS}	0.71 ± 0.25	1.3 ± 0.3^{NS}
Striatum	0.34 ± 0.04	1.1 ± 0.1^{NS}	0.42 ± 0.09	1.2 ± 0.2^{NS}
Thalamus	0.28 ± 0.05	1.1 ± 0.1^{NS}	0.32 ± 0.07	1.3 ± 0.2^{NS}

NS not significant

Absolute [^{18}F]FSPG uptake in brain regions as measured by PET, 75 min p.i. of radiotracer in EAE mice (n = 6–10, mean %ID/g ± SD) and fold differences ± SEM versus controls with indices indicating significance by Mann-Whitney test: $^{**}p$ = 0.001–0.01, $^{*}p$ = 0.01–0.05

xCT subunit of system xc- (responsible for the activity of this antiporter) is upregulated in postmortem CNS tissues from both MS patients and MS rodent models [6] and that it might be a promising PET imaging biomarker of disease progression in EAE rats [8].

Here, we show that [^{18}F]FSPG-PET enables the sensitive detection of alterations in xCT protein levels/ xc- activity in EAE mice at different stages of disease in vivo. Most notably, [^{18}F]FSPG-PET showed potential for the early detection of MS due to its increased uptake in

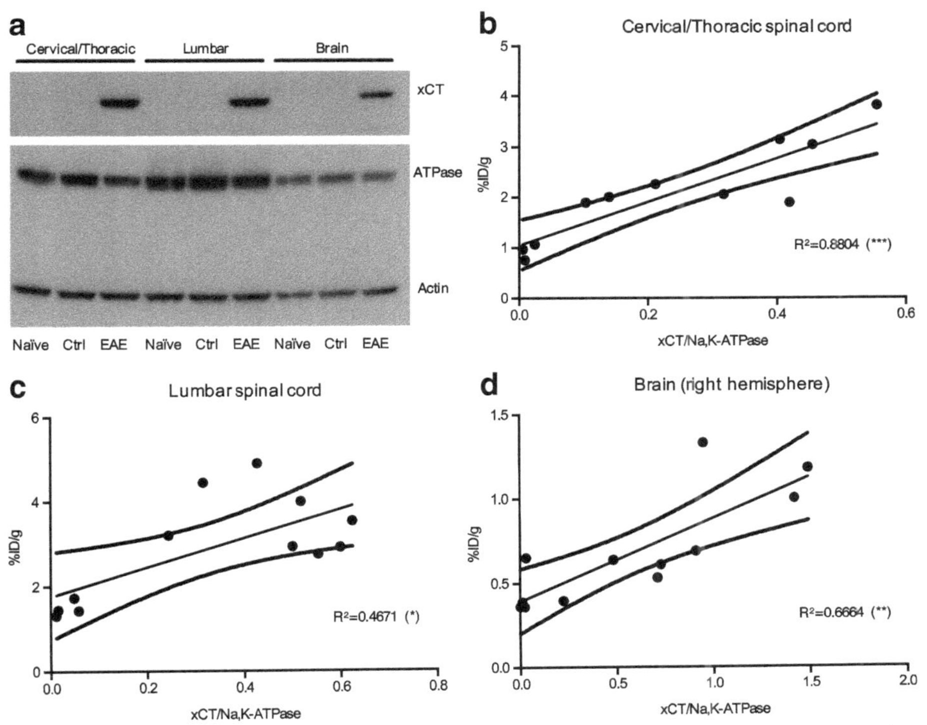

Fig. 4 Significant correlation between xCT protein levels in CNS tissues and in vivo PET signal. **a** Representative Western blot with actin and NaK-ATPase as loading controls (Ctrl). Correlation between xCT protein levels (determined by densitometric Western analysis) and [^{18}F]FSPG uptake (determined by PET quantification) in the **b** cervical/thoracic spinal cord (SC), **c** lumbar SC, and **d** brain. $^{***}p$ 0.0001–0.001, $^{**}p$ 0.001–0.01, $^{*}p$ 0.01–0.05

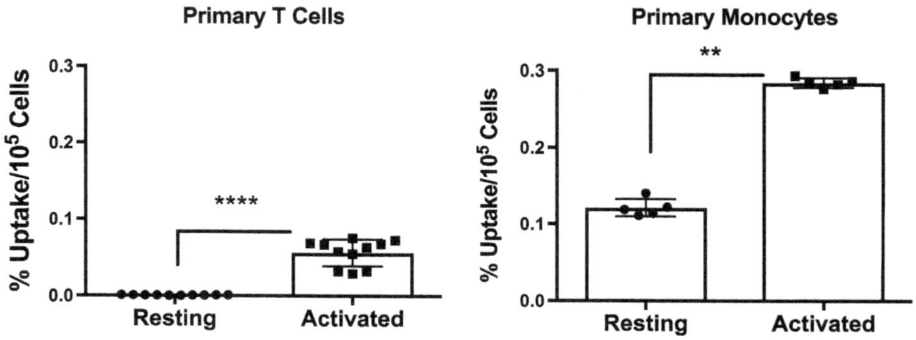

Fig. 5 [^{18}F]FSPG uptake in resting and activated primary human immune cells. In vitro accumulation of [^{18}F]FSPG in isolated primary human T cells and monocytes ($n = 5$–11, mean %ID/g ± SD). ****$p < 0.0001$, **$p < 0.01$

the spinal cord of EAE mice even at the pre-symptomatic stage of disease. This is the first report that [^{18}F]FSPG-PET signal is elevated at this early stage of EAE, thus emphasizing the utility of [^{18}F]FSPG-PET as a technique for characterizing the in vivo role of this anti-porter in the early stages of EAE disease development. Previously reported studies performed by Martin and colleagues using [^{18}F]FSPG-PET for imaging xc- in EAE rats did not detect increased PET signal at the pre-symptomatic stage of EAE; however, they did not image control or naïve rats for direct comparison [8].

Here, [^{18}F]FSPG showed greater sensitivity than [^{18}F]FDG in detecting metabolic changes in the EAE spinal cord, exhibiting a 21-fold difference in uptake in EAE vs naïve mice in ex vivo biodistribution studies. [^{18}F]FDG biodistribution results from EAE versus naïve and control mice were comparable to those previously reported by Radu et al. [18], Martin et al. [8], and Buck et al. [11]. As in our study, the latter found no statistical significance between groups. The heterogeneous pattern of [^{18}F]FDG uptake in distinct inflammatory infiltrates in the spinal cords of EAE mice and significant decrease in [^{18}F]FDG uptake in the brain, observed by autoradiography, was also consistent with previous findings [14, 15]. Grassiot and colleagues reported hypometabolism in MS patients and postulated that low [^{18}F]FDG brain uptake is likely due to reduced brain volume and disturbed glucose metabolism in these patients [19]. One reason for the difference in sensitivity between [^{18}F]FSPG and [^{18}F]FDG is likely due to their different uptake mechanisms, and therefore the different biological phenomena these tracers measure. [^{18}F]FDG is taken up via glucose transporters and subsequently trapped in cells following phosphorylation by hexokinase II, while [^{18}F]FSPG is taken up via xc- and retained in cells by an unconfirmed mechanism [15]. It is possible that alterations in xc- activity are more striking than alterations in glucose metabolism in rodent EAE.

Both PET and autoradiography images indicated higher accumulation of [^{18}F]FSPG in the cerebellum, hippocampus, medulla, and midbrain of EAE mice, all regions where demyelinating lesions and tissue damage can occur in MS patients [20] and EAE mice [21]. These findings correspond well with what is known about the spatial distribution of infiltrating immune cells, known to overexpress xCT, in the CNS of EAE rodents. For example, Brown and colleagues reported marked infiltration of CD3-positive T cells and also the presence of activated microglia in the sensory-related substructures of the medulla and cerebellar peduncles of EAE mice [21]. We additionally observed a region with tracer uptake of variable intensity just outside the brain. This signal could possibly be associated with [^{18}F]FSPG signal in CD3-positive T cells (or other infiltrating immune cells) in the meninges/subarachnoid space [22] or a meningeal lymphatic vessel [23]—all of which have been shown to be sites where T cells can reside as they mobilize and cross the BBB.

We observed significantly higher [^{18}F]FSPG levels in the blood and kidneys of EAE mice compared to naïve mice. The higher kidney uptake is likely due to impaired renal function in EAE mice, a co-morbidity with low prevalence in MS patients [24], leading to inferior excretion ability [25]. The increased level of [^{18}F]FSPG in the blood is most likely due to increased circulating activated monocytes in EAE mice, which are known to have elevated xCT protein levels [6]. It is important to note that the measured difference in [^{18}F]FSPG uptake levels in CNS tissues of EAE versus naïve/control mice became even more pronounced after removal of the blood via perfusion (as seen in ex vivo biodistribution data) compared to that in in vivo PET data. Hence, it appears that the increased blood pool activity observed in EAE mice partially obscures the specific signal increase. As previously demonstrated by Ayzenberg et al., the effect of EAE immunizations must be considered when interpreting bulk imaging signals by comparing to appropriate controls (i.e., control mice which undergo incomplete immunization with CFA emulsion and pertussis toxin while omitting MOG peptide, rather than using naïve mice) in order to prove specificity of the readout [26]. In this study, we demonstrated specificity of the observed in vivo [^{18}F]FSPG-PET signal by using such control mice and also by performing Western blotting of brain and cervical/thoracic and lumbar spinal cord to investigate how well the PET signal reflected alterations in xCT expression. A significant correlation was found between the levels of xCT protein and the PET signal in these tissues, thus verifying the utility of [^{18}F]FSPG-PET for investigating in vivo alterations in xCT over time in this mouse model.

As a prelude to clinical evaluation of [^{18}F]FSPG in MS patients, we investigated whether a single immune cell population might be primarily responsible for the elevated tissue uptake of [^{18}F]FSPG. A recent study by Evonuk and colleagues linked xCT expression on activated T cells with CNS infiltration and disease progression, highlighting the possible utility of xc- as a theranostic target in MS [27]. Numerous studies have highlighted considerable infiltration of CD68-positive cells (macrophages/microglia), monocytes, as well as T cells in spinal cord and brain lesions of EAE rodents [6]. We performed tracer uptake studies in isolated primary human T cells and monocytes to gain clarity on the relative accumulation of [^{18}F]FSPG in each cell type. Results from these studies revealed a dramatic 75-fold increase in [^{18}F]FSPG uptake in activated versus resting T cells and a comparatively modest, yet significant, 2.3-fold increase in activated versus resting monocytes. These results are in agreement with studies which have shown that T cells only express xCT in the activated state [28], while monocytes constitutively express xCT with upregulation upon activation [6]. CD11b/CD45-positive cells account for the majority of immune cells found in the CNS tissue of EAE mice (40–56% at all stages of disease), whereas cells of the T cell lineage represent a lower fraction (approximately 17%) [29]. Together with the higher absolute tracer uptake in monocytes compared to T cells, it is suspected that both types of immune cells likely contribute to the increased [^{18}F]FSPG tissue signal. Moreover, microglia/macrophages likely also contribute to the observed elevated [^{18}F]FSPG signal, as [^{18}F]FSPG-PET signal in EAE rats was significantly reduced after selectively depleting microglia via intracerebroventricular injection of liposome-encapsulated clodronate [8]. Further characterization of the immune cell populations (both murine and human) predominantly responsible for the increased [^{18}F]FSPG tissue uptake at different stages of disease progression are planned and will likely provide insight into the spatiotemporal dynamics of immune cells and their oxidative stress levels in MS.

Conclusion

In summary, we have shown that [^{18}F]FSPG-PET is a promising imaging technique for non-invasively monitoring xc- activity in EAE mice, both at very early stages of disease and throughout progression, and holds great potential as a sensitive tool for investigating the links between oxidative stress, immune cell trafficking, and clinical symptoms of MS. Using this technique, we gained new insights into the in vivo spatiotemporal dynamics of xc- activity in pre-symptomatic and symptomatic EAE. Future studies will involve evaluating the use of [^{18}F]FSPG-PET for predicting/monitoring response to novel antioxidant therapeutics, which are gaining interest as neuroprotective agents in MS.

Additional files

Additional file 1: Methods for defining regions of interest (ROIs) in CNS using VivoQuant image analysis software. (a) Spine/vertebrae (blue) was segmented out using Otsu Thresholding. (b) The spine ROI was made immutable, and the thoracic/cervical (orange) and lumbar (yellow) spinal cord ROIs were highlighted using the 3D ROI drawing tool. (c) The spine ROI was then removed, leaving only the ROIs for the lumbar and thoracic/cervical spinal cords. (d) Brain ROIs of interest were obtained using a 3D mouse brain atlas: medulla (yellow), cerebellum (light blue), midbrain (dark green), pons (light pink), cortex (gray), thalamus (red), hypothalamus (light purple), hippocampus (dark purple), striatum (magenta), pallidum (peach), and olfactory bulbs (maroon). After fitting the 3D mouse brain atlas ROI to the CT, the amount of activity in each region was obtained in nCi/cm^3 and then converted to %ID/g. (e) ROI of the right hemisphere was used for correlation with Western blot data, which was performed using only the right brain hemisphere for each mouse.

Additional file 2: Dynamic PET imaging of [^{18}F]FSPG uptake in the spinal cords (a) and brains (b). Time-activity curves represent average counts from a dynamic 90-min scan in EAE and naïve mice. Data are mean ± SEM ($n = 3$–7 animals per group).

Additional file 3: [^{18}F]FSPG and [^{18}F]FDG ex vivo autoradiography of EAE versus naïve mice. Representative autoradiography images of whole spinal cords and sagittal brain sections from EAE (score 3.0–3.5) versus naïve mice collected ~ 110 min after injection of (a) [^{18}F]FSPG and (b) [^{18}F]FDG. The same brain sections were stained with Nissl and overlayed with the corresponding autoradiographic images. Cb—cerebellum, Ctx—cortex, HC—hippocampus, Med—medulla, Ob—olfactory bulb, Thal—thalamus. Dotted lines highlight region containing the optic chiasm.

Additional file 4: Adjacent coronal brain PET/CT images of a representative EAE mouse. Images of EAE mouse (score 1.5) were acquired ~ 75 min after injection of [^{18}F]FSPG. Images are arranged beginning with caudal slices through to more rostral regions of the brain. Dotted lines highlight region of [^{18}F]FSPG accumulation in meninges and/or in possible meningeal vessel(s) or subarachnoid space.

Additional file 5: Ex vivo biodistribution of [^{18}F]FSPG in EAE versus control mice (a) with magnified views of the brain (b) and spinal cord (c) data ($n = 8$–10, mean %ID/g ± SD). Data was collected 110 min after injection of radiotracer and mean score of EAE mice was 2.4 ± 0.8. Significance determined Mann-Whitney test with ****$p < 0.0001$, ***p 0.0001–0.001, **p 0.001–0.01, *p 0.01–0.05.

Additional file 6: Complete raw/unedited images of Western blots shown in Fig. 4a. Blot after incubation with anti-xCT antibody (a) the same blot having been re-probed with loading controls anti-actin and anti-Na,K-ATPase antibody (b).

Additional file 7: xCT protein levels in CNS tissues do not differ between control and naïve mice. SC = spinal cord. Data are represented as mean xCT/Na,K-ATPase signal ± SD ($n = 3–5$). Significance determined by Mann-Whitney test with NS = not significant.

Abbreviations

[^{18}F]FDG: ^{18}F-Fluorodeoxyglucose; [^{18}F]FSPG: (4S)-4-(3-[^{18}F]Fluoropropyl)-L-glutamate; BCA: Bicinchoninic acid; Bl: Bladder; Br: Brain; Cb: Cerebellum; CFA: Complete Freund's adjuvant; CNS: Central nervous system; CT: Computed tomography; Ctrl: Control; Ctx: Cortex; EAE: Experimental autoimmune encephalomyelitis; ECL: Enhanced chemiluminescence; FBS: Fetal bovine serum; H: Haderian glands; HBSS: Hank's buffered salt solution; HC: Hippocampus; I: Immunization site; i.p.: Intraperitoneal; i.v.: Intravenous; ID: Injected dose; K: Kidneys; LPS: Lipopolysaccharide; MAP: Maximum a posteriori; Mb: Midbrain; Med: Medulla; MOG: Myelin oligodendrocyte glycoprotein; MS: multiple sclerosis; NS: Not significant; O.C.T.: Optimal cutting temperature; Ob: Olfactory bulb; p.i.: Post injection; PBS: Phosphate buffered saline; PET: Positron emission tomography; PMBC: Peripheral mononuclear blood cell; ROI: Region of interest; ROS: Reactive oxygen species; RPMI medium: Roswell Park Memorial Institute medium; S: Salivary glands; SC: Spinal cord; SD: Standard deviation; Thal: Thalamus; xc-: Cystine/glutamate antiporter; xCT: Light chain of xc-

Acknowledgements

We thank Piramal Imaging for providing the [^{18}F]FSPG precursor and synthesis equipment. We thank Robert E. Reeves, Ataya Sathirachinda, and Dr. Erwan Jouannot for their technical help, Dr. Frezghi Habte for the help with image processing, Dr. Timothy Doyle for the technical assistance with PET/CT, and Dr. Jarrett Rosenberg for statistical advice.

Funding

This work was funded in part by Piramal Imaging.

Author contributions

AH and MLJ conceived and designed the research studies, developed the methodology, conducted experiments, acquired and analyzed the data, and prepared the manuscript. ISA conducted the experiments, developed the methodology, acquired and analyzed data, and prepared the manuscript. JAR conducted the experiments, developed the methodology, acquired and analyzed the data. BS conducted the experiments and acquired and analyzed the data. AS conducted the experiments and acquired the data. THW developed the methodology and conducted the experiments. LA developed the methodology and analyzed data. HC conducted the experiments, analyzed the data, and reviewed the manuscript. DB developed the methodology, conducted the experiments, and analyzed data. GG conducted the experiments and reviewed the manuscript. ZD provided reagents and conducted the experiments. TWC provided the reagents and conceptual advice, alongside critical the help with the manuscript preparation and edits. FTC provided advice on radiosynthesis and reviewed the manuscript. SB provided advice on the study design and interpretation of results, and reviewed/edited the manuscript. SSG conceived and designed research studies, and prepared the manuscript. All authors read and approved the final manuscript.

Consent for publication

Not applicable.

Competing interests

The authors declare that they have no competing interests.

Author details

[1]Molecular Imaging Program at Stanford (MIPS), Department of Radiology, Stanford University, Stanford, CA 94305, USA. [2]Department of Neurology and Neurological Sciences, Stanford University, Stanford, CA 94305, USA. [3]Department of Bioengineering, Department of Materials Science & Engineering, Stanford University, Stanford, CA 94305, USA.

References

1. Stadelmann C. Multiple sclerosis as a neurodegenerative disease: pathology, mechanisms and therapeutic implications. Curr Opin Neurol. 2011;24:224–9.
2. Gilgun-Sherki Y, Melamed E, Offen D. The role of oxidative stress in the pathogenesis of multiple sclerosis: the need for effective antioxidant therapy. J Neurol. 2004;251:261–8.
3. Conrad M, Sato H. The oxidative stress-inducible cystine/glutamate antiporter, system x c-: cystine supplier and beyond. Amino Acids. 2012;42:231–46.
4. Domercq M, Sánchez-Gómez MV, Sherwin C, Etxebarria E, Fern R, Matute C. System xc- and glutamate transporter inhibition mediates microglial toxicity to oligodendrocytes. J Immunol. 2007;178:6549–56.
5. Kostic M, Zivkovic N, Stojanovic I. Multiple sclerosis and glutamate excitotoxicity. Rev Neurosci. 2013;24:71–88.
6. Pampliega O, Domercq M, Soria FN, Villoslada P, Rodríguez-Antigüedad A, Matute C. Increased expression of cystine/glutamate antiporter in multiple sclerosis. J Neuroinflammation BioMed Central Ltd. 2011;8:63.
7. Merckx E, Albertini G, Paterka M, Jensen C, Albrecht P, Dietrich M, et al. Absence of system xc—on immune cells invading the central nervous system alleviates experimental autoimmune encephalitis. J Neuroinflammation. 2017;14:9.
8. Martín A, Vázquez-Villoldo N, Gómez-Vallejo V, Padro D, Soria FN, Szczupak B, et al. In vivo imaging of system xc- as a novel approach to monitor multiple sclerosis. Eur J Nucl Med Mol Imaging. 2016;43:1124–38.
9. Hoehne A. A novel strategy for imaging multiple sclerosis with positron emission tomography. J Nucl Med. 2016;57:Abstract 112.
10. Croxford AL, Kurschus FC, Waisman A. Mouse models for multiple sclerosis: historical facts and future implications. Biochim Biophys Acta. 2011;1812: 177–83.
11. Buck D, Forschler A, Lapa C, Schuster T, Vollmar P, Korn T, et al. 18F-FDG PET detects inflammatory infiltrates in spinal cord experimental autoimmune encephalomyelitis lesions. J Nucl Med. 2012;53:1269–76.
12. Schiepers C, Van Hecke P, Vandenberghe R, Van Oostende S, Dupont P, Demaerel P, et al. Positron emission tomography, magnetic resonance imaging and proton NMR spectroscopy of white matter in multiple sclerosis. Mult Scler. 1997;3:8–17.
13. Kindred JH, Koo PJ, Rudroff T. Glucose uptake of the spinal cord in patients with multiple sclerosis detected by 18F-fluorodeoxyglucose PET/CT after walking. Spinal Cord. 2014;52:S11–3.
14. Poutiainen P, Jaronen M, Quintana FJ, Brownell A-L. Precision medicine in multiple sclerosis: future of PET imaging of inflammation and reactive astrocytes. Front Mol Neurosci. 2016;9
15. Koglin N, Mueller A, Berndt M, Schmitt-Willich H, Toschi L, Stephens AW, et al. Specific PET imaging of x C—transporter activity using a 18F-labeled glutamate derivative reveals a dominant pathway in tumor metabolism. Clin Cancer Res. 2011;17:6000–11.
16. Ramos KM, Lewis MT, Morgan KN, Crysdale NY, Kroll JL, Taylor FR, et al. Spinal upregulation of glutamate transporter GLT-1 by ceftriaxone: therapeutic efficacy in a range of experimental nervous system disorders. Neuroscience. 2010;169:1888–900.
17. Ronald JA, Kim B-S, Gowrishankar G, Namavari M, Alam IS, D'Souza A, et al. A PET imaging strategy to visualize activated T cells in acute graft-versus-host disease elicited by allogenic hematopoietic cell transplant. Cancer Res. 2017;77:2893–902.
18. Radu CG, Shu CJ, Shelly SM, Phelps ME, Witte ON. Positron emission tomography with computed tomography imaging of neuroinflammation in experimental autoimmune encephalomyelitis. Proc Natl Acad Sci. 2007;104: 1937–42.
19. Grassiot B, Desgranges B, Eustache F, Defer G. Quantification and clinical relevance of brain atrophy in multiple sclerosis: a review. J Neurol. 2009: 1397–412.
20. Kipp M, Wagenknecht N, Beyer C, Samer S, Wuerfel J, Nikoubashman O. Thalamus pathology in multiple sclerosis: from biology to clinical application. Cell Mol Life Sci. 2014;72:1127–47.
21. Brown DA, Sawchenko PE. Time course and distribution of inflammatory and neurodegenerative events suggest structural bases for the pathogenesis of experimental autoimmune encephalomyelitis. J Comp Neurol. 2007;502:236–60.
22. Kivisakk P, Imitola J, Rasmussen S, Elyaman W, Zhu B, Ransohoff RM, et al. Localizing central nervous system immune surveillance: meningeal antigen-presenting cells activate T cells during experimental autoimmune encephalomyelitis. Ann Neurol. 2009;65:457–69.

23. Louveau A, Smirnov I, Keyes TJ, Eccles JD, Rouhani SJ, Peske JD, et al. Structural and functional features of central nervous system lymphatic vessels. Nature. 2015;523:337–41.
24. Marrie RA, Reider N, Stuve O, Trojano M, Sorensen PS, Cutter GR, et al. The incidence and prevalence of comorbid gastrointestinal, musculoskeletal, ocular, pulmonary, and renal disorders in multiple sclerosis: a systematic review. Mult Scler. 2015;21:332–41.
25. Peterson LK, Masaki T, Wheelwright SR, Tsunoda I, Fujinami RS. Cross-reactive myelin antibody induces renal pathology. Autoimmunity. 2008;41:526–36.
26. Ayzenberg I, Schlevogt S, Metzdorf J, Stahlke S, Pedreitturia X, Hunfeld A, et al. Analysis of neurogenesis during experimental autoimmune encephalomyelitis reveals pitfalls of bioluminescence imaging. PLoS One. 2015;10:e0118550.
27. Evonuk KS, Baker BJ, Doyle RE, Moseley CE, Sestero CM, Johnston BP, et al. Inhibition of system Xc(−) transporter attenuates autoimmune inflammatory demyelination. J Immunol. 2015;195:450–63.
28. Levring TB, Hansen AK, Nielsen BL, Kongsbak M, von Essen MR, Woetmann A, et al. Activated human CD4+ T cells express transporters for both cysteine and cystine. Sci Rep. 2012;2:2–7.
29. Berard JL, Wolak K, Fournier S, David S. Characterization of relapsing-remitting and chronic forms of experimental autoimmune encephalomyelitis in C57BL/6 mice. Glia. 2010;58:434–45.

16

MicroRNA-142 regulates inflammation and T cell differentiation in an animal model of multiple sclerosis

Farideh Talebi[1,2], Samira Ghorbani[1], Wing Fuk Chan[3], Roobina Boghozian[1], Farimah Masoumi[1], Sedigheh Ghasemi[2], Mohammed Vojgani[1], Christopher Power[3,4] and Farshid Noorbakhsh[1*]

Abstract

Background: MicroRNAs have emerged as an important class of modulators of gene expression. These molecules influence protein synthesis through translational repression or degradation of mRNA transcripts. Herein, we investigated the potential role of miR-142a isoforms, miR-142a-3p and miR-142a-5p, in the context of autoimmune neuroinflammation.

Methods: The expression levels of two mature isoforms of miR-142 were measured in the brains of patients with multiple sclerosis (MS) and the CNS tissues from mice with experimental autoimmune encephalomyelitis (EAE), an animal model of MS. Expression analyses were also performed in mitogen and antigen-stimulated splenocytes, as well as macrophages and astrocytes using real-time RT-PCR. The role of the mature miRNAs was then investigated in T cell differentiation by transfection of $CD4^+$ T cells, followed by flow cytometric analysis of intracellular cytokines. Luciferase assays using vectors containing the 3′UTR of predicted targets were performed to confirm the interaction of miRNA sequences with transcripts. Expression of targets were then analyzed in activated splenocytes and MS/EAE tissues.

Results: Expression of miR-142-5p was significantly increased in the frontal white matter from MS patients compared with white matter from non-MS controls. Likewise, expression levels of miR-142a-5p and miR-142a-3p showed significant upregulation in the spinal cords of EAE mice at days 15 and 25 post disease induction. Splenocytes stimulated with myelin oligodendrocyte glycoprotein (MOG) peptide or anti-CD3/anti-CD28 antibodies showed upregulation of miR-142a-5p and miR-142a-3p isoforms, whereas stimulated bone marrow-derived macrophages and primary astrocytes did not show any significant changes in miRNA expression levels. miR-142a-5p overexpression in activated lymphocytes shifted the pattern of T cell differentiation towards Th1 cells. Luciferase assays revealed SOCS1 and TGFBR1 as direct targets of miR-142a-5p and miR-142a-3p, respectively, and overexpression of miRNA mimic sequences suppressed the expression of these target transcripts in lymphocytes. SOCS1 levels were also diminished in MS white matter and EAE spinal cords.

Conclusions: Our findings suggest that increased expression of miR-142 isoforms might be involved in the pathogenesis of autoimmune neuroinflammation by influencing T cell differentiation, and this effect could be mediated by interaction of miR-142 isoforms with SOCS1 and TGFBR-1 transcripts.

Keywords: MicroRNA, Neuroinflammation, Multiple sclerosis, Experimental autoimmune encephalomyelitis, T cell differentiation

* Correspondence: f-noorbakhsh@sina.tums.ac.ir
[1]Department of Immunology, School of Medicine, Tehran University of Medical Sciences, Tehran, Iran

Background

MicroRNAs (miRNAs) are a family of small noncoding RNAs that function as negative regulators of gene expression through sequence-specific binding to the 3′-untranslated region (3′-UTR) of their target messenger RNAs (mRNAs) [1, 2]. Numerous studies have demonstrated the role of miRNAs in different cell biological processes including cell proliferation, differentiation, apoptosis, and migration by targeting and downregulating the expression of various protein-coding genes [3]. Moreover, dysregulation of specific miRNAs have been associated with human disease, including cancers, infectious diseases, and inflammatory and immune-related disorders. In the context of immunological disorders, miRNAs have been shown to influence the activity and function of both innate and adaptive arms of the immune system [4], which makes them important pathogenic players as well as potential therapeutic targets in these disorders. Autoimmune diseases have been of particular interest to miRNA researchers over the last decade and various miRNAs have been shown to exert critical effects in major autoimmune disorders including diabetes, rheumatoid arthritis, systemic lupus erythematosus, and multiple sclerosis (MS) [5]. In the case of MS, studies on peripheral blood leukocytes and brain tissue have shown altered expression of various miRNAs [6–8]. In one of the first studies performed on peripheral blood leukocytes from MS patients, Otaegui et al. reported an association between miR-18b and miR-599 with disease relapses and miR-96 with remissions [6]. In another miRNA study on blood cells, Keller et al. identified a set of 48 miRNAs which could differentiate relapsing-remitting multiple sclerosis (RR-MS) patients from healthy controls with high specificity and sensitivity [9]. Studies focusing on miRNA expression in T cells have revealed altered expression of miRNAs which target genes with known role in T cell activation [10–12]. In addition to association with disease, studies have also shown direct involvement of miRNAs in MS disease pathogenesis. In a seminal work by Du et al., miR-326 was reported to regulate the differentiation of T cell towards the pathogenic Th17 phenotype in MS patients and experimental autoimmune encephalomyelitis (EAE) mice [13]. Investigating the expression of miRNAs in autopsy brain tissue derived from MS patients also supports the role of these molecules in disease process. miRNA profiling on active and inactive brain lesion by Junker et al. has revealed dysregulation of multiple miRNAs including miR-34a, miR-155, and miR-326, which target CD47 regulatory protein, in MS brains [14]. Other miRNA-profiling studies on brain tissue derived from MS patients have also shown dysregulation of multiple miRNA species in MS brain including normal-appearing white matter [15]. In addition to their role in pathogenesis, miRNAs might also be important as therapeutic targets in MS. In the study by Du et al., in vivo silencing of miR-326 resulted in fewer Th17 cells and milder EAE, and its overexpression led to more severe EAE disease [13]. Likewise, treatment of EAE mice with anti-miR-155 sequences have been reported to decrease the clinical severity of EAE, a finding which is consistent with the role of miR-155 in development of Th1 and Th17 cells [16].

In the current study, we focused on the role of miR-142 in autoimmune neuroinflammation that takes place in MS and the EAE. mir-142 is broadly conserved between different species, including human and mouse (Additional file 1: Figure S1). Immature mir-142 generates two mature isoforms; miR-142-3p and miR-142-5p which have both been implicated in regulation of leukocyte activity and also in inflammatory diseases [17–20]. In the context of autoimmune neuroinflammation, upregulation of miR-142-5p have been reported in MS brain tissue in miRNA-profiling studies [5, 8, 14]. Moreover, high expression of miR-142-3P in EAE brain tissue and CSF of patients with multiple sclerosis during active inflammation has been illustrated [21]. Nonetheless, the potential pathogenic or protective role that this miRNA might have in disease process is not fully known.

In this study, we first used human brain autopsy samples as well as central nervous system (CNS) tissue derived from EAE animals at different time points after disease induction to investigate the expression of miR-142-5p and miR-142-3p isoforms in disease tissues. Expression of miRNA isoforms were next measured in cultures of cells with potential roles in MS/EAE pathogenesis. Overexpression experiments in $CD4^+$ T cells were performed to examine the effect of miR-142 on T cell differentiation. 3′UTR cloning and luciferase assays were then carried out to identify direct mRNA targets of miR-142, followed by quantifying the expression of targets in CNS tissue and cultured cells.

Methods

Human brain studies

The use of autopsied brain tissues was approved by the University of Alberta Human Research Ethics Board (Biomedical, protocol number 2291), and written informed consent was obtained for all samples collected from age- and sex-matched subjects including non-MS patients (n = 6; mean age = 61 + 4.0 years; male:female, 3:3; diagnoses at death: sepsis, cancer, myocardial infarction, stroke, HIV-AIDS, Parkinson's disease) and patients with MS (n = 6; mean age = 56 + 3.2 years; male:female, 2:4; diagnoses at death: secondary progressive MS (n = 4), primary progressive MS (n = 1) and relapsing-remitting MS (n = 1). All tissue samples were stored at −80 °C as previously reported [22, 23]. In order to detect demyelinated lesions, luxol fast blue (LFB) staining was performed on brain sections and parts of the tissues which did not show evident demyelination were used for RNA preparation.

Mice and EAE induction

C57BL/6 wild-type (WT) female mice (8 weeks old) were purchased from The Pasteur Institute of Iran and maintained in the animal facility of Tehran University of Medical Sciences. After 4 weeks, EAE was induced in 12-week-old mice by using MOG35-55 peptide. While both recombinant myelin oligodendrocyte glycoprotein (MOG) protein and MOG35-55 have been used for EAE induction in C57BL/6 mice, in this study, MOG35-55 was used considering its role in inducing EAE by stimulating neuroantigen-reactive T cells [24, 25]. MOG35-55 peptide emulsified in complete Freund's adjuvant (CFA) was injected subcutaneously at two sites on the back (0.1 ml of emulsion/site) (EK-2110, Hooke Kit™ MOG35-55/CFA Emulsion PTX). On the same day, and on the following day, mice received intraperitoneal injections of pertussis toxin in PBS, at 200 ng/mouse/dose (0.1 ml). Control mice received subcutaneous CFA and intraperitoneal pertussis toxin injections with the same dose as the EAE mice. Animals were assessed daily for disease severity for up to 30 days following immunization using a 0–15-point scoring scale [15]. All experiments conformed to guidelines from the Research Ethics Committee of Tehran University of Medical Sciences. CNS tissues were removed from EAE and control mice at three different time points after disease induction (pre-onset, peak of disease, and post peak phase) and were stored at −80 freezers. Previous analyses of CNS tissue in this model of EAE have revealed that lumbar spinal cord is the location which shows higher levels of inflammation and demyelination more consistently [26, 27]. Hence, in this study, we focused on lumbar spinal cord tissue for further expression analysis.

Immunohistochemistry

To detect T cell infiltration and demyelination in EAE spinal cords, immunohistochemical staining for CD3 T cell marker and myelin basic protein (MBP) was performed on lumbar spinal cord sections, as previously described [22]. Briefly, formalin-fixed paraffin-embedded spinal cord sections were deparaffinized in xylene and rehydrated in decreasing concentrations of ethanol. Antigen retrieval was performed by boiling the sections in 0.01 M trisodium citrate buffer (pH = 6). Sections were next blocked in 10% normal goat serum containing 0.1% triton X-100 and then incubated overnight at 4° with antibodies against CD3 (1:100; Santa Cruz Biotechnology Inc.) and myelin basic protein (1:500; Sternberger Monoclonal) followed by washing. Sections were then incubated with HRP-conjugated secondary antibodies (1:500, Abcam) followed by color development using DAB substrate solution.

Splenocytes culture and treatment

Spleens were removed from MOG-immunized mice 7 days after EAE induction; tissues were homogenized; and splenocytes were isolated using Ficoll centrifugation (Inno-Train). 2×10^6 cells were cultured in the presence or absence of different concentrations of MOG-35-55 (MOG_{35-55}, Hooke labs) in 24-well plates in a final volume of 1 ml RPMI 1640 medium supplemented with 5% FBS. Treated cells were harvested after 12, 24, and 48 h of incubation at 37 °C. Mouse splenocytes were also cultured in 24-well plates and treated with mouse anti-CD3 (0.5 μg/ml) and anti-CD28 (0.2 μg/ ml) (eBioscience) for different durations from 1 to 72 h at 37 °C in a humidified CO_2 incubator.

Macrophage and astrocyte cell cultures and treatment

Bone marrow-derived macrophages and primary mouse astrocyte cultures were prepared, as previously described [28]. Briefly, femur and tibia were removed from euthanized C57BL/6 mice under sterile conditions. The two ends of bones were cut, and bone marrow was expelled with a syringe filled with culture medium. Cells from bone marrow were cultured for 7 days in the presence of 50 ng/ml recombinant macrophage colony-stimulating factor (M-CSF) (eBioscience) [28]. Differentiated macrophages were treated with lipopolysaccharide (LPS) (10 and 100 ng/ml) for 12 h at 37 °C before RNA extraction. For astrocyte cultures, neonatal mouse brain tissue was used. Brains were removed and placed in DMEM medium under sterile conditions. Brain tissues were dissected, and astrocyte cells were cultured in DMEM medium supplemented with 20% FBS. Astrocytes were stimulated with 10 and 100 ng/ml LPS (Sigma Aldrich) for 12 h at 37 °C [29]. To confirm the identity of the cells, we performed immunofluorescent staining using an anti-GFAP antibody (1:250, mouse polyclonal, Abcam).

RNA extraction and cDNA synthesis

Total RNA, containing microRNAs, was extracted from human brain tissue samples, EAE lumbar spinal cord tissues, stimulated splenocytes, cultured macrophages, and astrocytes using miRNeasy Mini Kit (Qiagen). RNA concentration was determined with a Nanodrop. First-strand cDNA synthesis was performed from 1 μg total RNA using miScript II RT Kit (Qiagen) for microRNA analyses and TAKARA kit for gene expression analyses, according to the manufacturers' instructions.

Real-time RT-PCR

MicroRNAs (miR-142-3p and miR-142-5p) and their predicted target levels were measured by real-time reverse transcription–PCR using SYBR Green dye on a Bio-Rad CFX96 system in cells and tissues. MicroRNA expression data were normalized against snord 68 and snord 72 expression levels (Qiagen). Expression of the other genes were normalized against β-actin mRNA levels.

Primer sequences used for mRNA expression analysis are shown in Additional file 1: Table S1.

Cell transfections with miRNA mimics

To analyze the effect of microRNA overexpression on endogenous levels of TGFBR-1, TGFBR-2, and SOCS-1 in cells, mouse splenocyte were transfected with miR-142a-3p and miR-142a-5p mimic sequences at 50nM/ml (Qiagen) using Hiperfect transfection reagent (Qiagen) according to the manufacturer's protocol. After 4 h, the transfected cells were treated with anti-CD3 (0.5 μg/ml) and anti-CD28 (0.2 μg/ml) (eBioscience) for 48 h at 37 °C. For transfection experiments, AllStars negative control siRNA sequence (Qiagen) was used as a control. Total RNA was extracted from transfected cells using miRNeasy Mini Kit (Qiagen), and the levels of predicted gene targets expression were measured by real-time RT–PCR.

Luciferase assays and miRNA target verification analyses

In order to verify the interaction of TGFBR1 transcripts with miR-142a-3p as well as TGFBR2 and suppressor of cytokine signaling 1 (SOCS1) transcripts with miR-142a-5p, we used luciferase-3′-UTR reporter system. TGFBR-1, TGFBR-2, and SOCS-1 3′ UTR entire fragments were cloned downstream of the Renilla luciferase coding sequence (NotI/XhoI sites) in the psiCheck-2 plasmid (Promega). 25×10^3 HEK293T cells were cultured in each well of 96-well plates, and the reporter plasmids psiCHECK 3′ UTR (100 ng) were co-transfected along with miR-142a-3p and miR-142a-5p mimic sequences (50 ng) into cultured cells using Attractene transfection reagent (Qiagen) according to the manufacturer's protocol. For each gene relevant psiCHECK 3′ UTR plus negative control siRNA (Qiagen), co-transfection was used as a control. Following 48 h of incubation at 37 °C, cells were harvested and both Firefly and Renilla luciferase activity were measured using the Dual-Glo dual luciferase assay system (Promega) according to the manufacturer's protocols. Firefly luciferase activity was normalized to Renilla luciferase expression for each sample [15].

T cell differentiation

Mouse naive $CD4^+$ T cells were isolated from C57/BL6 mice spleens using Ficoll followed by naïve $CD4^+$ T cell isolation by negative selection kit (mouse $CD4^+$ T cell isolation kit, Miltenyi Biotec). 1×10^5 cells were cultured in each well of 96-well plates and were then transfected with miR-142a-3p and miR-142a-5p mimic 50nM/ml (Qiagen) using Hiperfect transfection reagent (Qiagen) according to the manufacturer's protocol. After 4 h, the transfected cells were transferred to anti-CD3-coated wells (1 μg/ml) and were treated with soluble anti-CD28 (0.2 μg/ml) (eBioscience). AllStars negative control siRNA sequence (Qiagen) was used as a control. Transfected cells were differentiated to three subtypes of T cells, i.e., T regulatory cells, Th1, and Th17, using three different cytokine regimens. For regulatory T (Treg) cells, transfected cells were cultured in complete RPMI, plate-bound CD3 antibody, and soluble CD28 antibody (0.2 μg/ml), IL-2 (20 ng/ml), and TGF-β1 (50 ng/ml) (BioLegend) for 96 h. For Th1 cells, transfected cells were cultured in complete RPMI, plate-bound CD3 antibody, and soluble CD28 antibody (0.2 μg/ml), IL-2 (20 ng/ml), IL-12 (50 ng/ml), and anti-IL-4 antibody (10 ng/ml) (BioLegend) for 96 h. To differentiate the cells into Th17 cells, transfected cells were cultured in complete RPMI, plate-bound CD3 antibody, and soluble CD28 antibody (0.2 μg/ml), TGF-β (5 ng/ml), IL-6 (100 ng/ml), anti-IFN-γ (10 ng/ml), anti-IL-4 (10 ng/ml), and IL-23 (50 ng/ml) (BioLegend) for 96 h.

Intracellular staining and flow cytometry

To detect intracellular expression of interferon (IFN)-γ, interleukin (IL)-17A, and FoxP3 in transfected $CD4^+$ T cells, cells were surface-stained with anti-CD4 and anti-CD3 antibodies and then fixed with 1 ml/tube BioLegend's Fixation Buffer, at room temperature in the dark for 20 min. Cells were permeabilized with 1 ml BioLegend's Permeabilization Buffer (1×) and then stained with flurochrome-conjugated anti- IFN-γ, IL-17A, and Foxp3 antibodies (Biolegend). Stained cells were assayed with a BD FACSCalibur flow cytometer, and results were analyzed with FlowJo software. APC Rat IgG2b, κ Isotype Ctrl antibody, PerCP Rat IgG2b, κ Isotype Ctrl antibody, PE Rat IgG1, and κ Isotype Ctrl antibody were used as isotype controls.

Statistical analysis

Statistical analyses were performed using SPSS software, Version 20. Student's t and Mann–Whitney U tests were used for parametric and non-parametric mean comparisons between the two groups. One-way ANOVA or Kruskal–Wallis tests were performed for parametric and non-parametric mean comparisons between multiple groups. Data are shown as mean + SEM.

Results

miR-142 isoforms are upregulated in the CNS of MS patients and animals with EAE

To confirm altered expression of miR-142 in MS white matter, we analyzed the expression of miR-142-3p and miR-142-5p isoforms in normal-appearing cerebral white matter from MS and non-MS cases by real-time PCR. These studies showed that miR-142-5p expression levels were significantly increased in MS brains compared with non-MS brain tissues (Fig. 1a), as previously reported in miRNA-profiling studies [2, 14, 15]. Given these findings, we then investigated the expression of miRNAs in

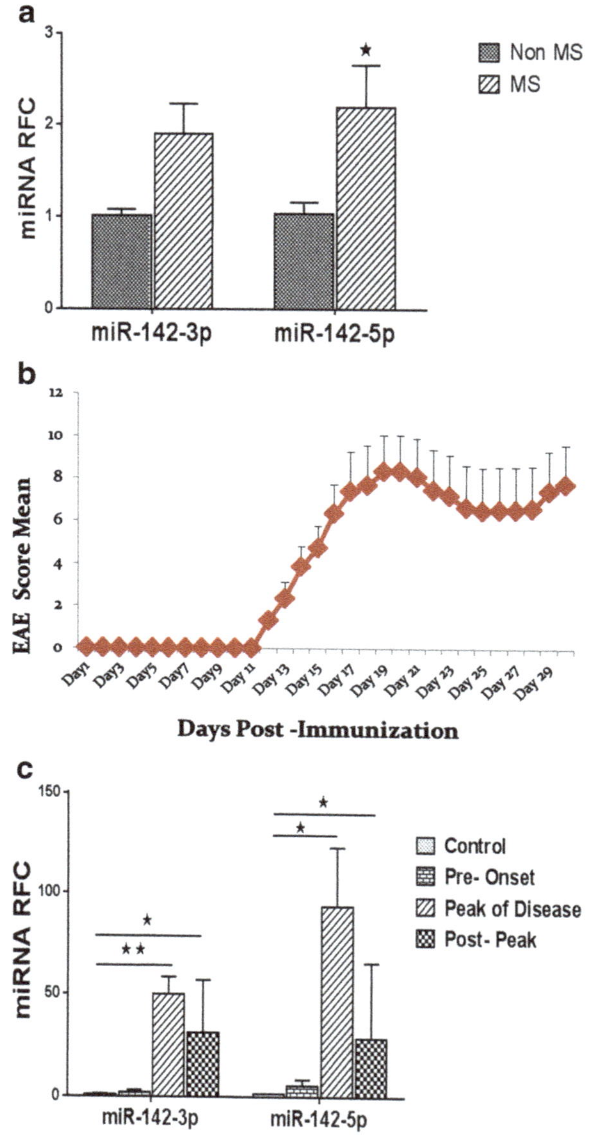

Fig. 1 miR-142-3p and miR-142-5p levels in human brain tissue samples and EAE spinal cords. Expression of microRNAs was measured in CNS tissues by real-time RT-PCR. The level of miR-142-5p was significantly increased in human MS samples compared with non-MS controls (**a**) ($n = 6$, Mann–Whitney *U* test, $*p \leq 0.05$). EAE was induced in C57BL6 mice and spinal cord tissues were extracted at three time points after disease induction (**b**). Expression levels of miR-142a-3p and miR-142a-5p were significantly increased in spinal cord during the peak of disease and post peak phases of EAE (**c**). Data are shown as mean ± SEM. Number of mice in each group = 10, $*p < 0.05$, $**p < 0.01$, Kruskal–Wallis tests

the MS animal model, EAE at different phases of disease. EAE was induced in 30 animals which were divided into three groups for tissue extraction at three time points after the induction of disease. The first time point was day 10 post-induction before the development of any neurological signs (pre-onset); the second time-point was at the peak of the disease that varied between days 18 and 20 for mice in the group ("peak of disease phase"); and the third time point was at day 25 post-induction ("post peak phase") (Fig. 1b). Immunohistochemical analysis of lumbar spinal cord tissue isolated from mice at the peak of disease showed infiltration of CD3 immunopositive T cells as well as reduced staining for myelin basic protein in EAE mice compared with CFA control animals (Additional file 1: Figure S2). Expression analysis for two miR-142 mature isoforms on the RNA extracted from spinal cord tissue showed substantial upregulation of miR-142a-5p and miR-142a-3p in the lumbar spinal cord in peak of disease and post peak phases of EAE compared with control mice (Fig. 1c).

miR-142a-3p and miR-142a-5p are induced in activated splenocytes

Different cell types are involved in the neuroinflammatory process in MS/EAE, with autoreactive T cells and monocytoid cells, i.e., infiltrating monocytes and locally activated microglia, being key players. Astrocytes have also been implicated in disease process by producing various inflammatory mediators. To examine the potential contribution of these cells to miR-142a upregulation during inflammation, different in vitro systems were used. First, the expression of miR-142a isoforms were analyzed in splenocytes isolated from mice immunized with MOG35–55. Cells were restimulated in culture with three concentrations of MOG peptide for different time points before lysis and RNA extraction. RT-PCR data showed that miR-142a-5p levels were significantly increased in MOG-treated splenocytes after 12 h at 20 and 40 ng/ml and after 24 and 48 h at 40 ng/ml concentrations of peptide. A significant upregulation was also detected for miR-142a-3p at 10 ng/ml concentration of peptide at 12 h of treatment (Fig. 2a, b). We next studied the expression of miRNAs in T cells polyclonally activated by anti-CD3 and anti-CD28 antibodies. To this end, RNA was extracted from the cells at a range of time points after activation. The analyses revealed a substantial increase in miR-142a-3p and miR-142a-5p levels in stimulated splenocytes after 48 and 72 h (Fig. 2c, d). Indeed, the miRNA upregulation was much stronger in anti-CD3/CD28-stimulated T cells compared with MOG-stimulated cells, an effect that was expected considering that only a small fraction of splenocytes in MOG-immunized animals is MOG-reactive. Primary cultures of bone marrow-derived macrophages (BMDM) and astrocytes were then established to study miRNA expression in these cell types. LPS stimulation of cells was used as a model that could recapitulate some of the features of monocyte/glial cell activation during disease [30, 31]. A mild increase in miR-142a-3p and miR-142a-5p levels was seen in LPS-stimulated macrophages, but it did not reach statistical significance (Fig. 2e). Likewise,

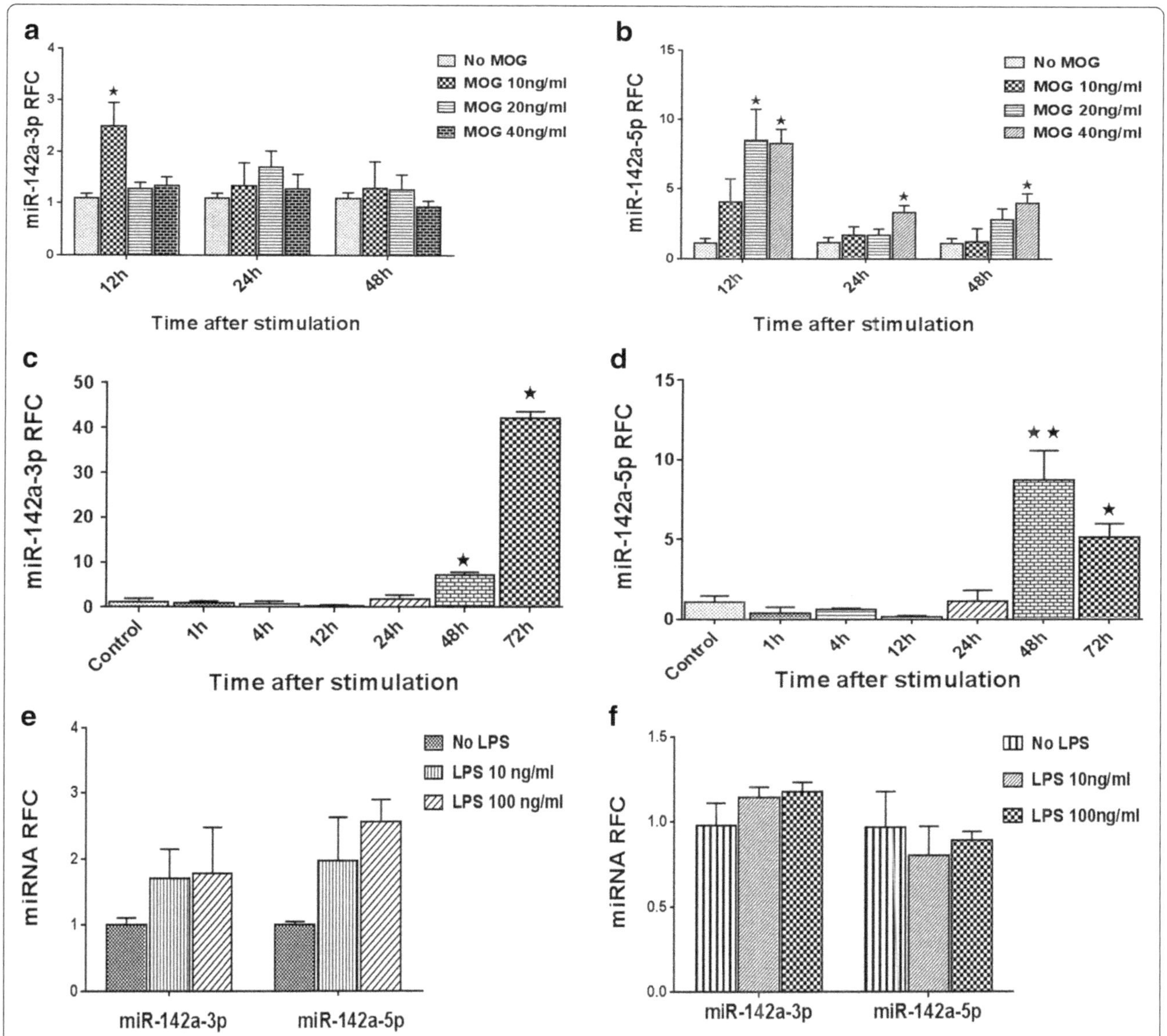

Fig. 2 miR-142a-3p and miR-142a-5p expression levels in splenocytes, macrophages, and astrocytes. Expression levels of miR-142a-3p and miR-142a-5p were analyzed in MOG-treated splenocytes from immunized animals (**a**, **b**) or splenocytes stimulated with anti-CD3 and anti-CD28 for different time points (**c**, **d**). Bone marrow-derived macrophages (**e**) and primary astrocytes (**f**) were stimulated with two concentrations of LPS for 12 h, before expression analysis by RT-PCR. Data are shown as mean ± SEM, $n = 3$. Experiment was repeated twice. *$p < 0.05$, **$p < 0.01$, Kruskal–Wallis test

activated primary astrocytes did not show any change in miR-142a-3p or miR-142a-5p levels following stimulation with LPS (Fig. 2f). Overall, these data indicate that splenocytes are able to enhance their expression of miR-142 isoforms after antigen-specific or polyclonal activation, and hence, they might be responsible for higher levels of miRNA transcripts identified in MS and EAE CNS tissues.

miR-142a-5p induces differentiation of naïve CD4$^+$ T cells towards Th1 subset

Considering the upregulation of miR-142 isoforms in antigen-stimulated or anti-CD3/CD28 activated splenocytes, we next investigated the effect of miR-142a isoforms on CD4 T cell differentiation. Naïve CD4$^+$ T cells were purified from the splenocytes of C57/BL6 mice, with a purity of more than 95% (Fig. 3a). Purified CD4$^+$ cells were transfected with miR-142a-3p and miR-142a-5p mimics and were then cultured in the presence of anti-CD3 and anti-CD28 in the presence of the required cytokines for differentiation to Th1, Th17, and Treg cells, as described in the "Methods" section. Intracellular cytokine staining and flow cytometric analysis after 4 days showed increased differentiation of miR-142a-5p-transfected cells towards IFN-γ producing Th1 subtype, compared with T cells transfected with a

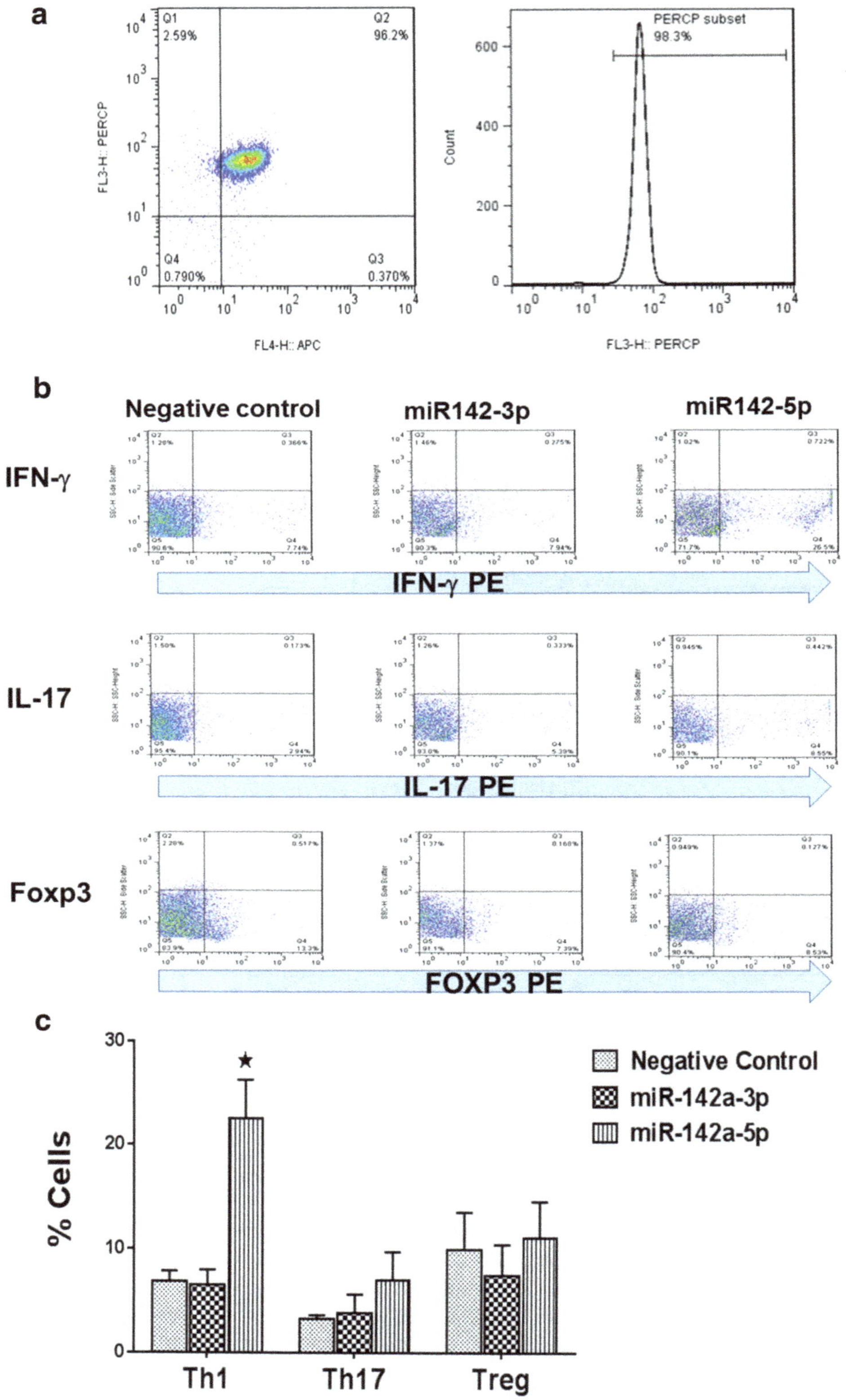

Fig. 3 (See legend on next page.)

(See figure on previous page.)
Fig. 3 Overexpression of miR-142a-5p affects the differentiation of CD4$^+$ T cells. Naïve CD4$^+$ T cells were isolated from mouse splenocytes to a purity of approximately 95% (**a**). miR-142a-3p, miR-142a-5p, and negative control sequences were transfected into CD4$^+$ T cells which were activated and polarized under relevant cytokine regimens. The frequencies of Th1, Th17, and Treg cells in CD4$^+$ T cells were determined by intracellular staining and flow cytometry after 4 days. Representative dot plots and the percentages of IFN-γ, IL-17, and FoxP3 immunopositive cells within the CD4$^+$ T cells (**b**). Average cell frequencies (**c**). Data are shown as mean ± SEM, $n = 3$. Data are from a single experiment representative of three independent experiments.(*$p < 0.05$, one-way ANOVA)

control miRNA sequence (Fig. 3b). There was also a mild increase in the frequency of IL-17-producing Th17 cells, but the increase did not reach statistical significance (Fig. 3c). The frequency of Treg cells did not reveal any difference following miR-142a-5p transfection. Similar experiments were performed for miR-142a-3p isoform. In contrast to miR-142a-5p, miR-142a-3p-transfected cells did not show any shifts in their differentiation towards Th1, Th17, or T regulatory cells, compared with T cells transfected with a scrambled miRNA control sequence. These data indicate that miR-142 isoforms can be upregulated in T cells following exposure to the antigen and activation of TCR signaling and their upregulation, at least for the 5p isoform, might be able to influence CD4 T cell status towards the more pathogenic Th1 phenotype (Fig. 3c).

Expression of inflammation-related transcripts are regulated by miR-142 isoforms

miRNAs exert their effects by targeting protein-coding transcripts. To investigate the potential mRNA transcripts which might be targeted by each of miR-142 isoforms, we extracted a list of predicted mRNA targets from TargetScan and miRDB databases. Considering the high number of potential targets, we focused on targets with known roles in cytokine signaling which also show conserved miRNA binding sites between human and mouse. We selected TGFBR-1 as a predicted target for miR-142a-3p and TGFBR-2 and SOCS-1 as predicted targets for mir-142a-5p. Adenylate cyclase 9 (ADCY9) was also selected as a confirmed target for miR-142a-5p (Additional file 1: Table S2). In addition to the mature miRNA sequences, the mRNA binding sites on the 3′ UTR of these genes (TGFBR1, ADCY9, TGFBR2, and SOCS1) are conserved between human and mouse (Additional file 1: Figure S1).

We first transfected miR-142a mimic sequences into mouse splenocytes and measured the target expression levels by real-time RT-PCR. TGFBR1 and ADCY9 transcript levels showed a significant reduction in miR-142a-3p-transfected cells in comparison with CD4$^+$ T cells transfected with a negative control sequence (Fig. 4a). Likewise, in cells transfected with miR-142a-5p sequences the levels of TGFBR2 and SOCS1 were decreased significantly in comparison with negative control transfected cells (Fig. 4b).

Expression of miR-142a isoform targets is dysregulated in activated splenocytes

As shown in Fig. 2, the expression of miR-142a isoforms increased in stimulated splenocytes after 48 and 72 h. Hence, to investigate whether altered miRNA expression is associated with any changes in the expression levels of potential targets, we analyzed the expression levels of miR-142a-3p predicted targets, TGFBR1, and ADCY9, as well as miR-142a-5p predicted targets, TGFBR2, and SOCS1 in stimulated splenocytes. TGFBR1 mRNA levels showed an initial upregulation after 1 h of stimulation compared with untreated cells; however, the expression quickly decreased in subsequent time points, to levels significantly below control cells after 24 h of stimulation

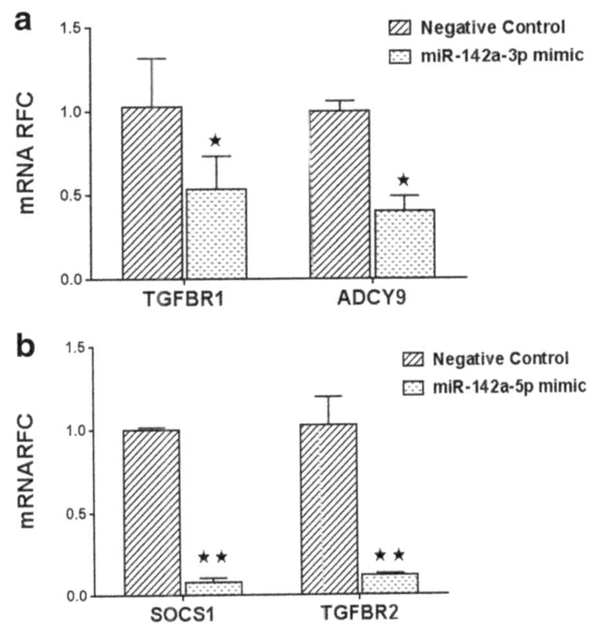

Fig. 4 Overexpression of miRNA sequences affects target gene expression in stimulated splenocytes. The expression of potential target genes was examined in cells transfected with miRNA sequences by real-time RT-PCR. TGFBR1 and ADCY9 transcripts were significantly suppressed in cells overexpressing miR-142a-3p compared with miRNA negative control transfected cells (**a**). SOCS1 and TGFBR2 transcripts were also significantly suppressed in cells overexpressing miR-142a-5p compared with miRNA negative control overexpressing cells (**b**). Data are shown as mean ± SEM, $n = 3$. Experiment was repeated twice. **$p < 0.01$, *$p < 0.05$, Student's t test

(Fig. 5a). ADCY9 levels also displayed a similar down-regulation after 24 h (Fig. 5b). TGFBR2 and SOCS1 showed an initial induction but were substantially down-regulated at time points after 24 h (Fig. 5c, d). Overall, these data show changes in expression of the targets which are "anti-parallel" with miRNA levels in the cells, further supporting their potential regulation by miRNAs.

Luciferase assays show direct interaction between miR-142a isoforms and mRNA transcripts

To examine whether miR-142a directly interacts with TGFBR1, TGFBR2, and SOCS1 transcripts, we used a luciferase reporter system. The 3′-UTR region of TGFBR1 mRNA was PCR amplified and cloned into psiCHECK-2 vector, downstream of firefly luciferase coding sequence. HEK293T cells were co-transfected with luciferase-3′UTR construct and miR-142a-3p mimics or a negative miRNA control. Quantification of luciferase activity after co-transfection revealed significant suppression of luciferase activity in cells co-transfected with miR-142a-3p mimics in comparison with cells transfected with the negative control miRNA (Fig. 6a). Similar experiments were performed for miR-142a-5p. The 3′-UTR region of TGFBR2 and SOCS1 mRNAs were cloned into psiCHECK-2 vector, separately. HEK293T cells were then co-transfected with vectors encoding the firefly luciferase open reading frame fused to the 3′-UTR region of TGFBR2 or SOCS1 and mimics of miR-142a-5p or negative control miRNA. Quantification of luciferase activity after co-transfection revealed significant reduction in luciferase activity in cells co-transfected with SOCS1-3′-UTR region and miR-142a-5p in comparison with cells transfected with a negative control miRNA (Fig. 6c). Nonetheless, in cells co-transfected with miR-142a-5p mimics and TGFBR2-3′-UTR constructs, luciferase activity did not show any significant suppression (Fig. 6b). Altogether, these data indicate that miR-142a-3p and miR-142a-5p isoforms directly target TGFBR1 and SOCS1 transcripts, respectively. In the case of TGFBR2 our data did not reveal evidence of direct interactions, however, considering the results of T cells transfection experiments, it seems that miR-142-3p might be able to affect TGFBR2 levels, perhaps by indirect means.

miR-142a isoforms target genes show dysregulation in the CNS of patients with multiple sclerosis and animals with EAE

Given the increased expression of miR-142 isoforms in human and miR-142a isoforms in EAE CNS tissues we next investigated the expression levels of each target transcript in MS and EAE tissues. We analyzed the transcript levels of TGFBR1 and ADCY9 as targets of miR-142a-3p, as well as SOCS1 as a target of miR-142a-5p in the human brain samples and in the lumbar spinal cord tissue from EAE mice in three phases of disease (pre-onset, peak of disease and post peak) using real-time PCR. Data in EAE tissue showed that the expression of TGFBR1 was

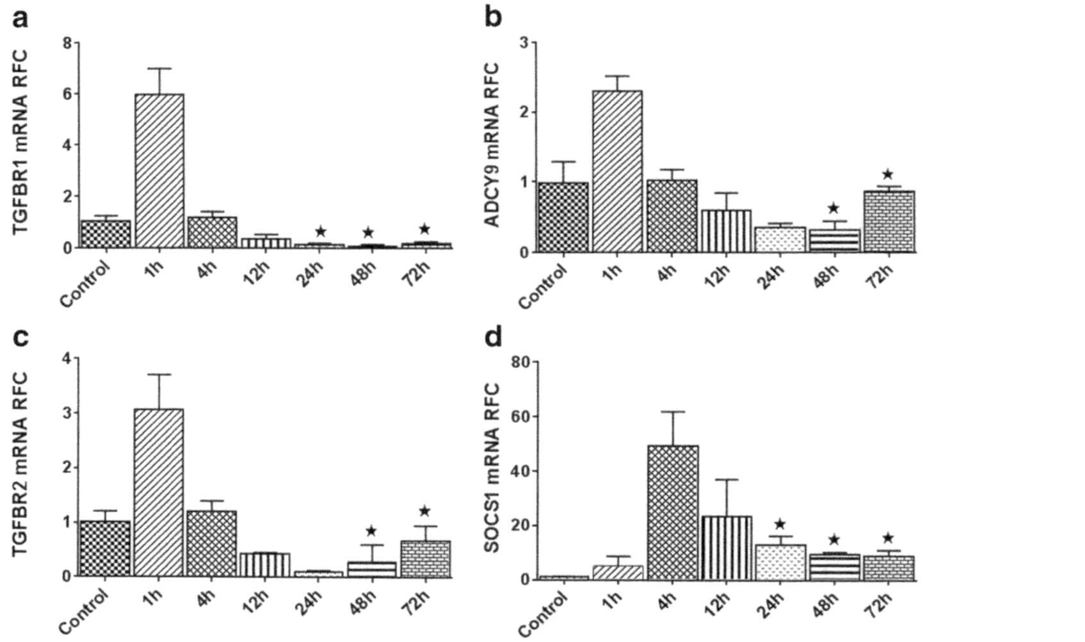

Fig. 5 miR-142a-3p and miR-142a-5p predicted target genes expression in activated splenocytes. Expression of miR-142 isoforms target genes in stimulated splenocytes was determined by real-time RT-PCR. The levels of TGFBR1 and ADCY9 genes in 24, 48, and 72 h (**a**, **b**). TGFBR2 in 24 and 48 h after stimulation were significantly decreased in stimulated splenocytes compared with unstimulated cells (**c**). SOCS1 levels were initially upregulated followed by a significant reduction (**d**). Data are shown as mean ± SEM, $n = 3$. Experiment was repeated twice. *$p < 0.05$, one-way ANOVA)

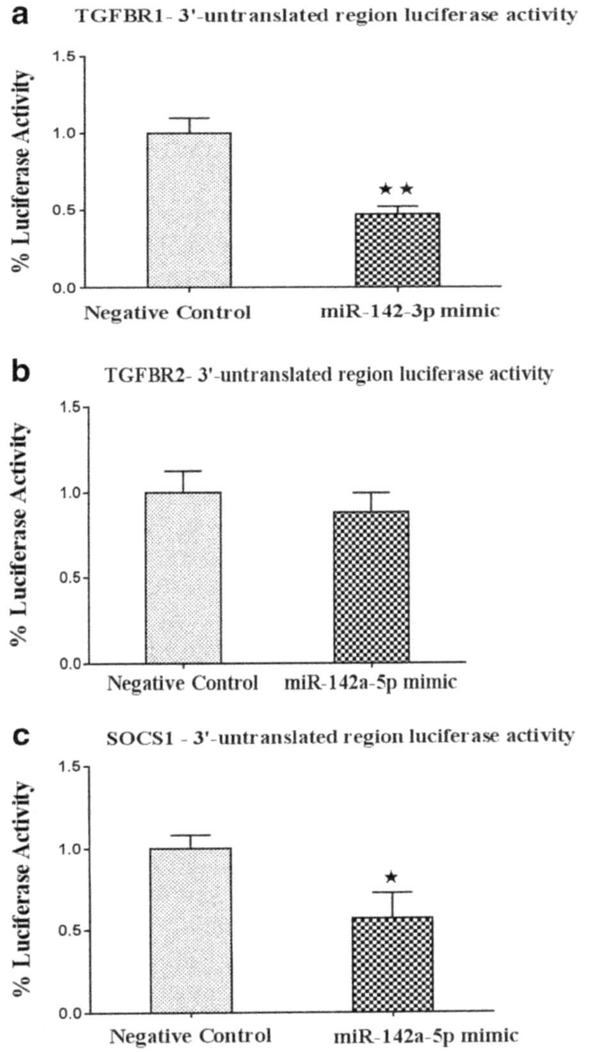

Fig. 6 Luciferase-3′-untranslated region reporter assay. Interaction of miR-142a-3p with TGFBR1 and miR-142a-5p with TGFBR2 and SOCS1 transcripts were assessed using luciferase assay system. Co-transfection of HEK293T cells containing luciferase-3′UTR construct from TGFBR1 together with miR-142a-3p mimics showed significant suppression of luciferase activity in comparison with cells transfected with a control miRNA sequence (**a**). miR-142a-5p transfection did not lead to significant suppression of luciferase activity in cells co-transfected with TGFBR2 3′UTR constructs (**b**). Similar experiments with luciferase-3′ UTR from SOCS1 and miR-142a-5p mimics showed suppression of luciferase activity compared with cells transfected a control sequence (**c**). Firefly luciferase levels were normalized against renilla luciferase, expressed as an internal control in the vector. Data are shown as mean ± SEM, $n = 5$. Data are from a single experiment representative of three independent experiments. *$p < 0.05$, **$p < 0.01$, Student's t test

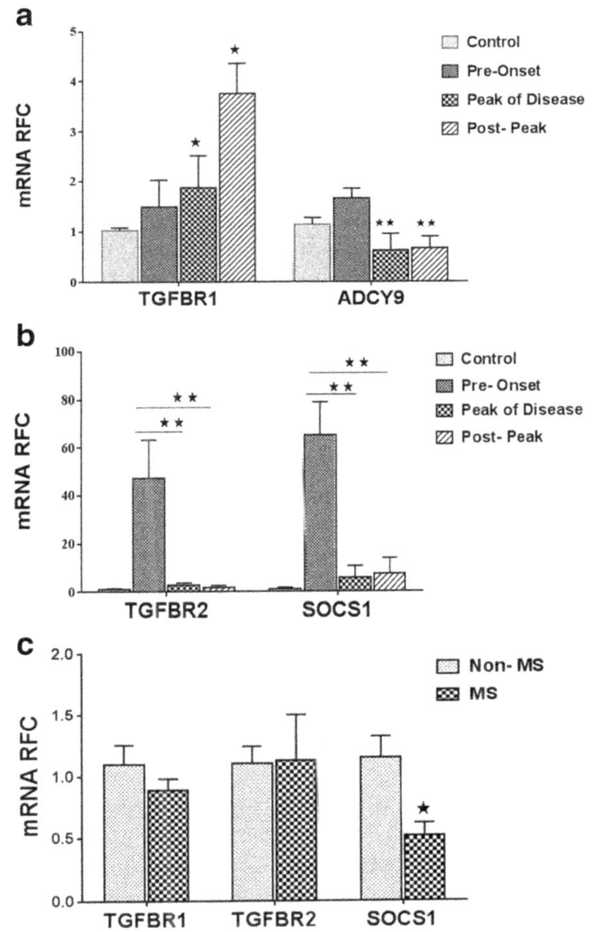

Fig. 7 miR-142a-3p and miR-142a-5p target gene expression in EAE tissue and human MS brain samples. miR-142a-3p target gene, TGFBR1, was significantly increased in peak of disease and post peak phase of EAE in spinal cord (**a**). SOCS1 and TGFBR2 were significantly decreased in peak of disease and post peak phases of EAE in comparison with pre-onset phase (**b**). In human autopsy samples, SOCS1 showed significant reduction in MS samples but the levels of TGFBR1 and TGFBR2 did not differ between MS and control tissues (**c**). Data are shown as mean ± SEM, **$p < 0.01$, *$p < 0.05$, one-way ANOVA

increased in peak of disease and post peak phases of disease (Fig. 7a), whereas the expression levels of ADCY9 was lower in peak of disease and post peak stages of disease compared with controls or the pre-onset phase (Fig. 7a). SOCS1 expression showed a significant upregulation before the onset of neurological signs but it was downregulated at later stages of the disease (Fig. 7b). Expression of TGFBR2, an indirect target of miR-142a-5p also showed a similar pattern (Fig. 7b). Analysis of the human white matter showed significant reduction in SOCS1 transcript levels in comparison with non-MS samples but TGFBR1 and TGFBR2 expression levels were similar between patient groups with a trend towards reduced TGFBR1 expression in MS white matter (Fig. 7c).

Discussion

In this study, we investigated the role of miR-142a isoforms (miR-142a-3p and miR-142a-5p) in autoimmune neuroinflammation. Using human brain autopsy samples and EAE CNS tissues, as well as different cell culture systems and molecular analyses, we show that miR-142 isoforms might be involved in the neuroinflammatory processes underlying MS/EAE. Our gene expression studies showed increased levels of both miR-142-5p and miR-142-3p isoforms in EAE spinal cord, and in MS brains miR-142-5p showed statistically significant increase. Consistent with previous reports [32], our in vitro gene expression studies showed expression of miR-142 mature isoforms in both T cells and primary macrophages. Both cell types contribute to neuroinflammation in MS/EAE. MS tissues used in this study were derived from the so-called normal-appearing white matter (NAWM) around lesions. It should be noted that while inflammation is most severe in classical MS lesions, studies on NAWM have shown diffuse axonal injury together with microglial activation and T cell infiltration in these areas [33–35]. Of note, T cell receptor expression analysis in different brain regions has shown that the same T cell clones that are present in lesions are also present in NAWM indicating that similar antigens are recognized by T cells in lesions and NAWM [36]. While the current study is chiefly focused on miR-142 expression in T cells, we believe that both T cells and activated microglia in the NAWM contribute to enhanced miRNA expression in the tissues from MS patients.

Some very recent studies have pointed to the role of miR-142 isoforms in MS pathogenesis. Mandolesi et al. have reported increased levels of miR-142-3p in the CSF of patients with active MS as well as brain tissue from EAE mice [21]. miR-142-3p was shown to regulate IL-1beta-dependent synaptic abnormalities that occur during neuroinflammation. Interestingly, inhibition of miR-142-3p prevented an increase in glutamergic transmission caused by exposure of cerebellar slices to CSF from MS patients [21]. Studies on blood cells have also linked miR-142-3p with MS disease process. Arruda et al. have recently reported enhanced miR-142-3p expression in $CD4^+$ and $CD8^+$ T cells from MS patients [37]. Conversely, some T cell studies have reported downregulation of miR-142-3p. In a study by Sanders et al., researchers performed next generation sequencing on $CD4^+$ T cells from secondary progressive multiple sclerosis (SP-MS) patients. The results revealed downregulation of multiple miRNAs including miR-142-3p in T cells derived from MS patients [38]. These discrepancies could likely be a reflection of disease heterogeneity as well as highly dynamic nature of miRNA expression during different phases of disease.

Our data suggest that the miR-142 isoforms could target transcripts which are involved in cytokine signaling and T cell differentiation, thereby affecting the phenotype of neuroantigen-reactive T cells infiltrating the nervous system during disease. We show that "suppressor of cytokine signaling 1", SOCS1, is a direct target of miR-142a-5p. SOCS1 is a member of the SOCS family of proteins which are negative regulators of cytokine signaling. Multiple cytokines recruit the Janus kinase (JAK)–signal transducers and activators of the transcription (STAT) molecules to exert their effects [39, 40]. The proteins of SOCS family which are induced by different cytokines including IL-2 and IFN-γ can impede the signal transduction by these and other cytokines through inhibition of JAKs or blockade of their recruitment to the cytokine receptors [41]. SOCS1, one the most widely studied members of the SOCS family, has been shown to be involved in regulating the differentiation of T cells, making the molecule a key player in T cell-mediated immunopathologies [42]. It is known that STAT1 and STAT5 contribute to Th1 differentiation by enhancing T-bet and IFN-γ expression [43, 44]. SOCS1 suppresses STAT1 [41] and blocks IFN-γ-mediated STAT1 activation by targeting JAK2 and IFN-cRa chain [45]. In addition to its role in Th1 development, SOCS1 is necessary for Treg stability and suppressor function through stabilizing Foxp3 expression [46] and by preventing the production of inflammatory cytokines by Tregs [47]. Normally, Tregs do not secret inflammatory cytokines but in the absence of SOCS1, these cells secret IFN-γ and IL-17 likely due to hyperactivation of STAT1 and STAT3 [48]. This phenomenon can lead to the loss of Foxp3 expression and the conversion of regulatory cells to a Th1/Th17 phenotype [49]. Indeed, studies of SOCS1 KO mice have shown that most SOCS1-deficient CD4 naïve T cells differentiate into Th1 [50, 51] and SOCS1-deficient mice develop autoimmune inflammatory diseases with age [31]. All these findings point to SOCS1 as a guardian of Tregs and a controller of Th1 development. In this study, we show that SOCS1 levels are diminished in MS tissues, and that it could be targeted by miR-142-5p, a finding that can be viewed important both from the perspectives of understanding MS pathogenesis and potential therapeutic interventions.

The other isoform of miR-142, i.e., miR-142-3p, has also been implicated in regulating T cell activity. Indeed, it has been reported that miR-142-3p reduces the production of cyclic 3′5′-adenosine monophosphate (cAMP), a molecule required for regulatory function of Tregs, by suppressing adenylyl cyclase (AC) 9 mRNA in T cells and macrophages. Apparently, miR-142-3p does not influence the expression of Foxp3, but Foxp3 regulates, directly or indirectly, the expression of miR-142-3p [19]. In this study, using overexpression experiments and luciferase assays, we showed that TGFBR1 is a target of miR-142a-3p. TGF-β is a cytokine with pleiotropic functions including regulation of inflammation as well as survival, growth and differentiation of many cell types [32]. TGF-β signaling is initiated by the binding of TGF-β to heteromeric complexes of type I (TGFbRI) and type II (TGFbRII) receptors on the cell membrane [52]. Several studies have shown the enhanced expression of TGF-β1 in the CNS in MS and EAE [53–57]. The effects of TGFβ1 in the context of MS/EAE are diverse and chiefly protective. These effects could be roughly categorized to two types: effects on neural cells and on leukocytes. TGF-β1's promotion of oligodendrocyte differentiation leading to enhanced remyelination in MS lesions is an example of the effects on neural cells [58, 59]. TGFβ1 also suppresses autoantigen-induced activation of lymphocytes, activation of monocytoid cells, and the production of pro-inflammatory cytokines [60]. This latter function is believed to be chiefly mediated by increasing Treg activity. The finding that miR-142a-3p can target TGFBR1 and thereby diminish TGFβ signaling might point to a novel pathogenic pathway that diminishes both neuroprotective and immunomodulatory effects of the cytokine simultaneously. Indeed, it has been demonstrated that the expression of miR-142a-3p in Treg cells is lower compared with non Treg $CD4^+$ T cells. While we did not observe a shift in T cell differentiation following miR-142a-3p transfection of these cells, the possibility still remains that miRNA-mediated reduction in TGFBR1 expression in T cells, monocytoid cells, or neural cells might play a role in neuroinflammation/degeneration.

Conclusions

Results of this study suggest that miR-142 isoforms are upregulated in the CNS of MS patients and animals with EAE. Increased expression of these microRNAs might be involved in the autoimmune neuroinflammation and pathogenesis of multiple sclerosis through changing the pattern of T cells differentiation towards IFN-γ-producing Th1 cells; an effect which might be mediated through targeting and suppression of protective genes such as TGFBR1 and SOCS1.

Abbreviations

ADCY9: Adenylate cyclase 9; BMDM: Bone marrow-derived macrophages; cAMP: Cyclic adenosine monophosphate; CNS: Central nervous system; EAE: Experimental autoimmune encephalomyelitis; IFN-γ: Interferon gamma; JAK: Janus kinase; LPS: Lipopolysaccharide; M-CSF: Macrophage colony-stimulating factor; MOG: Myelin oligodendrocyte glycoprotein; MS: Multiple sclerosis; RR-MS: Relapsing-remitting multiple sclerosis; RT-PCR: Reverse transcriptase polymerase chain reaction; SOCS1: Suppressor of cytokine signaling 1; SP-MS: Secondary progressive multiple sclerosis; STAT1: Signal transducer and activator of transcription 1; TGFBR: Transforming growth factor beta receptor; TGF-β: Transforming growth factor; Th cell: T helper cell; Treg cell: Regulatory T cell

Acknowledgements

The authors would like to thank all of the faculty members at Department of Immunology at School of Medicine at TUMS for helpful discussions regarding the work.

Funding

This work was supported by research grants from Iranian National Science Foundation (INSF) (Grant number: 93051855) and Tehran University of Medical Sciences (90-03-15048). Funding bodies had no role in the design of the study and collection, analysis, and interpretation of data and in writing the manuscript.

Authors' contributions

FT and SG (1) designed, optimized, and performed most of the experiments, including EAE studies, cell cultures, gene expressions, flow cytometries, and molecular analyses. FT analyzed all the data and wrote the manuscript. WFC performed gene expression experiments on human autopsy brains. RB performed immunohistochemistry experiments on spinal cord of EAE and control mice. FM and SG (2) helped with flow cytometries and cell cultures. MV and CP supervised and oversaw the research process. FN conceived the hypotheses and designed and supervised the research. CP and FN edited the final manuscript. All authors read and approved the final manuscript.

Competing interests

The authors declare that they have no competing interests.

Author details

[1]Department of Immunology, School of Medicine, Tehran University of Medical Sciences, Tehran, Iran. [2]Shefa Neuroscience Research Institute, Khatam Al-Anbia Hospital, Tehran, Iran. [3]Department of Medicine (Neurology), University of Alberta, Edmonton, AB, Canada. [4]Multiple Sclerosis Centre, University of Alberta, Edmonton, AB, Canada.

References

1. Nilsen TW. Mechanisms of microRNA-mediated gene regulation in animal cells. Trends Genet. 2007;23(5):243–9.
2. Pillai RS. MicroRNA function: multiple mechanisms for a tiny RNA? RNA. 2005;11(12):1753–61.
3. Ebert MS, Sharp PA. Roles for microRNAs in conferring robustness to biological processes. Cell. 2012;149(3):515–24.
4. Lodish HF, Zhou B, Liu G, Chen CZ. Micromanagement of the immune system by microRNAs. Nat Rev Immunol. 2008;8(2):120–30.
5. Pauley KM, Cha S, Chan EK. MicroRNA in autoimmunity and autoimmune diseases. J Autoimmun. 2009;32(3-4):189–94.
6. Otaegui D, Baranzini SE, Armananzas R, Calvo B, Munoz-Culla M, Khankhanian P, et al. Differential micro RNA expression in PBMC from multiple sclerosis patients. PLoS One. 2009;4(7):e6309.
7. Gandhi KS, McKay FC, Cox M, Riveros C, Armstrong N, Heard RN, et al. The multiple sclerosis whole blood mRNA transcriptome and genetic associations indicate dysregulation of specific T cell pathways in pathogenesis. Hum Mol Genet. 2010;19(11):2134–43.
8. Raddatz BB, Hansmann F, Spitzbarth I, Kalkuhl A, Deschl U, Baumgartner W, et al. Transcriptomic meta-analysis of multiple sclerosis and its experimental models. PLoS One. 2014;9(1):e86643.
9. Keller A, Leidinger P, Lange J, Borries A, Schroers H, Scheffler M, et al. Multiple sclerosis: microRNA expression profiles accurately differentiate patients with relapsing-remitting disease from healthy controls. PLoS One. 2009;4(10):e7440.
10. De Santis G, Ferracin M, Biondani A, Caniatti L, Rosaria Tola M, Castellazzi M, et al. Altered miRNA expression in T regulatory cells in course of multiple sclerosis. J Neuroimmunol. 2010;226(1-2):165–71.
11. Lindberg RL, Hoffmann F, Mehling M. Kuhle J, Kappos L. Altered expression of miR-17-5p in CD4+ lymphocytes of relapsing-remitting multiple sclerosis patients. Eur J Immunol. 2010;40(3):888–98.
12. Guerau-de-Arellano M, Smith KM, Godlewski J, Liu Y, Winger R, Lawler SE, et al. Micro-RNA dysregulation in multiple sclerosis favours pro-inflammatory T-cell-mediated autoimmunity. Brain. 2011;134(Pt 12):3578–89.
13. Du C, Liu C, Kang J, Zhao G, Ye Z, Huang S, et al. MicroRNA miR-326 regulates TH-17 differentiation and is associated with the pathogenesis of multiple sclerosis. Nat Immunol. 2009;10(12):1252–9.
14. Junker A, Krumbholz M, Eisele S, Mohan H, Augstein F, Bittner R, et al. MicroRNA profiling of multiple sclerosis lesions identifies modulators of the

regulatory protein CD47. Brain. 2009;132(Pt 12):3342–52.
15. Giuliani F, Metz LM, Wilson T, Fan Y, Bar-Or A, Yong VW. Additive effect of the combination of glatiramer acetate and minocycline in a model of MS. J Neuroimmunol. 2005;158(1–2):213–21.
16. Murugaiyan G, Beynon V, Mittal A, Joller N, Weiner HL. Silencing microRNA-155 ameliorates experimental autoimmune encephalomyelitis. J Immunol. 2011;187(5):2213–21.
17. Wu H, Neilson JR, Kumar P, Manocha M, Shankar P, Sharp PA, et al. miRNA profiling of naive, effector and memory CD8 T cells. PLoS One. 2007;2(10):e1020.
18. Zhou Q, Haupt S, Prots I, Thummler K, Kremmer E, Lipsky PE, et al. miR-142-3p is involved in CD25+ CD4 T cell proliferation by targeting the expression of glycoprotein A repetitions predominant. J Immunol. 2013;190(12):6579–88.
19. Huang B, Zhao J, Lei Z, Shen S, Li D, Shen GX, et al. miR-142-3p restricts cAMP production in CD4 + CD25- T cells and CD4 + CD25+ TREG cells by targeting AC9 mRNA. EMBO Rep. 2009;10(2):180–5.
20. Fordham JB, Naqvi AR, Nares S. Regulation of miR-24, miR-30b, and miR-142-3p during macrophage and dendritic cell differentiation potentiates innate immunity. J Leukoc Biol. 2015;98(2):195–207.
21. Mandolesi G, De Vito F, Musella A, Gentile A, Bullitta S, Fresegna D, et al. miR-142-3p is a key regulator of IL-1beta-dependent synaptopathy in neuroinflammation. J Neurosci. 2017;37(3):546–561.
22. Noorbakhsh F, Tsutsui S, Vergnolle N, Boven LA, Shariat N, Vodjgani M, et al. Proteinase-activated receptor 2 modulates neuroinflammation in experimental autoimmune encephalomyelitis and multiple sclerosis. J Exp Med. 2006;203(2):425–35.
23. Ellestad KK, Tsutsui S, Noorbakhsh F, Warren KG, Yong VW, Pittman QJ, et al. Early life exposure to lipopolysaccharide suppresses experimental autoimmune encephalomyelitis by promoting tolerogenic dendritic cells and regulatory T cells. J Immunol. 2009;183(1):298–309.
24. Delarasse C, Smith P, Baker D, Amor S. Novel pathogenic epitopes of myelin oligodendrocyte glycoprotein induce experimental autoimmune encephalomyelitis in C57BL/6 mice. Immunology. 2013;140(4):456–64.
25. Lyons JA, San M, Happ MP, Cross AH. B cells are critical to induction of experimental allergic encephalomyelitis by protein but not by a short encephalitogenic peptide. Eur J Immunol. 1999;29(11):3432–9.
26. Schellenberg AE, Buist R, Yong VW, Del Bigio MR, Peeling J. Magnetic resonance imaging of blood-spinal cord barrier disruption in mice with experimental autoimmune encephalomyelitis. Magn Reson Med. 2007;58(2):298–305.
27. Miller SD, Karpus WJ. Experimental autoimmune encephalomyelitis in the mouse. Curr Protoc Immunol. 2007;Chapter 15:Unit 15 1.
28. Tsutsui S, Schnermann J, Noorbakhsh F, Henry S, Yong VW, Winston BW, et al. A1 adenosine receptor upregulation and activation attenuates neuroinflammation and demyelination in a model of multiple sclerosis. J Neurosci. 2004;24(6):1521–9.
29. Schildge S, Bohrer C, Beck K, Schachtrup C. Isolation and culture of mouse cortical astrocytes. J Vis Exp. 2013;(71). doi:10.3791/50079.
30. Chen J, Bruns AH, Donnelly HK, Wunderink RG. Comparative in vitro stimulation with lipopolysaccharide to study TNFalpha gene expression in fresh whole blood, fresh and frozen peripheral blood mononuclear cells. J Immunol Methods. 2010;357(1-2):33–7.
31. Gresa-Arribas N, Vieitez C, Dentesano G, Serratosa J, Saura J, Sola C. Modelling neuroinflammation in vitro: a tool to test the potential neuroprotective effect of anti-inflammatory agents. PLoS One. 2012;7(9):e45227.
32. Sun Y, Oravecz-Wilson K, Mathewson N, Wang Y, McEachin R, Liu C, et al. Mature T cell responses are controlled by microRNA-142. J Clin Invest. 2015;125(7):2825–40.
33. Kutzelnigg A, Lucchinetti CF, Stadelmann C, Bruck W, Rauschka H, Bergmann M, et al. Cortical demyelination and diffuse white matter injury in multiple sclerosis. Brain. 2005;128(Pt 11):2705–12.
34. Metz I, Lucchinetti CF, Openshaw H, Garcia-Merino A, Lassmann H, Freedman MS, et al. Autologous haematopoietic stem cell transplantation fails to stop demyelination and neurodegeneration in multiple sclerosis. Brain. 2007;130(Pt 5):1254–62.
35. Traugott U, Reinherz EL, Raine CS. Multiple sclerosis. Distribution of T cells, T cell subsets and Ia-positive macrophages in lesions of different ages. J Neuroimmunol. 1983;4(3):201–21.
36. Junker A, Ivanidze J, Malotka J, Eiglmeier I, Lassmann H, Wekerle H, et al. Multiple sclerosis: T-cell receptor expression in distinct brain regions. Brain. 2007;130(Pt 11):2789–99.
37. Arruda LC, Lorenzi JC, Sousa AP, Zanette DL, Palma PV, Panepucci RA, et al. Autologous hematopoietic SCT normalizes miR-16, -155 and -142-3p expression in multiple sclerosis patients. Bone Marrow Transplant. 2015;50(3):380–9.
38. Sanders KA, Benton MC, Lea RA, Maltby VE, Agland S, Griffin N, et al. Next-generation sequencing reveals broad down-regulation of microRNAs in secondary progressive multiple sclerosis CD4+ T cells. Clin Epigenetics. 2016;8(1):87.
39. O'Shea JJ, Gadina M, Schreiber RD. Cytokine signaling in 2002: new surprises in the Jak/Stat pathway. Cell. 2002;109(Suppl):S121–31.
40. Adamson AS, Collins K, Laurence A, O'Shea JJ. The Current STATus of lymphocyte signaling: new roles for old players. Curr Opin Immunol. 2009;21(2):161–6.
41. Torisu T, Nakaya M, Watanabe S, Hashimoto M, Yoshida H, Chinen T, et al. Suppressor of cytokine signaling 1 protects mice against concanavalin A-induced hepatitis by inhibiting apoptosis. Hepatology. 2008;47(5):1644–54.
42. Bhattacharyya S, Zhao Y, Kay TW, Muglia LJ. Glucocorticoids target suppressor of cytokine signaling 1 (SOCS1) and type 1 interferons to regulate Toll-like receptor-induced STAT1 activation. Proc Natl Acad Sci U S A. 2011;108(23):9554–9.
43. Starr R, Metcalf D, Elefanty AG, Brysha M, Willson TA, Nicola NA, et al. Liver degeneration and lymphoid deficiencies in mice lacking suppressor of cytokine signaling-1. Proc Natl Acad Sci U S A. 1998;95(24):14395–9.
44. Alexander WS, Starr R, Fenner JE, Scott CL, Handman E, Sprigg NS, et al. SOCS1 is a critical inhibitor of interferon gamma signaling and prevents the potentially fatal neonatal actions of this cytokine. Cell. 1999;98(5):597–608.
45. Sakamoto H, Yasukawa H, Masuhara M, Tanimura S, Sasaki A, Yuge K, et al. A Janus kinase inhibitor, JAB, is an interferon-gamma-inducible gene and confers resistance to interferons. Blood. 1998;92(5):1668–76.
46. Takahashi R, Nishimoto S, Muto G, Sekiya T, Tamiya T, Kimura A, et al. SOCS1 is essential for regulatory T cell functions by preventing loss of Foxp3 expression as well as IFN-{gamma} and IL-17A production. J Exp Med. 2011;208(10):2055–67.
47. Zhou X, Bailey-Bucktrout SL, Jeker LT, Penaranda C, Martinez-Llordella M, Ashby M, et al. Instability of the transcription factor Foxp3 leads to the generation of pathogenic memory T cells in vivo. Nat Immunol. 2009;10(9):1000–7.
48. Tanaka K, Ichiyama K, Hashimoto M, Yoshida H, Takimoto T, Takaesu G, et al. Loss of suppressor of cytokine signaling 1 in helper T cells leads to defective Th17 differentiation by enhancing antagonistic effects of IFN-gamma on STAT3 and Smads. J Immunol. 2008;180(6):3746–56.
49. Lu LF, Thai TH, Calado DP, Chaudhry A, Kubo M, Tanaka K, et al. Foxp3-dependent microRNA155 confers competitive fitness to regulatory T cells by targeting SOCS1 protein. Immunity. 2009;30(1):80–91.
50. Pillemer BB, Xu H, Oriss TB, Qi Z, Ray A. Deficient SOCS3 expression in CD4 + CD25 + FoxP3+ regulatory T cells and SOCS3-mediated suppression of Treg function. Eur J Immunol. 2007;37(8):2082–9.
51. Lawrence DA. Transforming growth factor-beta: a general review. Eur Cytokine Netw. 1996;7(3):363–74.
52. Konig HG, Kogel D, Rami A, Prehn JH. TGF-{beta}1 activates two distinct type I receptors in neurons: implications for neuronal NF-{kappa}B signaling. J Cell Biol. 2005;168(7):1077–86.
53. Beck J, Rondot P, Jullien P, Wietzerbin J, Lawrence DA. TGF-beta-like activity produced during regression of exacerbations in multiple sclerosis. Acta Neurol Scand. 1991;84(5):452–5.
54. van Horssen J, Bo L, Dijkstra CD, de Vries HE. Extensive extracellular matrix depositions in active multiple sclerosis lesions. Neurobiol Dis. 2006;24(3):484–91.
55. Kiefer R, Schweitzer T, Jung S, Toyka KV, Hartung HP. Sequential expression of transforming growth factor-beta1 by T-cells, macrophages, and microglia in rat spinal cord during autoimmune inflammation. J Neuropathol Exp Neurol. 1998;57(5):385–95.
56. Link J, Soderstrom M, Olsson T, Hojeberg B, Ljungdahl A, Link H. Increased transforming growth factor-beta, interleukin-4, and interferon-gamma in multiple sclerosis. Ann Neurol. 1994;36(3):379–86.
57. Rollnik JD, Sindern E, Schweppe C, Malin JP. Biologically active TGF-beta 1 is increased in cerebrospinal fluid while it is reduced in serum in multiple sclerosis patients. Acta Neurol Scand. 1997;96(2):101–5.
58. Heupel K, Sargsyan V, Plomp JJ, Rickmann M, Varoqueaux F, Zhang W, et al. Loss of transforming growth factor-beta 2 leads to impairment of central synapse function. Neural Dev. 2008;3:25.
59. Diemel LT, Jackson SJ, Cuzner ML. Role for TGF-beta1, FGF-2 and PDGF-AA in a myelination of CNS aggregate cultures enriched with macrophages. J Neurosci Res. 2003;74(6):858–67.

17

Exome sequencing study in patients with multiple sclerosis reveals variants associated with disease course

Elia Gil-Varea[1], Elena Urcelay[2], Carles Vilariño-Güell[3], Carme Costa[1], Luciana Midaglia[1], Fuencisla Matesanz[4], Alfredo Rodríguez-Antigüedad[5], Jorge Oksenberg[6], Laura Espino-Paisan[2], A. Dessa Sadovnick[3], Albert Saiz[7], Luisa M. Villar[8], Juan Antonio García-Merino[9], Lluís Ramió-Torrentà[10], Juan Carlos Triviño[11], Ester Quintana[10], René Robles[10], Antonio Sánchez-López[9], Rafael Arroyo[12], Jose C. Alvarez-Cermeño[8], Angela Vidal-Jordana[1], Sunny Malhotra[1], Nicolas Fissolo[1], Xavier Montalban[1] and Manuel Comabella[1*]

Abstract

Background: It remains unclear whether disease course in multiple sclerosis (MS) is influenced by genetic polymorphisms. Here, we aimed to identify genetic variants associated with benign and aggressive disease courses in MS patients.

Methods: MS patients were classified into benign and aggressive phenotypes according to clinical criteria. We performed exome sequencing in a discovery cohort, which included 20 MS patients, 10 with benign and 10 with aggressive disease course, and genotyping in 2 independent validation cohorts. The first validation cohort encompassed 194 MS patients, 107 with benign and 87 with aggressive phenotypes. The second validation cohort comprised 257 patients, of whom 224 patients had benign phenotypes and 33 aggressive disease courses. Brain immunohistochemistries were performed using disease course associated genes antibodies.

Results: By means of single-nucleotide polymorphism (SNP) detection and comparison of allele frequencies between patients with benign and aggressive phenotypes, a total of 16 SNPs were selected for validation from the exome sequencing data in the discovery cohort. Meta-analysis of genotyping results in two validation cohorts revealed two polymorphisms, rs28469012 and rs10894768, significantly associated with disease course. SNP rs28469012 is located in *CPXM2* (carboxypeptidase X, M14 family, member 2) and was associated with aggressive disease course (uncorrected p value < 0.05). SNP rs10894768, which is positioned in *IGSF9B* (immunoglobulin superfamily member 9B) was associated with benign phenotype (uncorrected p value < 0.05). In addition, a trend for association with benign phenotype was observed for a third SNP, rs10423927, in *NLRP9* (NLR family pyrin domain containing 9). Brain immunohistochemistries in chronic active lesions from MS patients revealed expression of IGSF9B in astrocytes and macrophages/microglial cells, and expression of CPXM2 and NLRP9 restricted to brain macrophages/microglia.

Conclusions: Genetic variants located in *CPXM2*, *IGSF9B*, and *NLRP9* have the potential to modulate disease course in MS patients and may be used as disease activity biomarkers to identify patients with divergent disease courses. Altogether, the reported results from this study support the influence of genetic factors in MS disease course and may help to better understand the complex molecular mechanisms underlying disease pathogenesis.

Keywords: Multiple sclerosis, Immunology, Disease course, Exome sequencing, Polymorphisms, *CPXM2*, *IGSF9B*, *NLRP9*

* Correspondence: manuel.comabella@vhir.org
[1]Servei de Neurologia-Neuroimmunologia, Centre d'Esclerosi Múltiple de Catalunya (Cemcat), Institut de Recerca Vall d'Hebron (VHIR), Hospital Universitari Vall d'Hebron, Universitat Autònoma de Barcelona, Barcelona, Spain

Background

Multiple sclerosis (MS [MIM: 126200]) is a common disease of the central nervous system (CNS) of complex pathogenesis. Although the etiology of MS is unknown, it is assumed that both genetic and environmental factors, such as cigarette smoking, vitamin D deficiency, viral infections, or obesity, influence disease phenotype [1–3]. Additionally, there is increasing evidence that inherited epigenetic variation complements the role of the genetic predisposition in the susceptibility to develop MS [4]. Over the last years, genome-wide association studies (GWAS) have significantly contributed to the characterization of the MS genetic component, with the identification of more than 200 genetic variants outside the major histocompatibility complex (MHC) that influence the risk of developing MS [2–5]. Despite the growing knowledge of MS risk genes, still little is known about the disease-modifying genes that modulate MS course. Disease course in MS is extremely variable and patients may have relapse-onset or progressive clinical forms, and face benign or severe disease courses. Although the underlying cause of this disease variability remains elusive, evidence exists that it may be influenced by genetic factors [6, 7].

In the present study, we aimed to identify genes associated with MS disease course by first applying an exome sequencing approach to a discovery cohort of MS patients with benign and aggressive disease courses, followed by the validation of selected genetic variants in two independent cohorts of patients with divergent disease courses.

Methods

Discovery cohort

The discovery cohort comprised 20 MS patients classified according to their disease course into benign and aggressive phenotypes. Patients with benign phenotypes ($n = 10$) were defined as having an Expanded Disability Status Scale (EDSS) equal or lower than 3.0 after 15 or more years from disease onset [8] and never received MS therapies. Patients with aggressive disease courses ($n = 10$) reached an EDSS score equal or higher than 6.0 within the first 5 years after disease onset, regardless of treatment [9]. All patients included in the discovery cohort were recruited at the Centre d'Esclerosi Múltiple de Catalunya (Cemcat). Additional file 1: Table S1 summarizes demographic and main clinical characteristics of the discovery cohort.

Exome sequencing

Genomic DNA was extracted from peripheral blood using standard methods. An exome sequencing approach was applied to the discovery cohort in order to identify genes associated with benign and aggressive disease courses. Exome sequencing was based on an Illumina HiSeq2000 sequencing platform and an Agilent's SureSelect Target Enrichment System for 51 Mb. Sequencing was done with a 50× of coverage and reads were aligned against the human reference genome (GRCh37/hg19 assembly) using the Burrows-Wheeler Alignment tool (BWA) [10]. After reads mapping, low-quality reads and sequences flagged as PCR duplicates were removed from the BAM file using the Sequence Alignment/Map (SAM) [10] and Picard Tools. Unmasked variants were annotated considering all possible transcripts for each target gene, and in some cases variants located within a coding sequence when considering one isoform could be positioned within a non-coding region when considering another isoform, thus resulting also in the identification of intronic variants. Exome sequencing was performed in Sistemas Genómicos (Valencia, Spain).

Selection of candidate single-nucleotide polymorphisms for validation

For the variant calling process, different algorithms were applied, including VarScan [11] and the *Genome Analysis Toolkit* (GATK) [12]. Python scripts were developed to combine variants. Variants annotation was based on Ensembl and NCBI databases. For the selection of significant variants, a Fisher exact test was applied to the benign and aggressive phenotypes. For prioritization and selection of the most promising variants, the following criteria were applied: (i) presence of two or more statistically significant variants per gene; (ii) odds ratio difference of the prevalence for the variant between disease phenotypes equal or higher than 2; (iii) absence of the variant in one disease phenotype and presence of the variant in ≥ 50% of patients belonging to the counterpart phenotype; (iv) missense variants, splice region variants, and variants reported as possible deleterious mutations; and (v) biological and functional relevance of the target genes to MS, as reported in the literature. A total of 16 independent variants satisfying 2 or more of the aforementioned criteria were selected for validation.

Validation cohorts

Two independent cohorts with benign and aggressive disease courses were included in the study in order to validate the selected variants from the exome sequencing approach.

The first validation cohort included 194 MS patients from 7 MS centers [Bilbao ($n = 56$); UCSF ($n = 55$); Madrid—Hospital Clínico ($n = 32$); Barcelona—Hospital Clinic ($n = 23$); Madrid—Ramón y Cajal ($n = 16$); Madrid—Puerta de Hierro ($n = 9$); Girona ($n = 3$)]. Of these, 107 MS patients had benign phenotypes and 87 aggressive disease courses.

The second validation cohort consisted of 257 MS patients from Canada, 224 patients with benign phenotypes and 33 with aggressive disease courses. MS patients were ascertained through the Canadian Collaborative Project on the Genetic Susceptibility to Multiple Sclerosis (CCPGSMS) [13].

Clinical criteria to classify patients into benign and aggressive disease courses were the same as those applied to the discovery cohort, except for the second validation cohort in which treatment information on patients with benign disease course was not available. Similar to the discovery cohort, patients with benign phenotypes from the first validation cohort never received MS therapies. A summary of demographic and clinical characteristics of the first and second validation cohorts is shown in Additional file 1: Table S1.

The study was approved by the corresponding local ethics committees, and all participants provided informed consent.

TaqMan OpenArray genotyping

Genotyping of selected variants in the first validation cohort was performed using an OpenArray technology (Thermo Fisher Scientific, Massachusetts, USA) and following the manufacturer's instructions. Briefly, DNA samples were loaded into custom designed arrays using an OpenArray® AccuFill System (Thermo Fisher Scientific). QuantStudio™ 12K Flex system (Thermo Fisher Scientific) was used for sample amplification and fluorescent data collection. Hapmap samples with known genotype were included as internal controls of the process. Genotype was assigned using Taqman Genotyper Software (Thermo Fisher Scientific). Genotyping was performed by the Human Genotyping laboratory of the Spanish National Cancer Research Centre (CNIO).

Sequenom MassARRAY genotyping

In the second validation cohort, selected variants were genotyped using a MassArray iPLEX platform (Sequenom, San Diego, CA, USA) as previously described [14].

CPXM2, IGSF9B, and NLRP9 expression analysis in peripheral blood cells

Gene expression levels for *CPMX2*, *NLRP9*, and *IGSF9B* were determined by real-time PCR in peripheral blood mononuclear cells (PBMC) available from a subgroup of untreated MS patients from the first validation cohort. In order to avoid a confounding effect of disease course in the expression levels for these genes, analysis was restricted to the group of patients with aggressive disease course ($n = 8$ for *CPXM2*; $n = 9$ for *NLRP9*; $n = 7$ for *IGSF9B*). Briefly, PBMC were isolated by Ficoll-Isopaque density gradient centrifugation (Gibco BRL, Life Technologies LTD, Paisley, UK) and stored in liquid nitrogen until used. Total RNA was extracted from PBMC using TRIzol® reagent (Invitrogen, Carlsbad, CA) and cDNA synthesized using the High Capacity cDNA Archive kit (Applied Biosystems, Foster City, CA, USA). Messenger RNA expression levels for *CPMX2*, *NLRP9*, and *IGSF9B* were determined by real-time PCR using TaqMan® probes specific for each gene (Applied Biosystems, Foster City, CA, USA). The housekeeping gene glyceraldehyde-3-phosphate dehydrogenase (*GAPDH*) was used as an endogenous control (Applied Biosystems). Assays were run on the ABI PRISM® 7900HT system (Applied Biosystems) and data were analyzed using the $2^{-\Delta\Delta CT}$ method [15]. Results were expressed as fold change in gene expression in MS patients carrying the risk allele relative to non-carrier patients.

Immunohistochemistry for CPXM2, IGSF9B, and NLRP9 in MS brain tissue

Paraffin-embedded brain samples of chronic active lesions from four MS patients were provided by the UK Multiple Sclerosis Tissue Bank and stained with hematoxylin and eosin (HE) and Klüver-Barrera (KB) for inflammation and demyelination assessment. Four-micrometer-thick, paraffin-embedded serial sections were deparaffined in xylene and rehydrated in alcohol. Endogenous peroxidase activity was blocked with hydrogen peroxide (2%), methanol (70%), and PBS for 20 min. Antigen retrieval was performed in TE buffer (1 M TrismaBase and 1 mM EDTA) (pH = 9) in the microwave. Non-specific protein binding was blocked with 0.2% of bovine albumin (BSA) in PBS. Sections were incubated overnight at 4 °C with the following primary antibodies: rabbit anti-CPXM2 (Biorbyt), rabbit anti-NLRP9 (Abcam), and rabbit anti-IGSG9B (Abcam). Samples were incubated for 1 h at room temperature with goat-anti rabbit HRP secondary antibody (Dakocytomation) and stainings were visualized with 3,3′diaminobenzidine (Sigma, St Louis, MO, USA) as a chromogenic substrate.

Results

Exome sequencing in the discovery cohort of patients with benign and aggressive disease courses and selection of candidate genetic variants

A flowchart summarizing the main steps of the study design and analysis is depicted in Fig. 1. In order to identify genetic variants associated with disease course, we first performed exome sequencing in an initial cohort of 20 MS patients classified according to their disease course into benign ($n = 10$) and aggressive ($n = 10$). A total of 915 single-nucleotide polymorphisms (SNPs) were differentially distributed between MS patients with benign and aggressive disease courses (uncorrected p values < 0.05; data not shown). From the list of differentially distributed SNPs and after applying the selection criteria described in the "Methods" section, 16 SNPs were chosen for validation in two validation cohorts.

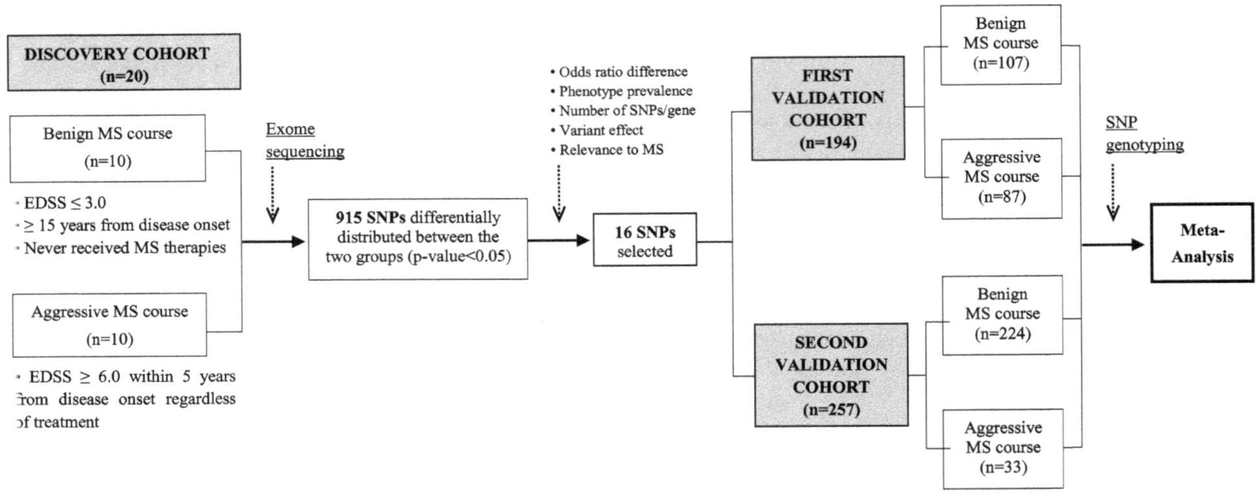

Fig. 1 Flowchart showing the study design and analysis. Patients were classified according to their disease course into benign and aggressive MS, as described in the Methods. By means of exome sequencing, a total of 915 single-nucleotide polymorphisms (SNPs) were identified from 10 MS patients with benign and 10 with aggressive disease courses as being differentially distributed between both groups (discovery cohort). After applying several selection criteria on the list of 915 SNPs including odds ratio difference, phenotype prevalence, number of statistically significant SNPs per gene, type and variant effects on the predicted protein, and relevance of target genes to MS, a total of 16 SNPs were chosen for further validation in two independent cohorts of patients also classified into benign and aggressive phenotypes. The first validation cohort comprised 194 MS patients, 107 with benign and 87 with aggressive disease courses, and genotyping was conducting using an OpenArray technology. The second validation cohort consisted of 257 MS patients, 224 with benign and 33 with aggressive disease courses, and genotyping was performed on a MassArray iPLEX platform. Finally, a meta-analysis was performed in the two validation cohorts

Table 1 shows a description of the 16 selected SNPs from the discovery cohort, and Table 2 provides the results of the exome sequencing analysis for these 16 SNPs.

Validation of selected SNPs in two independent cohorts of patients with benign and aggressive disease courses

Selected SNPs were genotyped in two independent validation cohorts composed of MS patients classified according to their disease course. A total of 194 MS patients were included in the first validation cohort and 257 MS patients in the second validation cohort. Meta-analysis of genotyping results in both cohorts identified two SNPs, rs28469012 and rs10894768, significantly associated with MS disease course. As shown in Fig. 2, the minor allele for rs28469012, an intronic SNP positioned in *CPXM2* (carboxypeptidase X, M14 family, member 2), was nominally significantly associated with more aggressive disease course [p-value; odds ratio (95% confidence interval): $p = 0.04$; 1.81 (1.03–3.18)] (Fig. 2). In this case, a modest degree of heterogeneity was found between both validation cohorts.

The minor allele for rs10894768, which corresponds to a synonymous SNP located in *IGSF9B* (immunoglobulin superfamily member 9B), was nominally significantly associated with benign disease course [$p = 0.04$; 0.70 (0.49–0.99)]. Meta-analysis of this variant supported the originally identified association with homogeneous outcomes for both cohorts ($I^2 = 0$).

A trend for significance was observed in a third SNP, rs10423927, an intronic variant located in *NLRP9* (NLR family pyrin domain containing 9), with the minor allele associated with benign disease course [$p = 0.09$; 0.58 (0.31–1.09)]. Similar to the *IGSF9B* variant, meta-analysis for rs10423927 also supported the association in the discovery cohort and resulted in similar outcomes in both validation cohorts ($I^2 = 0$).

It should be noted that rs2374639, a synonymous variant positioned in *VPS50* (VPS50, EARP/GARPII complex subunit), showed a significant association in the second validation cohort with the same protective effect observed in the discovery cohort [$p = 0.04$; 0.47 (0.23–0.95)]. However, the heterogeneity found between both validation cohorts did not allow to perform a joint analysis (Table 2; $I^2 = 80\%$).

Genotyping frequencies and results of statistical analysis in the two validation cohorts for all selected variants are provided in Table 2.

Tissue-specific expression of IGSF9B, CPXM2, and NLRP9

In order to explore the functional consequences of the polymorphisms associated with MS disease course, we first investigated whether mRNA expression levels for *IGSF9B*, *CPXM2*, and *NLRP9* in

Table 1 Description and functional consequences of SNPs selected for validation from exome sequencing

SNP	Location (hg19)	Gene	Official full name	Variant effect
rs17844444 (G/A)	chr5:140,532,165	*PCDHB6*	Protocadherin Beta 6	Missense variant
rs17082236 (C/A)	chr6:152,470,752	*SYNE1*	Spectrin repeat containing nuclear envelope prote n 1	Missense variant
rs10279499 (C/A)	chr7:92,733,766	*SAMD9*	Sterile alpha motif domain containing 9	Missense variant[a]
rs10488532 (C/T)	chr7:92,764,489	*SAMD9L*	Sterile alpha motif domain containing 9 like	Missense variant
rs2374639 (T/C)	chr7:92,985,252	*VPS50*	VPS50, EARP/GARPII complex subunit	Synonymous variant
rs17552167 (C/T)	chr7:148,529,922	*EZH2*	Enhancer of zeste 2 polycomb repressive complex 2 subunit	Intronic variant
rs28469012 (A/T)	chr10:125,622,263	*CPXM2*	Carboxypeptidase X, M14 family, member 2	Intronic variant
rs10894768 (C/G)	chr11:133,815,981	*IGSF9B*	Immunoglobulin superfamily member 9B	Synonymous variant
rs60252902 (G/A)	chr12:125,451,767	*DHX37*	DEAH-box helicase 37	Splice region variant[b]
rs3742130 (G/A)	chr13:99,907,341	*GPR18*	G protein-coupled receptor 18	Synonymous variant
rs9919887 (A/G)	chr14:95,911,008	*SYNE3*	Spectrin repeat containing nuclear envelope family member 3	Intronic variant
rs2230434 (C/T)	chr16:30,518,096	*ITGAL*	Integrin subunit alpha L	Synonymous variant
rs2070896 (T/C)	chr16:31,384,554	*ITGAX*	Integrin subunit alpha X	Intronic variant
rs35299026 (G/A)	chr19:49,318,380	*HSD17B14*	Hydroxysteroid 17-beta dehydrogenase 14	Missense variant[a]
rs10423927 (A/G)	chr19: 56,235,537	*NLRP9*	NLR family pyrin domain containing 9	Intronic variant
rs2254562 (T/C)	chr21:34,059,352	*SYNJ1*	Synaptojanin 1	Missense variant[a]

[a]Variants reported as possible deleterious mutations (based on SIFT and PolyPhen-2 algorithms)
[b]By definition, a splice region variant is a sequence variant in which a change has occurred within the region of the splice site, either within 1–3 bases of the exon or 3–8 bases of the intron [30]

PBMC differed between MS patients carrying the minor allele associated with disease course and non-carrier patients. *CPXM2* and *NLRP9* expression was not detected in PBMC from MS patients (data not shown). *IGSF9B* expression was detected in PBMC from MS patients, although no differences were observed between carriers and non-carriers of the minor allele associated with benign disease course (Additional file 1: Figure S1).

In order to determine whether the selected genetic variants associated with disease course could be modifying the expression of nearby genes in the region, we analyzed *cis*-expression quantitative trait loci (eQTLs) in 48 tissues from the Genotype-Tissue Expression (GTEx) project [16], lymphoblastoid cell lines in 465 individuals from the Geuvadis project [17], and trans-eQTLs from expression data of 9196 tumor samples in 33 cancer types from the PancanQTL study [18]. We observed correlation of the rs10894768 genotypes with *IGSF9B* expression in pancreatic tissue ($p = 3.6 \times 10^{-6}$) from 171 individuals and thyroid tissue ($p = 5.6 \times 10^{-11}$) from 323 individuals from the GTEx study [16]. The minor allele for this polymorphism, which was more represented in patients with benign disease course, was associated with lower *IGSF9B* expression (Additional file 1: Figure S2). Of note, *IGSF9B* was highly expressed in cerebellar hemisphere, cerebellum and also in cortex, hypothalamus, and spinal cord; however, no eQTLs were described for these tissues most likely due to the lower number of samples analyzed in brain tissue (105 samples from cerebellar hemisphere and 125 from cerebellum).

IGSF9B, CPXM2, and NLRP9 are expressed in brain chronic active lesions from MS patients

Based on the negative results observed for IGSF9B, CPXM2, and NLRP9 expression in peripheral blood, we wondered whether selected genes associated with MS disease course could play more specific roles at the CNS level by investigating their expression in brain tissue from patients. Figure 3 depicts the results of IGSF9B, CPXM2, and NLRP9 immunohistochemistries in brain tissue sections from chronic active lesions of MS patients. IGSF9B showed a diffuse neutrophil staining in both the gray and the white matter. The most intense IGSF9B staining was detected in the cytoplasm of microglia/macrophages and astrocytes located at the margins of MS lesions, where inflammatory activity is highest. IGSF9B immunostaining was also observed in less active areas of the lesions, albeit to a lesser degree compared to more active areas. CPXM2 and NLRP9 exhibited a similar and very discrete immunostaining. Their expression was restricted to the cytoplasm of few microglia/macrophages located at the margins of MS lesions showing the highest inflammatory activity (Fig. 3).

Table 2 Summary of statistical analysis of selected SNPs in the discovery and validation cohorts

Selected variants			Discovery cohort ($n = 20$)			First validation cohort ($n = 194$)		Second validation cohort ($n = 257$)		Meta-analysis	
SNP	Gene	Minor allele	MAF, Benign ($n = 10$)	MAF, Aggressive ($n = 10$)	p value	MAF, Benign ($n = 107$)	MAF, Aggressive ($n = 87$)	MAF, Benign ($n = 224$)	MAF, Aggressive ($n = 33$)	Joint p value	OR (95% CI)
rs17844444	*PCDHB6*	A	0.10	0.40	0.03	0.15	0.15	0.18	0.14	0.52	
rs17082236	*SYNE1*	A	0.00	0.35	0.003	0.09	0.1	0.05	0.07	0.54	
rs10279499	*SAMD9*	A	0.45	0.00	0.0006	0.12	0.12	0.10	0.04	0.29	
rs10488532	*SAMD9L*	T	0.45	0.00	0.0006	0.12	0.14	0.12	0.06	0.79	
rs2374639	*VPS50*	C	0.60	0.06	0.003	0.27	0.31	0.27	0.15	(*)	
rs17552167	*EZH2*	T	0.30	0.00	0.007	0.07	0.06	0.08	0.12	0.63	
rs28469012	*CPXM2*	T	0.05	0.45	0.003	0.04	0.10	0.10	0.12	0.04	1.81 [1.03–3.18]
rs10894768	*IGSF9B*	G	0.50	0.05	0.001	0.35	0.28	0.36	0.27	0.04	0.70 [0.49–0.99]
rs60252902	*DHX37*	A	0.30	0.00	0.007	0.11	0.11	0.09	0.07	0.76	
rs3742130	*GPR18*	A	0.55	0.05	0.0005	0.26	0.27	0.23	0.19	0.80	
rs9919887	*SYNE3*	G	0.05	0.45	0.003	0.20	0.16	0.20	0.19	0.43	
rs2230434	*ITGAL*	T	0.00	0.25	0.01	0.11	0.09	0.09	0.07	0.32	
rs2070896	*ITGAX*	C	0.56	0.05	0.0006	0.37	0.38	0.33	0.32	0.85	
rs35299026	*HSD17B14*	A	0.25	0.00	0.01	0.05	0.07	0.05	0.06	0.31	
rs10423927	*NLRP9*	G	0.25	0.00	0.01	0.11	0.06	0.08	0.06	0.09	0.58 [0.31–1.09]
rs2254562	*SYNJ1*	C	0.05	0.45	0.003	0.30	0.29	0.29	0.35	0.65	

The minor allele frequencies (MAF) and uncorrected p values for each SNP selected from the discovery cohort are presented. For validation, heterogeneity tests and subsequent meta-analysis was performed in the two replication cohorts whenever possible. MAF and joint p values (calculated with Mantel-Haenszel test) are depicted for each SNP. In addition, odds ratio (OR) with their corresponding 95% confidence intervals (95% CI) are presented for SNPs with statistically significant results. *For SNP rs2374639, validation cohorts cannot be meta-analyzed due to high heterogeneity ($I^2 = 80\%$, $p = 0.03$). On a separate analysis, the first validation cohort shows replication of the effect observed in the discovery cohort, with a lower frequency of the minor allele in aggressive MS compared to benign MS [$p = 0.04$, OR = 0.47 (0.23–0.95)]. The second validation cohort shows an increased frequency of the minor allele in aggressive MS that is not statistically significant [$p = 0.39$, OR = 1.22 (0.77–1.94)]

Discussion

Exome sequencing has significantly contributed to the characterization of the genetic component of a number of common complex diseases [19]. In the present study, we aimed to identify genetic variants associated with MS disease course by applying, as a first step, an exome sequencing approach to a small discovery cohort of patients stratified according to benign and aggressive phenotypes. This initial approach led to the identification of a ranked list of candidate polymorphisms associated either with benign or aggressive MS disease courses. Despite the statistically significant associations of a large number of SNPs with MS disease course, in small discovery cohorts only strong statistically significant associations are likely to be real, and hence original findings should be better replicated in additional cohorts to eliminate the chances of false positive results. Based on these observations, in our study selected SNPs identified in the discovery cohort were further genotyped in two independent validation cohorts of patients classified according to similar criteria into benign and aggressive phenotypes.

Meta-analysis in the two validation cohorts revealed two polymorphisms, rs28469012 and rs10894768, as potential MS phenotype modifiers. The SNP rs28469012 is an intronic variant located in the *CPXM2* gene whose minor allele was associated with worse disease evolution. *CPXM2* codes for a member of the metallocarboxypeptidase family with potential roles in synaptic integrity [20]. Previous studies have associated the *CPXM2* gene to Alzheimer disease [21], Parkinson's disease [20], and schizophrenia [22]. Although no studies of CPXM2 have been reported thus far in MS, it is interesting to mention that experimental autoimmune encephalomyelitis (EAE) mice deficient for another metallocarboxypeptidase that shares protein homology with CPXM2, carboxipeptidase N, had attenuated EAE disease course and reduced spinal cord inflammation and demyelination [23], data that indirectly support the association observed in our study between CPXM2 and aggressive MS phenotypes.

The synonymous exonic variant rs10894768 is positioned in the *IGSF9B* gene, and the minor allele for this polymorphism was more represented in MS

rs28469012 *(CPXM2)*

Study or Subgroup	Aggressive Events	Aggressive Total	Benign Events	Benign Total	Weight	Odds Ratio M-H, Fixed, 95% CI
First validation cohort	17	162	8	198	38.3%	2.78 [1.17, 6.63]
Second validation cohort	8	66	46	448	61.7%	1.21 [0.54, 2.68]
Total (95% CI)		**228**		**646**	**100.0%**	**1.81 [1.03, 3.18]**
Total events	25		54			

Heterogeneity: Chi² = 1.94, df = 1 (P = 0.16); I² = 48%
Test for overall effect: Z = 2.07 (P = 0.04)

rs10894768 *(IGSF9B)*

Study or Subgroup	Aggressive Events	Aggressive Total	Benign Events	Benign Total	Weight	Odds Ratio M-H, Fixed, 95% CI
First validation cohort	47	170	71	204	60.9%	0.72 [0.46, 1.11]
Second validation cohort	18	66	160	446	39.1%	0.67 [0.38, 1.19]
Total (95% CI)		**236**		**650**	**100.0%**	**0.70 [0.49, 0.99]**
Total events	65		231			

Heterogeneity: Chi² = 0.03, df = 1 (P = 0.86); I² = 0%
Test for overall effect: Z = 2.01 (P = 0.04)

rs10423927 *(NLRP9)*

Study or Subgroup	Aggressive Events	Aggressive Total	Benign Events	Benign Total	Weight	Odds Ratio M-H, Fixed, 95% CI
First validation cohort	10	172	23	214	69.0%	0.51 [0.24, 1.11]
Second validation cohort	4	66	36	448	31.0%	0.74 [0.25, 2.15]
Total (95% CI)		**238**		**662**	**100.0%**	**0.58 [0.31, 1.09]**
Total events	14		59			

Heterogeneity: Chi² = 0.30, df = 1 (P = 0.59); I² = 0%
Test for overall effect: Z = 1.68 (P = 0.09)

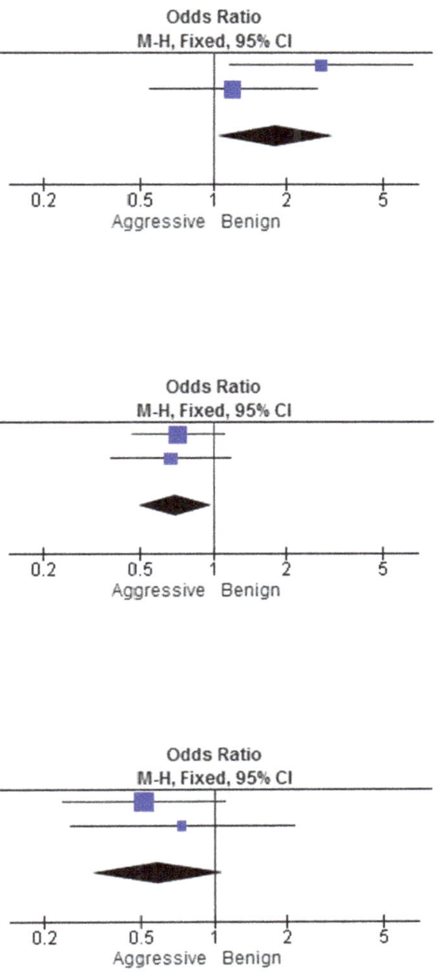

Fig. 2 Meta-analysis for rs28469012 (*CPXM2*), rs10894768 (*IGSF9B*), and rs10423927 (*NLRP9*) in the two validation cohorts of patients with aggressive and benign disease courses. The figure depicts joint analyses for the first and second validation cohorts in each SNP, with homogeneity tests (I^2) and tests for overall effects. The squares and horizontal lines correspond to the study specific odds ratios (ORs) and 95% confidence intervals (CI) respectively. The area of the squares reflects the study specific weight (inverse of the variance). The diamond represents the pooled ORs and 95% CI. *M-H* Mantel-Haenszel

patients with benign disease course. *IGSF9B* encodes a transmembrane immunoglobulin that has been reported to be highly expressed in GABAergic interneurons, where it may play a role promoting inhibitory synaptic development via the formation of a ternary complex with the postsynaptic scaffolding protein S-SCAM and the neuronal cell surface protein neuroligin 2 [24]. Similar to CPXM2, the role of IGSF9B in MS is unknown. However, considering that the GABAergic system is dysregulated in both MS and EAE and a selective loss of GABAergic interneurons has been reported in EAE [25], it is tempting to speculate that the finding of a higher frequency of genetic variants located in a gene that promotes maintenance of inhibitory synapses may result in more benign disease outcomes of MS patients. Noteworthy, MS brain tissue immunohistochemistry revealed IGSF9B expression in astrocytes, cells that are known to be involved in the formation and control of neuronal synapses [26].

Although rs28469012 and rs10894768 were the only polymorphisms whose association with MS disease course was validated, a trend for association with benign phenotypes was also observed for rs10423927, an

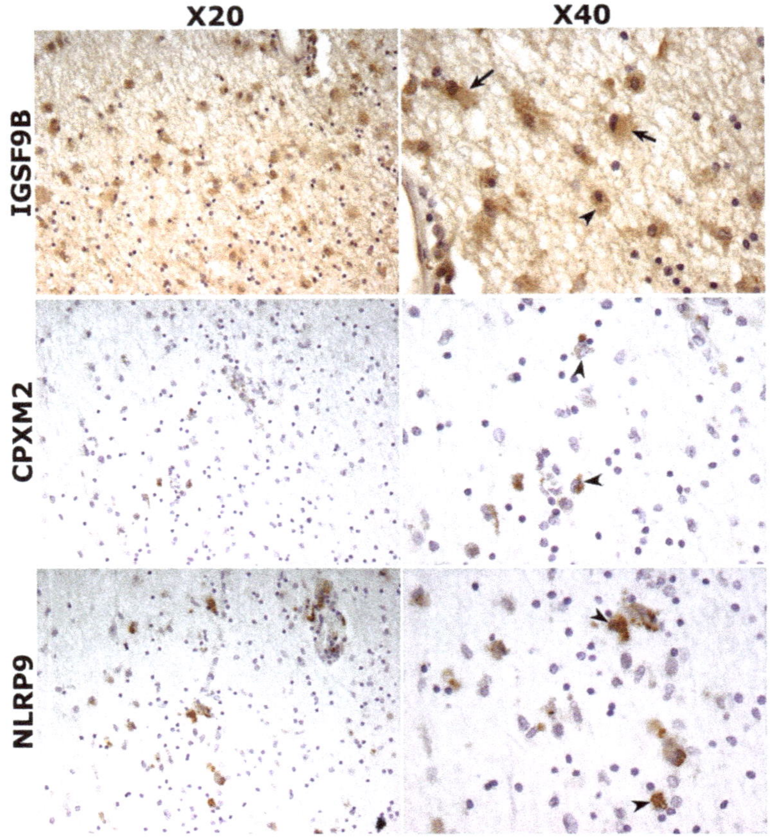

Fig. 3 IGSF9B, CPXM2, and NLRP9 expression in MS brain tissue. Immunostainings for IGSF9B, CPXM2, and NLRP9 in the margins of MS brain chronic active lesions, where inflammatory activity is highest. IGSF9B expression was observed in astrocytes (arrows) and macrophages/microglia (arrow heads), whereas CPMX2 and NLRP9 immunostaining was only detected in macrophages/microglia (arrow heads). Photos were taken at × 20 and × 40

intronic variant located in the *NLRP9* gene. Despite that little evidence exists in the literature regarding its function, NLRP9 belongs to the NOD-like receptor (NLR) family of inflammasomes, which are known to play critical roles both in innate and adaptive immunity and whose dysfunction has strongly been linked to autoimmune diseases [27]. Interestingly, a missense variant located in another member of the NLR family of inflammasomes, NLRP5, was recently found to be associated with higher disease severity scores, suggesting a role of NLR inflammasomes in MS disease course [28].

In an attempt to investigate the functional consequences of the genetic variants associated with benign and aggressive phenotypes, expression of IGSF9B, CPXM2, and NLRP9 was investigated at the gene and protein expression levels in PBMC and brain tissue respectively. Although not proven in the study, the negative results obtained in peripheral blood, with lack of expression of CPXM2 and NLRP9 in PBMC and no evidence of differences in *IGSF9B* expression between minor allele carriers and non-carriers for rs10894768, suggest that the genetic variants associated with disease course in MS may act by modulating the function of CNS cells such as macrophages/microglia and astrocytes, as supported by the immunohistochemistry studies in MS brain tissue showing expression for these genes in these particular cell types. Unfortunately, postmortem brain studies are not suitable for patient stratification to explore allele-specific gene expression differences. Furthermore, it could be possible that the MS course-associated allele of our reported SNPs confers increased ability to interact with certain environmental risk factors or impacts on chromatin structure by affecting epigenetic marks, including DNA methylation or histone modifications [29].

Finally, the finding that the minor allele of rs10894768, which is more represented in MS patients with benign outcomes, was associated with lower expression of *IGSF9B* in thyroid and pancreatic tissues supports the view that gene expression may be markedly different across tissues.

Conclusions

In summary, we identified genetic variants in the *IGSF9B*, *CPXM2*, and *NLRP9* genes associated with benign and aggressive disease phenotypes in MS patients. Interestingly, the two genes that were validated in two independent cohorts of MS patients, *IGSF9B* and *CPXM2*, are known to play roles in CNS synapse integrity, findings that warrant additional studies to explore at the CNS level the potential functional consequences of the reported polymorphisms associated with MS disease course. Finally, aiming to provide a personalized medicine in MS, the reported polymorphisms may become disease activity biomarkers to identify MS patients with diverging disease courses.

Abbreviations

BWA: Burrows-Wheeler Alignment tool; CCPGSMS: Canadian Collaborative Project on the Genetic Susceptibility to Multiple Sclerosis; Cemcat: Centre d'Esclerosi Múltiple de Catalunya; CNIO: Spanish National Cancer Research Centre; CPXM2: Carboxypeptidase X, M14 family member 2; EAE: Experimental autoimmune encephalomyelitis; EDSS: Expanded Disability Status Scale; eQTL: *Cis*-expression quantitative trait loci; GATK: Genome analysis toolkit; GRCh37: Genome Reference Consortium Human Build 37; GWAS: Genome-wide association studies; IGSF9B: Immunoglobulin superfamily member 9B; KB: Klüver-Barrera; MS: Multiple sclerosis; NLR: NOD-like receptor; NLRP5: NLR family pyrin domain containing 5; NLRP9: NLR family pyrin domain containing 9; SAM: Sequence Alignment/Map; SNP: Single-nucleotide polymorphism; TE: Tris-ethylenediaminetetraacetic acid; UCSF: University of California, San Francisco; VPS50: VPS50, EARP/GARPII complex subunit

Acknowledgements

The authors thank the "Red Española de Esclerosis Múltiple (REEM)" sponsored by the FEDER-FIS and the "Ajuts per donar Suport als Grups de Recerca de Catalunya," sponsored by the "Agència de Gestió d'Ajuts Universitaris i de Recerca" (AGAUR), Generalitat de Catalunya, Spain.

Funding

This work was supported by (a) grants PI10/02099, FIS PI13/0879, PI15/00513, PI15/00587, PI16/01259, RD16/0015/0001, RD16/0015/0002, RD16/0015/0004 integrated in the Plan Estatal de Investigación Científica y Técnica de Innovación I+D+I and co-funded by the Instituto de Salud Carlos III-Subdirección General de Evaluación and the Fondo Europeo de Desarrollo Regional (FEDER), and Red Española de Esclerosis Múltiple (REEM); (b) Junta de Andalucía (JA)-FEDER grant CTS2704, Ministerio de Economía y Competitividad (grant number SAF 2016-80595-C2-1-P); (c) MS Society of Canada Scientific Research Foundation as part of the CCPGSMS, and research undertaken thanks to funding from the Canada Research Chair (950-228408) program, Michael Smith Foundation for Health Research (16827) and Canadian Institutes of Health Research (MOP-137051). The authors wish to thank the donors, and the Biobank Hospital Universitario Puerta de Hierro Majadahonda (HUPHM)/Instituto de Investigación Sanitaria Puerta de Hierro-Segovia de Arana (IDIPHISA) for the human specimens used in this study.

Authors' contributions

EGV: manuscript drafting and revision, study concept and design, immunohistochemistry experiments, peripheral blood expression studies, analysis, and interpretation of the data. EU, CVG: manuscript drafting and revision, contribution of patients and clinical data, statistical analysis. FM, JCT: manuscript drafting and revision, statistical analysis. CC: manuscript drafting and revision, immunohistochemistry experiments, analysis and interpretation of the data. LM, ARA, JO, LEP, ADS, AS, LMV, JAGM, LRT, EQ, RR, ASL, RA, JCAC, AVJ, XM: manuscript revision, contribution of patients and clinical data, analysis, and interpretation of the data. SM, NF: manuscript drafting and revision, peripheral blood expression studies, analysis, and interpretation of the data. MC: manuscript drafting and revision, study concept and design, analysis and interpretation of the data, study supervision. All authors read and approved the final manuscript.

Consent for publication

Not applicable.

Competing interests

The authors declare that they have no competing interests.

Author details

[1]Servei de Neurologia-Neuroimmunologia, Centre d'Esclerosi Múltiple de Catalunya (Cemcat), Institut de Recerca Vall d'Hebron (VHIR), Hospital Universitari Vall d'Hebron, Universitat Autònoma de Barcelona, Barcelona, Spain. [2]Immunology Department, Hospital Clinico San Carlos, Instituto de Investigacion Sanitaria San Carlos (Id SSC), Madrid, Spain. [3]Department of Medical Genetics, University of British Columbia, Vancouver, Canada. [4]Department of Cell Biology and Immunology, Instituto de Parasitología y Biomedicina "López Neyra", Consejo Superior de Investigaciones Científicas (IPBLN-CSIC), Granada, Spain. [5]Servicio de Neurología, Hospital Universitario Basurto-Osakidetza, Bilbao, Spain. [6]Department of Neurology, University of California, San Francisco, CA, USA. [7]Neurology Service, Hospital Clinic and Institut d'Investigació Biomèdica Pi i Sunyer (IDIBAPS), Barcelona, Spain. [8]Departments of Immunology and Neurology, Multiple Sclerosis Unit, Hospital Ramon y Cajal, (IRYCIS), Madrid, Spain. [9]Neuroimmunology Unit, Puerta de Hierro University Hospital and Research Institute, Universidad Autónoma de Madrid, Madrid, Spain. [10]Neuroimmunology and Multiple Sclerosis Unit, Department of Neurology, Hospital Dr Josep Trueta, IDIBGI, University of Girona, Girona, Spain. [11]Genomic Systems, Valencia, Spain. [12]Servicio de Neurología, Hospital Universitario Quirón Salud, Madrid, Spain.

References

1. Ascherio A, Munger KL, Lünemann JD. The initiation and prevention of multiple sclerosis. Nat Rev Neurol. 2012;8:602–12.
2. Sawcer S, Hellenthal G, Pirinen M, Spencer CCA, Patsopoulos NA, Moutsianas L, et al. International multiple sclerosis genetics consortium (IMSGC) and Wellcome Trust case control consortium 2 (WTCCC2). Genetic risk and a primary role for cell-mediated immune mechanisms in multiple sclerosis. Nature. 2011;476:214–9.
3. Beecham AH, Patsopoulos NA, Xifara DK, Davis MF, Kemppinen A, Cotsapas C, et al. International multiple sclerosis genetics consortium (IMSGC), Wellcome Trust case control consortium 2 (WTCCC2), international IBD genetics consortium (IIBDGC). Analysis of immune-related loci identifies 48 new susceptibility variants for multiple sclerosis. Nat Genet. 2013;45:1353–60.
4. Küçükali Cİ, Kürtüncü M, Çoban A, Çebi M, Tüzün E. Epigenetics of multiple sclerosis: an updated review. Neuromolecular Med. 2015;17:83–96.
5. Patsopoulos N, Baranzini SE, Santaniello A, Shoostari P, Cotsapas C, Wong G, et al. International Multiple Sclerosis Genetics Consortium (IMSGC). The Multiple Sclerosis Genomic Map: role of peripheral immune cells and resident microglia in susceptibility. Available at: https://www.biorxiv.org/content/early/2017/07/13/143933. Accessed 24 May 2018.
6. Oksenberg JR, Barcellos LF. Multiple sclerosis genetics: leaving no stone unturned. Genes Immun. 2005;6:375–87.
7. Kantarci OH, de Andrade M, Weinshenker BG. Identifying disease modifying genes in multiple sclerosis. J Neuroimmunol. 2002;123:144–59.
8. Amato MP, Zipoli V, Goretti B, Portaccio E, De Caro MF, Ricchiuti L, et al. Benign multiple sclerosis: cognitive psychological and social aspects in a clinical cohort. J Neurol. 2006;253:1054–9.
9. Menon S, Shirani A, Zhao Y, Oger J, Traboulsee A, Freedman MS, et al. Characterising aggressive multiple sclerosis. J Neurol Neurosurg Psychiatry. 2013;84:1192–8.
10. Li H, Durbin R. Fast and accurate short read alignment with Burrows-Wheeler transform. Bioinformatics. 2009;25:1754–60.
11. Koboldt DC, Chen K, Wylie T, Larson DE, McLellan MD, Mardis ER, et al. VarScan: variant detection in massively parallel sequencing of individual and pooled samples. Bioinformatics. 2009;25:2283–5.

12. McKenna A, Hanna M, Banks E, Sivachenko A, Cibulskis K, Kernytsky A, et al. The genome analysis toolkit: a MapReduce framework for analyzing next-generation DNA sequencing data. Genome Res. 2010;20:1297–303.
13. Sadovnick AD, Risch NJ, Ebers GC. Canadian collaborative project on genetic susceptibility to MS, phase 2: rationale and method. Can J Neurol Sci. 1998; 25:216–21.
14. Nishioka K, Wider C, Vilariño-Güell C, Soto-Ortolaza AI, Lincoln SJ, Kachergus JM, et al. Association of alpha-, beta-, and gamma-Synuclein with diffuse lewy body disease. Arch Neurol. 2010;67:970–5.
15. Livak KJ, Schmittgen TD. Analysis of relative gene expression data using real-time quantitative PCR and the 2(−Delta Delta C(T)) method. Methods. 2001;25:402–8.
16. GTEx Consortium, Laboratory, Data Analysis &Coordinating Center (LDACC)—Analysis Working Group; Statistical Methods groups—Analysis Working Group; Enhancing GTEx (eGTEx) groups; NIH Common Fund; NIH/NCI; NIH/NHGRI, et al. Genetic effects on gene expression across human tissues. Nature. 2017;550:204–13.
17. Lappalainen T, Sammeth M, Friedländer MR, 't Hoen PA, Monlong J, Rivas MA, et al. Transcriptome and genome sequencing uncovers functional variation in humans. Nature. 2013;501:506–11.
18. Gong J, Mei S, Liu C, Xiang Y, Ye Y, Zhang Z, et al. PancanQTL: systematic identification of cis-eQTLs and trans-eQTLs in 33 cancer types. Nucleic Acids Res. 2018;46(D1):D971–6.
19. Goh G, Choi M. Application of whole exome sequencing to identify disease-causing variants in inherited human diseases. Genomics Inform. 2012;10:214–9.
20. Hoepken HH, Gispert S, Azizov M, Klinkenberg M, Ricciardi F, Kurz A, et al. Parkinson patient fibroblasts show increased alpha-synuclein expression. Exp Neurol. 2008;212:307–13.
21. Chen YC, Hsiao CJ, Jung CC, Hu HH, Chen JH, Lee WC, et al. Performance metrics for selecting single nucleotide polymorphisms in late-onset Alzheimer's disease. Sci Rep. 2016;6:36155.
22. Hashimoto R, Ikeda M, Ohi K, Yasuda Y, Yamamori H, Fukumoto M, et al. Genome-wide association study of cognitive decline in schizophrenia. Am J Psychiatry. 2013;170:683–4.
23. Hu X, Wetsel RA, Ramos TN. Carboxypeptidase N-deficient mice present with polymorphic disease phenotypes on induction of experimental autoimmune encephalomyelitis. Immunobiology. 2014;219:104–8.
24. Woo J, Kwon SK, Nam J, Choi S, Takahashi H, Krueger D, et al. The adhesion protein IgSF9b is coupled to neuroligin 2 via S-SCAM to promote inhibitory synapse development. J Cell Biol. 2013;201:929–44.
25. Mandolesi G, Gentile A, Musella A. Synaptopathy connects inflammation and neurodegeneration in multiple sclerosis. Nat Rev Neurol. 2015;11:711–24.
26. Eroglu C, Barres BA. Regulation of synaptic connectivity by glia. Nature. 2010;468:223–31.
27. Shaw PJ, Lamkanfi M, Kanneganti TD. NOD-like receptor (NLR) signaling beyond the inflammasome. Eur J Immunol. 2010;40:624–7.
28. Sadovnick AD, Traboulsee AL, Zhao Y, Bernales CQ, Encarnacion M, Ross JP, et al. Genetic modifiers of multiple sclerosis progression, severity and onset. Clin Immunol. 2017;180:100–5.
29. Eilbeck K, Lewis SE, Mungall CJ, Yandell M, Stein L, Durbin R, et al. The sequence ontology: a tool for the unification of genome annotations. Genome Biol. 2005;6:R44.
30. Cazaly E, Charlesworth J, Dickinson JL, Holloway AF. Genetic determinants of epigenetic patterns: providing insight into disease. Mol Med. 2015;21: 400–9.

18

In vivo assessment of neuroinflammation in progressive multiple sclerosis: a proof of concept study with [^{18}F]DPA714 PET

Marloes H. J. Hagens[1,2*], Sandeep V. Golla[3], Martijn T. Wijburg[1,2], Maqsood Yaqub[3], Dennis Heijtel[3,4], Martijn D. Steenwijk[1,5], Patrick Schober[6], John J. P. Brevé[5], Robert C. Schuit[3], Tristan A. Reekie[7], Michael Kassiou[7], Anne-Marie van Dam[1,5], Albert D. Windhorst[3], Joep Killestein[1,2], Frederik Barkhof[1,3,8], Bart N. M. van Berckel[3] and Adriaan A. Lammertsma[3]

Abstract

Background: Over the past decades, positron emission tomography (PET) imaging has become an increasingly useful research modality in the field of multiple sclerosis (MS) research, as PET can visualise molecular processes, such as neuroinflammation, in vivo. The second generation PET radioligand [^{18}F]DPA714 binds with high affinity to the 18-kDa translocator-protein (TSPO), which is mainly expressed on activated microglia. The aim of this proof of concept study was to evaluate this in vivo marker of neuroinflammation in primary and secondary progressive MS.

Methods: All subjects were genotyped for the rs6971 polymorphism within the TSPO gene, and low-affinity binders were excluded from participation in this study. Eight patients with progressive MS and seven age and genetic binding status matched healthy controls underwent a 60 min dynamic PET scan using [^{18}F]DPA714, including both continuous on-line and manual arterial blood sampling to obtain metabolite-corrected arterial plasma input functions.

Results: The optimal model for quantification of [^{18}F]DPA714 kinetics was a reversible two-tissue compartment model with additional blood volume parameter. For genetic high-affinity binders, a clear increase in binding potential was observed in patients with MS compared with age-matched controls. For both high and medium affinity binders, a further increase in binding potential was observed in T2 white matter lesions compared with non-lesional white matter. Volume of distribution, however, did not differentiate patients from healthy controls, as the large non-displaceable compartment of [^{18}F]DPA714 masks its relatively small specific signal.

Conclusion: The TSPO radioligand [^{18}F]DPA714 can reliably identify increased focal and diffuse neuroinflammation in progressive MS when using plasma input-derived binding potential, but observed differences were predominantly visible in high-affinity binders.

Keywords: [^{18}F]DPA714, Multiple sclerosis, Neuroinflammation, Positron emission tomography, TSPO

* Correspondence: m.hagens1@vumc.nl
[1]VUmc MS Center Amsterdam, VU University Medical Center, De Boelelaan 1117, 1081 HV Amsterdam, the Netherlands
[2]Department of Neurology, VU University Medical Center, De Boelelaan 1117, 1081 HV Amsterdam, the Netherlands

Background

Conventional magnetic resonance imaging [1] has a central role in the diagnosis of multiple sclerosis (MS), based on its high sensitivity for identifying MS-specific demyelinating lesions in the brain and spinal cord [2]. In patients with a relapsing-remitting disease course, radiological monitoring is based on the development of new MS lesions on T2-weighted MRI and the presence of gadolinium-enhancing lesions on T1-weighted MRI, demonstrating disruption of the blood-brain barrier which is indicative of active neuroinflammation [3]. However, these focal lesions as seen on MRI cannot fully explain the neurological and cognitive deficits in patients with MS [4]. In addition, in both primary and secondary progressive MS, neuroinflammation usually is not characterised by focal active demyelinating lesions [5]. Animal model and human post-mortem studies have identified a more diffuse and low-grade neuroinflammation behind an intact blood-brain barrier, not depicted by conventional MRI [6, 7]. Consequently, there is a need for novel imaging techniques.

Over the past decades, positron emission tomography (PET) imaging has become an increasingly useful research modality in the field of MS research, as PET can visualise molecular processes, such as neuroinflammation, in vivo [8, 9]. Specifically, the 18-kDa translocator-protein (TSPO) receptor, which is present on the mitochondrial membrane of microglial cells, with additional binding sites in monocytes, astrocytes and vascular endothelium, has shown potential as a target for imaging neuroinflammation with PET [10]. Using the first-generation TSPO PET tracer *(R)*-[^{11}C]PK11195, increased TSPO expression has been demonstrated in both MS lesions and normal appearing brain tissue of patients with MS, which was associated with increased disability and disease progression in all phases of the disease [11–16]. Unfortunately, *(R)*-[^{11}C]PK11195 suffers from poor brain penetration and high nonspecific binding in the brain, hindering accurate quantification [12]. Over the years, a large number of second-generation TSPO tracers have been developed, such as [^{11}C]PBR28, [^{18}F]PBR111, [^{11}C]DPA713, [^{18}F]GE180 and [18F]FEDAA1106. These novel tracers have an improved signal-to-noise ratio, resulting from lower lipophilicity and therefore less non-specific binding to e.g. plasma proteins and improved blood-brain barrier passage [17–21]. It has been shown that the second-generation radioligand [^{18}F]DPA714 provides increased bioavailability to brain tissue and indeed has a higher signal-to-noise ratio [22, 23]. One limitation of second-generation tracers, including [^{18}F]DPA714, is their genetically determined binding affinity, resulting from a single nuclide polymorphism rs6971 within the TSPO gene. Approximately 50% of the general population is a genetically determined high-affinity binder (HAB), 30–40% a medium-affinity binder (MAB) and 10–20% a low-affinity binder (LAB) [24].

To date, quantification of cerebral [^{18}F]DPA714 binding has been described in healthy controls [25] and in patients with Alzheimer's disease [26], with both studies agreeing on a reversible two-tissue compartment model with blood volume parameter (2T4k_V_B) as the optimal kinetic model. In addition, pseudo-quantitative analyses have been performed in post-stroke [27] and Alzheimer's disease patients [28]. Moreover, the simplified reference tissue model, using cerebellar grey matter as a reference region, has been found to reliably assess binding potential in Alzheimer's disease [26]. However, the pathophysiology of MS violates the assumptions underlying reference tissue models: firstly, no single brain region can be used as a reference region in MS, as no region can be assumed to be devoid of specific TSPO binding, and secondly, the blood volume contribution is not negligible throughout the MS brain due to potential disruption of the blood-brain barrier [29]. The latter will also influence the kinetics of the tracer making reference tissue models unreliable [30].

The aim of this proof of concept study was to identify the optimal plasma input tracer kinetic model for characterising in vivo [^{18}F]DPA714 kinetics in patients with primary and secondary progressive MS and to evaluate whether the kinetic parameters estimated from this model can be used to quantify TSPO binding in this patient group.

Methods

Participants

Patients diagnosed with primary or secondary progressive MS, according to the 2010 revisions of the McDonald criteria, and healthy controls were recruited from the MS Center, VU University Medical Center, Amsterdam, between January 2015 and February 2016. All subjects were genotyped for the rs6971 polymorphism within the TSPO gene, which predicts binding affinity to the second generation TSPO tracers [24]. Only genetically high and medium affinity binders (HAB and MAB) were included, and genetically low-affinity binders (LAB) were excluded. Further exclusion criteria for all subjects were a medical history of relevant neurological or auto-immune disease (other than MS); known cardiac, haematological, oncological or renal diseases; current or previous alcohol or drug abuse; recent treatment with immunomodulating drugs; or the use of benzodiazepines. None of the patients with progressive MS were on disease-modifying therapy, and no patients were treated with intravenous methylprednisolone for the last 3 months prior to the PET scans. All subjects had normal physical examination and all healthy controls a normal neurological examination.

This study was approved by the Medical Ethics Review Board of the VU University Medical Center and was registered under number 2014.356. All subjects gave written informed consent prior to participation.

MRI acquisition

MR imaging was performed on a 3 Tesla Ingenuity TF PET-MR system (Philips Medical Systems, Best, The Netherlands) on the same day as the PET-CT acquisition. MRI analysis included 3D T1 (repetition time 7.9 ms, echo time 4.5 ms, flip angle 8°, measured voxel size $1 \times 1 \times 1$ mm^3) for region of interest (ROI) definition and 3D T2 Fluid Attenuated Inversion Recovery (FLAIR) (repetition time 4800 ms, echo time 279 ms, inversion time 1650 ms, measured voxel size $0.9 \times 0.9 \times 1.1$ mm^3) for lesion segmentation. In patients, additional post-contrast 2D T1 sequences (repetition time 600 ms, echo time 10 ms, measured voxel size $0.56 \times 0.44 \times 5$ mm^3) were acquired.

PET acquisition and reconstruction

Radiosynthesis of [^{18}F]DPA714 was performed with an in-house built automatic apparatus using procedures described previously [26]. PET scans were acquired on an Ingenuity TF PET-CT scanner (Philips Medical Systems, Best, The Netherlands). Following a low-dose CT scan for attenuation correction, a bolus of 263 ± 13 MBq [^{18}F]DPA714, with a mean molar activity of 39 ± 20 GBq/μmol, was injected intravenously at 0.8 mL/sec with an automated infusion pump. Simultaneously, a 60-min PET dynamic emission scan was started. The emission scan was collected in list mode and rebinned into 19 frames (1×15, 3×5, 3×10, 4×60, 2×150, 2×300, 4×600 s). PET data were reconstructed to a final voxel size of $2 \times 2 \times 2$ mm^3 using standard scanner software (BLOB-OS-TF), which incorporates standard corrections for attenuation, scatter and randoms.

Arterial blood was withdrawn continuously from the radial artery during the entire scan (using an automated pump for the first 5 min at 5 mL/min and from 5 to 60 min at 2.5 mL/min), and in addition, manual samples were collected at six time points (5, 10, 20, 30, 40 and 60 min) [31]. Continuous whole blood time activity curves (TACs) were corrected for plasma to whole blood ratios, metabolites and time delay to obtain metabolite-corrected arterial plasma input functions.

Data analysis

MS white matter lesions were automatically segmented on the FLAIR and T1-weighted images using kNN-TTP [32]. Lesion filling of the T1-weighted image was obtained using LEAP [33], after which the filled T1-weighted image was registered to the PET scan using the VINCI software package [34, 35]. Grey matter, white matter and cerebral spinal fluid segmentation was performed automatically using SPM8 implemented in PVElab [36]. ROIs were defined according to the Hammers template on the co-registered 3D T1 MRI [37]. Regional TACs were extracted by superimposing the MR-derived ROIs onto the dynamic PET images. Volume weighted larger ROIs were also defined to assess the impact of ROI size on quantitative analyses. The lesion masks were subtracted from segmented white matter to define non-lesional white matter.

Kinetic modelling was performed using standard single-tissue (1T2k) together with reversible and irreversible two-tissue (2T3k and 2T4k) compartment models, both with and without blood volume parameter (V_B) [38]. It has been hypothesised that some binding to the vascular endothelium exists for TSPO tracers, which can be characterised by slow irreversible binding (K_b) [39, 40]. Therefore, a 2T4k_V_B with an irreversible vascular binding component (1T1k) was also tested. Akaike information criterion (AIC) was used to compare model fits and to identify the optimal tracer kinetic model. Reliability of parameter estimates was determined by the percentage standard deviation (%SD) of these estimates, with a cut-off of 25% for the generally robust K_1, and 50% for the other parameters. Estimates for K_1, BP_{ND} (k_3/k_4), V_T and K_b from the optimal model were used to assess group differences between patients and controls, and between genetically high and medium affinity binders (HAB and MAB).

Statistical analysis

Group differences were evaluated using the Mann-Whitney U test in SPSS 22.0 (IBM Corp., Armonk, NY). Due to the explorative nature of this proof of concept study, we did not correct for multiple comparisons. To evaluate regional differences within the patient group, a Wilcoxon signed-rank test was used.

Results

Demographics

At screening, all subjects were genotyped for the rs6971 polymorphism within the TSPO gene and low-affinity binders were excluded from participation in this study. In total, eight patients diagnosed with primary or secondary progressive MS and seven healthy controls completed the whole study protocol. Demographic information is reported in Table 1. Patients included were four HAB and four MAB, with a mean age of 53 ± 3 years and a wide variation in T2 lesion load, ranging from a few solitary lesions to widespread confluent lesions (3.6 to 60.6 cm^2). In only two patients, one small enhancing lesion could be identified, not uncommon in primary or secondary progressive MS. In healthy controls, genetic binding status was similarly distributed: three HAB and four MAB. The mean age for healthy controls was 52 ± 4 years, which was not significantly different from the patients with MS ($p = 0.413$).

Table 1 Demographical characteristics

	Patients ($n = 8$)	Healthy controls ($n = 7$)
Age, mean and SD (years)	53.1 ± 2.7	52.0 ± 4.1
Gender, male/female	3/5	3/4
Genotype, HAB/MAB	4/4	3/4
Subtype MS, PPMS/SPMS	5/3	N/A
Disease duration, mean and SD (years)	13.1 ± 9.4	N/A
EDSS, median and range	5.0 (4.0–6.0)	N/A
PASAT-3 score, mean and SD	45.8 ± 10.8	49.6 ± 12.5
SDMT score, mean and SD	44.0 ± 11.9	55.0 ± 13.5
T2 lesion volume, median and range (cm^3)	14.3 (3.6–60.6)	N/A

Abbreviations: *EDSS* Expanded Disability Status Scale, *HAB* genetic high-affinity binder, *MAB* genetic medium-affinity binder, *PASAT* Paced Auditory Serial Addition Test, *PPMS* primary progressive multiple sclerosis, *SDMT* Symbol Digit Modalities Test, *SPMS* secondary progressive multiple sclerosis

Tracer kinetics

Based on the AIC, for the majority of subjects, the preferred model for quantification of [^{18}F]DPA714 was 2T4k_V_B_1T1k, see Fig. 1. However, when evaluating reliability of the parameter estimates, for a large number of regions, K_1, BP_{ND} and/or K_b could not be reliably estimated, with either a high %SD or values touching the boundaries (see Additional files 1 and 2). This was even the case for subjects in which 2T4k_V_B_1T1k was the preferred model according to AIC, and it was true not only for small, but also for large ROIs. As model fits for 2T4k_V_B_1T1k and 2T4k_V_B were comparable (see Fig. 2) and 2T4k_V_B did result in reliable parameter estimates, the latter model was used for further analyses.

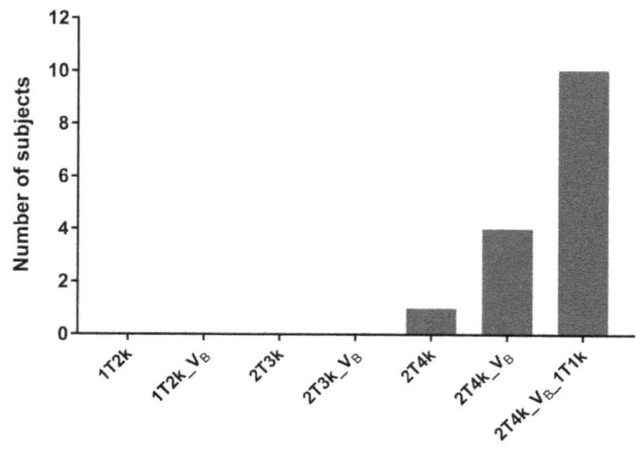

Fig. 1 Model preference. Number of subjects per preferred model according to the Akaike information criterion. All subjects preferred a reversible two-tissue compartment model (2T4k), primarily for the model including blood volume parameter [38] and a vascular binding component (1T1k)

Volume of distribution

Mean regional V_T values were on average 1.6 times higher in HABs than in MABs (Fig. 3a). There was no clear regional difference in V_T between patients and healthy controls for both HABs and MABs, as Fig. 3a illustrates for the MS white matter lesions, non-lesional white matter and whole brain grey matter. Moreover, very limited within-subject variation in V_T was observed, even for the patients with MS. Figure 3b illustrates that all subjects showed a similar distribution pattern for V_T throughout the brain. In addition, a strong correlation between V_T and K_1 was seen (Fig. 4a), whereas no correlations were found between V_T and both k_2 and k_3/k_4.

Finally, regional V_T values for the 2T4k_V_B_1T1k model were evaluated (Fig. 3c). As expected, the added vascular binding component decreased the V_T. As the regional V_T values for the two models were strongly correlated for the large ROIs, there was also no difference in 2T4k_V_B_1T1k V_T between patients and healthy controls for both the HABs and MABs (Fig. 3c). It is of interest to know that also the correlation between V_T and K_1 as seen for the simpler model remained the same for this model incorporating a vascular binding component (Fig. 4b).

Binding potential

BP_{ND} (k_3/k_4) estimates for the larger ROIs were reliable using the 2T4k_V_B model, as for almost all regions, the standard deviation was well below 50% for both HABs and MABs (in both patients and controls), see Additional file 3. This indicates that plasma input-derived BP_{ND} can be used as outcome parameter for these larger brain regions. Like V_T, regional BP_{ND} was on average 1.6 times higher in HAB than in MAB subjects (Fig. 5). For the regions shown in Fig. 5, this difference was statistically significant for frontal cortex ($p = 0.001$), cingulate cortex ($p = 0.006$), thalamic grey matter ($p = 0.002$) and brainstem white matter ($p = 0.004$). In contrast to the V_T findings, regional BP_{ND} in both grey and white matter of HAB patients was higher than in HAB healthy controls. This difference was statistically significant for cingulate cortex ($p = 0.034$), cerebellar white matter ($p = 0.034$) and non-lesional white matter ($p = 0.034$). This difference was not observed in the MAB group.

Multiple sclerosis lesions

In both HAB and MAB patients with MS, MRI-defined T2 white matter lesions showed a significant increase in BP_{ND} compared with non-lesional white matter of the same subject ($p = 0.017$) (Fig. 6a). There was a strong correlation between the BP_{ND} values, except for one patient. When including all the subjects, the correlation coefficient (R^2) was 0.246 (slope 1.04 ± 0.744), excluding

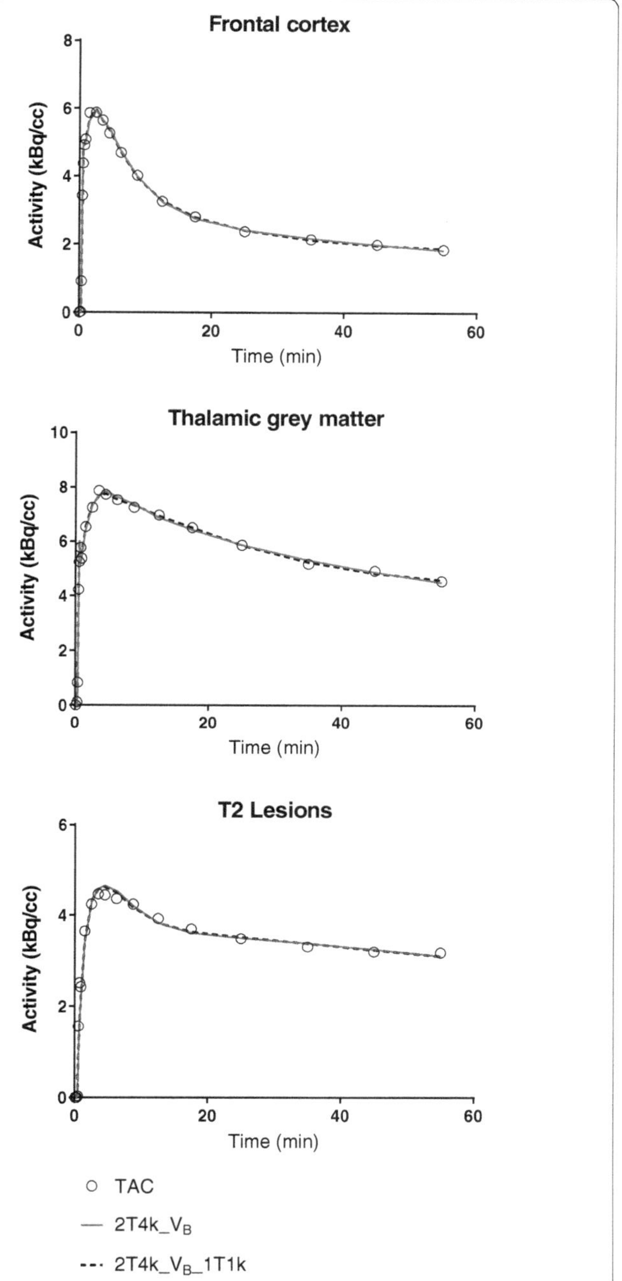

Fig. 2 Model fit comparisons. Representative model fits for the frontal cortex of a medium affinity binding healthy control, the thalamic grey matter of a high-affinity binding MS patient and the T2 lesions of a medium-affinity binding MS patient. The open circles represent the measured time-activity curves (TAC) and the solid grey and dashed black lines represent the fits for the reversible two-tissue compartment model without and with vascular binding component (2T4k_V_B and 2T4k_V_B_1T1k)

the one outlier improved the R^2 to 0.861 (slope 2.39 ± 0.429). For V_T, values were similar for lesions and non-lesional white matter of each MS patient, with an R^2 of 0.844 and slope 1.02 ± 0.178 (Fig. 6b).

Discussion

This proof of concept study in patients with progressive MS showed that quantitative assessment of the second-generation TSPO radiotracer [^{18}F]DPA714 can identify an increased binding potential not only in MS-specific lesions, but for HAB patients also in grey matter and non-lesional white matter. Although the results from this study need to be replicated in a larger cohort, they suggest that [18F]DPA714-PET could be used as an in vivo imaging technique for measuring neuroinflammation in progressive MS.

Neuroinflammation in MS is characterised by complex and dynamic processes, including the activation of microglia [6, 7]. This is most distinct in active MS lesions, identified by gadolinium enhancement on T1-weighted MRI, and chronic MS lesions as seen on T2-weighted MRI [3]. In line with this, an increase in [^{18}F]DPA714 BP_{ND} was seen in the focal lesions compared with non-lesional white matter for all patients except one, independent of the patient's genetic binding status (HAB or MAB). As MRI-defined lesions for these patients with progressive MS were almost exclusively non-enhancing chronic lesions, this increase TSPO binding indicates that these are chronic active lesions [41]. The classification of different stages of MS lesions, such as chronic active and chronic inactive lesions, results from pathological studies. Current conventional MRI techniques can identify active inflammatory lesions, with the use of gadolinium-enhanced T1-weighted scans; however, they cannot further differentiate non-enhancing lesions. Results from the present study suggest that [^{18}F]DPA714 PET can identify different stages of MS lesions in vivo, which could be clinically relevant, e.g. in relation to treatment options and monitoring.

Even more importantly, increased [^{18}F]DPA714 BP_{ND} was also seen in non-lesional brain parenchyma, both in white and grey matter, for HAB patients. In relapsing-remitting MS, neuroinflammation is evident from the development of new focal (gadolinium enhancing) lesions, but in primary and secondary progressive MS, neuroinflammation is often more diffuse and low-grade [5]. Therefore, it is highly relevant that a biomarker of neuroinflammation in MS demonstrates not only focal changes, but also more diffuse pathology. As [^{18}F]DPA714 BP_{ND} can identify both, this marker of TSPO expression can be used as a biomarker to further investigate neuroinflammation in MS in vivo.

As plasma input-derived BP_{ND} was estimated reliably using the 2T4k_V_B model, BP_{ND} should be preferred over the less specific V_T. As V_T contains both free, non-specific and specific signals, it is an inferior outcome measured compared with BP_{ND} (=k_3/k_4), which only reflects specific binding. Contrary to BP_{ND} analysis, group analysis using V_T showed no difference between patients and controls for both HAB and MAB subjects.

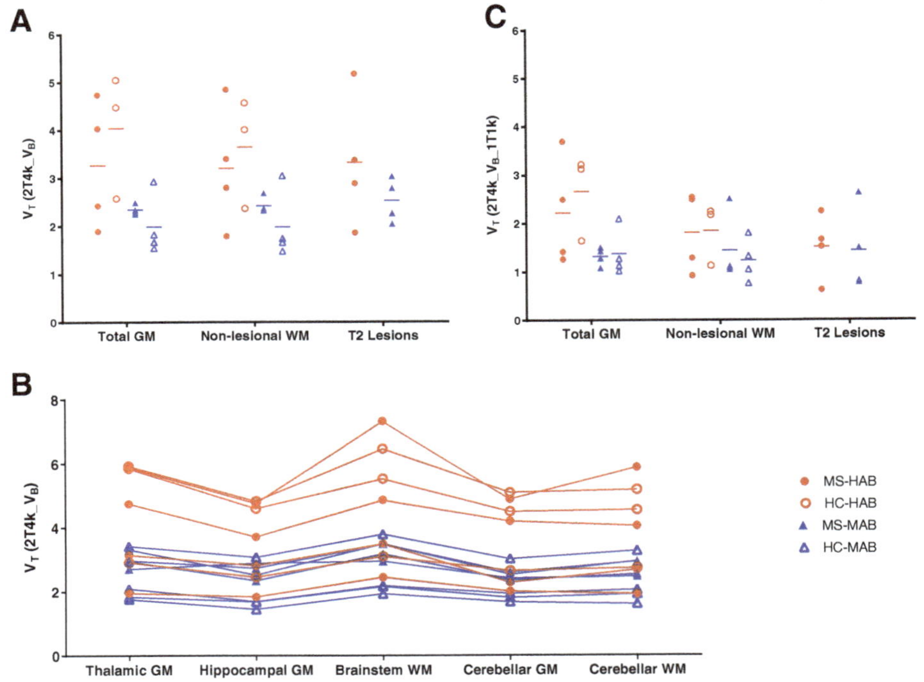

Fig. 3 Volume of distribution. **a** Volume of distribution (V_T) for total grey matter non-lesional white matter (WM) and T2 defined white matter lesions for the reversible two-tissue compartment model (2T4k_V_B). High-affinity binding (HAB) subjects in red have a 1.5 to 2-fold higher V_T than medium affinity binding (MAB) subjects in blue. No difference in V_T was seen between multiple sclerosis patients (MS; closed symbols) and healthy controls (HC; open symbols) for both HABs and MABs. **b** V_T across various regions of all patients and controls. The intra-subject variation appears to be much smaller than the inter-subject variation. **c** The reversible two-tissue compartment model with vascular binding component (2T4k_V_B_1T1k) also identified an increase in V_T for HAB subjects compared with MAB subjects, but no difference in mean regional V_T for patients compared to controls for either HABs or MABs

In addition, V_T appeared to be almost similar between different ROIs within each subject, resulting from a nearly homogeneous distribution of DPA714 throughout the brain of an individual. As V_T includes the large non-displaceable compartment of [^{18}F]DPA714, this effectively obscured any changes in the disease-specific neuroinflammatory signal. This is also seen in the analysis of the T2 MS lesions in Fig. 6, illustrating that the increase in specific [^{18}F]DPA714 signal in MS lesions depicted by BP_{ND} is diluted in the V_T values due to the non-displaceable component.

Interestingly, V_T was strongly correlated with K_1. Although a change in K_1 can be related to neuroinflammation, as K_1 is a function of blood flow and vascular permeability, a correlation between V_T and K_1 was unexpected as V_T should be independent of K_1. A possible explanation for this finding could be related to binding of [^{18}F]DPA714 to the endothelium of blood vessels in the brain [42, 43]. However, the model incorporating a vascular binding component still provided correlated K_1 and V_T values (Fig. 4b).

Although the 2T4k_V_B_1T1k model was preferred according to AIC, it decreased the reliability of the parameter estimates compared with the simpler 2T4k_V_B model. Moreover, K_b estimates were inaccurate for many regions, even in subjects where this model was preferred. A proposed method of decreasing the number of parameters, attempting to increase their reliability, is fixing V_B to 5%. However, due to the large inter- and intra-subject variation in V_B, this seems inappropriate.

Although we used the simpler model in our analysis, the results are similar, as the regional V_T values for the two models correlate.

In line with other TSPO studies, assessment of the rs6971 polymorphism defined binding status is important also for quantitative analysis of [^{18}F]DPA714. Although observed differences between HABs and MABs were smaller than those observed for some other second-generation TSPO tracers [24], both mean V_T and BP_{ND} values were on average 1.6 times higher for HABs compared with MABs for the different brain regions. This indicates that the selection of subjects based on binding status is essential. Furthermore, group differences between HABs were only observed when using BP_{ND}, suggesting that [^{18}F]DPA714 in MS could best be studied in HABs only. Due to basal expression of TSPO, the contrast for [^{18}F]DPA714 appears to be too low for MAB subjects to identify patients from controls. Strikingly, the increase in

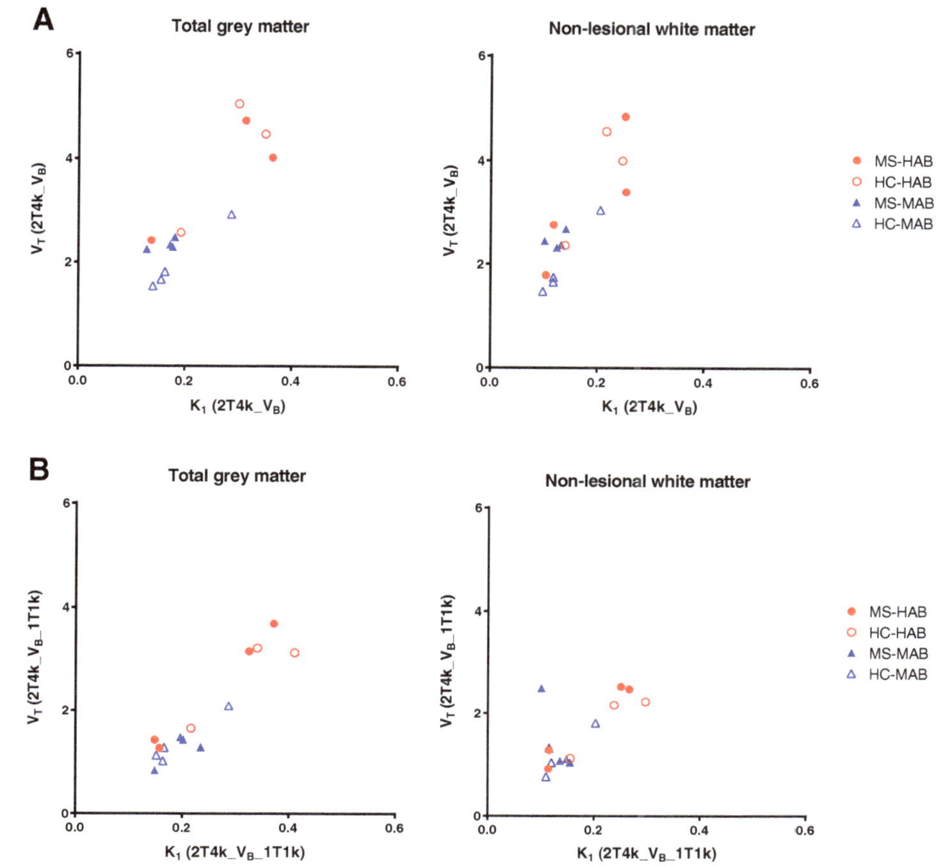

Fig. 4 Correlation for V_T and K_1. For both the reversible two-tissue compartment model **a** without and **b** with vascular binding component (2T4k_V_B and 2T4k_V_B_1T1k), there was a strong correlation between V_T and K_1 in both grey and white matter, independent of binding status

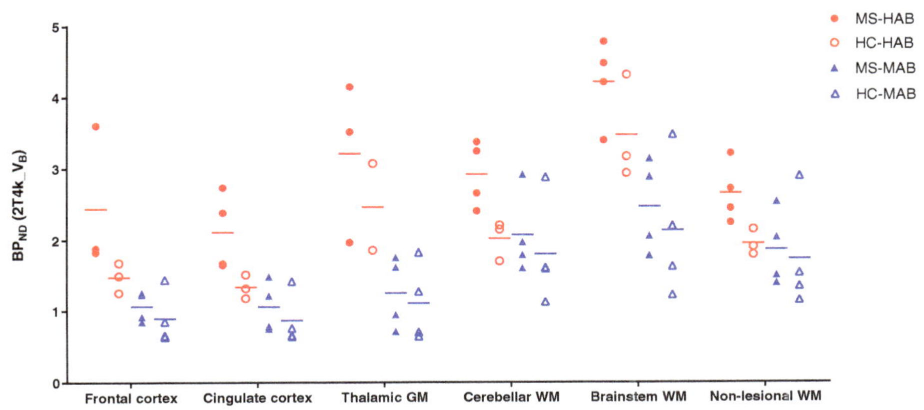

Fig. 5 Binding potential for different regions of interest. For high-affinity binders, a higher binding potential (BP_{ND}) was seen in multiple sclerosis patients (MS-HAB) than in healthy controls (HC-HAB) for different regions of interest. This difference was not seen in medium-affinity binding (MAB) subjects

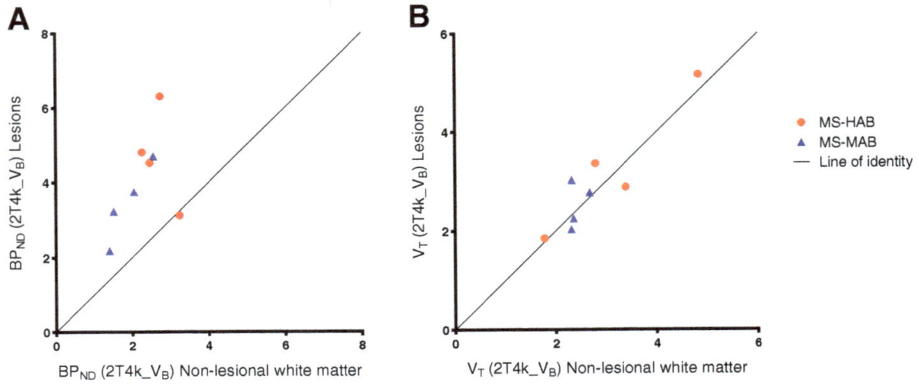

Fig. 6 Kinetic parameter values for the multiple sclerosis lesions. Independent of binding status, **a** binding potential (BP_{ND}) identified increased [^{18}F]DPA714 binding in MS-specific brain lesions compared with non-lesional white matter in the same patients, **b** whereas volume of distribution (V_T) did not depict this difference

BP_{ND} in MS lesions was also seen in MAB patients, indicating that [^{18}F]DPA714 can identify neuroinflammation in MAB subjects in MS lesions, but due to high non-specific binding of the tracer, it is not evident in other ROIs with more low-grade neuroinflammation. As only approximately half of the general population is HAB, this is a limitation of second-generation TSPO studies.

This study is limited mainly by its small sample size. Because of the limited number of subjects in each group, only limited statistical analysis was performed. Nevertheless, based on the promising results of this pilot project, further studies using a larger sample size are warranted. This would allow for evaluation of possible correlations between [^{18}F]DPA714 BP_{ND} and clinical outcome scores, such as Expanded Disability Status Scale and Symbol Digit Modalities Test. Finally, assessment of a possible relationship with MRI-derived outcome measures, such as atrophy of cortical and deep grey matter structures, would be of great interest in understanding progressive MS.

Conclusions

Plasma input-derived BP_{ND} can reliably be estimated for [^{18}F]DPA714, and a $2T4k\_V_B$ model [^{18}F]DPA714 BP_{ND} can identify increased neuroinflammation in both grey and non-lesional white matter of patients with progressive MS, with a further increase in T2 MS lesions. As these differences cannot be seen using V_T due to inclusion of non-displaceable uptake, BP_{ND} is recommended for analysis of [^{18}F]DPA714 studies in patients with MS. Similar to other second-generation TSPO tracers, the effect of genetically defined binding status limits the clinical use of [^{18}F]DPA714. Nevertheless, further studies are warranted to confirm the results of the present proof of concept study.

Additional files

Additional file 1: $2T4k\_V_B\_1T1k$ - Percentage standard deviation for BP_{ND} (k_3/k_4). Additional file provides the percentage of standard deviation for the for $2T4k\_V_B\_1T1k$ BP_{ND} (k_3/k_4) for the different large regions of interest.

Additional file 2: $2T4k\_V_B\_1T1k$ - Percentage standard deviation for k_b. Additional file provides the percentage of standard deviation for the for $2T4k\_V_B\_1T1k$ k_b for the different large regions of interest.

Additional file 3: $2T4k\_V_B$ - Percentage standard deviation for BP_{ND} (k_3/k_4). Additional file provides the percentage of standard deviation for the arterial input-derived BP_{ND} (k_3/k_4) for the different large regions of interest.

Abbreviations

1T2k: Single-tissue compartment model; 2T3k: Irreversible two-tissue compartment model; 2T4k: Reversible two-tissue compartment model; BP_{ND}: Binding potential (k_3/k_4); FLAIR: Fluid Attenuated Inversion Recovery; HAB: High-affinity binder; k_b: Vascular binding component; LAB: Low-affinity binder; MAB: Medium-affinity binder; MRI: Magnetic resonance imaging; MS: Multiple sclerosis; PET: Positron emission tomography; ROI: Region of interest; TAC: Time activity curve; TSPO: 18-kDa translocator-protein; V_B: Blood volume parameter; V_T: Volume of distribution

Acknowledgements

The authors would like to thank Mattia Veronese (Department of Neuroimaging, King's College London) for his help on the implementation of the kinetic model including a vascular binding component.

Funding

This research has received funding from Amsterdam Neuroscience and the Dutch MS Research Foundation (programme grant 14-358e). Both organisations had no role in the design of the study or the collection, analysis and interpretation of data.

Authors' contributions

The study was designed by MH, AMvD, JK, ADW, FB and BvB. Tracer development was done by TAR, MK and ADW. Data were collected by MH, MTW, PS and JB. Analysis of the data was performed by MH, SVG, MY, DH, MDS, RCS and AAL and data were interpreted by MH, SVG, MY, BvB and AAL. The manuscript was drafted by MH and SVG. All authors read and approved the final manuscript.

Consent for publication
Not applicable.

Competing interests
DH is employed by Philips Healthcare. JK has accepted speaker and consultancy fees from Merck-Serono, Teva, Biogen, Genzyme, Roche and Novartis. FB is supported by the NIHR UCLH Biomedical Research Centre and serves as a consultant for Bayer-Schering Pharma, Sanofi-Aventis, Genzyme, Biogen-Idec, Teva, Novartis, Roche, Synthon BV and Jansen Research. All other authors declare that they have no competing interests.

Author details
[1]VUmc MS Center Amsterdam, VU University Medical Center, De Boelelaan 1117, 1081 HV Amsterdam, the Netherlands. [2]Department of Neurology, VU University Medical Center, De Boelelaan 1117, 1081 HV Amsterdam, the Netherlands. [3]Department of Radiology and Nuclear Medicine, VU University Medical Center Amsterdam, De Boelelaan 1117, 1081 HV Amsterdam, the Netherlands. [4]Philips Healthcare, Best, the Netherlands, Veenpluis 4, 5684 PC Best, the Netherlands. [5]Department of Anatomy and Neurosciences, VU University Medical Center Amsterdam, De Boelelaan 1117, 1081 HV Amsterdam, the Netherlands. [6]Department of Anaesthesiology, VU University Medical Center Amsterdam, De Boelelaan 1117, 1081 HV Amsterdam, the Netherlands. [7]School of Chemistry, University of Sydney, F11, Eastern Ave, Sydney, NSW 2006, Australia. [8]Institutes of Neurology and Healthcare Engineering, UCL Institute of Neurology, Queen Square, London WC1N 3BG, UK.

References
1. O'Connor P, Comi G, Freedman MS, Miller AE, Kappos L, Bouchard JP, et al. Long-term safety and efficacy of teriflunomide: nine-year follow-up of the randomized TEMSO study. Neurology. 2016;86:10.
2. Rovira A, Wattjes MP, Tintore M, Tur C, Yousry TA, Sormani MP, et al. Evidence-based guidelines: MAGNIMS consensus guidelines on the use of MRI in multiple sclerosis-clinical implementation in the diagnostic process. Nat Rev Neurol. 2015;11:8.
3. Wattjes MP, Rovira A, Miller D, Yousry TA, Sormani MP, de Stefano MP, et al. Evidence-based guidelines: MAGNIMS consensus guidelines on the use of MRI in multiple sclerosis--establishing disease prognosis and monitoring patients. Nat Rev Neurol. 2015;11:10.
4. Barkhof F. The clinico-radiological paradox in multiple sclerosis revisited. Curr Opin Neurol. 2002;15:3.
5. Lassmann H, van Horssen J, Mahad D. Progressive multiple sclerosis: pathology and pathogenesis. Nat Rev Neurol. 2012;8:11.
6. Hemmer B, Kerschensteiner M, Korn T. Role of the innate and adaptive immune responses in the course of multiple sclerosis. Lancet Neurol. 2015;14:4.
7. Mahad DH, Trapp BD, Lassmann H. Pathological mechanisms in progressive multiple sclerosis. Lancet Neurol. 2015;14:2.
8. Airas L, Rissanen E, Rinne J. Imaging of microglial activation in MS using PET: research use and potential future clinical application. Mult Scler. 2017;23:4.
9. Hagens M, van Berckel B, Barkhof F. Novel MRI and PET markers of neuroinflammation in multiple sclerosis. Curr Opin Neurol. 2016;29:3.
10. Cumming P, Burgher B, Patkar O, Breakspear M, Vasdev N, Thomas P, et al. Sifting through the surfeit of neuroinflammation tracers. J Cereb Blood Flow Metab. 2018;38:2.
11. Vowinckel E, Reutens D, Becher B, Verge G, Evans A, Owens T, et al. PK11195 binding to the peripheral benzodiazepine receptor as a marker of microglia activation in multiple sclerosis and experimental autoimmune encephalomyelitis. J Neurosci Res. 1997;50:2.
12. Banati RB, Newcombe J, Gunn RN, Cagnin A, Turkheimer F, Heppner F, et al. The peripheral benzodiazepine binding site in the brain in multiple sclerosis: quantitative in vivo imaging of microglia as a measure of disease activity. Brain. 2000;123(Pt 11):2321–37.
13. Politis M, Giannetti P, Su P, Turkheimer F, Keihaninejad S, Wu K, et al. Increased PK11195 PET binding in the cortex of patients with MS correlates with disability. Neurology. 2012;79:6.
14. Rissanen E, Tuisku J, Rokka J, Paavilainen T, Parkkola R, Rinne JO, et al. In vivo detection of diffuse inflammation in secondary progressive multiple sclerosis using PET imaging and the radioligand ^{11}C-PK11195. J Nucl Med. 2014;55:6.
15. Giannetti P, Politis M, Su P, Turkheimer F, Malik O, Keihaninejad S, et al. Microglia activation in multiple sclerosis black holes predicts outcome in progressive patients: an in vivo [^{1}C](R)-PK11195-PET pilot study. Neurobiol Dis. 2014;65:203–10.
16. Giannetti P, Politis M, Su P, Turkheimer FE, Malik O, Keihaninejad S, et al. Increased PK11195-PET binding in normal-appearing white matter in clinically isolated syndrome. Brain. 2015;138:Pt 1.
17. Boutin H, Chauveau F, Thominiaux C, Gregoire MC, James ML, Trebossen R, et al. 11C-DPA-713: a novel peripheral benzodiazepine receptor PET ligand for in vivo imaging of neuroinflammation. J Nucl Med. 2007;48:4.
18. Fookes CJ, Pham TQ, Mattner F, Greguric I, Loc'h C, Liu X, et al. Synthesis and biological evaluation of substituted [^{18}F]imidazo[1,2-a]pyridines and [^{18}F]pyrazolo[1,5-a]pyrimidines for the study of the peripheral benzodiazepine receptor using positron emission tomography. J Med Chem. 2008;51:13.
19. Kreisl WC, Fujita M, Fujimura Y, Kimura N, Jenko KJ, Kannan P, et al. Comparison of [^{11}C]-(R)-PK 11195 and [^{11}C]PBR28, two radioligands for translocator protein (18 kDa) in human and monkey: implications for positron emission tomographic imaging of this inflammation biomarker. NeuroImage. 2010;49:4.
20. Wadsworth H, Jones PA, Chau WF, Durrant C, Fouladi N, Passmore J, et al. [^{18}F]GE-180: a novel fluorine-18 labelled PET tracer for imaging Translocator protein 18 kDa (TSPO). Bioorg Med Chem Lett. 2012;22:3.
21. Zhang MR, Maeda J, Ogawa M, Noguchi J, Ito T, Yoshida Y, et al. Development of a new radioligand, N-(5-fluoro-2-phenoxyphenyl)-N-(2-[^{18}F]fluoroethyl-5-methoxybenzyl)acetamide, for pet imaging of peripheral benzodiazepine receptor in primate brain. J Med Chem. 2004;47:9.
22. James ML, Fulton RR, Vercoullie J, Henderson DJ, Garreau L, Chalon S, et al. DPA-714, a new translocator protein-specific ligand: synthesis, radiofluorination, and pharmacologic characterization. J Nucl Med. 2008;49:5.
23. Peyronneau MA, Saba W, Goutal S, Damont A, Dolle F, Kassiou M, et al. Metabolism and quantification of [^{18}F]DPA-714, a new TSPO positron emission tomography radioligand. Drug Metab Dispos. 2013;41:1.
24. Owen DR, Gunn RN, Rabiner EA, Bennacef I, Fujita M, Kreisl WC, et al. Mixed-affinity binding in humans with 18-kDa translocator protein ligands. J Nucl Med. 2011;52:1.
25. Lavisse S, Garcia-Lorenzo D, Peyronneau MA, Bodini B, Thiriez C, Kuhnast B, et al. Optimized quantification of translocator protein radioligand ^{18}F-DPA-714 uptake in the brain of genotyped healthy volunteers. J Nucl Med. 2015;56:7.
26. Golla SS, Boellaard R, Oikonen V, Hoffmann A, van Berckel BN, Windhorst AD, et al. Quantification of [^{18}F]DPA-714 binding in the human brain: initial studies in healthy controls and Alzheimer's disease patients. J Cereb Blood Flow Metab. 2015;35:5.
27. Ribeiro MJ, Vercouillie J, Debiais S, Cottier JP, Bonnaud I, Camus V, et al. Could ^{18}F-DPA-714 PET imaging be interesting to use in the early post-stroke period? EJNMMI Res. 2014;4:28.
28. Hamelin L, Lagarde J, Dorothee G, Leroy C, Labit M, Comley RA, et al. Early and protective microglial activation in Alzheimer's disease: a prospective study using ^{18}F-DPA-714 PET imaging. Brain. 2016;139:Pt 4.
29. Salinas CA, Searle GE, Gunn RN. The simplified reference tissue model: model assumption violations and their impact on binding potential. J Cereb Blood Flow Metab. 2015;35:2.
30. Folkersma H, Boellaard R, Vandertop WP, Kloet RW, Lubberink M, Lammertsma AA, et al. Reference tissue models and blood-brain barrier disruption: lessons from (R)-[^{11}C]PK11195 in traumatic brain injury. J Nucl Med. 2009;50:12.
31. Boellaard R, van Lingen A, van Balen SC, Hoving BG, Lammertsma AA. Characteristics of a new fully programmable blood sampling device for monitoring blood radioactivity during PET. Eur J Nucl Med. 2001;28:1.
32. Steenwijk MD, Pouwels PJ, Daams M, van Dalen JW, Caan MW, Richard E, et al. Accurate white matter lesion segmentation by k nearest neighbor classification with tissue type priors (kNN-TTPs). Neuroimage Clin. 2013;3:462–9.
33. Chard DT, Jackson JS, Miller DH, Wheeler-Kingshott CA. Reducing the impact of white matter lesions on automated measures of brain gray and

white matter volumes. J Magn Reson Imaging. 2010;32:1.
34. Cizek J, Herholz K, Vollmar S, Schrader R, Klein J, Heiss WD. Fast and robust registration of PET and MR images of human brain. NeuroImage. 2004;22:1.
35. Vollmar S, Cizek J, Sue J, Klein A, Jacbos K, Herholz K. VINCI-volume imaging in neurological research, co-registration and ROIs included. Forschung und wissenschaftliches Rechnen 2003 (Kremer K, Macho V, eds); 2004.
36. Svarer C, Madsen K, Hasselbalch SG, Pinborg LH, Haugbol S, Frokjaer VG, et al. MR-based automatic delineation of volumes of interest in human brain PET images using probability maps. NeuroImage. 2005;24:4.
37. Hammers A, Allom R, Koepp MJ, Free SL, Myers R, Lemieux L, et al. Three-dimensional maximum probability atlas of the human brain, with particular reference to the temporal lobe. Hum Brain Mapp. 2003;19:4.
38. Frisoni GB, Boccardi M, Barkhof F, Blennow K, Cappa S, Chiotis K, et al. Strategic roadmap for an early diagnosis of Alzheimer's disease based on biomarkers. Lancet Neurol. 2017;16:8.
39. Rizzo G, Veronese M, Tonietto M, Zanotti-Fregonara P, Turkheimer FE, Bertoldo A. Kinetic modeling without accounting for the vascular component impairs the quantification of [^{11}C]PBR28 brain PET data. J Cereb Blood Flow Metab. 2014;34:6.
40. Wimberley C, Lavisse S, Brulon V, Peyronneau MA, Leroy C, Bodini B, et al. Impact of endothelial TSPO on the quantification of 18F-DPA-714. J Nucl Med. 2018;59:307–14.
41. van der Valk P, De Groot CJ. Staging of multiple sclerosis (MS) lesions: pathology of the time frame of MS. Neuropathol Appl Neurobiol. 2000;26:1.
42. Tomasi G, Edison P, Bertoldo A, Roncaroli F, Singh P, Gerhard A, et al. Novel reference region model reveals increased microglial and reduced vascular binding of ^{11}C-(R)-PK11195 in patients with Alzheimer's disease. J Nucl Med. 2008;49:8.
43. Turkheimer FE, Edison P, Pavese N, Roncaroli F, Anderson AN, Hammers A, et al. Reference and target region modeling of [^{11}C]-(R)-PK11195 brain studies. J Nucl Med. 2007;48:1.

Restoration of regulatory B cell deficiency following alemtuzumab therapy in patients with relapsing multiple sclerosis

Yeseul Kim[1,3], Gayoung Kim[1], Hyun-June Shin[2], Jae-Won Hyun[2], Su-Hyun Kim[2], Eunjig Lee[3] and Ho Jin Kim[1,2*]

Abstract

Background: Regulatory B cells (Bregs), which protect from autoimmunity, are deficient in multiple sclerosis (MS). Novel regulatory B cell subsets $CD19^{+}CD24^{hi}CD38^{hi}$ cells and $CD19^{+}PD\text{-}L1^{hi}$ cells, with disparate regulatory mechanisms have been defined. Alemtuzumab provides a long-lasting suppression of disease activity in MS. In contrast to its documented efficacy, alemtuzumab's mechanism of action is not fully understood and information about the composition of repopulating B cell pool is scarce.

Aim: To characterize repopulated B cell subsets and elucidate alemtuzumab's mechanism of action in B cell perspective.

Methods: The frequency and the absolute number of Bregs were studied in peripheral blood mononuclear cells (PBMC) of 37 MS patients and 11 healthy controls (HC). Longitudinal analysis of the frequency and the absolute number of Bregs in PBMC of 11 MS patients was evaluated, before and at 6, 9, and 12 months post alemtuzumab.

Results: We found deficiency of $CD19^{+}CD24^{hi}CD38^{hi}$ cells during relapse compared to remission and HC (relapse vs remission: $p = 0.0006$, relapse vs HC: $p = 0.0004$). $CD19^{+}PD\text{-}L1^{hi}$ cells were deficient during relapse than remission and HC (relapse vs remission: $p = 0.0113$, relapse vs HC: $p = 0.0007$). Following alemtuzumab, the distribution of B cells shifts towards naïve phenotype and Breg deficiency is restored. The frequency of $CD19^{+}CD24^{hi}CD38^{hi}$ cells was significantly increased at 6 M and 9 M compared to 0 M (6 M vs 0 M: $p = 0.0004$, 9 M vs 0 M: $p = 0.0079$). At 9 M, the frequency of $CD19^{+}CD24^{hi}CD38^{hi}$ cells started to decrease and by 12 M the frequency was reduced compared to 6 M, although it was significantly higher than baseline level (12 M vs 0 M: $p = 0.0257$). The absolute number was significantly increased at 6 M and 9 M post-alemtuzumab (6 M vs 0 M: $p = 0.0063$, 9 M vs 0 M: $p = 0.02$). The frequency of $CD19^{+}PD\text{-}L1^{hi}$ cells significantly increased until 12 M (6 M vs 0 M: $p = 0.0004$, 12 M vs 0 M: $p = 0.0036$). The frequency of $CD19^{+}PD\text{-}L1^{hi}$ cells at 12 M was significantly higher than 9 M ($p = 0.0311$). We further pinpoint that $CD19^{+}CD24^{hi}CD38^{hi}$ cells were deficient at severe relapses following alemtuzumab infusion and restored during recovery.

Conclusions: Our results highlight the preferential reconstitution of Bregs as a possible mechanism of action of alemtuzumab and $CD19^{+}CD24^{hi}CD38^{hi}$ cells as a potential biomarker for disease activity.

Keywords: Multiple sclerosis, Regulatory B cells, Alemtuzumab, Relapse

* Correspondence: hojinkim@ncc.re.kr
[1]Division of Clinical Research, Research institute, National Cancer Center, Goyang, Korea
[2]Department of Neurology, Research Institute and Hospital of National Cancer Center, Goyang, Korea

Background

The concept that multiple sclerosis (MS) is a T-cell-mediated disease has been changed and it is now widely accepted that B cells play a part in the pathogenesis of MS. [1–3] Multiple roles of B cells have been elucidated emphasizing that B cells have dual contribution to autoimmunity [1, 4–6]. Hence, the concept of regulatory B cells (Breg) has emerged, proving that B cell subset distribution is far more complex than the original concept. A novel Breg subset that was originally known as immature transitional B cells ($CD19^+CD24^{hi}CD38^{hi}$) has been described to have regulatory capacity through interleukin-10 production [7]. Another study has found B cells highly expressing programmed death ligand-1 ($CD19^+PD\text{-}L1^{hi}$ cells) that exert regulatory function through cell-to-cell contact via interaction of $CD19^+PD\text{-}L1^{hi}$ cells with PD-1 on T cells, resulting in suppression of T follicular helper (Tfh) cell differentiation and expansion, which are the cell type known to be involved in the relapse of MS patients [8, 9].

Alemtuzumab is a highly effective treatment in relapsing MS. It provides a long-lasting suppression of disease activity by altering the proportion of lymphocyte subsets with preferential increase of regulatory T cells (Treg) [10, 11]. In contrast to alemtuzumab's documented efficacy, alemtuzumab's mechanism of action is not fully understood and information about the composition of the repopulating B cell pool, especially Breg, is scarce.

Here, we pinpoint deficiency of $CD19^+CD24^{hi}CD38^{hi}$ and $CD19^+PD\text{-}L1^{hi}$ cells during relapse and subsequent expansion following alemtuzumab infusion. We also highlight the possible clinical implication of $CD19^+CD24^{hi}CD38^{hi}$ cells.

Methods

Study population

For cross-sectional study, 20 MS patients during relapse (MS-relapse) and 17 MS patients in remission (MS-remission) and 11 healthy controls (HC) were included. For longitudinal analysis, 11 patients who were treated with alemtuzumab were included. All MS patients fulfilled the 2010 McDonald's criteria [12]. Current study was approved by the Institutional Review Board, and informed consent was obtained from each subject. Demographic and clinical characteristics of participants are summarized in Table 1.

Flow cytometry

For cross-sectional study, fresh peripheral blood mononuclear cells (PBMCs) were surface stained with monoclonal antibodies against CD19-APC-cy7, CD27-FITC, CD24-BV421, CD38-BV510, and PD-L1(CD274)-PE-cy7 (BD Biosciences). For longitudinal study, frozen PBMCs, collected from 11 RRMS patients undergoing alemtuzumab at baseline and 6, 9, and 12 months, were surface stained with monoclonal antibodies as stated above.

Table 1 Demographic and clinical characteristics of MS patients in relapse and remission

Characteristic	MS relapse	MS remission
Age (years, mean ± SD)	34.5 ± 9.4	36.9 ± 5.2
Women:men (*n*:*n*)	16:4	10:7
Onset age (years, mean ± SD)	30.4 ± 22.0	29.8 ± 7.3
Disease duration (years, mean ± SD)	12 ± 24.9	6 ± 5.9
EDSS (mean ± SD)	2.9 ± 1.9	1.8 ± 1.9

Statistical analysis

We performed analysis of significance in Prism (GraphPad, La Jolla, USA). For cross-sectional data, one-way ANOVA analysis with Tukey's multiple comparison post hoc analysis was performed to compare the frequency of Bregs between HC, MS-relapse, and MS-remission. Unpaired *t* test was used to compare the absolute number of Bregs between MS-relapse and MS-remission. Repeated measures ANOVA with Tukey's multiple comparison post hoc analysis was performed for longitudinal analysis. A p value of < 0.05 was considered statistically significant. All values show mean ± SEM.

Result

Regulatory B cells are deficient in MS patients during relapse

In order to evaluate the relationship between the frequency of $CD19^+CD24^{hi}CD38^{hi}$ cells and $CD19^+PD\text{-}L1^{hi}$ cells with disease activity of MS, the frequency and the absolute number were measured in total $CD19^+$ B cells in MS-relapse and MS-remission and HC. The frequency of both $CD19^+CD24^{hi}CD38^{hi}$ cells (Fig. 1a, b) and $CD19^+PD\text{-}L1^{hi}$ cells (Fig. 2a, b) was significantly reduced in MS-relapse compared to MS-remission and HC. The average frequency of Bregs in MS-remission was lower than those of HC, but no statistical difference was observed. The absolute number of $CD19^+CD24^{hi}CD38^{hi}$ cells was significantly reduced in MS-relapse compared to MS-remission (Fig. 1c). Although no significant difference was observed, the absolute number of $CD19^+PD\text{-}L1^{hi}$ cells was reduced in MS-relapse compared to MS-remission (Fig. 2c).

Preferential reconstitution of naïve B cells following alemtuzumab

As expected, the frequency and absolute number of total lymphocytes was decreased at 6 months and gradually increased up to 12 months post alemtuzumab (Fig. 3a). The frequency and the absolute number of memory B cells and plasmablasts were significantly decreased compared to pre-treatment level, and naïve B cells comprised the majority of repopulated $CD19^+$ B cells (Fig. 3b).

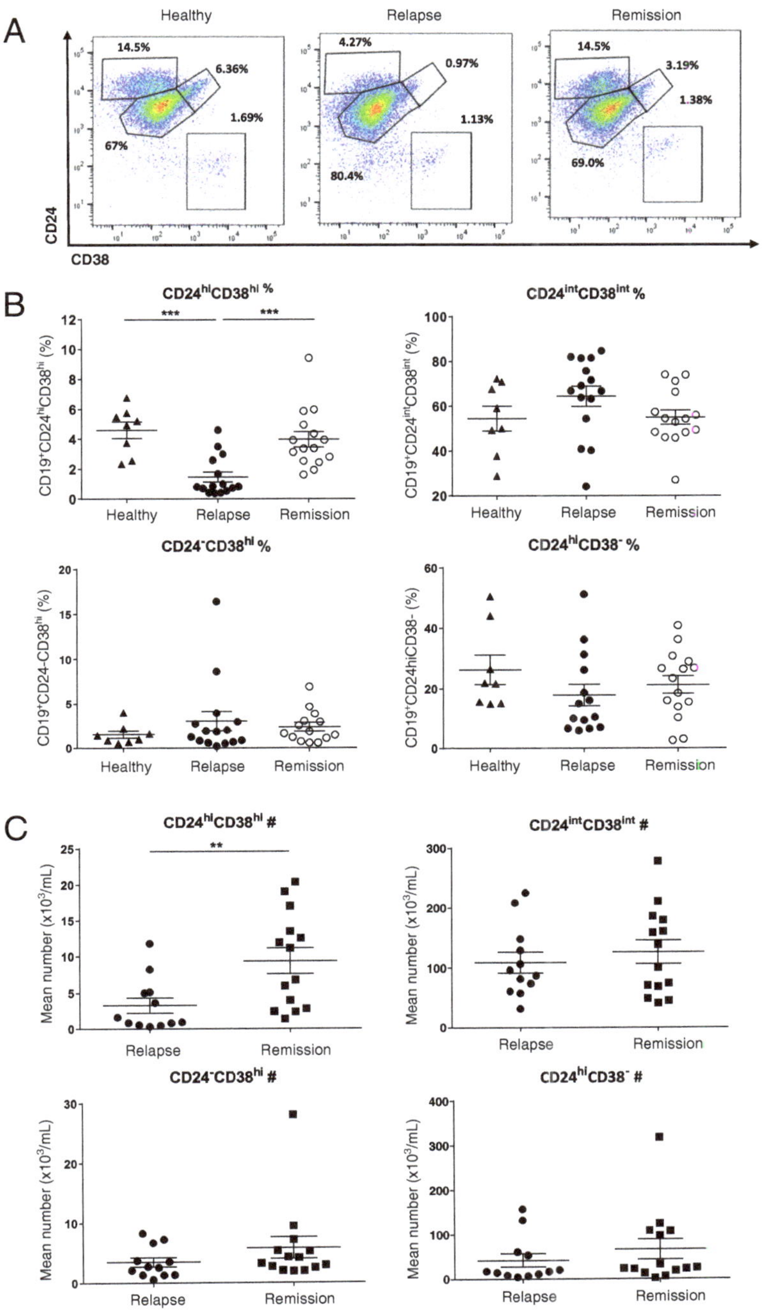

Fig. 1 MS patients show deficiency of $CD19^+CD24^{hi}CD38^{hi}$ cells during relapse. The percentage and the absolute number of $CD19^+CD24^{hi}CD38^{hi}$ B cells were measured in MS patients undergoing relapse ($n = 15$) and patients in remission ($n = 15$) and healthy controls ($n = 8$). PBMC was isolated from fresh peripheral blood and surface stained for flow cytometry. **a** Representative flow cytometry dot plot of CD24 and CD38 expression in total CD19+ B cells. **b** Scatter plots showing the percentage of $CD19^+CD24^{hi}CD38^{hi}$ B cells in MS-relapse, MS-remission, and HC. A significant reduction in the frequency of $CD19^+CD24^{hi}CD38^{hi}$ B cells was observed in MS-relapse compared to MS-remission and HC (relapse vs remission: $p = 0.0006$, relapse vs healthy: $p = 0.0004$). All values show mean ± SEM. Data were analyzed by one-way analysis of variance (ANOVA) with Tukey's multiple comparison post hoc analysis. ***$p < 0.001$. **c** The absolute number of $CD19^+CD24^{hi}CD38^{hi}$ B cells in MS-relapse was significantly reduced compared to MS-remission ($p = 0.009$). All values show mean ± SEM. Data were analyzed by unpaired t test. **$p < 0.01$. Ex vivo data were collected from peripheral blood samples taken during the time course of this study

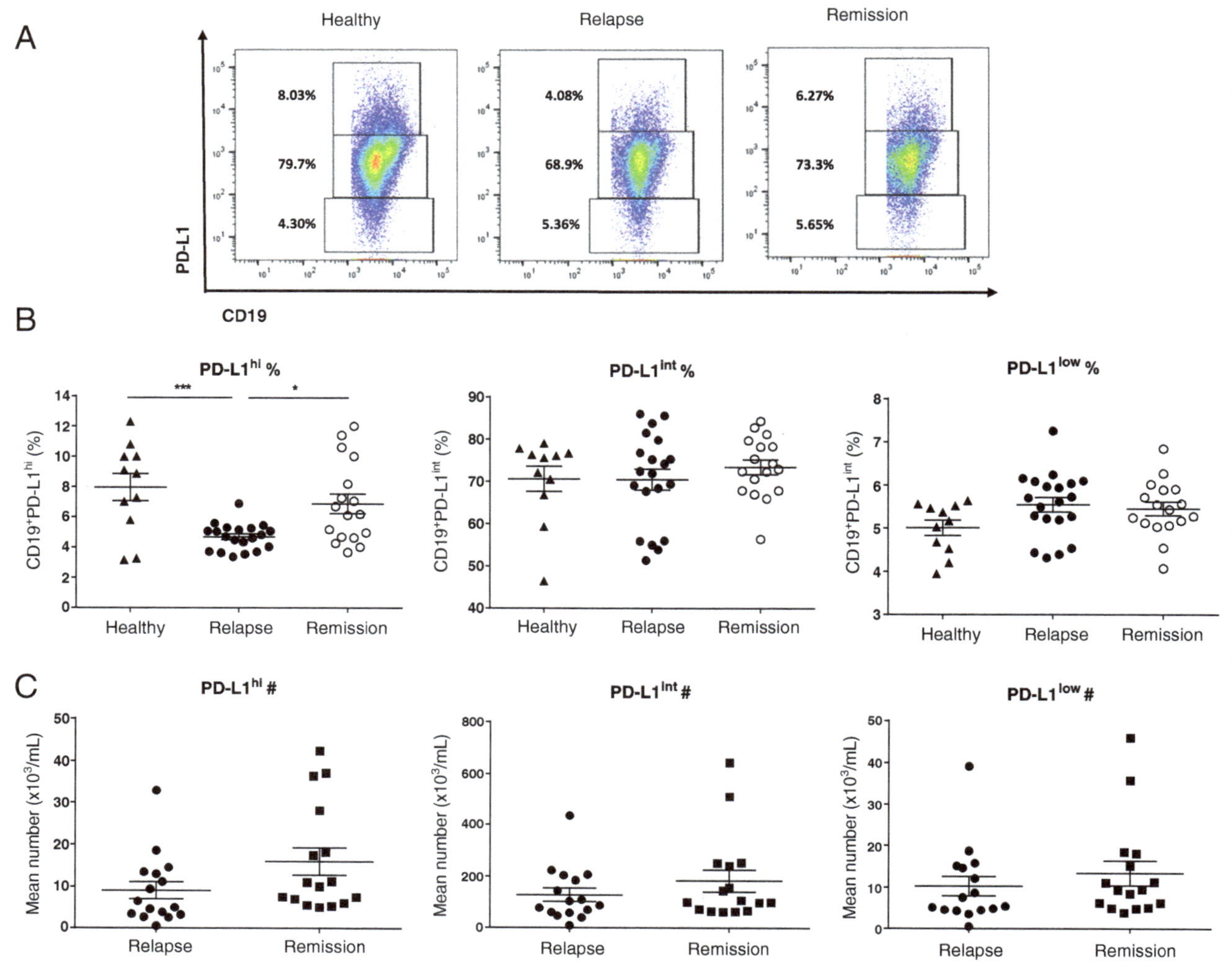

Fig. 2 MS patients have deficiency of $CD19^{+}PD\text{-}L1^{hi}$ cells during relapse. The percentage and the absolute number of $CD19^{+}PD\text{-}L1^{hi}$ cells were measured in MS patients undergoing relapse ($n = 20$) and patients in remission ($n = 17$) and healthy controls ($n = 11$). Fresh PBMC was isolated from peripheral blood and surface stained for flow cytometry. **a** Representative flow-cytometry dot plot of PD-L1 and CD19 expression in total CD19+ B cells. **b** Scatter plots showing the percentage of $CD19^{+}PD\text{-}L1^{hi}$ cells in MS-relapse, MS-remission, and HC. The frequency of $CD19^{+}PD\text{-}L1^{hi}$ cells was significantly reduced in MS-relapse compared to MS-remission and HC (relapse vs remission: $p = 0.0113$, relapse vs healthy: $p = 0.0007$). All values show mean ± SEM. Data were analyzed by one-way analysis of variance (ANOVA) with Tukey's multiple comparison post hoc analysis. $^{*}p < 0.05$; $^{***}p < 0.001$. **c** Scatter plots showing the absolute number of $CD19^{+}PD\text{-}L1^{hi}$ cells in MS-relapse and MS-remission. All values show mean ± SEM. Data were analyzed by unpaired t test. Ex vivo data were collected from peripheral blood samples taken during the time course of this study

Breg deficiency in MS is restored following alemtuzumab

The frequency and the absolute number of $CD19^{+}CD24^{hi}CD38^{hi}$ cells were markedly increased at 6 and 9 months following alemtuzumab treatment compared to pre-treatment level. By the end of the cycle (12 M), both the frequency and number were decreased, although did not reach pre-treatment level. The frequency and absolute number of $CD19^{+}CD24^{int}CD38^{int}$ mature naïve B cells were increased at 6 and 9 months post-alemtuzumab, and at 12 months post-alemtuzumab, the frequency of $CD19^{+}CD24^{int}CD38^{int}$ cells was lower than baseline level. A significant decrease in the frequency and absolute number of $CD19^{+}CD24^{hi}CD38^{-}$ memory B cells was observed following alemtuzumab treatment (Fig. 4a–c).

The frequency and absolute number of $CD19^{+}PD\text{-}L1^{hi}$ cells were increased at 6 and 9 months and maintained until the end of the cycle. The frequency of $CD19^{+}PD\text{-}L1^{int}$ cells was significantly decreased at 6, 9, and 12 months following alemtuzumab. The absolute number of $CD19^{+}PD\text{-}L1^{int}$ cells showed no significant difference. The frequency and absolute number of $CD19^{+}PD\text{-}L1^{low}$ cells showed no significant difference (Fig. 5a–c).

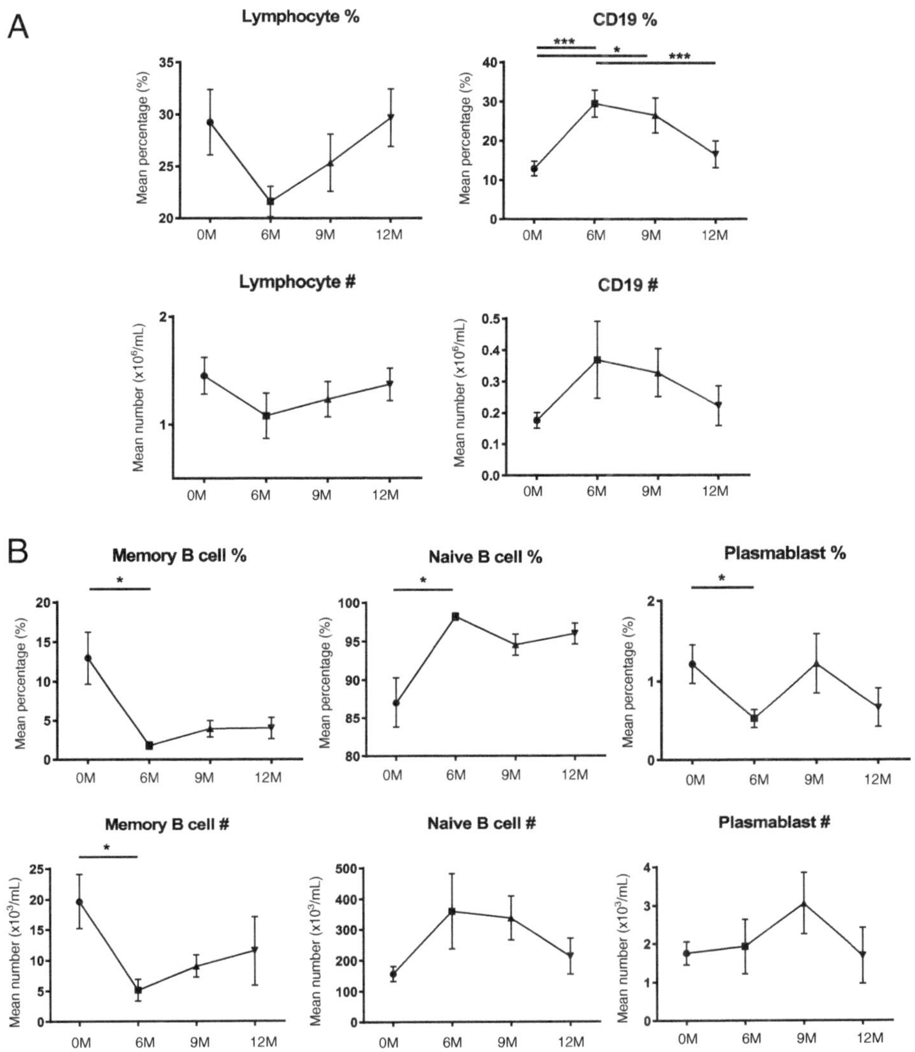

Fig. 3 Naive B cells predominate repopulated CD19+ cells following alemtuzumab treatment. In order to evaluate the B cell subset distribution post-alemtuzuamb, thawed PBMCs of alemtuzumab-treated patients ($n = 11$) were evaluated up to 12 months after induction. **a** Cumulative data for the frequency and the absolute number of total lymphocytes and $CD19^+$ B cells. Successful depletion and reconstitution of lymphocytes and $CD19^+$ B cells was confirmed. **b** Cumulative data for the frequency and the absolute number of $CD19^+CD27^+$ memory B cells, $CD19^+CD27^-$ naïve B cells, and $CD19^+CD27^+CD38^{hi}$ plasmablasts. Following alemtuzumab, significant reduction in the frequency of memory B cells (6 M vs 0 M: $p = 0.0278$) and plasmablasts (6 M vs 0 M: $p = 0.0448$) was observed and dominance of naïve B cells was observed (6 M vs 0 M: $p = 0.0269$). The absolute number of memory B cells was significantly decreased compared to 0 M (6 M vs 0 M: $p = 0.0112$). All values show mean ± SEM. Data were analyzed by repeated measures ANOVA with Tukey's multiple comparison post hoc analysis

Clinical implications

Among 11 patients treated with alemtuzumab, one patient experienced two severe relapses within 2 cycles of alemtuzumab infusion (Fig. 6a, b). During his first attack, overshoot of total B cells was observed while the frequency of $CD19^+CD24^{hi}CD38^{hi}$ cells was remarkably decreased to 0.45% compared to previous follow-up (6 M: 11.1%). 4 months later, the frequency of $CD19^+CD24^{hi}CD38^{hi}$ cells increased to 6.5%. 3 months post second alemtuzumab infusion, the frequency of $CD19^+CD24^{hi}CD38^{hi}$ cells was 10.5%. However, at his second attack, 10 M after second cycle infusion, the frequency of $CD19^+C D24^{hi}CD38^{hi}$ cells was again markedly decreased to 1.93% accompanied by overshooting B cell response. Interestingly, the reduction in the frequency of CDa, $b19^+CD24^{hi}CD38^{hi}$ cells (3.98%) 20 days preceding second attack was observed, which is an immense reduction from previous follow-up (15 M: 10.5%). In contrast to $CD19^+CD24^{hi}CD38^{hi}$ cells, no change in the frequency of $CD19^+PD\text{-}L1^{hi}$ cells was observed during both relapses. The absolute number of $CD19^+CD24^{hi}CD38^{hi}$ cells was also reduced during relapses.

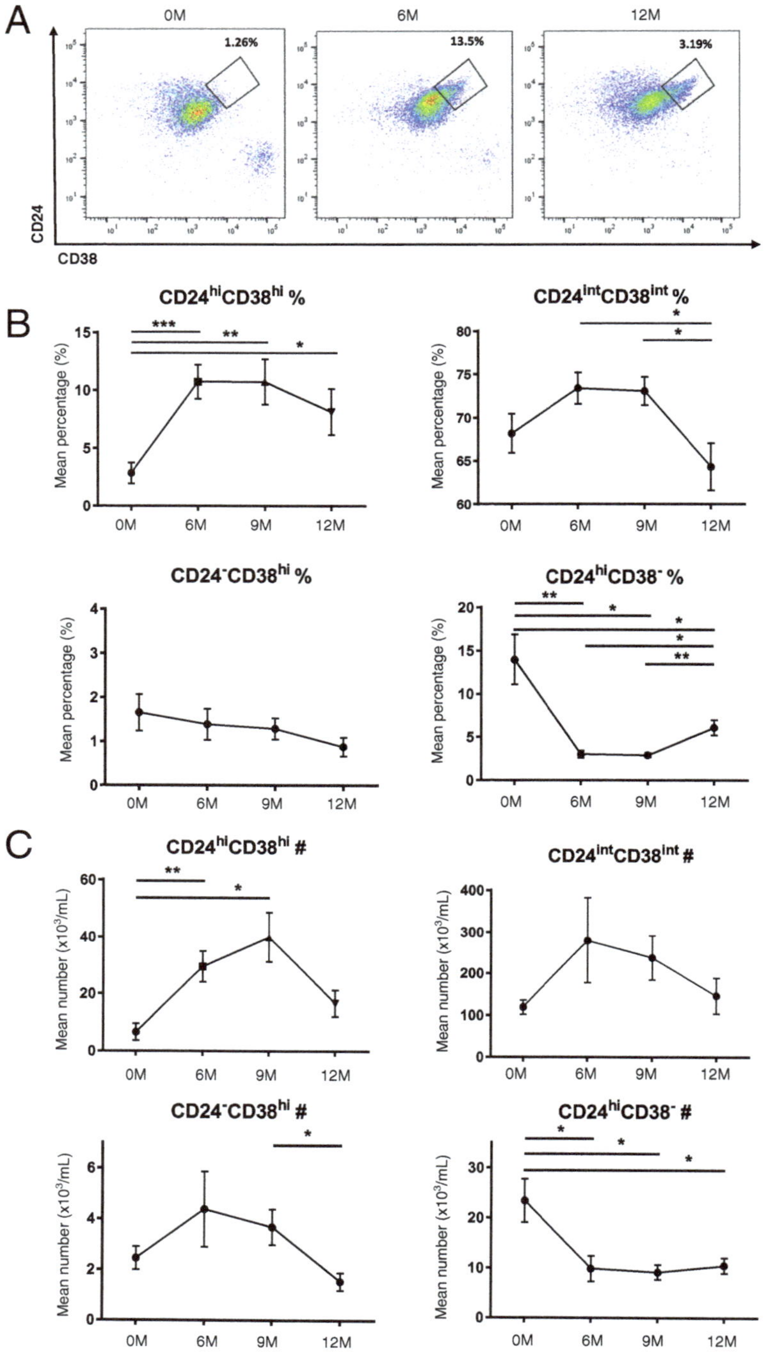

Fig. 4 Alemtuzumab treatment restores $CD19^+CD24^{hi}CD38^{hi}$ cells. In order to evaluate the B cell subset distribution post-alemtuzuamb, thawed PBMCs of alemtuzumab-treated patients ($n = 11$) were evaluated up to 12 months after induction. **a** Representative flow-cytometry dot plot of CD24 and CD38 in total $CD19^+$ B cells. **b**. Cumulative data for the frequency of $CD19^+CD24^{hi}CD38^{hi}$ B cells. The frequency of $CD19^+CD24^{hi}CD38^{hi}$ cells were significantly increased at 6 M and 9 M compared to pre-treatment level (6 M vs 0 M: $p = 0.0004$, 9 M vs 0 M: $p = 0.0079$). At 9 M, the frequency of $CD19^+CD24^{hi}CD38^{hi}$ cells started to decrease and by 12 M, the frequency was reduced compared to 6 M, although it was significantly increased than baseline level (12 M vs 0 M: $p = 0.0257$). **c** The absolute number was significantly increased at 6 M and 9 M post-alemtuzumab (6 M vs 0 M: $p = 0.0063$, 9 M vs 0 M: $p = 0.02$). All values show mean ± SEM. Data were analyzed by repeated measures ANOVA with Tukey's multiple comparison post-hoc analysis. *$p < 0.05$; **$p < 0.01$; ***$p < 0.001$

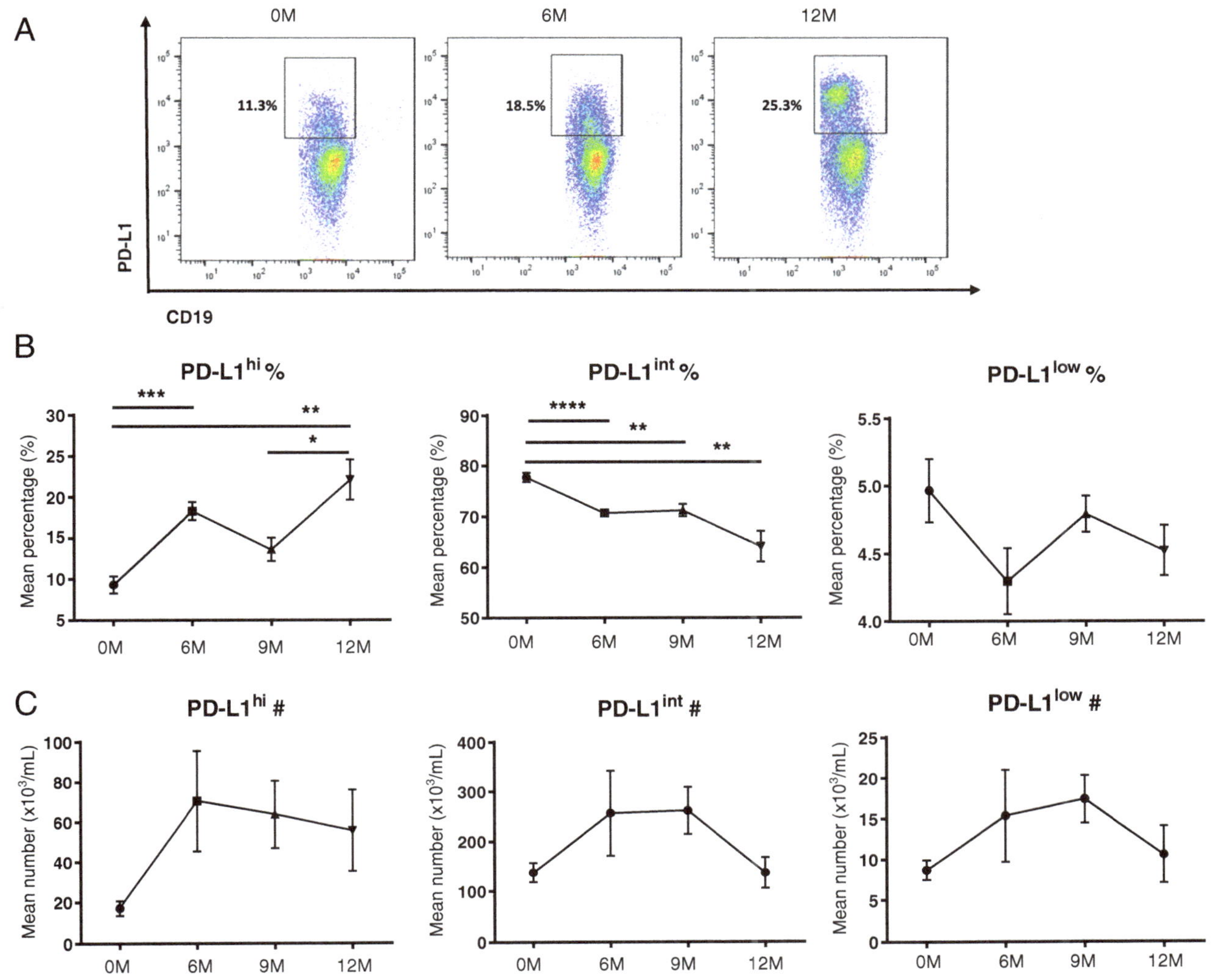

Fig. 5 Alemtuzumab treatment restores CD19^{+}PD-L1^{hi} cells. In order to evaluate the B cell subset distribution post-alemtuzuamb, thawed PBMCs of alemtuzumab-treated patients ($n = 11$) were evaluated up to 12 months after induction. **a** Representative flow-cytometry dot plot of PD-L1 in total CD19^{+} B cells. **b** Cumulative data for the frequency of CD19^{+}PD-L1^{hi} cells. The frequency of CD19^{+}PD-L1^{hi} cells increased significantly until 12 M (6 M vs 0 M: $p = 0.0004$, 12 M vs 0 M: $p = 0.0036$). **c** Cumulative data for the absolute number of CD19^{+}PD-L1^{hi} cells. No significant difference was observed in the absolute number of CD19^{+}PD-L1^{hi}, CD19^{+}PD-L1^{int}, and CD19^{+}PD-L1^{low} cells. All values show mean ± SEM. All values show mean ± SEM. Data were analyzed by repeated measures ANOVA with Tukey's multiple comparison post hoc analysis.*$p < 0.05$; **$p < 0.01$; ***$p < 0.001$; ****$p < 0.0001$

Discussion

Little is known about the repopulating B cell pool following alemtuzumab. Cases of severely exacerbated central nervous system inflammation in alemtuzumab-treated MS patients have reported B-cell driven pathology, further emphasizing the importance of B cell study in alemtuzumab-treated patients [13–15]. We show that deficiency of CD19^{+}CD24^{hi}CD38^{hi} cells and CD19^{+}PD-L1^{hi} cells in the peripheral blood of relapsing MS patients are restored following alemtuzumab and that B cell distribution shifts towards naïve phenotype. In fact, the frequency of Bregs with disparate regulatory mechanisms exceeded baseline level, which may underlie the long-lasting suppression of disease activity.

Interestingly, both frequency and absolute number of CD19^{+}CD24^{hi}CD38^{hi} cells are reduced during and prior to relapse in an alemtuzumab-treated patient. CD19^{+}CD24^{hi}CD38^{hi} cells are known to maintain Tregs and limit the differentiation of T helper 1 (Th1) and T helper 17 (Th17) cells [16]. The deficiency of CD19^{+}CD24^{hi}CD38^{hi} cells could have a significant impact on the regulation of pathology. Indeed, recent studies have found that transitional B cells are impaired in various immune-related disorders [7, 16–18], although conflicting results were observed in MS. [19, 20] In the early phase of alemtuzumab therapy, CD19^{+} B cells repopulate earlier than CD4+ T cells and immature B cells dominate the repopulated CD19+ B cells [21]; the

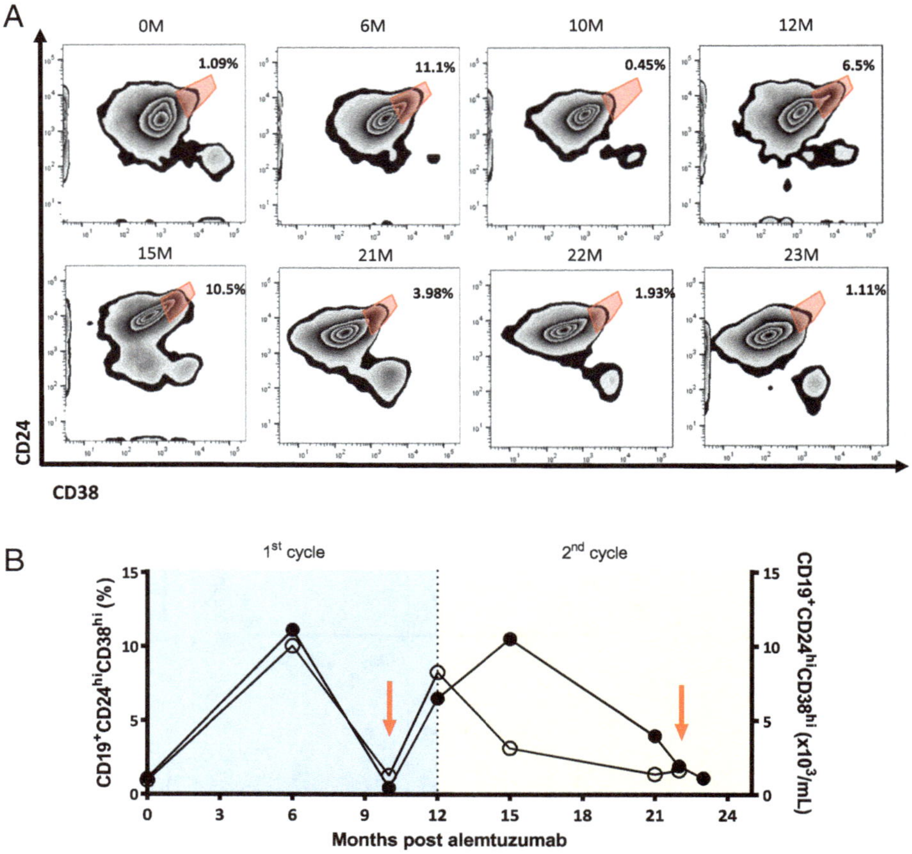

Fig. 6 The frequency of $CD19^+CD24^{hi}CD38^{hi}$ cells is decreased during relapse post alemtuzumab treatment. **a** Flow-cytometry plot of expression of CD24 and CD38 in total $CD19^+$ B cells. **b** Graph showing the clinical course. The frequency and the absolute number of $CD19^+CD24^{hi}CD38^{hi}$ B cells and infusion of 2 cycles of alemtuzumab are shown. Filled circles indicate the frequency of $CD19^+CD24^{hi}CD38^{hi}$ B cells, and hollow circles indicate the absolute number of $CD19^+CD24^{hi}CD38^{hi}$ B cells. Red arrow indicates relapse

extensive repopulation of $CD19^+CD24^{hi}CD38^{hi}$ cells following alemtuzumab may contribute to the expansion of Tregs while suppressing differentiation of naïve $CD4^+$ T cells into Th1 and Th17 cells and hence, contributing to the efficacy of alemtuzumab.

A recent study described that $CD19^+PD\text{-}L1^{hi}$ cells are capable of suppressing Tfh cell differentiation and expansion through interaction with PD-1 on activated T cells [8]. Interaction causes an increase in signal transducer and activator of transcription 5 expression, a known suppressor of Tfh-cell development and expansion. Since Tfh cells aid germinal center formation and hence, involved in the formation of memory B cells and plasma cells, Tfh cells were thought to have pathogenic role in the B-cell-mediated autoimmune diseases. There has been several reports on Tfh cell involvement in MS. [22–25] Most of all, there has been report that $CCR7^+$ $ICOS^+$ circulating memory Tfh cells are increased in MS patients during relapse, but decreased in patients during remission [9]. This finding is in line with our results, where $CD19^+PD\text{-}L1^{hi}$ cells are decreased in MS patients during relapse, but restored during remission. Hence, suppression of Tfh cell differentiation and proliferation by $CD19^+PD\text{-}L1^{hi}$ cells may be impaired due to CD19 + PD-L1hi cell deficiency, contributing to enhancement of disease activity.

This study is limited by its small sample size. In addition, we report that the marked reduction of $CD19^+CD24^{hi}CD38^{hi}$ cells during relapse in an alemtuzumab-treated patient was observed in only 2 relapses of a single case. Therefore, in order to decipher the critical role of $CD19^+CD24^{hi}CD38^{hi}$ cells in the long-term disease suppression of MS and in the mechanism of action of alemtuzumab, further longitudinal study with larger number of patients on how $CD19^+CD24^{hi}CD38^{hi}$ cells and other lymphocytes (including Tregs) change during relapse, is required. The extensive expansion of $CD19^+CD24^{hi}CD38^{hi}$ cells was maintained until 9 months post-alemtuzumab, whereas $CD19^+PD\text{-}L1^{hi}$ cells were maintained until the end of the cycle. Further work needs to be established to explain the difference in the results. In addition, a recent study has reported that hyperrepopulation of immature B cells post-alemtuzumab in the absence of adequate regulation by T cells increases the risk of secondary autoimmunity [21]. Due to vast composition of immature B cells and lack of understanding of their function, it remains to be further elucidated which specific immature B cell subset would be responsible for the secondary autoimmunity. Lastly, further functional study on the $CD19^{+}CD24^{hi}CD38^{hi}$ cells would clarify the mechanism of action of alemtuzumab.

Conclusion

Our results highlight the preferential reconstitution of Bregs as a possible mechanism of action of alemtuzumab and $CD19^{+}CD24^{hi}CD38^{hi}$ cells as a potential biomarker for disease activity.

Abbreviations

Bregs: Regulatory B cells; $CD19^{+}CD24^{hi}CD38^{hi}$: Transitional B cells; HC: Healthy controls; MS: Multiple sclerosis; MS-relapse: MS patients during relapse; MS-remission: MS patients in remission; PBMC: Peripheral blood mononuclear cells; PD-L1: Programmed death-ligand 1; Tfh: T follicular helper cells; Th1: T helper 1; Th17: T helper 17; Tregs: Regulatory T cells

Acknowledgements

Not applicable.

Funding

This study was supported by the Bio & Medical Technology Development Program (NRF-M3A9B6069339) and the Advanced Research Center Program (NRF-2018R1A5A2023127) of the National Research Foundation funded by the Ministry of Science & ICT.

Authors' contributions

KYS had full access to all of the data in the study and take responsibility for the integrity of the data and the accuracy of the data analysis. KYS and KHJ contributed to the study concept and design, and drafting of the manuscript. KYS and SHJ helped in the acquisition of data. All authors helped in the analysis and interpretation of data, and critical revision of the manuscript for intellectual content. KYS carried out the statistical analysis. KHJ supervised the study. All authors read and approved the final manuscript.

Consent for publication

Not applicable.

Competing interests

Kim YS, Kim GY, Hyun JW, Kim SH, and Shin HJ report no conflicts of interest. Kim HJ has lectured, consulted, and received honoraria from Bayer Schering Pharma, Biogen, Celltrion, Eisai, Genzyme, HanAll BioPharma, MedImmune, Merck Serono, Novartis, Teva-Handok, and UCB; received a grant from National Research Foundation of the Ministry of Science and ICT; and accepted research funding from Genzyme, Merck Serono, Teva-Handok, and UCB; serves on a steering committee for MedImmune; is a co-editor for the Multiple Sclerosis Journal—Experimental, Translational, and Clinical, and an associated editor for the Journal of Clinical Neurology.

Author details

[1]Division of Clinical Research, Research institute, National Cancer Center, Goyang, Korea. [2]Department of Neurology, Research Institute and Hospital of National Cancer Center, Goyang, Korea. [3]Yonsei University College of Medicine, Seoul, Korea.

References

1. Bar-Or A, Fawaz L, Fan B, Darlington PJ, Rieger A, Ghorayeb C, Calabresi PA, Waubant E, Hauser SL, Zhang J, Smith CH. Abnormal B-cell cytokine responses a trigger of T-cell-mediated disease in MS? Ann Neurol. 2010;67:452–61.
2. Owens GP, Bennett JL, Gilden DH, Burgoon MP. The B cell response in multiple sclerosis. Neurol Res. 2006;28:236–44.
3. Hauser SL, Waubant E, Arnold DL, Vollmer T, Antel J, Fox RJ, Bar-Or A, Panzara M, Sarkar N, Agarwal S, et al. B-cell depletion with rituximab in relapsing-remitting multiple sclerosis. N Engl J Med. 2008;358:676–88.
4. Weber MS, Hemmer B, Cepok S. The role of antibodies in multiple sclerosis. Biochim Biophys Acta. 1812;2011:239–45.
5. Duddy M, Niino M, Adatia F, Hebert S, Freedman M, Atkins H, Kim HJ, Bar-Or A. Distinct effector cytokine profiles of memory and naive human B cell subsets and implication in multiple sclerosis. J Immunol. 2007;178:6092–9.
6. Knippenberg S, Peelen E, Smolders J, Thewissen M, Menheere P, Cohen Tervaert JW, Hupperts R, Damoiseaux J. Reduction in IL-10 producing B cells (Breg) in multiple sclerosis is accompanied by a reduced naive/memory Breg ratio during a relapse but not in remission. J Neuroimmunol. 2011;239:80–6.
7. Blair PA, Norena LY, Flores-Borja F, Rawlings DJ, Isenberg DA, Ehrenstein MR, Mauri C. CD19(+)CD24(hi)CD38(hi) B cells exhibit regulatory capacity in healthy individuals but are functionally impaired in systemic lupus erythematosus patients. Immunity. 2010;32:129–40.
8. Khan AR, Hams E, Floudas A, Sparwasser T, Weaver CT, Fallon PG. PD-L1hi B cells are critical regulators of humoral immunity. Nat Commun. 2015;6:5997.
9. Fan X, Jin T, Zhao S, et al. Circulating CCR7+ICOS+ Memory T Follicular Helper Cells in Patients with Multiple Sclerosis. PLoS One. 2015;10(7):e0134523.
10. Zhang X, Tao Y, Chopra M, Ahn M, Marcus KL, Choudhary N, Zhu H, Markovic-Plese S. Differential reconstitution of T cell subsets following immunodepleting treatment with alemtuzumab (anti-CD52 monoclonal antibody) in patients with relapsing-remitting multiple sclerosis. J Immunol. 2013;191:5867–74.
11. Havari E, Turner MJ, Campos-Rivera J, Shankara S, Nguyen TH, Roberts B, Siders W, Kaplan JM. Impact of alemtuzumab treatment on the survival and function of human regulatory T cells in vitro. Immunology. 2014;141:123–31.
12. Polman CH, Reingold SC, Banwell B, Clanet M, Cohen JA, Filippi M, Fujihara K, Havrdova E, Hutchinson M, Kappos L, et al. Diagnostic criteria for multiple sclerosis: 2010 revisions to the McDonald criteria. Ann Neurol. 2011;69:292–302.
13. Haghikia A, Dendrou CA, Schneider R, Gruter T, Postert T, Matzke M, Stephanik H, Fugger L, Gold R. Severe B-cell-mediated CNS disease secondary to alemtuzumab therapy. Lancet Neurol. 2017;16:104–6.
14. Wehrum T, Beume LA, Stich O, Mader I, Maurer M, Czaplinski A, Weiller C, Rauer S. Activation of disease during therapy with alemtuzumab in 3 patients with multiple sclerosis. Neurology. 2018;90:e601–5.
15. Rinaldi F, Federle L, Puthenparampil M, Perini P, Grassivaro F, Gallo P. Evidence of B-cell dysregulation in severe CNS inflammation after alemtuzumab therapy. Neurol Neuroimmunol Neuroinflamm. 2018;5:e420.
16. Flores-Borja F, Bosma A, Ng D, Reddy V, Ehrenstein MR, Isenberg DA, Mauri C. CD19+CD24hiCD38hi B cells maintain regulatory T cells while limiting TH1 and TH17 differentiation. Sci Transl Med. 2013;5:173ra123.
17. Newell KA, Asare A, Kirk AD, Gisler TD, Bourcier K, Suthanthiran M, Burlingham WJ, Marks WH, Sanz I, Lechler RI, et al. Identification of a B cell signature associated with renal transplant tolerance in humans. J Clin Invest. 2010;120:1836–47.
18. Lee-Chang C, Top I, Zephir H, Dubucquoi S, Trauet J, Dussart P, Prin L, Vermersch P. Primed status of transitional B cells associated with their presence in the cerebrospinal fluid in early phases of multiple sclerosis. Clin Immunol. 2011;139:12–20.
19. Haas J, Bekeredjian-Ding I, Milkova M, Balint B, Schwarz A, Korporal M, Jarius S, Fritz B, Lorenz HM, Wildemann B. B cells undergo unique compartmentalized redistribution in multiple sclerosis. J Autoimmun. 2011;37:289–99.
20. Guerrier T, Labalette M, Launay D, Lee-Chang C, Outteryck O, Lefevre G, Vermersch P, Dubucquoi S, Zephir H. Proinflammatory B-cell profile in the early phases of MS predicts an active disease. Neurol Neuroimmunol Neuroinflamm. 2018;5:e431.

21. Baker D, Herrod SS, Alvarez-Gonzalez C, Giovannoni G, Schmierer K. Interpreting lymphocyte reconstitution data from the pivotal phase 3 trials of Alemtuzumab. JAMA Neurol. 2017;74:961–9.
22. Piccio L, Naismith RT, Trinkaus K, Klein RS, Parks BJ, Lyons JA, Cross AH. Changes in B- and T-lymphocyte and chemokine levels with rituximab treatment in multiple sclerosis. Arch Neurol. 2010;67:707–14.
23. Krumbholz M, Theil D, Cepok S, Hemmer B, Kivisakk P, Ransohoff RM, Hofbauer M, Farina C, Derfuss T, Hartle C, et al. Chemokines in multiple sclerosis: CXCL12 and CXCL13 up-regulation is differentially linked to CNS immune cell recruitment. Brain. 2006;129:200–11.
24. Magliozzi R, Howell O, Vora A, Serafini B, Nicholas R, Puopolo M, Reynolds R, Aloisi F. Meningeal B-cell follicles in secondary progressive multiple sclerosis associate with early onset of disease and severe cortical pathology. Brain. 2007;130:1089–104.
25. Serafini B, Rosicarelli B, Magliozzi R, Stigliano E, Aloisi F. Detection of ectopic B-cell follicles with germinal centers in the meninges of patients with secondary progressive multiple sclerosis. Brain Pathol. 2004;14:164–74.

Permissions

All chapters in this book were first published in JN, by BioMed Central; hereby published with permission under the Creative Commons Attribution License or equivalent. Every chapter published in this book has been scrutinized by our experts. Their significance has been extensively debated. The topics covered herein carry significant findings which will fuel the growth of the discipline. They may even be implemented as practical applications or may be referred to as a beginning point for another development.

The contributors of this book come from diverse backgrounds, making this book a truly international effort. This book will bring forth new frontiers with its revolutionizing research information and detailed analysis of the nascent developments around the world.

We would like to thank all the contributing authors for lending their expertise to make the book truly unique. They have played a crucial role in the development of this book. Without their invaluable contributions this book wouldn't have been possible. They have made vital efforts to compile up to date information on the varied aspects of this subject to make this book a valuable addition to the collection of many professionals and students.

This book was conceptualized with the vision of imparting up-to-date information and advanced data in this field. To ensure the same, a matchless editorial board was set up. Every individual on the board went through rigorous rounds of assessment to prove their worth. After which they invested a large part of their time researching and compiling the most relevant data for our readers.

The editorial board has been involved in producing this book since its inception. They have spent rigorous hours researching and exploring the diverse topics which have resulted in the successful publishing of this book. They have passed on their knowledge of decades through this book. To expedite this challenging task, the publisher supported the team at every step. A small team of assistant editors was also appointed to further simplify the editing procedure and attain best results for the readers.

Apart from the editorial board, the designing team has also invested a significant amount of their time in understanding the subject and creating the most relevant covers. They scrutinized every image to scout for the most suitable representation of the subject and create an appropriate cover for the book.

The publishing team has been an ardent support to the editorial, designing and production team. Their endless efforts to recruit the best for this project, has resulted in the accomplishment of this book. They are a veteran in the field of academics and their pool of knowledge is as vast as their experience in printing. Their expertise and guidance has proved useful at every step. Their uncompromising quality standards have made this book an exceptional effort. Their encouragement from time to time has been an inspiration for everyone.

The publisher and the editorial board hope that this book will prove to be a valuable piece of knowledge for researchers, students, practitioners and scholars across the globe.

List of Contributors

M. Puthenparampil, L. Federle, S. Miante, A. Zito, D. Poggiali, P. Perini, F. Rinaldi and P. Gallo
Multiple Sclerosis Centre, Department of Neurosciences DNS, University Hospital-Medical School, via Giustiniani 5, 3518 Padova, Italy

E. Toffanin, S. Ruggero, M. Ermani and S. Pravato
Department of Neurosciences DNS, University Hospital-Medical School, via Giustiniani 5, 3518 Padova, Italy

Irene Håkansson, Charlotte Dahle and Magnus Vrethem
Department of Neurology and Department of Clinical and Experimental Medicine, Linköping University, Linköping, Sweden

Anders Tisell and Peter Lundberg
Radiation Physics, Department of Medical and Health Sciences, Linköping University, Linköping, Sweden
Center for Medical Image Science and Visualization (CMIV), Linköping University, Linköping, Sweden

Petra Cassel, Jan Ernerudh and Charlotte Dahle
Department of Clinical Immunology and Transfusion Medicine and Department of Clinical and Experimental Medicine, Linköping University, Linköping, Sweden

Kaj Blennow and Henrik Zetterberg
Inst. of Neuroscience and Physiology, Department of Psychiatry and Neurochemistry, The Sahlgrenska Academy at the University of Gothenburg, Gothenburg, Sweden
Clinical Neurochemistry Laboratory, Sahlgrenska University Hospital, Mölndal, Sweden

Henrik Zetterberg
Department of Molecular Neuroscience, UCL Institute of Neurology, Queen Square, London, UK
UK Dementia Research Institute at UCL, London, UK

Peter Lundberg
Radiology, Department of Medical and Health Sciences, Linköping University, Linköping, Sweden

S. Hahn, M. Scharf, Y. Denno, S. Brakopp, B. Teegen, C. Probst, M. Buttmann, A. Haarmann, W. Stöcker and L. Komorowski
Institute of Experimental Immunology, Euroimmun AG, Seekamp 31, 23560 Lübeck, Germany

G. Trendelenburg
Department of Neurology, University Medical Center Göttingen, Göttingen, Germany

B. Teegen and W. Stöcker
Clinical Immunological Laboratory Prof. Dr. med Stöcker, Lübeck, Germany

K. P. Wandinger
Department of Neurology, University Medical Center Schleswig Holstein (UKSH), Lübeck, Germany

M. Buttmann and A. Haarmann
Department of Neurology, University of Würzburg, Würzburg, Germany

M. Buttmann
Department of Neurology, Caritas Hospital, Bad Mergentheim, Germany

F. Szabados
Medical Laboratory Osnabrück, Georgsmarienhütte, Germany

M. vom Dahl
Department of Neurology, Ammerland Klinik, Westerstede, Germany

T. Kümpfel
Institute of Clinical Neuroimmunology, Ludwig Maximilian University, Munich, Germany

P. Eichhorn
Institute of Clinical Chemistry, Ludwig Maximilian University, Munich, Germany

P, H. Gold
Department of Neurology, Klinikum am Gesundbrunnen, Heilbronn, Germany

F. Paul
NeuroCure Clinical Research Center and Clinical and Experimental Multiple Sclerosis Research Center, Department of Neurology, Charité Universitätsmedizin, Berlin, Germany
Experimental and Clinical Research Center, Max Delbrück Center for Molecular Medicine and Charité Universitätsmedizin, Berlin, Germany

S. Jarius
Department of Neurology, University of Heidelberg, Heidelberg, Germany

N. Melzer
Department of Neurology, University of Münster, Münster, Germany

Silvy Mardiguian, Emma Ladds, Roberta Turner, Hazel Shepherd, Sandra J. Campbell and Daniel C. Anthony
Department of Pharmacology, University of Oxford, Oxford OX1 4QT, UK

Emma Ladds
Department of Primary Care Health Sciences, University of Oxford, Oxford OX2 6GG, UK

Claudia Sestito, John J. P. Brevé, Micha M. M. Wilhelmus, Benjamin Drukarch and Anne-Marie van Dam
Department of Anatomy and Neurosciences, Amsterdam Neuroscience, VU University Medical Center, Postbus 7057, 1007 MB Amsterdam, the Netherlands

Marja C. J. A. van Eggermond and Peter J. van den Elsen
Department of Immunohematology and Blood Transfusion, Leiden University Medical Center, Leiden, the Netherlands

Joep Killestein and Joram van Rossum
Department of Neurology, VU University Medical Center, Amsterdam, the Netherlands

Charlotte E. Teunissen
Department of Clinical Chemistry, VU University Medical Center, Amsterdam, the Netherlands

Peter J. van den Elsen
Department of Pathology, VU University Medical Center, Amsterdam, the Netherlands

Claudia Sestito
Brain Plasticity Group, Center for Neuroscience, Swammerdam Institute for Life Sciences, University of Amsterdam, Science Park 904, Amsterdam, the Netherlands

Gabriele Farina, Roberta Magliozzi, Marco Pitteri, Stefania Rossi, Alberto Gajofatto, Maria Donata Benedetti, Salvatore Monaco and Massimiliano Calabrese
Neurology B, Department of Neurological, Biomedical and Movement Sciences, University of Verona, Policlinico "G.B. Rossi" Borgo Roma, Piazzale L.A. Scuro, 10, 37134 Verona, Italy

Gabriele Farina
Unit of Neurology, Department of Clinical and Experimental Medicine, University of Sassari, Sassari, Italy

Roberta Magliozzi and Richard Reynolds
Division of Brain Sciences, Faculty of Medicine, Imperial College London, London, UK

Francesco Facchiano
Department EOMM, Istituto Superiore di Sanità, Rome, Italy

Micha Simon, Rojda Ipek, Damiano M. Rovituso, Andrea Schampel and Stefanie Kuerten
Department of Anatomy and Cell Biology, University of Würzburg, Würzburg, Germany

György A. Homola
Department of Diagnostic and Interventional Neuroradiology, University Hospital Würzburg, Würzburg, Germany

Christoph Kleinschnitz
Department of Neurology, University Hospital Würzburg, Würzburg, Germany
Department of Neurology, University Hospital Essen, Essen, Germany

Stefanie Kuerten
Institute of Anatomy and Cell Biology, Friedrich Alexander University Erlangen-Nürnberg (FAU), Krankenhausstr. 9, 91054 Erlangen, Bavaria, Germany

Wissam Beaino, Bieneke Janssen and Albert D. Windhorst
Department of Radiology and Nuclear Medicine, VU University Medical Center, Amsterdam, The Netherlands

Gijs Kooij, Susanne M. A. van der Pol, B. van Het Hof, Jack van Horssen and Helga E. de Vries
Department of Molecular Cell Biology and Immunology, VUmc MS Center Amsterdam, Amsterdam Neuroscience, VU University Medical Center, Amsterdam, The Netherlands

Tissa Rahim, Pierre Becquart, Maria-Elizabeth Baeva and Jacqueline Quandt
Department of Pathology and Laboratory Medicine, University of British Columbia, G227-2211 Wesbrook Mall, Vancouver, BC V6T 2B5, Canada

Patrice H. Lalive and Caroline Pot
Unit of Neuroimmunology and Neuromuscular Diseases, Division of Neurology, Department of Clinical Neurosciences, Geneva University Hospital, 1211 Geneva 4, Switzerland
Department of Pathology and Immunology, Geneva University Hospital and University of Geneva, 1211 Geneva 4, Switzerland

Mario Kreutzfeldt and Doron Merkler
Department of Pathology and Immunology, Clinical Pathology Division, Geneva University Hospital and University of Geneva, 1211 Geneva 4, Switzerland

Odile Devergne
Institut Necker Enfants Malades, INSERM U1151 CNRS UMR 8253, Université Paris Descartes, Sorbonne Paris Cité, 75 015 Paris, France

Imke Metz and Wolfgang Bruck
Institute of Neuropathology, University Medical Center Göttingen, 37075 Göttingen, Germany

Caroline Pot
Laboratories of Neuroimmunology, Division of Neurology and Neuroscience Research Center, Department of Clinical Neurosciences, Lausanne University Hospital, 1011 Lausanne, Switzerland

Yohannes Haile, Carolina Ortiz-Sandoval, Nasser Tahbaz, Aleksandra Janowicz, Fabrizio Giuliani and Thomas Simmen
Department of Cell Biology, University of Alberta, Edmonton, Canada

Xiaodan Deng
Department of Medicine, Division of Neurology, University of Alberta, Edmonton, Canada

Jian-Qiang Lu
Department of Laboratory Medicine and Pathology, University of Alberta, Edmonton, Canada

Bradley J. Kerr
Department of Anesthesiology and Pain Medicine, University of Alberta, Edmonton, Canada

Nicholas J. Gutowski, Janet E. Holley and Paul Eggletons
University of Exeter Medical School and Neurology Department, Royal Devon and Exeter Hospital, Exeter, UK

Yohannes Haile
Alberta Diabetes Institute, University of Alberta, Edmonton, Canada

Yuri Nakamura, Takuya Matsushita, Koji Shinoda, Ryo Yamasaki and Jun-ichi Kira
Department of Neurology, Neurological Institute, Graduate School of Medical Sciences, Kyushu University, 3-1-1 Maidashi, Higashi-ku, Fukuoka 812-8582, Japan

Laura Gaetano, Altermatt Anna, Jens Wuerfel, Lorena Bauer and Michael Amann
Medical Image Analysis Center (MIAC AG), Marktgasse 8, 4051 Basel, Switzerland

Laura Gaetano and Michael Amann
Neurology and Department of Biomedicine, University Hospital Basel, Spitalstrasse 21, 4031 Basel, Switzerland

Altermatt Anna and Jens Wuerfel
Department of Biomedical Engineering, University of Basel, Marktgasse 8, 4051 Basel, Switzerland

Till Sprenger
DKD Helios Klinik Wiesbaden, Aukammallee 33, 65191 Wiesbaden, Germany

Ernst-Wilhelm Radue
Biomedical Research and Education GmbH, Mittlere Strasse 91, 4031 Basel, Switzerland

Lorena Bauer
Klinikum rechts der Isar, Department of Neurology, Technical University of Munich, Ismaninger Str. 22, 81675 Munich, Germany

Michael Amann
Division of Diagnostic and Interventional Neuroradiology, Department of Radiology, University Hospital Basel, Spitalstrasse 21, 4031 Basel, Switzerland

Noriko Isobe
Department of Neurological Therapeutics, Neurological Institute, Graduate School of Medical Sciences, Kyushu University, 3-1-1 Maidashi, Higashi-ku, Fukuoka 812-8582, Japan

Takahiko Saida
Institute of Neurotherapeutics, 16-1 Nishinokyoukasugachou, Nakagyo-ku, Kyoto 604-8453, Japan
Department of Neurology, Kyoto Min-Iren-Central Hospital, 16-1 Nishinokyoukasugachou, Nakagyo-ku, Kyoto 604-8453, Japan

Kathrin Bail, Quirin Notz, Damiano M. Rovituso, Andrea Schampel, Marie Wunsch, Tobias Koeniger and Stefanie Kuerten
Department of Anatomy and Cell Biology, University of Würzburg, Würzburg, Germany

Richa Bharti, Claus-Juergen Scholz and Konrad U. Foerstner
Core Unit Systems Medicine, University Hospitals of Würzburg, Würzburg, Germany

Claus-Juergen Scholz
LIMES Institute, University of Bonn, Bonn, Germany

Christoph Kleinschnitz
Department of Neurology, University Hospital Würzburg, Würzburg, Germany Department of Neurology, University Hospital Essen, Essen, Germany

Verena Schropp and Stefanie Kuerten
Institute of Anatomy and Cell Biology, Friedrich-Alexander University Erlangen-Nürnberg, Erlangen, Germany

Shailender Singh, Tobias Dallenga, Anne Winkler, Shanu Roemer, Brigitte Maruschak, Heike Siebert, Wolfgang Brück and Christine Stadelmann
Institute of Neuropathology, University Medical Center, Göttingen, Germany

Tobias Dallenga
Cellular Microbiology, Research Center Borstel, Borstel, Germany

Shanu Roemer
Department of Neurology, Rigshospitalet, Copenhagen, Denmark

Aileen Hoehne, Michelle L. James, Israt S. Alam, John A. Ronald, Bernadette Schneider, Aloma D'Souza, Timothy H. Witney, Lauren E. Andrews, Haley C. Cropper, Deepak Behera, Gayatri Gowrishankar, Frederick T. Chin, Sandip Biswal and Sanjiv S. Gambhir
Molecular Imaging Program at Stanford (MIPS), Department of Radiology, Stanford University, Stanford, CA 94305, USA

Michelle L. James, Zhaoqing Ding and Tony Wyss-Coray
Department of Neurology and Neurological Sciences, Stanford University, Stanford, CA 94305, USA

Sanjiv S. Gambhir
Department of Bioengineering, Department of Materials Science and Engineering, Stanford University, Stanford, CA 94305, USA

Farideh Talebi, Samira Ghorbani, Roobina Boghozian, Farimah Masoumi, Mohammed Vojgani and Farshid Noorbakhsh
Department of Immunology, School of Medicine, Tehran University of Medical Sciences, Tehran, Iran

Farideh Talebi and Sedigheh Ghasemi
Shefa Neuroscience Research Institute, Khatam Al-Anbia Hospital, Tehran, Iran

Wing Fuk Chan and Christopher Power
Department of Medicine (Neurology), University of Alberta, Edmonton, AB, Canada

Christopher Power
Multiple Sclerosis Centre, University of Alberta, Edmonton, AB, Canada

Elia Gil-Varea, Carme Costa, Luciana Midaglia, Angela Vidal-Jordana, Sunny Malhotra, Nicolas Fissolo, Xavier Montalban and Manuel Comabella
Servei de Neurologia-Neuroimmunologia, Centre d'Esclerosi Múltiple de Catalunya (Cemcat), Institut de Recerca Vall d'Hebron (VHIR), Hospital Universitari Vall d'Hebron, Universitat Autònoma de Barcelona, Barcelona, Spain

Elena Urcelay and Laura Espino-Paisan
Immunology Department, Hospital Clinico San Carlos, Instituto de Investigacion Sanitaria San Carlos (IdISSC), Madrid, Spain

Carles Vilariño-Güell and A. Dessa Sadovnick
Department of Medical Genetics, University of British Columbia, Vancouver, Canada

Fuencisla Matesanz
Department of Cell Biology and Immunology, Instituto de Parasitología y Biomedicina "López Neyra", Consejo Superior de Investigaciones Científicas (IPBLN-CSIC), Granada, Spain

Alfredo Rodríguez-Antigüedad
Servicio de Neurología, Hospital Universitario Basurto-Osakidetza, Bilbao, Spain

Jorge Oksenberg
Department of Neurology, University of California, San Francisco, CA, USA

Albert Saiz
Neurology Service, Hospital Clinic and Institut d'Investigació Biomèdica Pi i Sunyer (IDIBAPS), Barcelona, Spain

Luisa M. Villar and Jose C. Alvarez-Cermeño
Departments of Immunology and Neurology, Multiple Sclerosis Unit, Hospital Ramon y Cajal, (IRYCIS), Madrid, Spain

Juan Antonio García-Merino and Antonio Sánchez-López
Neuroimmunology Unit, Puerta de Hierro University Hospital and Research Institute, Universidad Autónoma de Madrid, Madrid, Spain

Lluís Ramió-Torrentà, Ester Quintana and René Robles
Neuroimmunology and Multiple Sclerosis Unit, Department of Neurology, Hospital Dr Josep Trueta, IDIBGI, University of Girona, Girona, Spain

Juan Carlos Triviño
Genomic Systems, Valencia, Spain

Rafael Arroyo
Servicio de Neurología, Hospital Universitario Quirón Salud, Madrid, Spain

Marloes H. J. Hagens, Martijn T. Wijburg, Martijn D. Steenwijk, Anne-Marie van Dam, Joep Killestein and Frederik Barkhof
VUmc MS Center Amsterdam, VU University Medical Center, De Boelelaan 1117, 1081 HV Amsterdam, the Netherlands

Marloes H. J. Hagens, Martijn T. Wijburg and Joep Killestein
Department of Neurology, VU University Medical Center, De Boelelaan 1117, 1081 HV Amsterdam, the Netherlands

Sandeep V. Golla, Maqsood Yaqub, Dennis Heijtel, Robert C. Schuit, Frederik Barkhof, Bart N. M. van Berckel and Adriaan A. Lammertsma
Department of Radiology and Nuclear Medicine, VU University Medical Center Amsterdam, De Boelelaan 1117, 1081 HV Amsterdam, the Netherlands

Dennis Heijtel
Philips Healthcare, Best, the Netherlands, Veenpluis 4, 5684 PC Best, the Netherlands

Martijn D. Steenwijk, Martijn D. Steenwijk, John J. P. Brevé and Anne-Marie van Dam
Department of Anatomy and Neurosciences, VU University Medical Center Amsterdam, De Boelelaan 1117, 1081 HV Amsterdam, the Netherlands

Patrick Schober
Department of Anaesthesiology, VU University Medical Center Amsterdam, De Boelelaan 1117, 1081 HV Amsterdam, the Netherlands

Tristan A. Reekie and Michael Kassiou
School of Chemistry, University of Sydney, F11, Eastern Ave, Sydney, NSW 2006, Australia

Frederik Barkhof
Institutes of Neurology and Healthcare Engineering, UCL Institute of Neurology, Queen Square, London WC1N 3BG, UK

Yeseul Kim, Gayoung Kim and Ho Jin Kim
Division of Clinical Research, Research institute, National Cancer Center, Goyang, Korea

Hyun-June Shin, Jae-Won Hyun, Su-Hyun Kim and Ho Jin Kim
Department of Neurology, Research Institute and Hospital of National Cancer Center, Goyang, Korea

Yeseul Kim and Eunjig Lee
Yonsei University College of Medicine, Seoul, Korea

Index